OPHTHALMIC CARE OF THE COMBAT CASUALTY

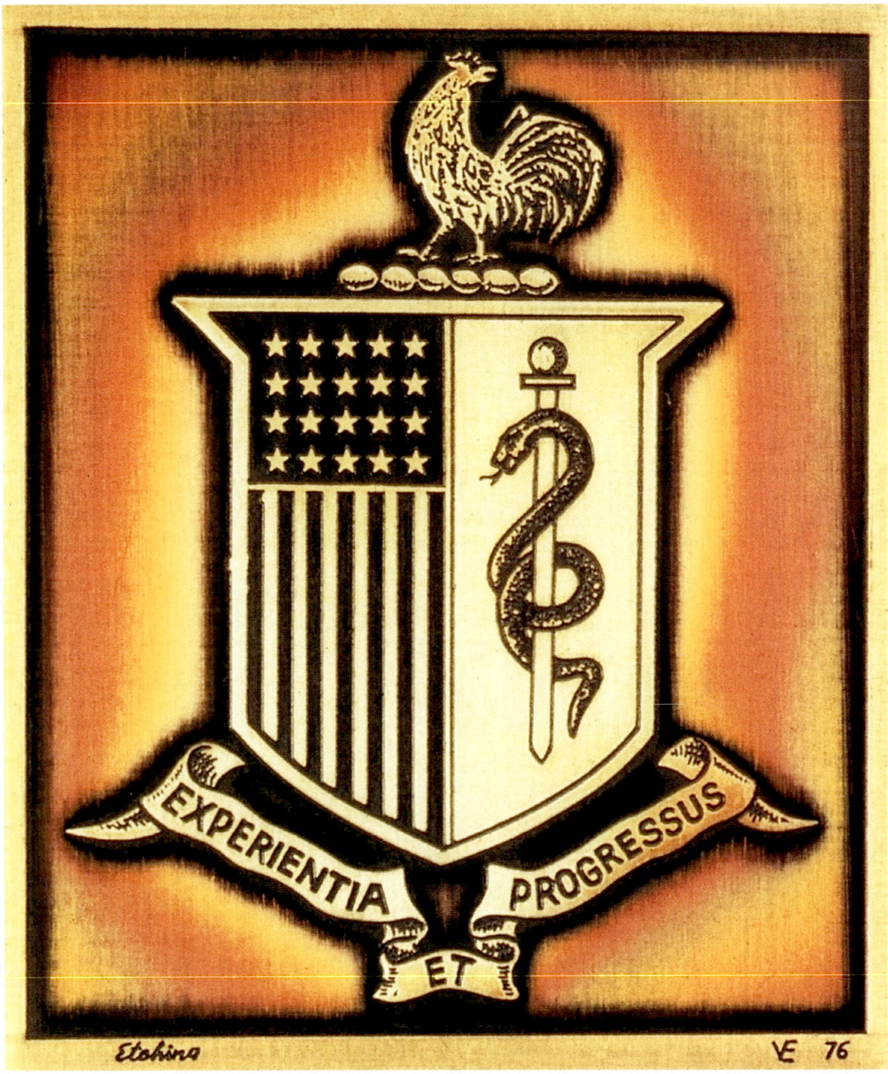

The Coat of Arms
1818
Medical Department of the Army

A 1976 etching by Vassil Ekimov of an
original color print that appeared in
The Military Surgeon, Vol XLI, No 2, 1917

The first line of medical defense in wartime is the combat medic. Although in ancient times medics carried the caduceus into battle to signify the neutral, humanitarian nature of their tasks, they have never been immune to the perils of war. They have made the highest sacrifices to save the lives of others, and their dedication to the wounded soldier is the foundation of military medical care.

Textbooks of Military Medicine

Published by the

Office of The Surgeon General
Department of the Army, United States of America

Editor in Chief and Director
Dave E. Lounsbury, MD, FACP
Colonel, MC, US Army
Borden Institute
Assistant Professor of Medicine
F. Edward Hébert School of Medicine
Uniformed Services University of the Health Sciences

Military Medical Editor
Ronald F. Bellamy, MD
Colonel, US Army, Retired
Borden Institute
Associate Professor of Military Medicine
Associate Professor of Surgery
F. Edward Hébert School of Medicine
Uniformed Services University of the Health Sciences

Editor in Chief Emeritus
Russ Zajtchuk, MD
Brigadier General, US Army, Retired
Former Commanding General
US Army Medical Research and Materiel Command
Professor of Surgery
F. Edward Hébert School of Medicine
Uniformed Services University of the Health Sciences
Bethesda, Maryland

The TMM Series

Published Textbooks

Medical Consequences of Nuclear Warfare (1989)

Conventional Warfare: Ballistic, Blast, and Burn Injuries (1991)

Occupational Health: The Soldier and the Industrial Base (1993)

Military Dermatology (1994)

Military Psychiatry: Preparing in Peace for War (1994)

Anesthesia and Perioperative Care of the Combat Casualty (1995)

War Psychiatry (1995)

Medical Aspects of Chemical and Biological Warfare (1997)

Rehabilitation of the Injured Soldier, Volume 1 (1998)

Rehabilitation of the Injured Soldier, Volume 2 (1999)

Medical Aspects of Harsh Environments, Volume 1 (2002)

Medical Aspects of Harsh Environments, Volume 2 (2002)

Ophthalmic Care of the Combat Casualty (2003)

Upcoming Textbooks

Medical Aspects of Harsh Environments, Volume 3 (2003)

Military Preventive Medicine: Mobilization and Deployment, Volume 1 (2003)

Military Preventive Medicine: Mobilization and Deployment, Volume 2 (2003)

Military Medical Ethics, Volume 1 (2003)

Military Medical Ethics, Volume 2 (2003)

Combat Injuries to the Head

Combat Injuries to the Extremities

Surgery for Victims of Conflict

Military Medicine in Peace and War

Recruit Medicine

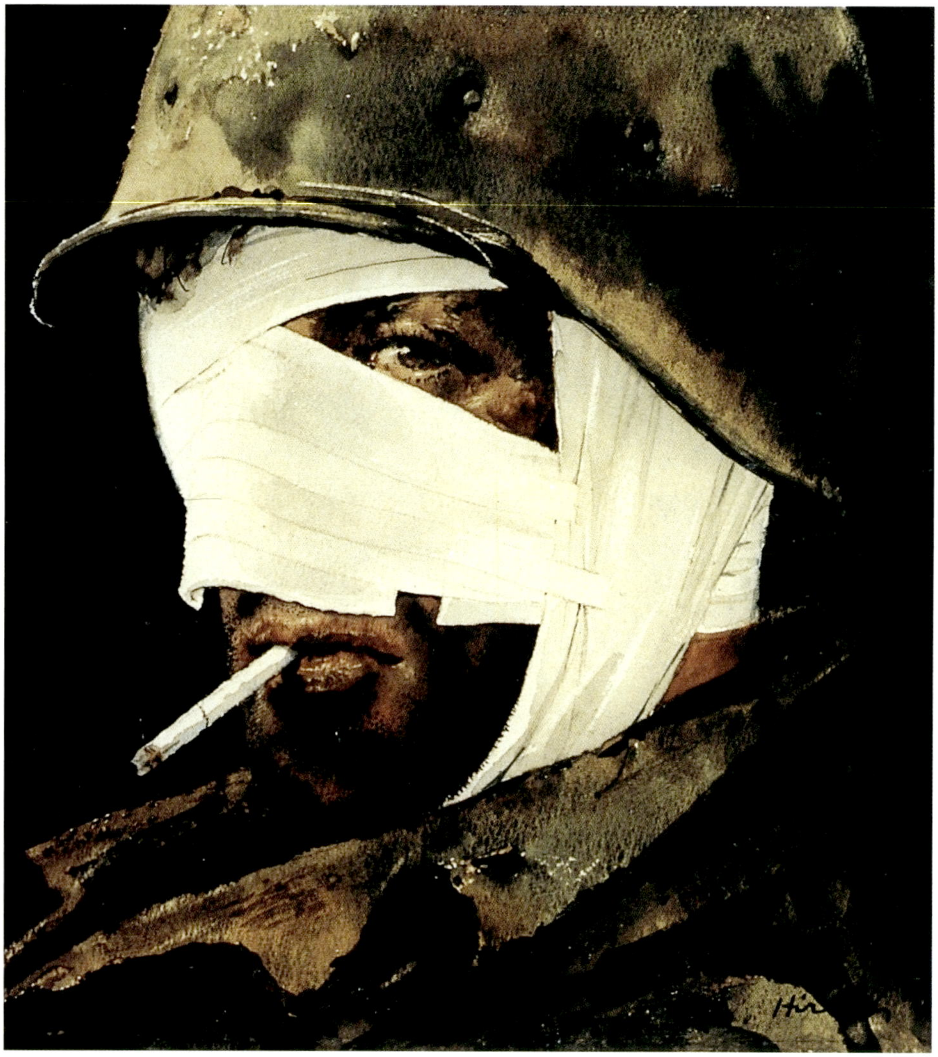

Joseph Hirsch *High Visibility Wrap* Watercolor on Paper, 1944

Although the formidable dressing seen here conceals a wound of the right globe and orbit, it cannot hide the indomitable spirit of this wounded American soldier. One wonders, however, to what extent artistic license was exercised in illustrating this elaborate and robust dressing, which would almost certainly have had a deleterious effect on intraocular pressure. The watercolor first appeared as the frontispiece to Volume 1 of *Neurosurgery* in the *Surgery in World War II* series, part of the official history of the Medical Department, US Army. We are pleased to reproduce the painting here, as its inclusion symbolizes the continuity between the current Textbooks of Military Medicine series and our illustrious predecessor. First printed in Spurling GR, Woodhall B, eds. *Neurosurgery.* Vol 1. In: Hays SB, Coates JB Jr, eds. *Surgery in World War II.* Washington, DC: Department of the Army, Medical Department, Office of The Surgeon General; 1958: frontispiece. Watercolor: Reproduced courtesy of Army Art Collection, US Army Center of Military History, Washington, DC.

OPHTHALMIC CARE
OF THE
COMBAT CASUALTY

Specialty Editor

ALLEN B. THACH, MD
Colonel, Medical Corps, US Army Reserve
Associate Professor of Surgery
Uniformed Services University of the Health Sciences
Bethesda, Maryland
Retinal Consultants of Arizona
Phoenix, Arizona

Office of The Surgeon General
United States Army
Falls Church, Virginia

Borden Institute
Walter Reed Army Medical Center
Washington, DC

United States Army Medical Department Center and School
Fort Sam Houston, Texas

Uniformed Services University of the Health Sciences
Bethesda, Maryland

2003

Featuring Original Drawings
Created Especially for This Textbook by

Gary Wind, MD, FACS

Uniformed Services University of the Health Sciences
Bethesda, Maryland

Editorial Staff: Lorraine B. Davis
Senior Production Manager
Colleen Mathews Quick
Volume Editor

This volume was prepared for military medical educational use. The focus of the information is to foster discussion that may form the basis of doctrine and policy. The opinions or assertions contained herein are the private views of the authors and are not to be construed as official or as reflecting the views of the Department of the Army or the Department of Defense.

Dosage Selection:

The authors and publisher have made every effort to ensure the accuracy of dosages cited herein. However, it is the responsibility of every practitioner to consult appropriate information sources to ascertain correct dosages for each clinical situation, especially for new or unfamiliar drugs and procedures. The authors, editors, publisher, and the Department of Defense cannot be held responsible for any errors found in this book.

Use of Trade or Brand Names:

Use of trade or brand names in this publication is for illustrative purposes only and does not imply endorsement by the Department of Defense.

Neutral Language:

Unless this publication states otherwise, masculine nouns and pronouns do not refer exclusively to men.

Published by the Office of The Surgeon General at TMM Publications
Borden Institute
Walter Reed Army Medical Center
Washington, DC 20307-5001

Library of Congress Cataloging-in-Publication Data

Ophthalmic care of the combat casualty / specialty editor, Allen B. Thach.
p. ; cm. — (Textbooks of military medicine)
Includes bibliographical references and index.
1. Eye—Wounds and injuries. 2. Medicine, Military. 3. Battle casualties. I. Thach, Allen B. II. United States. Dept. of the Army. Office of the Surgeon General. III. Series.
[DNLM: 1. Eye Injuries—therapy. 2. Eye Injuries—history. 3. Military Medicine. WW 525 O605 2003]
RE831 .O64 2003
617.7'1306—dc21

2002038489

PRINTED IN THE UNITED STATES OF AMERICA

10, 09, 08, 07, 06, 05, 04, 03 5 4 3 2 1

For sale by the Superintendent of Documents, U.S. Government Printing Office
Internet: bookstore.gpo.gov Phone: toll free (866) 512-1800; DC area (202) 512-1800
Fax: (202) 512-2250 Mail: Stop SSOP, Washington, DC 20402-0001

ISBN 0-16-051364-2

Contents

Contributors

DARRYL J. AINBINDER, MD
Lieutenant Colonel, Medical Corps, US Army; Director, Ophthalmic Oncology and Pathology; Staff, Ophthalmic Plastic, Reconstructive, and Orbital Surgery, Madigan Army Medical Center, Tacoma, Wash; Assistant Professor of Surgery (Ophthalmology), Uniformed Services University of the Health Sciences, Bethesda, Md

WENDALL C. BAUMAN, JR, MD
Colonel, US Air Force, Medical Corps; Assistant Chief, Department of Surgery; Chief, Retina Service, Brooke Army Medical Center, Fort Sam Houston, Tex; Staff, Retina Service, Lackland Air Force Base, Tex

JEFFREY P. BLICE, MD
Commander, Medical Corps, US Navy, National Naval Medical Center, Department of Ophthalmology, Bethesda, Md

KRAIG S. BOWER, MD
Lieutenant Colonel, Medical Corps, US Army; Cornea and External Disease Section, Ophthalmology Service, Walter Reed Army Medical Center, Washington, DC

GORDON A. BYRNES, MD
Captain, Medical Corps, US Navy; Department of Ophthalmology, National Naval Medical Center, Bethesda, Md

NEIL T. CHOPLIN, MD
Captain, US Navy (Ret); Eye Care of San Diego, San Diego, Calif; Adjunct Clinical Professor of Surgery, Uniformed Services University of Health Sciences, Bethesda, Md

GLENN C. COCKERHAM, MD
Colonel, US Air Force, (Ret); Cornea Service, Allegheny General Hospital, Pittsburgh, Pa

KIMBERLY PEELE COCKERHAM, MD
Director, Ophthalmic Plastics, Orbital Disease and Neuro-Ophthalmology, Allegheny General Hospital, Pittsburgh; Assistant Professor, Department of Ophthalmology, Drexel University College of Medicine, Philadelphia, Pa

PETER H. CUSTIS, MD
Captain, US Navy; Director, Retina Service, Department of Ophthalmology, Naval Medical Center San Diego, San Diego, Calif; and Clinical Assistant Professor, Department of Surgery, Uniformed Services University of Health Sciences, Bethesda, Md

ANDREW S. EISEMAN, MD
Lieutenant Colonel, Medical Corps, US Army; Chief, Oculoplastics and Orbit Service, Walter Reed Army Medical Center, Washington, DC

ELIZABETH A. HANSEN, MD
Colonel, Medical Corps, US Army; Director, Comprehensive Ophthalmology, Madigan Army Medical Center, Tacoma, Wash; Assistant Professor of Surgery (Ophthalmology), Uniformed Services University of the Health Sciences, Bethesda, Md

CRAIG D. HARTRANFT, MD
Lieutenant Colonel, Medical Corps, US Army; Chief, Vitreoretinal Service, Madigan Army Medical Center, Fort Lewis, Wash

DAVID E. E. HOLCK, MD
Lieutenant Colonel, US Air Force, Medical Corps; Flight Surgeon; Director, Oculoplastic, Orbital and Reconstructive Surgery Service, Wilford Hall Medical Center, Lackland Air Force Base, Tex

RODNEY D. HOLLIFIELD, MD
Vitreoretinal Surgeon, Retina Consultants of Nevada, Las Vegas, Nev

TIM B. HOPKINS, MD
Lieutenant Commander, Medical Corps, US Navy; Department of Ophthalmology, US Naval Hospital Great Lakes, Great Lakes, Ill

DANIEL J. JANIK, MD
Lieutenant Colonel, US Air Force (Ret); Associate Professor of Anesthesiology and Associate Medical Director of Operating Room Services, University of Colorado Health Sciences Center, Denver, Colo

THADDEUS J. KROLICKI, MD
Vitreoretinal Surgeon, Eye Clinic of Wisconsin, Wausau, Wis

FRANCIS G. LA PIANA, MD, FACS
Colonel, US Army (Ret); Professor of Surgery, Uniformed Services University of the Health Sciences, Bethesda, Md; Ophthalmology Residency Program Director, Department of Ophthalmology, Washington Hospital Center, Washington, DC

SCOTT K. MCCLATCHEY, MD
Commander, Medical Corps, US Navy; Director, Motility Service, Department of Ophthalmology, Naval Medical Center San Diego, San Diego, Calif; Assistant Professor, Department of Surgery, Uniformed Services University of Health Sciences, Bethesda, Md

THOMAS H. MADER, MD
Colonel, Medical Corps, US Army (Ret); Alaska Native Medical Center, Anchorage, Alaska

WILLIAM P. MADIGAN, JR, MD
Colonel, Medical Corps, US Army; Chief, Ophthalmology Service, Walter Reed Army Medical Center, Washington, DC; Associate Professor and Chief, Division of Ophthalmology, Department of Surgery, Uniformed Services University of the Health Sciences, Bethesda, Maryland

DAVID O. MAZUR, MD
Captain, Medical Corps, US Navy; Chairman, Department of Ophthalmology, National Naval Medical Center, Bethesda, Md

ROBERT A. MAZZOLI, MD
Colonel, Medical Corps, US Army; Chief, Department of Ophthalmology; Director, Ophthalmic Plastic, Reconstructive, and Orbital Surgery, Madigan Army Medical Center, Tacoma, Wash; Associate Professor of Surgery (Ophthalmology), Uniformed Services University of the Health Sciences, Bethesda, Md

ASA D. MORTON, MD
Commander, Medical Corps, US Navy; Chief, Oculoplastics Section, Naval Medical Center San Diego, San Diego, Calif

JOHN D. NG, MD
Assistant Professor of Ophthalmology, Division of Oculoplastics, Orbit, Lacrimal, and Reconstructive Surgery, Casey Eye Institute, Oregon Health and Sciences University, Portland, Ore

MATTHEW J. NUTAITIS, MD
Commander, Medical Corps, US Navy; Head, Glaucoma Service, Department of Ophthalmology, National Naval Medical Center, Bethesda, Md

JOSEPH PASTERNAK, MD
Commander, Medical Corps, US Navy; National Naval Medical Center, Bethesda, Md

WILLIAM R. RAYMOND IV, MD
Colonel, Medical Corps, US Army; Director, Pediatric Ophthalmology and Strabismus, Madigan Army Medical Center, Tacoma, Wash; Clinical Assistant Professor of Surgery (Ophthalmology), Uniformed Services University of the Health Sciences, Bethesda, Md

WILLIAM RIMM, MD
Colonel, Medical Corps, US Army; Ophthalmology Service, Walter Reed Army Medical Center, Washington, DC

E. GLENN SANFORD, MD
Major, Medical Corps, US Army; Chief, Department of Ophthalmology, Blanchfield Army Community Hospital, Fort Campbell, Ky

RICHARD D. STUTZMAN, MD
Major, Medical Corps, US Army; Staff Ophthalmologist, Department of Ophthalmology, Walter Reed Army Medical Center, Washington, DC

ALLEN B. THACH, MD
Colonel, Medical Corps, US Army Reserve; Retinal Consultants of Arizona, Phoenix, Arizona; Associate Professor of Surgery, Uniformed Services University of the Health Sciences, Bethesda, Md

EDWARD W. TRUDO, JR, MD
Lieutenant Colonel, Medical Corps, US Army Reserve; Assistant Professor of Surgery (Ophthalmology), Uniformed Services University of the Health Sciences, Bethesda, Md; Azar Eye Institute, Salisbury, Md

THOMAS P. WARD, MD
Colonel, Medical Corps, US Army; Ophthalmology Residency Program Director, Ophthalmology Service, Walter Reed Army Medical Center, Washington, DC; Associate Professor of Surgery, Uniformed Services University of the Health Sciences, Bethesda, Md

FLOYD L. WERGELAND, JR, MD
Colonel, US Army (Ret); Adjunct Clinical Professor of Surgery, Division of Ophthalmology, Uniformed Services University of the Health Services, Bethesda, Md; Eye Physicians Medical/Surgical Center, Chula Vista, Calif

Foreword

Since the end of the Cold War, the role of the US military has changed from one of fighting a massive war of prolonged duration to one involved in smaller conflicts requiring rapidly mobile forces. Forces are sent overseas on peacekeeping missions and special operations, yet must also remain prepared to fight larger conflicts. The US Army Medical Department has also changed in response to the demands of these new roles. The vicissitudes of these new missions no longer require large, stationary medical facilities to which the injured soldier will be transported. Instead, our facilities now include smaller, mobile medical units that are able to deploy rapidly and move with our soldiers. Despite these significant organizational changes, giving the best care to our troops as close to the front as possible remains of utmost importance. Previous conflicts have shown that rapid evaluation and treatment improves the ability to save injured soldiers' lives, limbs, and sight. Based in part on the lessons learned in past wars, the Textbooks of Military Medicine series presents the insights, discusses the issues, and provides the requirements of combat casualty care.

Given the trends in current warfare, conventional munitions—especially fragmentation devices—will continue to cause a significant percentage of all injuries to our soldiers, and a large number of those casualties will sustain eye injuries. Lasers (used both in current instrumentation and in offensive weapons) also have the potential to cause numerous eye injuries. Because the preservation of the eye and eyesight is of utmost importance, this volume, *Ophthalmic Care of the Combat Casualty*, was written for the Textbooks of Military Medicine series. This volume's goals are to aid in the early diagnosis and treatment of ocular injuries and to prevent unnecessary blindness—pertinent topics to the soldier giving buddy care at the unit level, to the medic and physician at the battalion aid station, and to the ophthalmologist in the higher echelons of care. The information provided includes lessons learned from the Revolutionary War to the Persian Gulf War, and military ophthalmologists from the Army, Navy, and Air Force have shared their expertise in preparing this thorough, up-to-date textbook.

Lieutenant General James B. Peake
The Surgeon General
US Army

Washington, DC
January 2003

Introduction

Along with saving the lives and limbs of our soldiers, sailors, and airmen injured in battle, the preservation of their eyes and eyesight is an extremely important goal. Despite comprising as little as 0.1% of the total body surface area and 0.27% of the frontal silhouette, the proportion of eye injuries in nonfatal casualties has been escalating in recent conflicts (Table). Several reasons account for the increasing risk of eye injuries:

1. preferential exposure of the eyes during combat (eg, foxholes, tank turrets);
2. improved body armor protecting the head, thorax, and abdomen, leading to fewer fatal injuries to these regions of the body;
3. improved surgical techniques and rapid evacuation of the wounded, which allow physicians to repair wounds that at one time would have resulted in the death of a soldier; and
4. improved munitions, which create more and smaller fragments that can cause severe, even blinding, injuries.

TABLE
INCIDENCE OF WARTIME EYE INJURIES

War (Dates)	Eye Injuries (% of Total Injuries)	References
American Civil War (1861–1865)	0.57[1]	(1) Duke-Elder S, MacFaul PA. War injuries. In: *Mechanical Injuries*. Part 1. In: *Injuries*. Vol 14. In: Duke-Elder S, ed. *System of Ophthalmology*. St Louis, Mo: C. V. Mosby; 1972; 49–56. (2) Steindorf K. Die Kreigschirurgie des schorgans. *Berlin Klin Wochensch*. 1914;51:1787–1789. (3) Parsons J. Protection of the eyes from war injuries. *Trans Ophthalmol Soc UK*. 1941;61:157–178. (4) Shimkin NI. Ophthalmic injuries in war. *Br J Ophthalmol*. 1940;24:265–285. (5) Stone W. Ocular injuries in the armed forces. *JAMA*. 1950;142:151–152. (6) Gunderson T. Surgery of intraocular foreign bodies. *Trans Am Acad Ophthalmol Otolaryngol*. 1947;52:604–613. (7) Hornblass A. Eye injuries in South Vietnam. *Surg Forum*. 1973;24:500–502. (8) Lowrey A, Shaffer F. Eye, ear, nose and throat injuries sustained in Korean theater. *Trans Pac Coast Ophthalmol Soc Ann Meet*. 1954;35:39–49. (9) Treister G. Ocular casualties in the 6 Day War. *Am J Ophthalmol*. 1969;68:669–675. (10) Hornblass A. Eye injuries in the military. *Int Ophthalmol Clin*. 1981;21:121–138. (11) Hoefle FB. Initial treatment of eye injuries. *Arch Ophthalmol*. 1968;79:33–35. (12) Belkin M. Ocular injuries in the Yom Kippur War. *J Ocul Therapy Surg*. 1983;2:40–49. (13) Belkin M, Treister G, Dotan S. Eye injuries and ocular protection in the Lebanon War, 1982. *Isr J Med Sci*. 1984;20:333–338. (14) Heier JS, Enzenauer RW, Wintermeyer SF, Delaney M, La Piana FG. Ocular injuries and diseases at a combat support hospital in support of Operation Desert Shield and Desert Storm. *Arch Ophthalmol*. 1993;111:795–798. (15) Jankovic S, Zuljan I, Sapunar D, Buca A, Plestina-Borjan I. Clinical and radiological management of wartime eye and orbit injuries. *Mil Med*. 1998;163:423–426.
Franco–Prussian War (1870–1871)	0.81–0.86[2]	
Sino–Japanese War (1894)	1.2[1]	
Russo–Japanese War (1904–1905)	2–2.22[2]	
World War I (1914–1918)	1.54[3]	
	2.25[4]	
World War II (1939–1945)	2.0[5]	
	2.57–3.38[6]	
Korean War (1950–1953)	4.1[7]	
	8.1[8]	
Arab–Israeli 6-Day War (1967)	5.6[9]	
Vietnam War (1962–1972)	5.0–9.0[10]	
	9.0[11]	
Arab–Israeli Yom Kippur War (1973)	6.7[12]	
Lebanon War (1982)	6.8[13]	
Persian Gulf War (1991)	13.0[14]	
Serbian–Croatian War (1991–1995)	9.8[15]	

Given the trends in modern warfare, as well as the expected increased use of laser devices, the percentage of ocular injuries will continue to increase. Because of advances in the care of eye trauma, however, injuries to the eye that once were deemed unsalvageable can now be repaired—often with the return of useful vision to the soldier. There are five echelons of care for troops injured on the modern battlefield, although their battlefield locations and the number of ophthalmologists at each echelon constantly change to meet the demands of our mobile fighting force.

Echelon 1 is in the unit area, and medics and a battalion aid station will provide initial care. Patients with minor eye injuries may be treated and returned to duty. Patients with more-severe injuries will be stabilized and sent to a higher echelon for more-definitive care.

Echelon 2 is at the division level and consists of a clearing station that can (*a*) provide emergency care (general anesthesia is usually not available) and (*b*) serve as a holding station for those troops who will return to duty, usually within the next 24 to 72 hours.

Echelon 3, at the corps level, is the most forward position in which an ophthalmologist will usually be located. In the Army, this will be at the combat hospital (previously known as the combat support hospital, an evacuation hospital, and the mobile army surgical hospital [MASH]); for the Marines, it is the fleet hospital; and for the Navy, it is the hospital ships (currently, the USNS *Comfort* and USNS *Mercy*). At this level, the ophthalmologist will be equipped with the Deployable Medical Systems (DEPMEDS), which should include all the equipment necessary to examine an injured patient, a diagnostic set (including ultrasound and, in some locations, a computerized tomography device), and equipment to repair most eye injuries (operating room microscope, phacoemulsification/vitrectomy unit, surgical instruments and sutures, and an external magnet). Ophthalmic surgeons at this level (in the Army and with the Marines) must be prepared to move forward with the fighting forces; thus, this equipment is packaged to facilitate movement. Injured troops may receive definitive care at Echelon 3 and either be (*a*) evacuated to a higher level for further treatment or rehabilitation, or (*b*) returned to duty.

Echelon 4 is usually found overseas in a fixed facility, such as a general hospital, which can provide full, definitive care and is equipped to treat any injury.

Echelon 5 is located in the United States at military and civilian hospitals. These hospitals are usually supplied with the latest equipment and can treat the most-severe problems, perform secondary repair and reconstructive surgery, and should have rehabilitative services available.

With the evolution of small fighting teams and rapid mobilization, the medical services must be able to deploy medical assets at a moment's notice. The Navy has instituted a Medical Mobilization Augmentation Readiness Team (MMARTS) for these types of operations. The Air Force has initiated the Expeditionary Medical Support (EMEDS) teams, which replace the Air Transportable Hospital (ATH). The EMEDS are scalable, depending on theater requirements, and support the Small Portable Expeditionary Aeromedical Rapid Response (SPEARR) teams. Ophthalmology as a subspecialty supports the EMEDS + 25 (25-bed) configuration. These teams must be able to deploy rapidly (within 2–48 h) and are to provide short-term (< 180 d) medical augmentation for peacetime and rapid-contingency operations.

The first section of this textbook provides a history of military eye care, including the lessons learned from the Vietnam and Persian Gulf wars. The second section describes some of the basic techniques needed to evaluate an eye injury (history, examination, and ancillary studies) and the techniques available to provide anesthesia to a patient with an eye injury. Included in this section is a discussion of an ocular trauma score (similar to the Glasgow Coma Scale). This trauma score was developed to assist the frontline medics and physicians with an easy-to-use guide for triaging and providing emergency treatment to the injured soldier. The third section deals with injuries to the anterior segment of the eye (ie, the cornea, lens, and conjunctiva), and includes a discussion of injuries to the eye from industrial chemicals and chemical warfare agents. The fourth section covers injuries of the posterior segment, with chapters on intraocular foreign bodies, sympathetic ophthalmia, and endophthalmitis. The fifth section describes the evaluation and treatment of injuries to the orbit, optic nerve, extraocular muscles, and ocular adnexa. The final section covers a variety of issues important to the military ophthalmologist such as terrorist blasts, laser injuries, eye protection, and geographical ophthalmology.

Although not an all-inclusive treatise on the subject, we hope that this textbook will provide a ready reference for all medical personnel dealing with eye-injured soldiers. Unlike the ophthalmologist in the civilian sector, who usually sees patients with a single injury in a relatively sterile environment, the military ophthalmologist will be faced with numerous casualties who have multisystem injuries in a setting that may be less than ideal. This textbook deals with some of these key issues that will face the military ophthalmologist in wartime situations.

It seems that with each conflict in the 20th century, every new generation of medics and physicians has had to learn—on its own—the lessons from earlier conflicts. We hope that the wisdom, experience, and lessons learned reported in this volume of the *Textbooks of Military Medicine* will enable optimal care to be provided in a timely manner to our eye-injured service members on the battlefield in future conflicts.

William P. Madigan, Jr, MD
Colonel, Medical Corps, US Army
Chief, Ophthalmology Service
Walter Reed Army Medical Center
Washington, DC
Consultant to The Surgeon General,
US Army, Ophthalmology
Associate Professor and
Chief, Division of Ophthalmology, Department of Surgery
Uniformed Services University of the Health Sciences
Bethesda, Maryland

Allen B. Thach, MD
Colonel, Medical Corps, US Army Reserve
Associate Professor of Surgery
Uniformed Services University of the Health Sciences
Bethesda, Maryland
Retinal Consultants of Arizona
Phoenix, Arizona

January 2003

Chapter 1

HISTORY OF MILITARY EYE CARE

FLOYD L. WERGELAND, Jr, MD*

*Colonel, Medical Corps, US Army (Ret); Adjunct Clinical Professor of Surgery, Division of Ophthalmology, Uniformed Services University of the Health Sciences, 4301 Jones Bridge Road, Bethesda, Maryland 20814-4799, and Eye Physicians Medical/Surgical Center, 681 Third Avenue, Chula Vista, California 92010; formerly, Consultant to The Surgeon General in Ophthalmology and Chief, Ophthalmology Service, Walter Reed Army Medical Center, Washington, DC 20307-5001

INTRODUCTION

The practice of ophthalmic care in the US military has evolved during peacetime and wartime. Beginning with the Revolutionary War, military medicine was the responsibility of general physicians, only some of whom had some training in the provision of eye care. Some surgeons performed cataract surgery but not as a specialty. By the American Civil War, however, ophthalmology had become recognized as a specialty in its own right by national organizations.

The demands of World War I and World War II made evident the need to maintain well-trained military ophthalmologists on continual active duty to provide care for military personnel. To meet this demand, residency training programs were established. The development of the ophthalmoscope and retinoscopy further improved methods of examination and treatment of trauma and medical eye disorders. Other improvements in surgery (not specific to ophthalmology but including enhancements in anesthesia, asepsis, and drug development) propelled the specialty forward.

The tradition of providing high-quality care to the military (active and retired), their dependents, and selected civilians has continued to this day. Military conflicts, peacekeeping efforts, and civilian medical assistance programs have challenged Army ophthalmologists, but as their history reveals, they have met these challenges and will continue to do so.

EVOLUTION OF OPHTHALMIC CARE IN THE US ARMY

Revolutionary War

The history of the US Army Medical Department begins with the outbreak of the American Revolution (1775) and particularly with the siege of Boston. The Army formed at Cambridge after the Battle of Lexington had little semblance of organization. Among those gathered were many physicians, none of whom held commissions or had any means of establishing hospitals. During the early phase of the Revolution, the sick and wounded were treated in their regiments or companies.

General George Washington, after taking command of the Army, recommended to the Colonial Congress the establishment of a hospital service with a director and necessary assistants. In July 1775, Congress passed a bill that established a medical service for the Army of 20,000 men by creating a hospital department and named Dr Benjamin Church of Boston, Massachusetts, as its first director general and chief physician.[1]

Army ophthalmology, as a part-time specialty, had its beginning at the start of the Revolutionary War. Several surgeons who were skilled in ophthalmic surgery became prominent during this period. Dr William Shippen (Figure 1-1), a noted surgeon from Philadelphia who performed cataract surgery, served as superintendent of the Army hospitals in New Jersey and later (1777–1781) as Director General of Military Hospitals of the Army.[2] Dr John Jones, a surgeon's mate who served during the French War of 1758 and the American Revolution, did eye surgery and wrote the first American medical book, *Plain, Concise, Practical Remarks on the Treatment of Wounds and Fractures*, published in New York in 1775 (Figure 1-2). This book became the Revolutionary War surgeon's text on military surgery.[3] Another ophthalmic surgeon of the day, Dr John Warren (Figure 1-3), served in the Army and later founded the Harvard Medical School. Lastly, Dr Hall Jackson, an Army surgeon, was noted for his ability in couching cataracts and curing the blind.[4]

A common eye injury during the Revolutionary War was related to the type of weapon used—the flintlock musket and the Kentucky rifle—which, on firing, would occasionally cause burns to the face and eyelids.

War of 1812

No formal Army medical department existed at the beginning of the War of 1812, but on 3 March 1813, one was established. During the War of 1812, many noted part-time ophthalmologists served with the Army, including doctors William E. Horner, Professor of Anatomy at the University of Pennsylvania (Figure 1-4), Horatio Jameson, Hosea Rich, and William Gibson.[4]

Anesthetics were not known, medical training was poor, and asepsis was unheard of at this time. Treatment of many eye conditions was the same as that for other wounds: "blistering and bleeding." Minimal surgery was performed for eye wounds, the only exception being enucleation.[3]

After the war, Congress passed an act in 1818 that provided for an Army Medical Department, this time to be headed by a Surgeon General. Of interest, in December 1822 at Fort Pitt, Pennsylvania,

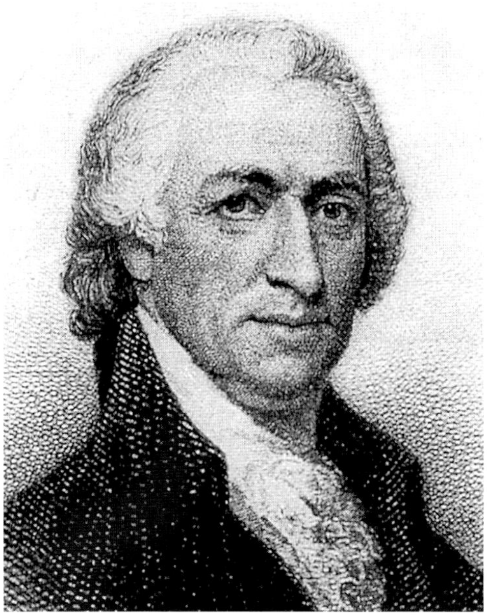

Fig. 1-1. William Shippen, Jr (1736–1808). Reproduced with permission from Packard FR. *History of Medicine in the United States.* Vol 1. New York, NY: Paul B. Haeberdic; 1931: 289.

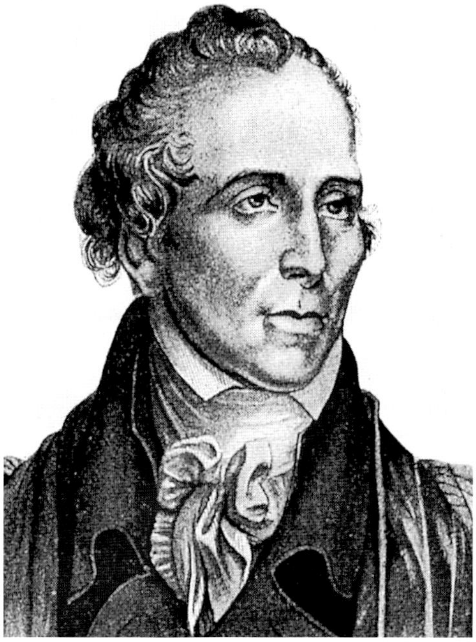

Fig. 1-3. John Warren (1753–1815). Reproduced with permission from Packard FR. *History of Medicine in the United States.* Vol 1. New York, NY: Paul B. Haeberdic; 1931: 431.

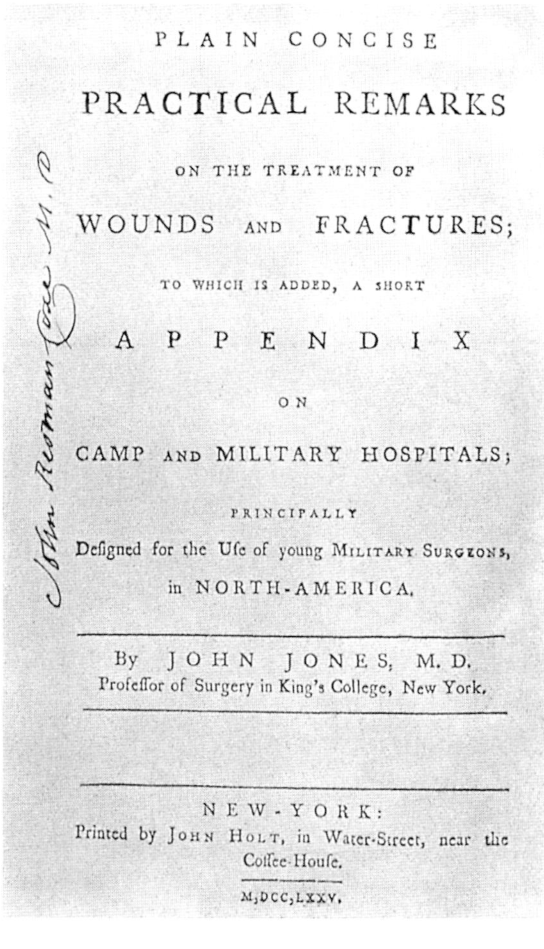

PLAIN CONCISE

PRACTICAL REMARKS

ON THE TREATMENT OF

WOUNDS AND FRACTURES;

TO WHICH IS ADDED, A SHORT

APPENDIX

ON

CAMP AND MILITARY HOSPITALS;

PRINCIPALLY

Deſigned for the Uſe of young MILITARY SURGEONS, in NORTH-AMERICA.

By JOHN JONES, M. D.
Profeſſor of Surgery in King's College, New York.

NEW-YORK:
Printed by JOHN HOLT, in Water-Street, near the Coffee-Houſe.
M,DCC,LXXV.

Fig. 1-2. The title page of the first medical book published in the colonies, entitled *Plain Concise Practical Remarks on the Treatment of Wounds and Fractures,* by John Jones, MD. Reproduced with permission from Ashburn PM. *A History of the Medical Department of the United States Army*. New York, NY: Houghton Mifflin (Cambridge, Mass: The Riverside Press); 1929: facing page 13.

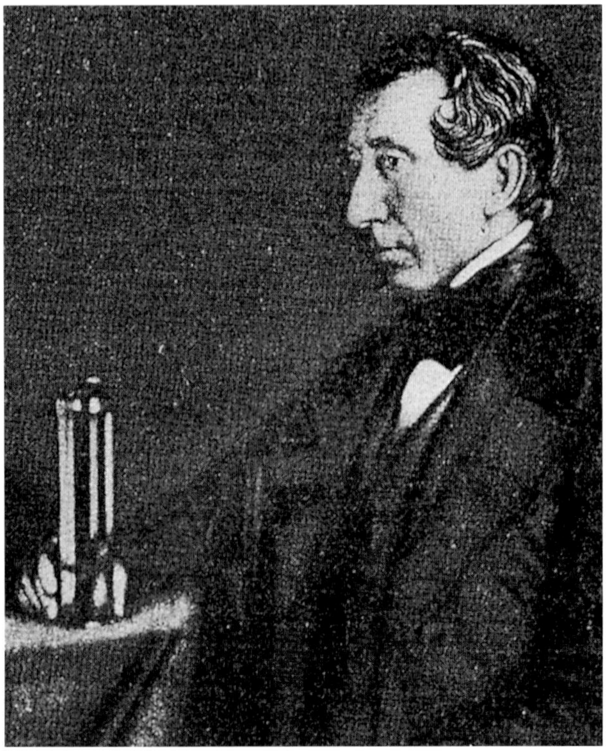

Fig. 1-4. William Edmonds Horner (1773–1853). Reproduced with permission from Packard FR. *History of Medicine in the United States.* Vol 1. New York, NY: Paul B. Haeberdic; 1931: 385.

patients with ophthalmia at the general hospital were treated with silver nitrate in a solution of "lunar caustic in the distilled waters."[5] On 11 February 1847, Congress passed an act that gave military rank to medical officers for the first time.

American Civil War

The onset of the American Civil War found the Army and its Medical Department unprepared for the numerous battlefield casualties. Fortunately, an efficient system of evacuation from the battlefields was developed by Dr Jonathan Letterman, Medical Director of the Army of Potomac[4] (Figure 1-5). Eye injuries in the Civil War constituted about 0.9% (1,190 eyes) of the injuries due to direct hits by missiles and hand-to-hand fighting. However, between 1861 and 1866 in the Union Army, 84,986 cases of purulent ophthalmia and inflammation of the conjunctiva were reported, with four deaths resulting.[6] Although the retinoscope and ophthalmoscope invented by Helmhottz came into use during this time, they were not used in field hospitals on either side of the war.[6] Ether was available, but local anesthesia was not.

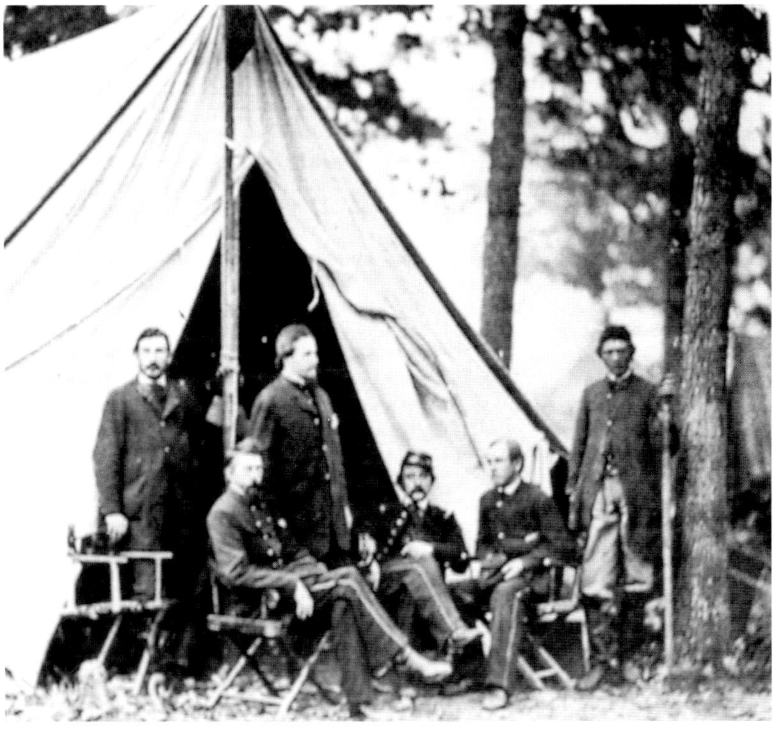

Fig. 1-5. Jonathan Letterman (seated, left). Reproduced with permission from Melin GR. The Army Medical Department, 1818–1865. *The American Medical Recorder.* 1862;8:193.

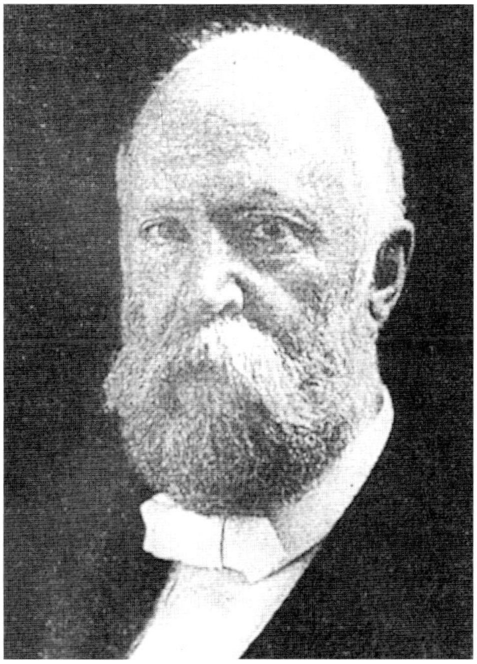

Fig. 1-6. William Fisher Norris. Reproduced with permission from Albert DM, Edward DD. *The History of Ophthalmology*. Cambridge, Mass: Blackwell Science, 1996: 151.

During the American Civil War, many ophthalmic surgeons served in the military, both part time and full time. Doctors Louis Dugas, Francis Cunningham, and Moses de Rosset served in the Confederate Army. Of note, the University of Pennsylvania, the Jefferson Hospital, and the Wills Hospital contributed many well-known ophthalmologists from their staffs to the Union Army, including doctors D. Hayes Agnew, William Henry Pancoast, Charles Robertson, William Norris, Richard Levis, Peter D. Keyser, William Hunt, Addinell Hewson, and Ezra Dyer.

Ophthalmology was established as a full-time specialty in the United States during the American Civil War, and in 1863 the American Medical Association recognized it as a specialty. Likewise, modern ophthalmology had its beginning in the Army Medical Department during the American Civil War. Many of the staff at the Wills Hospital of Philadelphia, one of the first general hospitals that paid particular attention to the diseases of the eye, went as a group into the Army. For example, Dr S. Weir Mitchell of Philadelphia, a neurologist, did his well-known work on eyestrain as a cause of headache and promoted the use of proper eyeglasses. Although not an ophthalmologist, Mitchell realized the importance of systemic ocular examinations as part of a general examination and developed a step-by-step method for ocular examinations that is still used today. Doctors William Norris and William Thomson made valuable microscopic studies that greatly added to the knowledge of the profession. In addition, Norris (Figure 1-6) established an eye-and-ear department at the University of Pennsylvania, and Thomson provided ocular micrographs for the Army Medical Museum.[7]

The period from 1865 to 1898—from the close of the American Civil War to the outbreak of the Spanish–American War—has been alluded to as "the day of small things" in the US Army. However, the Army Medical Museum (Figure 1-7) was established in 1863 for the purpose of preparing the text *Medical and Surgical History of the War of the Rebellion* and to collect all war-related specimens of interest to the study of military medicine and surgery.[8] In addition, the American Ophthalmology Society was established in 1864 and the American Academy of Ophthalmology and Otolaryngology in 1896.

Little is known of Army ophthalmology at the many small Army posts established after the American Civil War, except that cases of snow blindness filled the wards on the Texas frontier in 1876 and that cocaine was used in two eye operations in 1886[3] (Figure 1-8). The only eye disease reported from the more than 130 outposts in the Southwest was "army ophthalmia" from Fort Douglas, Utah. This condition was probably trachoma, which was promoted by the alkali dust that was common to the area.[9]

In 1893, US Army Surgeon General George M. Sternberg established the Army Medical School (the

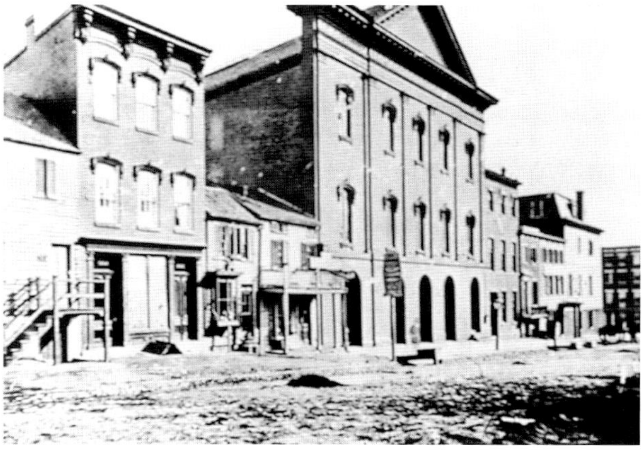

Fig. 1-7. The large building in the center of this photograph is Ford's Theater, which was the fourth home of the Army Medical Museum and which it occupied from 1866 until 1887. Photograph: Courtesy of National Museum of Health and Medicine, Armed Forces Institute of Pathology, Washington, DC; Reeve Negative 32782.

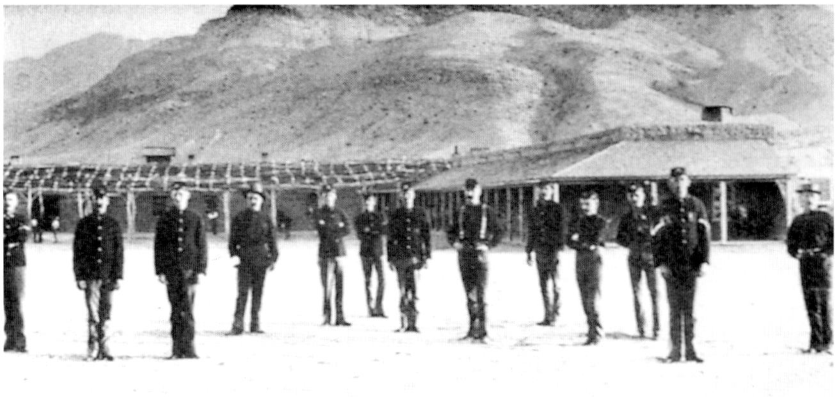

Fig. 1-8. Fort Seldon, Texas, 1865–1892. Eye care could be provided at this frontier hospital, seen here behind troops. Reproduced with permission from Hart HM. *Old Forts of the Southwest*. Seattle, Wash: Superior Publishing Company; 1964: 133.

forerunner of the modern Walter Reed Army Institute of Research), which offered courses in ophthalmology for Army surgeons. Army medical officers could receive advanced training in ophthalmology in Army general hospitals, medical schools, and even in foreign studies. A large number of Army medical officers became proficient in ophthalmology after the American Civil War; some of the most prominent were doctors John M. Bannister, H. A. Shaw, John L. Sheppard, Theodore C. Lyster, W. D. Crosby, P. S. Halloran, James Bourke, and Louis A. La Garde.

Colonel La Garde (Figure 1-9), who spent many years as a frontier surgeon and participated in several Indian campaigns, was one of the first medical officers to become expert in eye diseases after studying at the New York Postgraduate Medical School from 1889 to 1890. Although he filled many administrative posts during his long military service, La Garde's first interest was the practice of medicine, with special emphasis on surgery and diseases of the eye. He had a wide knowledge of surgical pathology and was a skillful surgeon. He is best remembered, however, for his work on wound infections from missiles and on the effects of high-velocity bullets on the human body. He published widely and lectured extensively on the subject, and during World War I he helped train physicians on the treatment of gunshot wounds at various medical training camps.[10]

Spanish–American War

Only 35 eye injuries were reported during the Spanish–American War, which accounted for 2.2% of the total 1,561 who were wounded in combat. With the occupation of Cuba and the Spanish colonies of Puerto Rico and the Philippines, tropical ophthalmology became very important. This made the need for specialization even more important in the military medical services, and after the war, for the first time, the Army concentrated its specialists and special equipment in its general hospitals.

World War I

Soon after the United States entered World War I, it became apparent that the Army Medical Depart-

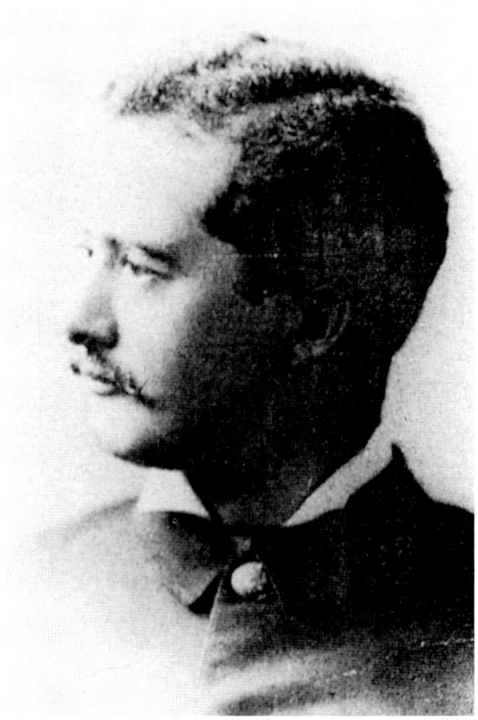

Fig. 1-9. Colonel Louis A. La Garde, a member of the US Army Medical Department. Reproduced from Mary C. Gillett. *Army Medical Department, 1865–1917*. Washington, DC: Center of Military History, US Army; 1995: 158.

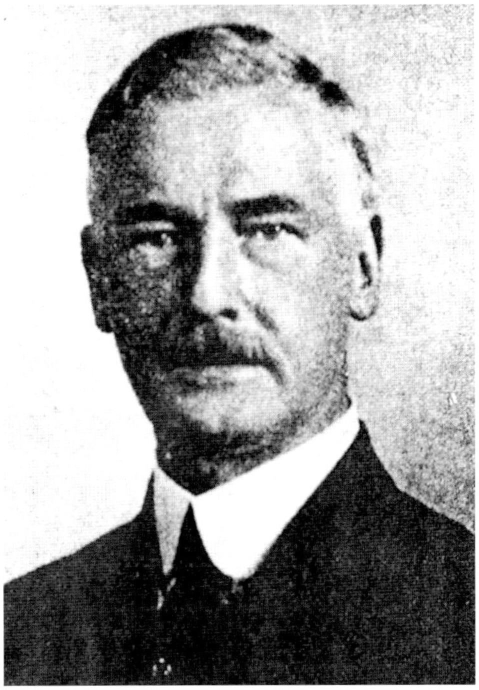

Fig. 1-10. Colonel George E. DeSchweinitz. Reproduced with permission from Albert DM, Edward DD. *The History of Ophthalmology*. Cambridge, Mass: Blackwell Science; 1996: 153.

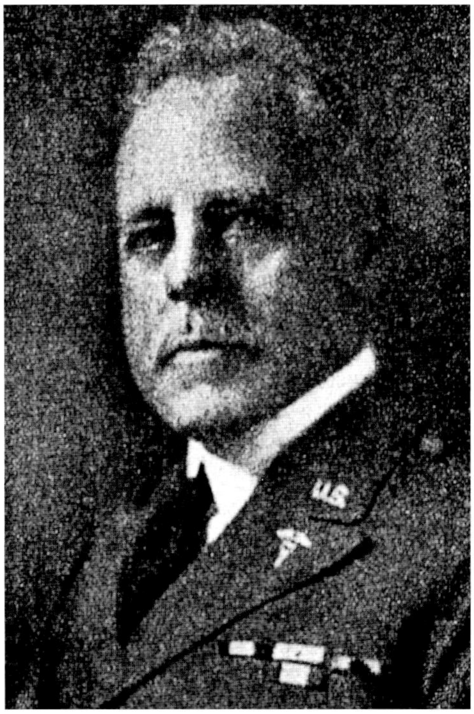

Fig. 1-11. Brigadier General William Holland Wilmer (circa 1920). Reproduced with permission from Hume EE. *The Golden Jubilee of the Association of Military Surgeons of the United States. A Brief History of its First Half Century 1891–1941*. Washington, DC: The Association of the Military Surgeons, 1941: 128.

ment would have to call to service many physicians and surgeons who were specialists in their particular branches. It was estimated that 500 trained ophthalmologists would be necessary to provide the military ophthalmic work required in the United States and abroad.[11(p659)] Army ophthalmology was established as a section under the Division of Head Surgery.[12] Colonel George E. de Schweinitz (Figure 1-10), a reserve officer and Professor of Ophthalmology at the University of Pennsylvania, served as Chief of the Ophthalmic Section. Colonel Allan Greenwood was appointed the Chief Consultant in Ophthalmology to the American Expeditionary Force (AEF); later, he wrote the ophthalmology section (AEF) of the official history of the US Army Medical Department in World War I.[11]

Colonel William Holland Wilmer (Figure 1-11), a clinical and research professor at Georgetown University Medical School in 1917, laid the foundation for the development of aviation medicine. Wilmer helped map out standards for the US Army Air Medical Service, the Medical Research Board, and the Air Medical Research Laboratory. He served as the first director of the laboratory, which eventually became the parent school for flight surgeons and later became known as the School of Aviation Medicine.[13]

Before the organization of the AEF, a number of Army ophthalmologists were sent to France for duty there with the British Expeditionary Force. The British medical profession, depleted in ranks because of the length of the war, needed medical officers to fill the gaps. These American surgeons gained great experience in the clinical and pathological ophthalmic problems in France and England before the US Army base hospital units arrived in Europe.[1] In addition, eminent men in civilian medicine were sent to France as consultants. This was the beginning of the Civilian Consultant Service, as it is known today. A total of 612 ophthalmologists were assigned to duty during World War I. An example of the type of men who served was Dr George Strong Derby, a professor at Massachusetts Eye and Ear Infirmary in Boston, who was stationed at Hospital 5 in France.[14] After the war, he was instrumental in appointing the first woman, Dr Maud Carvill, to his infirmary staff.[7]

The ophthalmological statistics of World War I plainly indicate the scope of this field in the mili-

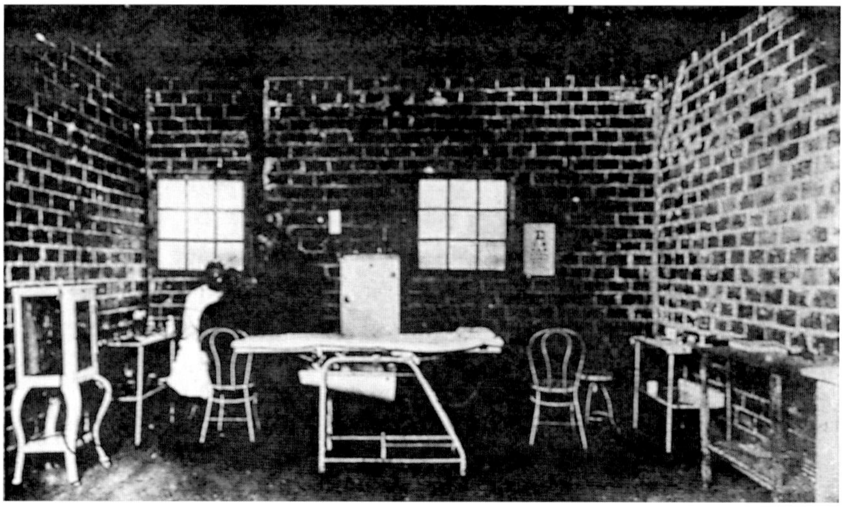

Fig. 1-12. Eye Clinic, Base Hospital 68. Reproduced from Greenwood A, ed. Ophthalmology in the American Expeditionary Forces. Section 4. In: Ireland MW, ed. *Medical Department of the US Army in World War I*. Vol 11, Part 2. Washington, DC: War Department, US Government Printing Office; 1924: 670.

tary service. Eye injuries averaged 2% of all the casualties, but a peak of 8% was reached during the static phases of trench warfare.[15] Some 6,400 operations on the eye were reported, such surgical interventions being limited to those (*a*) made necessary by injuries or (*b*) wherein the effectiveness of the soldier could be improved (Figure 1-12).

Of patients in base hospitals, 10% required eye examinations and treatment (Figure 1-13).[16] Syphilis was a frequent cause of iritis or iridocyclitis. Influenza was often complicated by ocular lesions, chiefly conjunctivitis. Most eye injuries were produced by flying fragments of shell casing, bits of exploding hand grenades, or gravel blown into the eyes by explosion of shells among sandbags around trenches. The most destructive injuries were caused by high-velocity bullets and shrapnel balls. Careful X-ray localization of intraocular foreign bodies (IOFBs) was stressed. Despite their large size, the use of the Haab giant magnets became routine; the extraction of nonmagnetic foreign bodies (FBs) in the vitreous, however, was more challenging. Forceps were introduced through a scleral incision and the object was visualized with an ophthalmoscope. Colonel Harvey Cushing, a noted neurosurgeon in the AEF, correlated traumatic brain injuries with their visual fields. This was of great importance to the field of neuroophthalmology, as it provided valuable diagnostic information to physicians in determining the site of visual tract lesions in the brain.[14]

One of the striking developments during the war was the effect that certain chemical agents had on

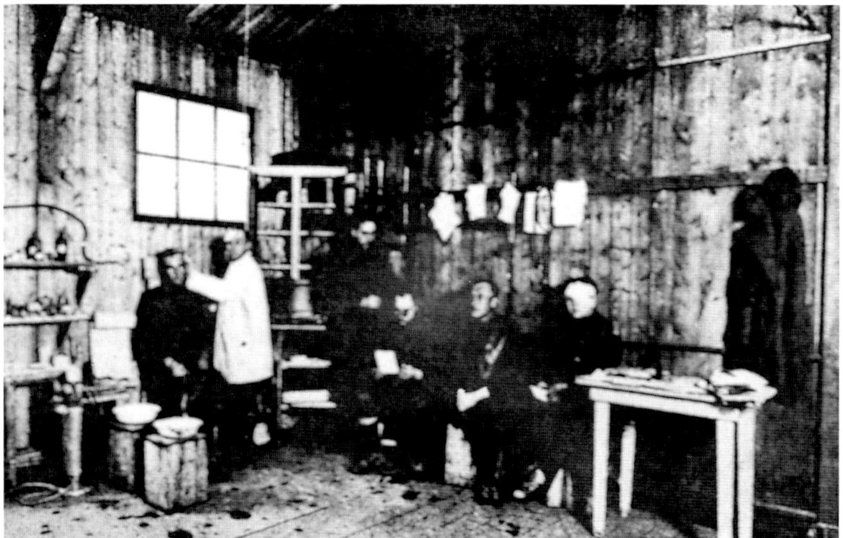

Fig. 1-13. Eye Clinic Camp Hospital 9. Reproduced from Greenwood A, ed. Ophthalmology in the American Expeditionary Forces. Section 4. In: Ireland MW, ed. *Medical Department of the US Army in World War I*. Vol 11, Part 2. Washington, DC: War Department, US Government Printing Office; 1924: 671.

the eyes. Mustard agent (2,2'-dichlorethyl sulfide), which was used by the Germans, produced many Allied casualties who often required prolonged hospitalization in special gas hospitals such as Field Hospital 16 in Luzancy, France. Experienced ophthalmologists were assigned to the staffs of these hospitals to treat chemical conjunctivitis, episcleritis, and keratitis. Acute cases were treated with mild solutions of boric acid or sodium bicarbonate and atropine, then during convalescence with zinc sulfate.[14]

Before casualties began to be returned from overseas, six hospitals in the United States were selected as eye centers and another was designated for the care of blinded casualties. Approximately 300 soldiers were blinded in the war,[17] and many of them received care and rehabilitation at the Army General Hospital 7 in Baltimore, Maryland. Major General Merritte W. Ireland (who was The Surgeon General, US Army, in 1918) had practiced some ophthalmology early in his career, which accounted for his intense interest in the care of blind soldiers during and after the war.[18] However, since 1921, the Veterans Administration (now known as the US Department of Veterans Affairs) has assumed the care and instruction of blinded soldiers.

The most notable advance in training during the war was the establishment in August 1918 of the Army School of Ophthalmology at Fort Oglethorpe, Georgia, although it functioned for only a few months. The course of instruction provided review and postgraduate work for experienced ophthalmologists, with special training in military ophthalmology.[19]

Between World Wars I and II

After World War I, the value of specialists in the proper care of the wounded and in the conservation of manpower was clearly defined. Between World Wars I and II, there were more than 30 men in the Regular Army who were well qualified in the specialty of ophthalmology, including doctors Roderic P. O'Connor, W. T. Davis, and Pfeffer, Keeler, Royalls, and Dale. Younger military ophthalmologists were detailed as understudies in the service and as students in leading postgraduate schools. Some were sent to Vienna, Austria, for postgraduate training.[14]

Two Army institutions that are of great importance to the profession of ophthalmology are the Army Medical Library and the Army Medical Museum. The place in medical science held by the Army Medical Museum was recognized by the leading ophthalmologists in the United States in 1922, when the Registry of Ophthalmic Pathology was established under the guidance of Lieutenant Colonel George R. Callender. The Registry quickly enlarged, and by 1933, civilian and military ophthalmologists had submitted 2,385 specimens. Together with succeeding specimens and records, these have assisted greatly in the publication—in close collaboration with the American Academy of Ophthalmology and Otolaryngology—of several classic textbooks in ocular pathology since 1929 to the present. These titles include Jonas Friedenwald's *The Pathology of the Eye* and his *Ophthalmic Pathology: An Atlas and Textbook;* De Coursey and Ash's *The Pathology of the Eye;* Hogan and Zimmerman's *Ophthalmic Pathology: An Atlas and Textbook;* and Spencer's *Ophthalmic Pathology.*

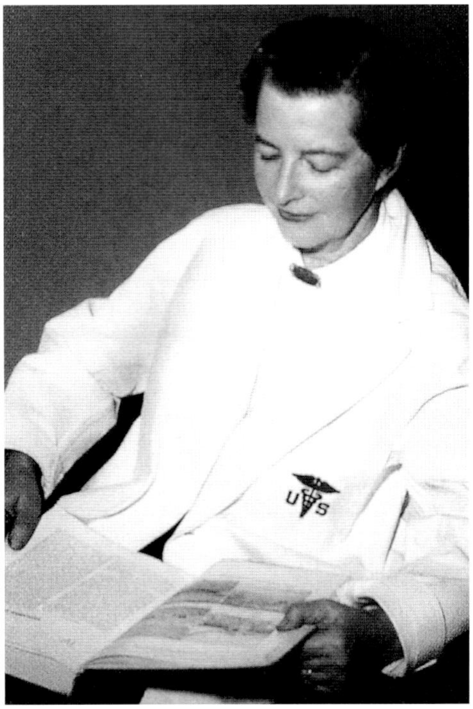

Fig. 1-14. Helen Campbell Wilder Foerster. Photograph: Courtesy of Armed Forces Institute of Pathology, Washington, DC.

Several individuals contributed to the outstanding success of the ophthalmic pathology section of the Army Medical Museum and its eventual development into the Armed Forces Institute of Pathology (AFIP) in 1949. In addition to Lieutenant Colonel George R. Callender (mentioned above), they also included Major General Elbert De Coursey, Lieutenant Colonel James Ash, Lieutenant Colonel Lorenz E. Zimmerman, and civilian Helen Campbell Wilder Foerster. Foerster (Figure 1-14), a histopa-

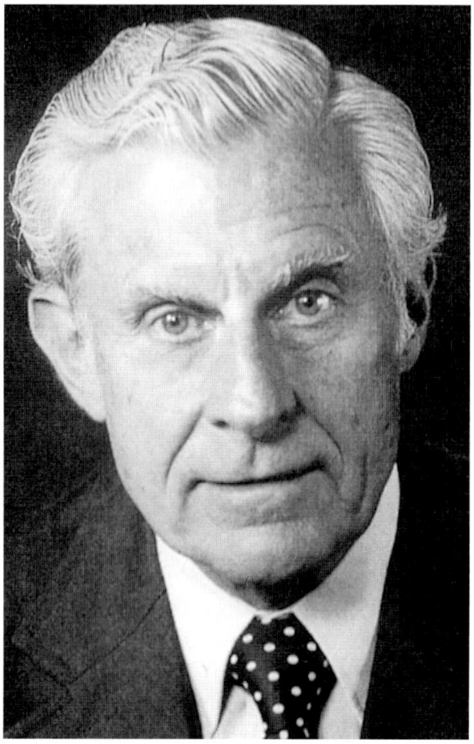

Fig. 1-15. Lorenz E. Zimmerman. Reproduced with permission from Albert DM, Edward DD. *The History of Ophthalmology*. Cambridge, Mass: Blackwell Science; 1996: 99.

thology technician at the museum for 33 years (from the establishment of the Registry), was an outstanding contributor and collaborator in ophthalmic pathology. She published many scholarly writings, especially studies of chorioretinitis caused by *Toxoplasma gondii* and *Toxocara canis*. Zimmerman (Figure 1-15), who became Chief of the Ophthalmic Pathology Section at AFIP in 1953, made significant contributions in ocular pathology with multiple publications and is a great teacher and excellent lecturer. He trained many ocular pathologists in the United States and abroad.

Graduate medical education in ophthalmology was begun in 1920 with the establishment of Army internship programs at several Army medical centers. Practical training was offered at Walter Reed General Hospital Clinic for medical officers designated to receive special instruction in ophthalmology. On 1 September 1923, to further the educational system of the Medical Department of the Army, the Department of Ophthalmology was established at Walter Reed General Hospital. Colonel Ralph H. Goldwaite served as the ophthalmologist at Walter Reed during the war, but Colonel Edward B. Spaeth became the first Chief of the Department of Ophthalmology (Figure 1-16).

a b

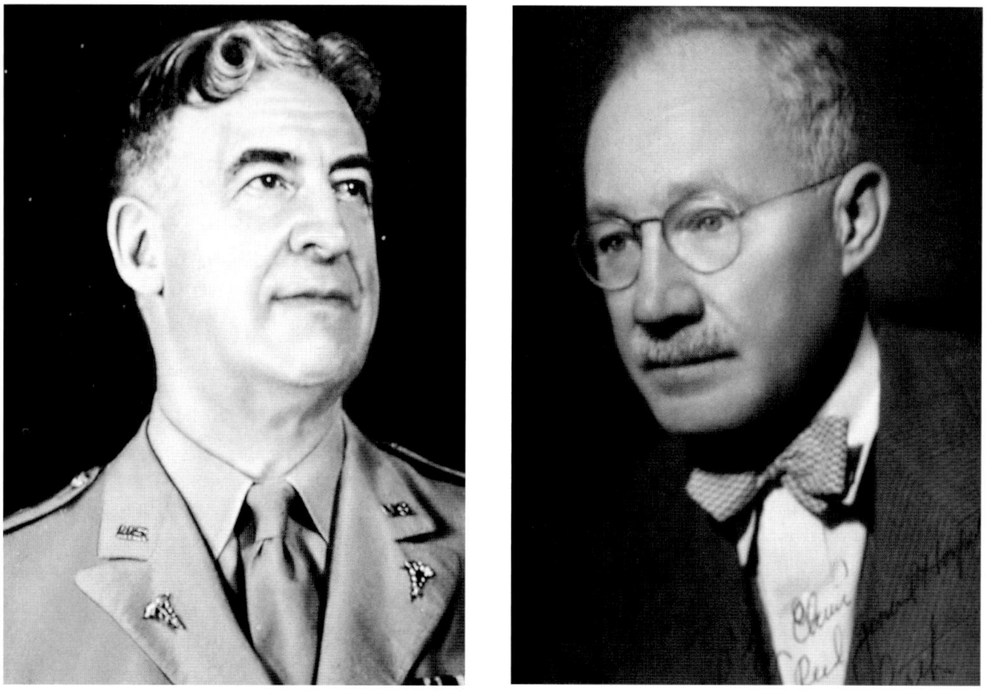

Fig. 1-16. (**a**) Colonel Ralph H. Goldwaite. (**b**) Colonel Edward B. Spaeth. Photographs: Courtesy of Walter Reed Army Medical Center, Washington, DC.

World War II

Military ophthalmology reached a new high during World War II, and its accomplishments were many. The bulk of the medical care and practically all specialists were obtained from civilian resources, with most of the members of the Regular Army Medical Corps acting in administrative capacities. The medical and surgical advances in ophthalmology, with modern drugs and better techniques and equipment, were well applied. The increased skill and training of the ophthalmologists, together with better evaluating methods for eye casualties, reduced eye loss.

Consultants in ophthalmology coordinated the care of eye casualties in the various theaters, and specialized centers for the treatment of eye injuries were established throughout the United States. Colonel Derrick T. Vail, Jr, Professor of Ophthalmology at Northwestern University, served as Senior Consultant in the European theater in 1942 through 1944 and briefly as Chief of the Ophthalmology Branch, Office of The Surgeon General (Figure 1-17). In that position in 1945, he participated in the examinations of the American Board of Ophthalmology to observe the performance of candidates for the Army.

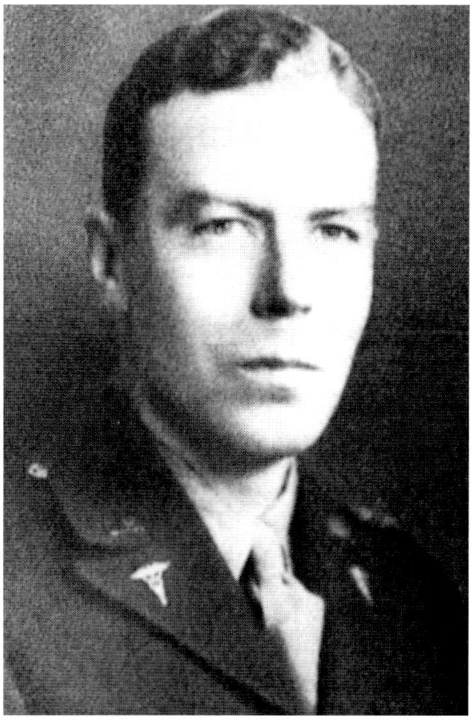

Fig. 1-18. Lieutenant Colonel M. Elliott Randolph. Reproduced from Carter BN, ed. *Activities of Surgical Consultants*. Vol 1. In: Coates JB Jr, ed. *Surgery in World War II*. Washington, DC: US Department of the Army, Medical Department, Office of The Surgeon General; 1962: 96.

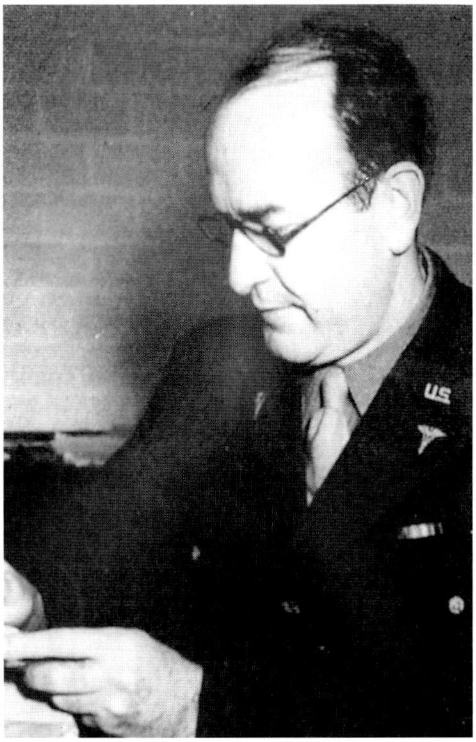

Fig. 1-17. Colonel Derrick T. Vail, Jr. Reproduced from Carter BN, ed. *Activities of Surgical Consultants*. Vol 2. In: Coates JB Jr, ed. *Surgery in World War II*. Washington, DC: US Department of the Army, Medical Department, Office of The Surgeon General; 1964: 444.

The Ophthalmology Branch of the Surgical Consultants Division, Office of The Surgeon General, was activated on 15 April 1944, with Lieutenant Colonel M. Elliott Randolph as its first Chief (Figure 1-18). Its function was to establish policies, procedures, and consultations in the management of general ophthalmology and the care of the blind in the Army.[19]

In most Army hospitals in the Zone of the Interior, the patient load in the eye centers was heavy, and, especially as the war advanced, staff numbers were limited. Many patients required some type of plastic or reconstructive work or treatment for IOFBs, intraocular neoplasms, and retinal detachments (Figure 1-19). Eye injuries in this war again reached an average of about 2% of all injuries, with a peak of 4%.[15] Approximately 1,700 were totally blinded.[20]

Centers for blind soldiers were established for early care and basic education at Valley Forge General Hospital, Pennsylvania; Diablo General Hospital, California; and the Naval Hospital in Phila-

a

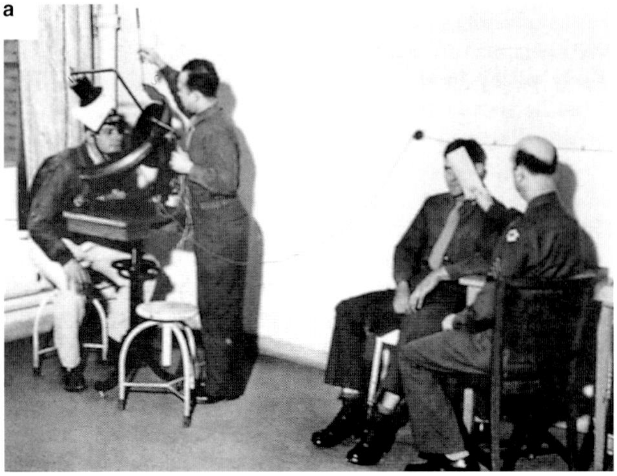

b

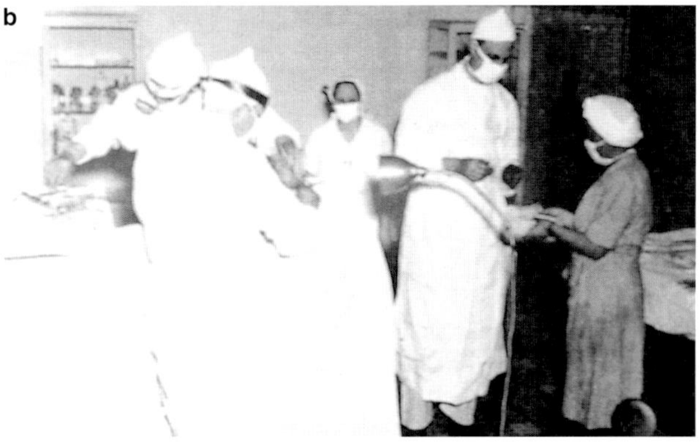

Fig. 1-19. (**a**) The Ophthalmology Service in a General Hospital (England, 1944). (**b**) Eye surgery in a General Hospital (England, 1944). Photographs: Reproduced from Carter BN, ed. *Activities of Surgical Consultants*. Vol 2. In: Coates JB Jr, ed. *Surgery in World War II*. Washington, DC: US Department of the Army, Medical Department, Office of The Surgeon General; 1964: 448, 449.

delphia. If no further medical and surgical treatment would be beneficial, these patients were transferred to Old Farm at Avon, Connecticut, for social rehabilitation and prevocational guidance and training. At the close of the war, a training center for the blind was established at Hines Veterans Administration Hospital, Illinois, which still fills that role today.

One major contribution that wartime medicine made to the ophthalmologic treatment was the development of an artificial eye. In 1944, Captain Stanley F. Erpf, Dental Corps, working at the Army Dental Section with the 30th General Hospital in England, created an artificial eye from acrylic plastic. The eye was unbreakable and closely resembled the coloring of the human eye. After development of a manufacturing process within the Army, approximately 10,000 eyes were produced.

Korean War

The Army Medical Department was in dire need of specialists after World War II ended. Medical officers who practiced specialties or who had some training received refresher courses at various general hospitals and short courses in civilian institutions. At that time, only seven officers were board certified. To help resolve this problem, Army residency programs in the medical and surgical specialties were established on 11 February 1946. This was the beginning of advanced postgraduate clinical education in Army teaching hospitals. This training provided a cadre of teachers, consultants, and specialty practitioners to the Army Medical Department.

The establishment of ophthalmology residency training programs began in 1947 at Brooke Army Hospital, Walter Reed Army Medical Center, Letterman Army Hospital, and Fitzsimons Army Hospital. By the time the Korean War started, 17 board-certified ophthalmologists were in the Regular Army, and 9 Reserve Army officers were on extended active duty.[17]

At the time hostilities began in Korea in June 1950, the Army had 2 ophthalmologists in the Far East, both at the Tokyo Army Hospital. Eventually, 25 ophthalmologists were assigned to the evacuation hospitals in Japan and Korea and some were assigned to mobile army surgical hospitals (MASHs) and neurosurgical teams on the front lines.[17]

In the first 2 years of the Korean War, eye cases represented 12% of all patients admitted to Tokyo Army Hospital.[17] Of the casualties sustained during the first year of the war, 4.6% had eye injuries. Approximately 150 became totally blind.

With the introduction of the helicopter, many eye patients could be evacuated quickly from the battlefield or frontline medical station to a MASH or an evacuation hospital, where definitive surgery could be performed. The seriously injured were sent to one of the five general hospitals in Japan. If hospitalization was expected to exceed 120 days, the patients were returned to the United States.

All types of eye injuries were seen in the Korean War, including perforating wounds, IOFBs, retinal detachments and hemorrhages, and some burns. The burns were more common among the prisoners of war who were accidentally bombed with napalm. The use of the Lancaster hand magnet and the Berman FB locator were invaluable in the treatment of IOFBs.

Despite the pressure of the war in the Far East,

in 1951 Colonel Forrest E. Hull, Chief of the Eye Service at Tokyo Army Hospital and Consultant to the Surgeon of the Far East Command, organized a course in the basic science of ophthalmology in Japan for ophthalmologists who had not completed their training because of the sudden onset of the war. Also, the American Board of Ophthalmology gave the written examinations in Tokyo in 1951 and 1952.[21]

One of the great advances in Army ophthalmology was in ocular research, which was practically nonexistent until Colonel Austin Lowrey, Jr (Figure 1-20), started a research unit in 1948 at what is now Walter Reed Army Medical Center, Washington, DC. The unit, under the Research and Development Board of The Surgeon General's office commanded by Colonel John H. King (Figure 1-21), Chief of Ophthalmology at Walter Reed and Consultant in Ophthalmology to The Surgeon General, US Army, performed active research and coordinated research projects in progress at other Army general hospitals, military installations, and key civilian institutions. Among many others, studies were conducted on ocular toxoplasmosis and leptospirosis, and, in addition, on problems with atomic radiation, new equipment both for field and stationary clinics, a survey on new drugs, development of protective combat goggles, the use of contact lenses in combat conditions, and vision and muscle balance in accidents.[17]

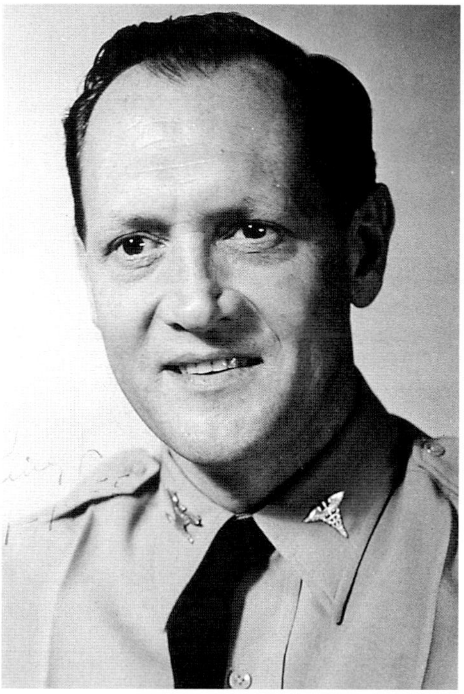

Fig. 1-21. Colonel John H. King. Photograph: Courtesy of Walter Reed Army Medical Center, Washington, DC.

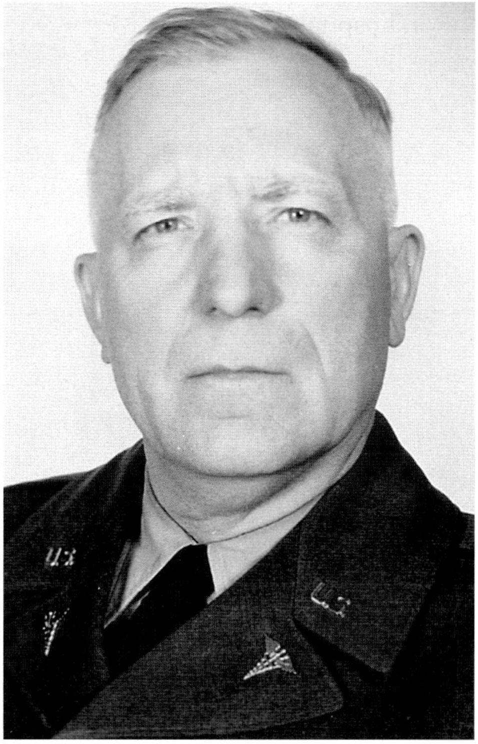

Fig. 1-20. Colonel Austin Lowrey, Jr. Photograph: Courtesy of Walter Reed Army Medical Center, Washington, DC.

Vietnam War

Although US troops were in Vietnam assisting the South Vietnamese regime as early as 1962, casualties with eye injuries were either taken care of by a US-trained Vietnamese ophthalmologist in Saigon or they were evacuated to the United States. In August 1965, the first US Army ophthalmologist was assigned to the 85th Evacuation Hospital in Qui Nhon. As the war escalated, eight additional ophthalmologists arrived in Vietnam and were stationed at evacuation and field hospitals (Figure 1-22).[22] The ophthalmologist at the 24th Evacuation Hospital in Long Binh was designated the Consultant in Ophthalmology to the Senior Medical Commander. However, he had limited authority to correct any deficiencies in ocular care in Vietnam.

Usually only one ophthalmologist was assigned to a hospital unit to provide surgical and medical care to inpatients and outpatients. Because there were not enough fully trained ophthalmologists to staff evacuation and field hospitals, general medi-

Fig. 1-22. US Army Hospitals in Vietnam, December 1968. Reproduced from Neel S. *Medical Support of the US Army in Vietnam 1965–1970.* Washington, DC: US Government Printing Office, 1973: 62.

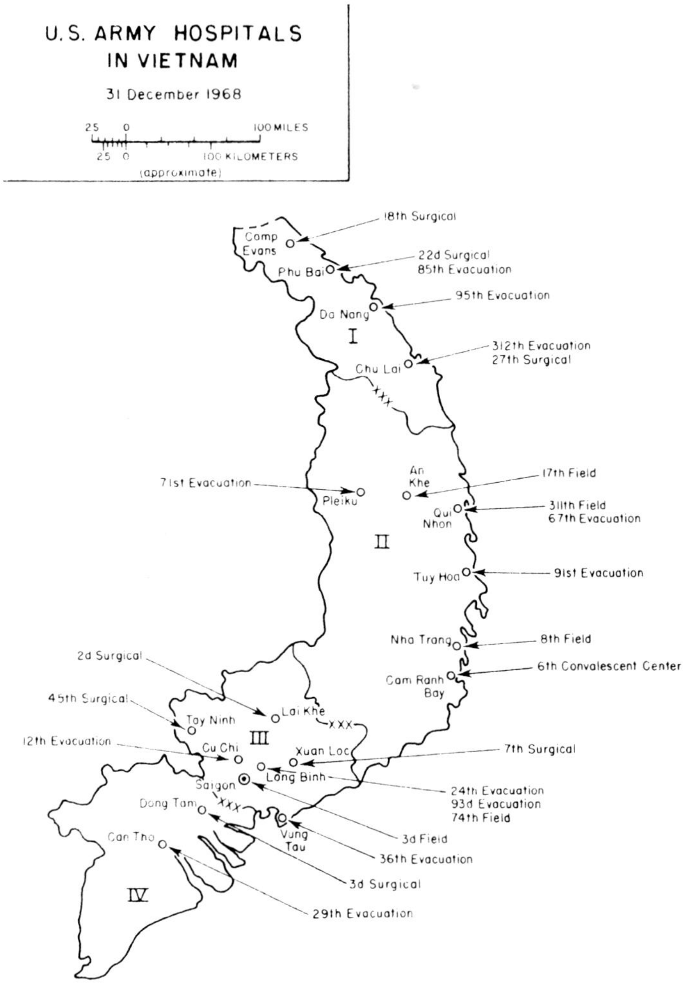

cine officers were given on-the-job training at the 24th Evacuation Hospital to provide some care. The absence of senior Army eye surgeons in theater made it difficult to obtain needed consultation and assistance to manage difficult cases.

Another prevalent problem was that the Army hospitals were designated and equipped to provide care only for specific combat units, and they were expected to evacuate casualties quickly. Moreover, these hospitals were required to provide care for all patients, including Allied military personnel and some civilians of all ages. Unfortunately, the hospitals had no ophthalmic equipment for outpatient care and had only minimal inpatient surgical supplies and instruments. These shortages necessitated the evacuation of many patients back to the Communication Zone in Japan and the Philippines, where delayed definitive care produced poorer outcomes. The ophthalmic supply problem was partially resolved when the ophthalmologists personally contacted civilian and military sources in the United States to obtain needed items such as standard medications and surgical instruments.

Regardless of the shortcomings experienced during the Vietnam War, the overall standard of eye care was high, and no documented cases of sympathetic uveitis were reported. Of casualties in Vietnam, 9% sustained ocular injuries, the highest in any American war or conflict. Only 25% of the ocular casualties studied could return to active duty, whereas 83% of all surviving wounded could do so. Further analysis also indicated that 39% of the eye injuries could have been prevented by the use of some form of eye armor.[22]

When not involved in their military duties, most Army ophthalmologists provided medical and surgical care for Vietnamese civilians and military in both Vietnamese and US Army hospitals. Several military ophthalmologists were able to actively participate in the Medical Civil Action Program

a b

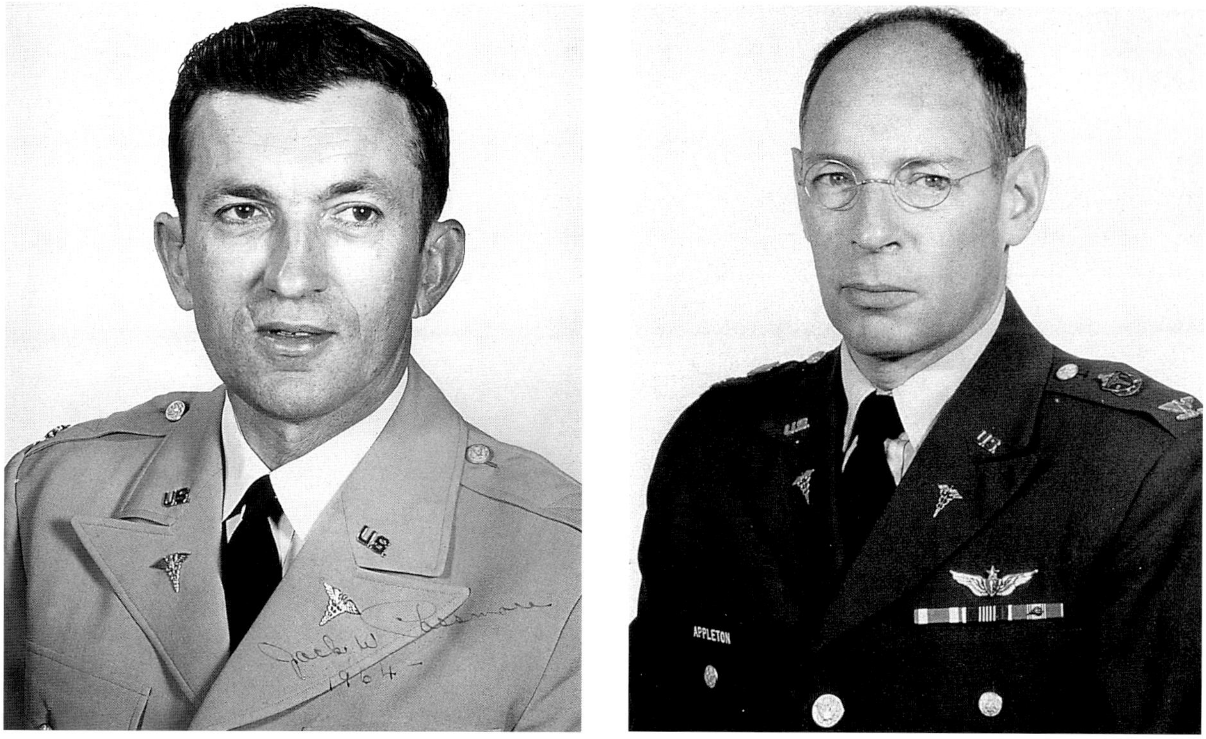

Fig. 1-23. (**a**) Colonel Jack W. Passmore. (**b**) Colonel Budd Appleton. Photographs: Courtesy of Walter Reed Army Medical Center, Washington, DC.

(MEDCAP), providing medical care and surgery to Vietnamese and Montagnard patients. In addition, they trained ophthalmologists in the Vietnamese army in cataract and ocular plastic surgery.

During the Vietnam War, Army ophthalmology worldwide was led by the Consultants in Ophthalmology to The Surgeon General: Colonel Jack W. Passmore (1964–1967) and Colonel Budd Appleton (1968–1978), both of whom also served as Chief of the Ophthalmology Service at Walter Reed Army Medical Center (Figure 1-23). Many ophthalmologists served well in Vietnam, including William Dale Anderson, Arnulf F. Ehmer, Francis G. La Piana, Albert Hornblass, Richard M. Leavitt, Lewis L. Lauring, F. B. Hoefle, and Bruce E. Spivey.

Errors in the provision of care to ophthalmic casualties in Vietnam could have been prevented if the lessons learned in previous wars had been better known and applied. Efforts are being directed toward improving the treatment of ocular injuries in any future conflict, (eg, blast and laser injuries).

Since the Vietnam War, the US Army has been involved with several conflicts around the world: in Panama, Grenada, Haiti, Somalia, the Persian Gulf, and the Balkans. Military ophthalmic care was important during the Persian Gulf War; Army and Navy ophthalmologists provided care for 221 casualties. Most of the injuries were caused by blast fragments (78%) from munitions.[23]

IMPLICATIONS FOR MILITARY OPHTHALMOLOGISTS

After the downsizing of the Army, the US Army Medical Department currently has training centers for ophthalmologists at three Army Medical Centers: Walter Reed, Brooke, and Madigan. Several centers also provide training for Air Force and Naval officers. In addition, postgraduate courses in ocular trauma and ocular pathology are offered to military ophthalmologists every year. The present role of military medicine and Army ophthalmology is to be prepared for battle and noncombat situations. Military ophthalmologists must now be equipped to provide humanitarian and civic assistance, global disaster preparedness, and combat ophthalmic care. Readiness for all assigned and unexpected missions is the present goal of military medicine.

REFERENCES

1. Tuttle AD. *Handbook for the Medical Soldier*. New York, NY: William Wood & Co; 1927.

2. Gillett MC. *Army Medical Department, 1775–1818*. Washington, DC: Center of Military History, US Army; 1981.

3. Ashburn PM. *History of the Medical Department of the US Army*. Boston, Mass: Houghton Mifflin; 1929.

4. Kelley HA. *Cyclopedia of the American Medical Biography*. Philadelphia, Pa: WB Saunders; 1912.

5. Melin GR. The Army Medical Department, 1818–1865. *The American Medical Recorder*. 1825;8:193.

6. Otis GA, Huntington DL. *Medical and Surgical History of the War of the Rebellion*. Washington, DC: US Government Printing Office; 1883.

7. Albert DM, Edward DD. *The History of Ophthalmology*. Cambridge, Mass: Blackwell Science; 1996.

8. Office of The Surgeon General. Circular 8. 26 May 1862.

9. Parkes A. *Manual of Practical Hygiene*. Vol 2. No date: 153.

10. US Army. *Army Medical Bulletin*. July 1939; 88–93. No. 49.

11. Greenwood A. Ophthalmology in the American Expeditionary Forces. Introduction. Section 4. In: Ireland MW, ed. *Medical Department of the US Army in World War I*. Vol 11, Part 2. Washington DC: War Department, US Government Printing Office; 1924: 659–676.

12. Greenwood A, de Schweinitz GD. *Medical Department of the US Army in World War I*. Vol 11, Part 2. Washington DC: War Department, US Government Printing Office; 1924.

13. Maumenee AE. History of the Wilmer Institute. *Am J Ophthalmol*. 1965;60:770–778.

14. Patterson RU. Address of The Surgeon General. Presented at: Annual Meeting of the American Academy of Ophthalmology and Otolaryngology; September 16, 1933; Boston, Mass.

15. Vail DT. Military ophthalmology. *Trans Am Acad Ophthalmol Otolaryngol*. 1951;55:709–715.

16. Greenwood A, de Schweinitz GD. *Medical War Manual 3, Military Ophthalmic Surgery*. New York, NY: L Febiger; 1918.

17. King JH. Army ophthalmology, past and present. *The Military Surgeon*. 1953;112:88–96.

18. Ireland E. Personal communication, 1952.

19. Coates JB Jr, Randolph ME, Canfield N, eds. *Ophthalmology and Otolaryngology*. In: Hays SB, Coates JB Jr, eds. *Surgery in World War II*. Washington, DC: US Department of the Army, Medical Department, Office of The Surgeon General; 1957.

20. Gruber KF. Assistant director, American Foundation for the Blind. Personal communication, 1952.

21. Hull FE. Consultant in Ophthalmology, Far East Command. Personal communication, 1952.

22. La Piana FG, Hornblass A. Military ophthalmology in the Vietnam War. *Doc Ophthalmol*. 1997;93:29–48.

23. Mader TH, Aragones JV, Chandler AC, et al. Ocular and ocular adnexal injuries treated by United States military ophthalmologists during Operations Desert Shield and Desert Storm. *Ophthalmology*. 1993;100:1462–1467.

Chapter 2

LESSONS LEARNED

FRANCIS G. LA PIANA, MD*; AND THOMAS H. MADER, MD†

*Colonel, US Army (Ret); Ophthalmology Residency Program Director, Department of Ophthalmology, The Washington Hospital Center, Washington, DC 20010; and Professor of Surgery, Uniformed Services University of the Health Sciences, 4301 Jones Bridge Road, Bethesda, Maryland 20814-4799; formerly, Consultant in Ophthalmology to The Surgeon General, US Army, and Ophthalmology Residency Program Director, Ophthalmology Service, Walter Reed Army Medical Center, Washington, DC

†Colonel, US Army (Ret); Alaska Native Medical Center, Anchorage, Alaska 99508; formerly, Chief of Ophthalmology, Madigan Army Medical Center, Tacoma, Washington

INTRODUCTION

This chapter summarizes some of the lessons learned from experiences in the Vietnam War (F. G. La P.) and the Persian Gulf War (T. H. M.). Our combined expertise in military ophthalmology—both the treatment of injured soldiers and the workings of the military medical system—leads us to believe that some of the same difficulties that the US military medical establishment experienced early in our nation's history continue to be repeated. Some of the hard-won lessons from our own experience and those from previous wars, which should be remembered by current and future generations of military ophthalmologists, include the following:

- Having experienced ophthalmologists at the forward echelons will ensure that our soldiers get the best possible initial and definitive care.
- Having a senior ophthalmologist in theater may ensure that (*a*) the concerns of all eye-care professionals are heard and (*b*) training of nonophthalmologists is accomplished.
- Hands-on inspection of supplies prior to deployment is mandatory to ensure that modern and usable equipment is available to treat the injured soldier.

If we do not learn from our predecessors, we will continue to make the same mistakes they did.

Allen Greenwood, MD (1866–1942), a prominent US ophthalmologist, volunteered his services in the Spanish–American War, volunteered again to serve in France during World War I, and became Senior Ophthalmic Consultant for the American Expeditionary Forces. At the end of that war, General Pershing cited him for exceptionally meritorious and conspicuous services. Greenwood's description of hospital conditions in France in 1918 underscores our first lesson, that experienced ophthalmologists must be deployed to forward echelons:

> I want to take a minute to draw a word-picture of an evacuation hospital in time of stress. During the height of the Argonne offensive I went to the most forward of the evacuation hospitals, at the tip of the forest, which had been opened only two days. It had been raining a week, was still raining when I arrived, and the roads were a sea of mud. The hospital was in an old chateau, with tents arranged around it, and practically every ambulance wheel went up to the hub in the mud. The nurses and officers were wearing rubber boots, and those that were there to help out or to see how things were going wore overshoes. I entered the hospital at three o'clock in the afternoon. Every ward was crowded. Ambulances were coming at the rate of one every two or three minutes. The officer who had charge of the shock ward had four tent wards filled with shock cases. Among these were ten or fifteen men whose faces were partly destroyed. I wish I had the gift of easy speech and the ability to draw word-pictures, so as to draw for you a real picture of that hospital—the rain coming down in torrents, the sea of mud, the shock ward filled, a little heater at the foot of each bed, with men looking at their last gasp, ambulances coming in every two or three minutes, and the drivers exhausted. About thirty miles away we had a special hospital for head cases, but it seemed a crime to ask the drivers and the patients to go the extra thirty miles to reach this eye hospital. This shows the *necessity of having a competent ophthalmic surgeon right at the spot to take care of such cases*" [emphasis added].[1]

What was true and vitally important in World War I remains even more so today, because—given the resources—today's ophthalmic surgeon with subspecialty expertise can salvage eyes that in past wars were inevitably lost, and therefore can increase the number of casualties returned to duty. As Spalding and Sternberg commented in 1990:

> The advent of microsurgery in the 1960's, leading to better closure of ocular lacerations, and the development of vitrectomy techniques in the 1970's, allowing successful repair of posterior segment wounds, have resulted in a dramatic improvement in the prognosis for patients with penetrating ocular injuries.[2]

The objective of this chapter is to specify exactly what theater of operations eye care (TOEC) should be and why. Its genesis lies in the preparation of the history of Army ophthalmology in the Vietnam War[3] and of the history of eye armor development,[4] in the review of reports of military ophthalmologists following World War I, World War II, the Korean War, and the Persian Gulf War, and in discussions with present and former military ophthalmologists of the Army, Navy, and Air Force. A radical revision of eye care provided at all four echelons within the theater of operations (TO) is required if the wounded are to receive optimal care.

The soldier who cannot see, cannot fight. Tiny fragments that produce minor if any disability when impacting elsewhere often produce incapacitating visual disability and, through sympathetic spasm of the orbicularis oculi of the fellow uninjured eye, functional bilateral blindness. The incidence of eye injuries has increased from 0.5% in the American Civil War to 9% in the Vietnam War mainly because of the increasing use of munitions that produce myriad, small, metallic and nonmetallic fragments on detonation. Battlefield eye injuries frequently coexist with other serious and even life-threatening injuries. Other threats to the eye include blunt forces (eg, tree branches, rifle butts and barrels), blown sand and dirt, flechettes, laser wavelengths, blistering agents, heat, and, in the future, probably microwaves and particle beams.

In Vietnam, a soldier struck in the eye in combat had a 50% chance of losing the eye.[3] Only 25% of the Vietnam eye casualties studied by Tredici[5] could return to active duty, while 83% of all surviving wounded could do so.[6] Eye injuries are expensive for society at large as well as for the casualty, in that these patients will have a permanent disability and will need rehabilitation and job training.

Polycarbonate eye armor (Ballistic Laser Protective Spectacles [BLPS] and Special Protective Eyewear Cylindrical Surface [SPECS]) has been developed and improved over the last several decades. Studies have indicated that 2-mm-thick polycarbonate will prevent almost all blunt-force injuries and 39% of injuries caused by missiles.[7] Two of the threatening laser wavelengths will be defeated by a laser-protective attachment, and polycarbonate intrinsically provides significant protection from the carbon dioxide laser emitted wavelength. Unfortunately for the soldier's eye, conventional munitions are being improved, tunable dye lasers are in development, flechettes penetrate 2-mm-thick polycarbonate, and current eye armor provides no specific protection against microwaves or particle beams, so that eye injuries can be expected to occur, to be of great seriousness, and to demand expert and immediate care.

EYE CARE IN THE THEATER OF OPERATIONS

The principles that should govern the provision of medical care in the TO to the eye-injured and -diseased can be divided into two groups: the general and the specific. The general principles are expertise, immediacy, control, assertiveness, complexity, cooperation, integration, reassessment, innovation, and education, and are discussed below. The specific principles apply to the care of the injuries and diseases of the anterior and posterior segments of the globe, the ocular adnexa, and the bony orbit, and are expressed in the Practice of TOEC section of this chapter.

General Principles

There is no delayed primary closure in ophthalmic surgery. The first surgical procedure performed on the injured eye and/or its adnexa is almost always the definitive one, and it must be performed as soon after injury as possible. It therefore follows that we must be prepared to practice such definitive ophthalmic surgery in the TO. To do so requires the presence of ophthalmologists with subspecialty expertise in certain hospitals in the TO. Ophthalmology residents and physicians who have received on-the-job training (OJT) are never qualified to practice independently as ophthalmologists in the TO. Some argue that eye casualties who require vitrectomy and other sophisticated posterior segment surgical procedures can and should receive such care after being evacuated from the TO. They are wrong, because (1) we may not be able to evacuate our casualties from a TO soon enough to provide such care at the appropriate time after injury because of other nonocular injuries that render the patient nontransportable, or (2) the means for such evacuation may not be available. We cannot assume that we will always have air superiority. Therefore, we must be prepared to practice definitive vitreoretinal surgery in the general hospital (GH) (see the section on Practice of TOEC). Ophthalmologists in the TO hospitals must (1) be supported by nurses and corpsmen specially trained to assist in ophthalmic surgery and (2) be provided with necessary diagnostic and therapeutic instruments and supplies.

These principles were first enunciated in 1918 by American ophthalmologists who had served in Europe in World War I and have been reiterated by their successors following World War II, the Korean War, the Vietnam War, and the Persian Gulf War. If we continue to fail to provide early definitive ophthalmic surgery for our casualties, as occurred in World War II and the Korean, Vietnam, and Persian Gulf wars, we will continue to condemn them to preventable blindness.

Expertise

Army ophthalmologists who served in World War I, World War II, the Korean War, the Vietnam War, and the Persian Gulf War agree that the major elements in the successful care of the eye injured are twofold: the expertise of the ophthalmologist providing such care, and the promptness with which it is provided. The US Army ophthalmologist who surveyed the provision of eye care by the British and French medical departments in 1917 and 1918 called for specially trained ophthalmic surgeons to serve in forward hospitals.[8]

As Wood stated in 1921, regarding the need for expert ophthalmological care near the front:

> In the American Expeditionary Forces ophthalmologists were finally stationed in most of the front line hospitals (casualty clearing hospitals) so that every ocular wound should receive attention at the earliest possible moment, the principle having become generally recognized by time of our entry into the war, that the golden opportunity in the treatment of traumatic corneal ulcers, penetrating and other wounds of the eye, as with all general wounds, lay between the moment of injury with its usual contamination and the time when simple contamination flamed into active infection. Further it has long been an ophthalmic axiom that the earlier the removal of intraocular foreign bodies the greater the chances of ultimate vision, and placing of these skilled men behind the front, backed by base hospitals and placed as far forward as possible and having radial control through their specialist chiefs, led accordingly to incalculable saving of vision and of life, as well as to the lessening of the final deformities in thousands of wounds.[9]

Vail expressed a similar thought in the official history of World War II:

> Experience showed that it would have been a wiser policy to *staff evacuation hospitals with the best ophthalmic talent available* rather than to concentrate it in the communication zone where, when the casualty was eventually received, there was not a great deal that even the most experienced ophthalmologist could do for him [emphasis added].[10]

In the early days of World War I, before ophthalmologists were fully functional in the combat zone, a great wastage of sight resulted from the enucleation of every perforated eye by general surgeons.[9] And the identical problem occurred at the onset of World War II.[11]

In the same vein, regarding the experience in World War II, Stone stated:

> [M]any traumatisms of the eye were unduly complicated by failure to treat the conditions properly at the time of the injury and in the period immediately thereafter.[12]

And King succinctly commented:

> The primary operation upon an eye is usually the definitive one and the surgeon seldom has a second chance. ... [T]he complete examination which is necessary before surgery demands specialized equipment; this equipment and the small delicate instruments which are required for ocular surgery are not usually available to the general surgeon.[13]

To provide our wounded with the quality of care to which they are entitled, it is mandatory that ophthalmologists who possess subspecialty expertise provide such care at 3rd- and 4th-echelon hospitals in the TO. Ophthalmology has advanced so rapidly since the 1980s that clearly defined subspecialties have emerged, each requiring 1 or more years of fellowship training and near-exclusive concentration on them by their practitioners. The results of subspecialization have been (1) a dramatic improvement in the diagnosis and management of ocular and ocular adnexal injury and disease, and (2) the disappearance of the general ophthalmic surgeon, for no one can master all types of ophthalmic surgery. The ophthalmic subspecialties most needed in the TO are those of the

- anterior segment (cornea/lens),
- posterior segment (vitreoretinal), and
- ocular adnexa (ocular plastic surgeon).

This matter will be considered in detail in the Practice of TOEC section. We must plan to put our best ophthalmic surgeons (Regular Army and Reserve) who possess subspecialty expertise in the TO and not keep them, for the most part, within the continental United States (CONUS), as was done during the Vietnam War.

Immediacy of Treatment

Any number of people have recognized that the sooner combat casualty care is given, the better the outcome for the patient, including the American College of Surgeons' Committee on Trauma:

> The most significant ingredient necessary for optimal care of the trauma patient is commitment, both personal and institutional. For the institution, optimal care means providing capable personnel who are immediately available. It also implies using sophisticated equipment and services that are frequently expensive to purchase and maintain. It means there must be a priority of access to sophisticated laboratory and radiologic facilities as well as to the operating suites and intensive care units.[14]

As with all serious injuries, the outcome following eye injury is directly related to the rapidity with which expert care is provided. Bellamy's comments regarding lifesaving surgery in World War II apply to sight-saving surgery, as well:

> [E]mphasis ... [was] ... placed upon providing lifesaving surgery far forward on the battlefield. During the North African campaign of 1942–1943 it was recognized that evacuation of the seriously wounded to hospitals in the rear without first performing needed surgery was associated with an unacceptably high mortality. The problem was successfully solved by attaching to clearing companies and evacuation hospitals near the front ad hoc units able to provide surgical care for casualties with trunk and serious extremity wounds.[15]

This principle of immediacy is most applicable in the management of severe posterior segment (retina, vitreous, choroid, and sclera) injuries, for it is now established that such injuries must be managed surgically as soon as possible,[16,17] and that the speedy repair of a retinal detachment decreases the incidence of proliferative vitreoretinopathy—a major cause of treatment failure. Corpsmen and general medical officers must be capable of detecting eye and ocular adnexal injuries, making an initial assessment of their significance, rendering appropriate care, and arranging for evacuation to the ophthalmologist (Figures 2-1 and 2-2). Skilled ophthalmologists must be available at 3rd-and 4th-echelon hospitals to provide expert definitive care as soon as possible after injury (Figures 2-3 and 2-4).

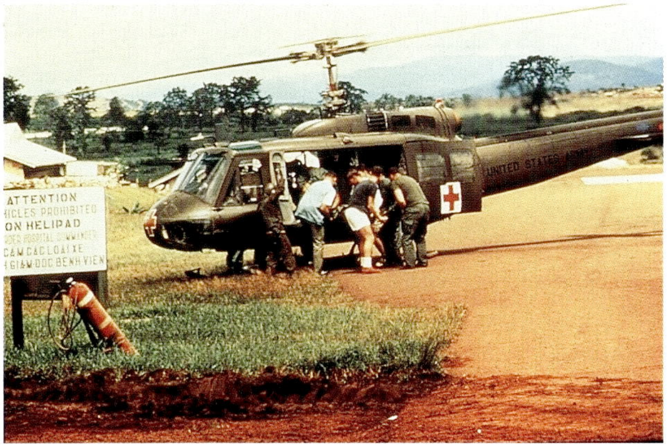

Fig. 2-1. Aeromedical evacuation helicopter. Air superiority and the ability to evacuate critically injured patients by air has resulted in faster delivery of definitive repair to our soldiers on the modern battlefield. Photograph: Courtesy of Albert Hornblass, MD, Major, Medical Corps, US Army (Ret), New York, NY.

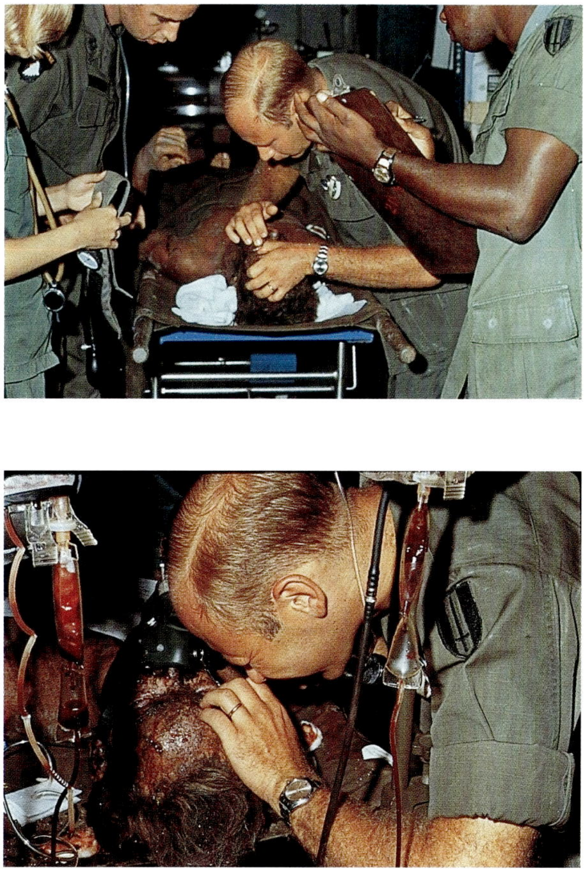

Fig. 2-2. (**a**) After performing the evaluation of airway, breathing, and circulation, the triage officer evaluates all body systems. (**b**) Examination of the eye, adnexa, and orbit must be done by the ophthalmologist in an expeditious but thorough manner to determine the extent of ocular injuries and establish the priority of surgical repair of these injuries. This information is then conveyed back to the triage officer. Reproduced with permission from La Piana FG, Hornblass A. Military ophthalmology in the Vietnam War. *Doc Ophthalmol*. 1997;93:39.

Such care may include, in addition to a full ophthalmic examination, additional diagnostic procedures (eg, ultrasonography, computed tomography [CT] scan), surgical repair, and initiation of antibiotic therapy. The ophthalmic surgeon will frequently work as a member of a head and maxillofacial trauma team and should be as familiar as possible with the procedures of neurosurgeons and maxillofacial surgeons (Table 2-1 and Figures 2-5 through 2-7). Edwards's comments, published in 1954, are highly relevant:

> At the beginning of the [Korean] war, definitive surgery was done mostly at Tokyo Army Hospital and some at the hospital ship in Pusan. The time elapsed between injury and arrival at Tokyo was

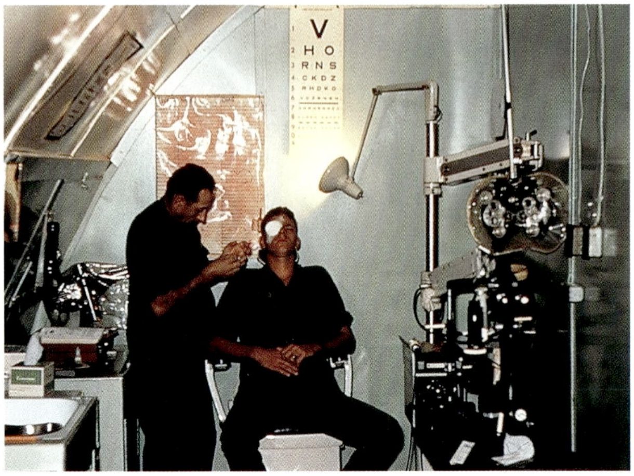

Fig. 2-3. Eye Clinic, 24th Evacuation Hospital, Long Binh, Vietnam. A complete ophthalmology lane allows for definitive evaluation of eye injuries. The complete eye lane must have at a minimum a slitlamp and an indirect ophthalmoscope. Reproduced with permission from La Piana FG, Hornblass A. Military ophthalmology in the Vietnam War. *Doc Ophthalmol.* 1997;93:40.

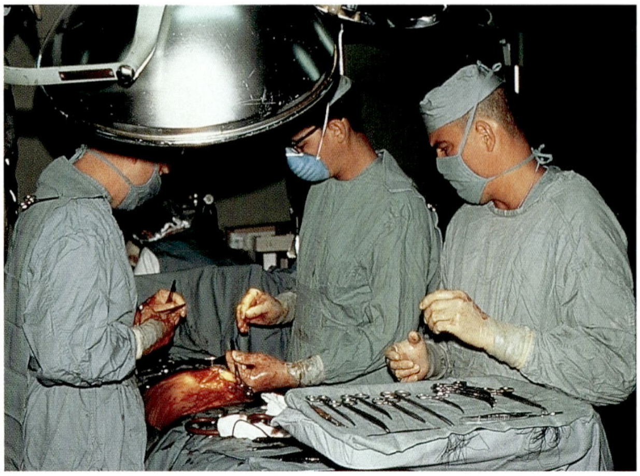

Fig. 2-4. Third- and 4th-echelon facilities have operating room capabilities. Often, the ophthalmologist will have to manage the patients with multiple injuries in coordination with a neurosurgeon or otolaryngologist. Photograph: Courtesy of William Dale Anderson, MD, Major, Medical Corps, US Army (Ret), Colorado Springs, Colo.

> often in excess of 24 hours. We found that the patients operated on by an ophthalmologist aboard the ship arrived in better condition at Tokyo than those who came directly, thus indicating the need for earlier surgery. For this reason, ophthalmologists were pushed forward into evacuation hospitals in Korea. Thereafter, definitive treatment could be given in 6 to 8 hours from even the most distant portions of the front line. In the opinion of everyone, the end-results justified this system. Thus, in the light of the experience in both wars, it is recommended that ophthalmologists be placed as far forward as possible, depending on their availability, to enable preoperative time lags of less than 12 to 18 hours.[13]

A major objective of TOEC is to maximize the number of casualties who can return to duty within the theater. Many eye and ocular adnexal injuries are initially incapacitating but—if managed expertly and promptly by ophthalmologists, with the requisite personnel, support, and equipment—can heal or at least stabilize rapidly enough to permit the patient's return to duty. If inappropriately managed, however, many will progress to a condition necessitating evacuation from the TO and perhaps ultimate retirement for medical disability. Corneal lacerations, hyphemas, blowout fractures of the orbit, and major lid and tear-duct lacerations are examples of such injuries.

TABLE 2-1

CONCOMITANT INJURIES ASSOCIATED WITH OCULAR TRAUMA* DURING THE KOREAN WAR

Other Injuries	Number and Percentage of Associated Ocular Injuries
Facial	42 (15%)
Maxillofacial	47 (16%)
Neurosurgical	32 (11%)
Thorax	6 (2%)
Abdomen	3 (1%)
Extremities	48 (17%)
None	59 (21%)
Unknown	49 (17%)
TOTAL	286 (100%)

*Attention is invited particularly to the 32 eye injuries that were seen in conjunction with neurosurgical injuries and to the 47 eye injuries with associated maxillofacial wounds.
Reproduced from King, Edwards. *Recent Advances in Medicine and Surgery*. US Army Medical Service Graduate School, Army Medical Center [now Walter Reed Army Medical Center], Washington, DC: 1954: 477–478, 481.

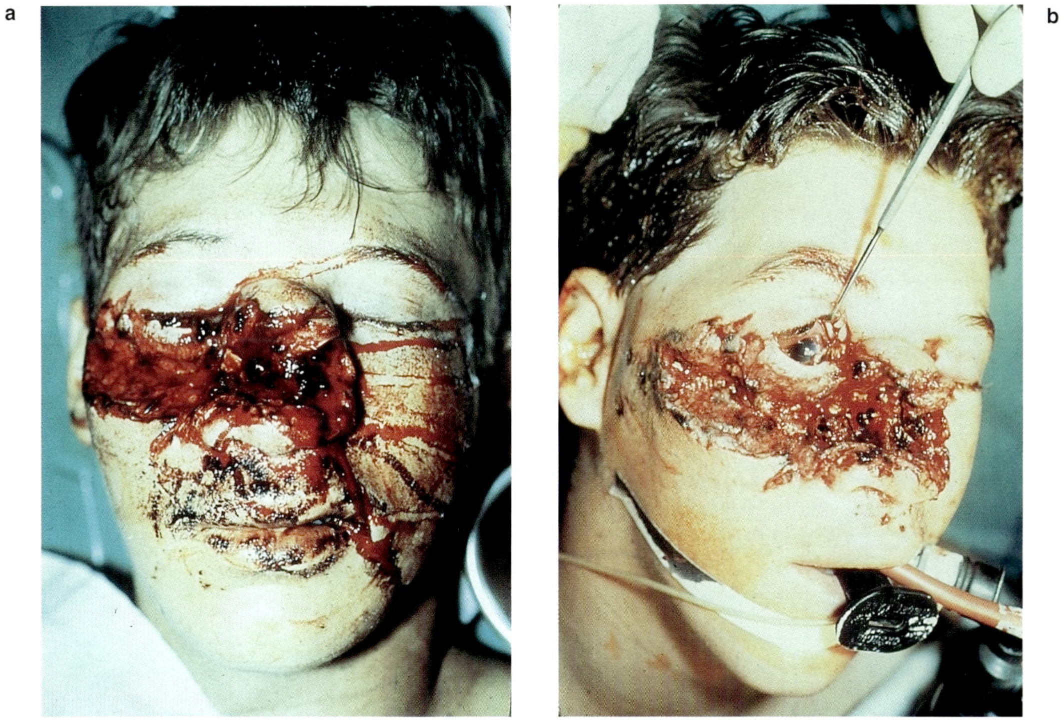

Fig. 2-5. During the Vietnam War, this soldier, having suffered severe midface and eye injuries, was seen (**a**) at the time of triage and (**b**) in the operating room.

Control of Medical Resources

The need for control of Army Medical Department (AMEDD) resources by AMEDD personnel is agreed on by all. An extension of this principle to the conduct of ophthalmology in the TO is necessary, because only a senior ophthalmology consultant possesses the understanding required for the appropriate allocation and utilization of resources. There is ample historical support for this principle. Based on experiences gained in World War I, it was recommended that the chief consultant in a specialty should not only supervise treatment but also

> give wise advice, instruction and actual demonstrations as to the best and most efficacious methods of treatment, in order that the work of his department may *conform to the recognized and accepted standards of the best civil and military practice* [emphasis added].[8]

This report also commended the Eye Centers of the British Expeditionary Forces under the British Medical Service for their efficiency, equipment, and organization, especially the appointment of one ophthalmic surgeon to supervise and coordinate

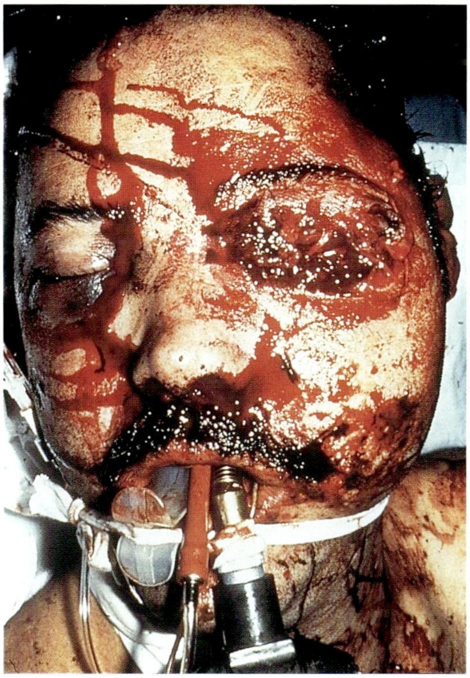

Fig. 2-6. A gunshot wound to the orbit has caused severe damage to this soldier's globe and adnexa during the Vietnam War. Ophthalmologists at the 3rd and 4th echelons must be prepared to treat patients with severe injuries of the globe and surrounding structures.

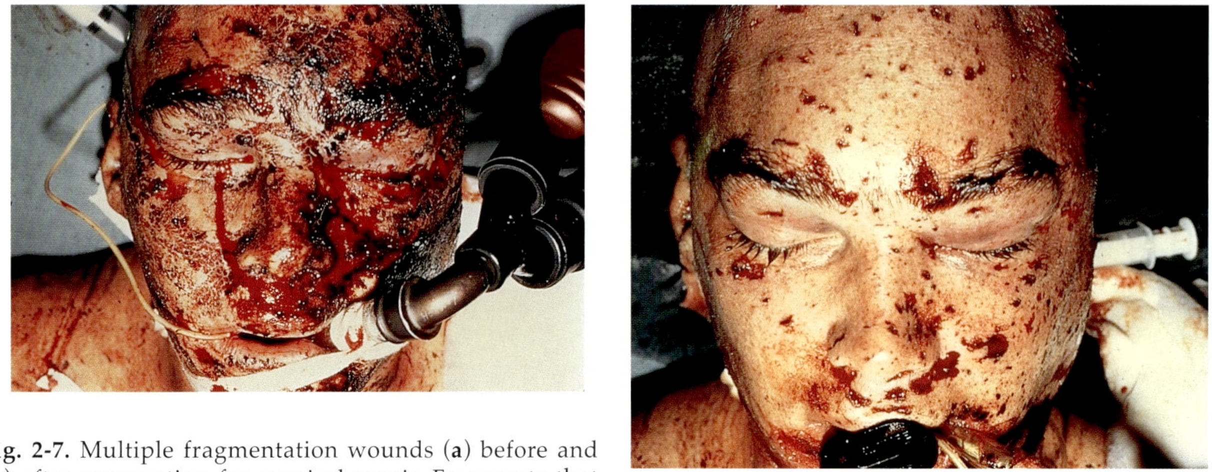

Fig. 2-7. Multiple fragmentation wounds (**a**) before and (**b**) after preparation for surgical repair. Fragments that may barely penetrate the superficial layers of the skin have the potential to cause severe damage to the eye. Photograph a: Reproduced with permission from Wong TY, Seet B, Ang CL. Eye injuries in twentieth century warfare: A historical perspective. *Surv Ophthalmol*. 1997;41:452. Photograph b: Courtesy of William Dale Anderson, MD, Major, Medical Corps, US Army (Ret), Colorado Springs, Colo.

services for the entire force.

Based on experience gained in World War II, the US Army official history recommends that in the event of the outbreak of future hostilities,

> 1. [a] Consultant in Ophthalmology should at once be placed on active duty in the Office of the Surgeon General, and
> 2. [u]pon the activation of each Overseas Theatre, a Consultant in Ophthalmology should at once be placed on duty and made responsible for ophthalmic programs within the theatre.[18]

Speaking of the lack of a consultant in ophthalmology throughout the US military in World War II, Vail stated:

> The chief fault of the past was the delay in setting up the position of chief consultant in ophthalmology in the office of the Surgeon General of the Army. The Navy never has such an officer; and the Air Force, even in those days, was a law unto itself. All of these errors and much of the waste could have been prevented by a skilled and experienced ophthalmologist with appropriate rank and authority placed in the offices of the Surgeon General of the various forces. At the present time there is no such officer any place.[19]

Apparently, however, some improvement was evident during the Korean War:

> The advice of Consultants was given great weight in matters of assigning personnel as well as of maintaining high caliber of medical care. The system worked out very well in Korea and should be continued in the future.[13]

In Vietnam, the Consultant in Ophthalmology to the Military Assistance Command Vietnam (MACV) Surgeon was usually the ophthalmologist of the 24th Evacuation Hospital (EH) (Figure 2-8). This ophthalmologist was, most of the time, a relatively junior officer and too busy to function as a true senior consultant and to effect necessary changes. On the outbreak of hostilities, a senior Army ophthalmologist should be assigned as the Consultant in Ophthalmology on the Theater Army Surgeon's/ Medical Brigade Commander's staff. This individual should directly and personally oversee all aspects of planning for and practice of ophthalmology within the theater. This individual and the Con-

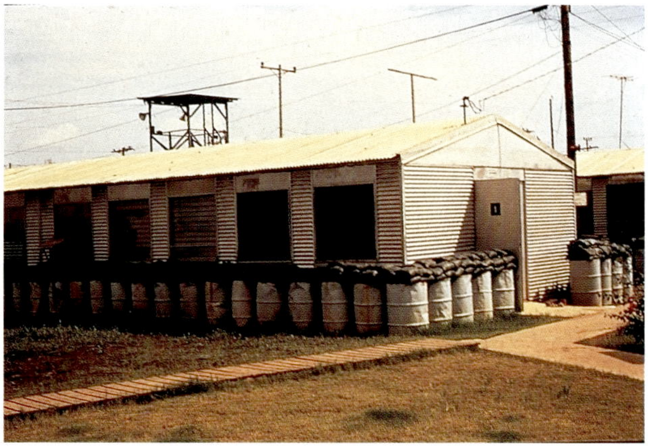

Fig. 2-8. Doctor's quarters at the 24th Evacuation Hospital in the Republic of Vietnam (1968–1969). Photograph: Courtesy of William Dale Anderson, MD, Major, Medical Corps, US Army (Ret), Colorado Springs, Colo.

sultant in Ophthalmology to The Surgeon General must be experienced in both military medicine and ophthalmology, and work closely together.

The senior Army ophthalmology consultants should be selected on the basis of their proven ability to perform their jobs (as are chiefs of staff of the Army and hospital commanders) and not simply on the basis of seniority. The consultant should

- have operational control of all ophthalmic and optometric resources within the TO;
- be responsible for, and personally supervise the care of, the eye-injured and diseased—not only by the ophthalmologists and optometrists but also by all who render such care (other medical corps officers, corpsmen, and nurses);
- understand the pertinent aspects of geographic ophthalmology in the theater (endemic/epidemic diseases);
- interact effectively with his Navy and Air Force counterparts in patient care and evacuation matters;
- see to the proper orientation of new arrivals to the theater and proper utilization of OJTs;
- control the distribution and use of K-teams (potentially the ophthalmic equivalent of the Auxiliary Surgical Groups of World War II), if employed[15]; and
- oversee the operation of a registry of eye diseases and injury that should immediately be established on formation of the theater force.

The importance of the establishment and maintenance of such a registry is evidenced by the great value of data concerning eye injuries and disease collected during World War II[20] and by the costs of the relative failure to acquire such data for eye injuries in Vietnam.

Assertiveness

AMEDD considers ophthalmology to be a constituent of surgery, and this subordination is expressed at all levels. Because many Army surgeons—like most physicians—know little and care less about the eye and think of ophthalmologists as little more than optometrists who perform cataract surgery, ophthalmology has often not been provided the attention and resources it requires to most effectively execute its missions. Therefore, Army ophthalmologists must assertively compete for resources, educate their fellow physicians, and plan for the provision of eye care to the war casualty—who otherwise will continue to be condemned to preventable blindness. Military ophthalmologists must make themselves the preventive medicine officers for the eye, working to diminish risks of injury by promoting (*a*) safe practices both on and off duty and (*b*) the wearing of eye armor during the conduct of all eye-hazardous activities (see Chapter 26, The Development of Eye Armor for the American Infantryman). In general, the wearing of hard and soft contact lenses in the combat zone must be discouraged, because contact lenses enhance the likelihood of eye infections.[21] Military ophthalmologists must also be assertive in the prevention and management of ocular malingering, as manifested by gazing at the sun (solar maculopathy) or breaking the eyeglasses.

Complexity of Injuries

Eye injuries in a civilian setting in peacetime can profitably be compared with those produced by war. Whereas in peacetime, few ocular structures are injured and few coexisting injuries occur, the picture is quite different in wartime (Table 2-2), when eye injuries tend to be multiple, averaging about two per eye. Cohen[22] analyzed 281 cases of severe globe injury sustained in Vietnam and subsequently treated at Fitzsimons Army Medical Center (FAMC) between 1967 and 1970. He found that the 133 eyes (47% of the total) that remained in situ on presentation to FAMC had a total of 277 injuries, for an average of 2.1 injuries per eye. Likewise, analysis of 57 patients evacuated from Vietnam to Walter Reed Army Medical Center Ophthalmology Service from May 1968 to September 1969 showed that those patients sustained 100 injuries to the globe and/or ocular adnexa, an average of 1.8 injuries per eye.[3]

TABLE 2-2

OCULAR INJURIES SEEN IN WARTIME VS IN A PEACETIME EMERGENCY DEPARTMENT

Injuries	Wartime	Peacetime
Ocular Structures Injured	Several	Few
Number of Patients	Multiple	Usually one
Coexisting Injuries	Very often	Usually not
Time Available to Provide Care	Limited	Unlimited
Stress on the Surgeon	Severe	Moderate

Cooperation Among Specialists

Most ophthalmic surgery in peacetime is performed without the need for support from other surgeons. Military ophthalmologists caring for war casualties, however, must often work intimately with other surgeons because of many casualties' multiplicity of injuries. Because of such combined injuries, ophthalmologists should be co-located with neurosurgeons and maxillofacial surgeons. The ophthalmologist will work not only with neurosurgeons, otolaryngologists, and plastic surgeons, but also with orthopedic and general surgeons. Thus, military ophthalmologists should participate in courses dealing with the management of war casualties (eg, the Combat Casualty Care course, which includes both the C-4 course and the American College of Surgeons' Advanced Trauma Life Support [ATLS] course) and seize every opportunity to participate in the care of patients with midface trauma.

Reassessing, Updating, and Integrating With Other Plans

Plans for TOEC must be periodically reassessed because (*a*) weaponry, tactics, and, therefore, threats change and (*b*) better means of preventing and caring for eye injuries and disease will be developed and need to be integrated into the plan. Breakthroughs in both prevention and therapy must be immediately identified by military ophthalmologists and exploited for the benefit of service personnel.

Planning for TOEC must be fully integrated with general AMEDD planning to ensure that the mission is accomplished while resources are conserved. Military ophthalmologists must participate actively at all levels in AMEDD planning for TO casualty care.

Continuing Military Medical Education for Ophthalmologists

Education of all those who practice TOEC is a continuing obligation of the military ophthalmologist. Civilian ophthalmologists must also be kept aware of the plans for TOEC so they can help implement them, if necessary. The Tri-Service Ocular Trauma Course currently provides such education for active duty military ophthalmologists of the Army, Navy, and Air Force and could be expanded to include civilian ophthalmologists. All military ophthalmologists should attend the Tri-Service Ocular Trauma Course, preferably first in their senior year of residency and then at 3-year intervals. Through lectures and practical sessions, this course attempts to familiarize the student with the realities of practice in a TO and also facilitates exchange of information and joint planning by representatives of the Army, Navy, and Air Force.

In addition, a 4-hour block of instruction in the detection, diagnosis, and management of ocular and ocular adnexal trauma is given the fourth-year medical students at the Uniformed Services University of the Health Sciences. This course provides a base of knowledge that medical officers can build on.

Instruction of all eye-care providers is a major and continuing responsibility of all military ophthalmologists and its accomplishment should be a direct responsibility of the theater Army ophthalmologist. Nonophthalmologists (physicians, physician assistants, and corpsmen) should receive instruction that is similar to or, if possible, identical to that presented in the ATLS manual.

Specific Principles

The practice of TOEC, including evacuation of eye casualties, takes place at each of the four echelons of care.

1st and 2nd Echelons: Initial Care of Ocular and Ocular Adnexal Injuries

It is mandatory that eye injuries be properly managed by those caring for the patient *before* he or she reaches an ophthalmologist. The "patch and ship" policy exacerbates morbidity. Corpsmen, physician assistants, and physicians at all echelons of care within the theater must be taught what *must* and *must not* be done for the eye-injured patient at the site of injury, during evacuation, at the battalion aid station, and at hospitals not having an ophthalmologist assigned. The person providing the casualty's initial care must inspect the eyes and adnexal structures for injuries, and detect such injuries; at least develop a differential diagnosis and make a diagnosis, if possible; and render appropriate management. All of this must be performed in such a manner that no additional injury is induced either by the care provider himself or by those who render subsequent care (eg, during ground ambulance or helicopter evacuation). The relevant instruction included in the 1988 revision of *Emergency War Surgery,*[23] the *ATLS Manual*[24] and the 1991 *Combat Casualty Guidelines: Operation Desert Storm*[25] is a

EXHIBIT 2-1

RECOMMENDATIONS FOR INITIAL CARE OF OCULAR AND ADNEXAL INJURIES AT THE 1ST AND 2ND ECHELONS

1. Do not "patch and ship." Get visual acuity and history of the injury.
2. Inspect eyes and adnexal structures using bent paper clips, if necessary.
3. Detect injuries without further injuring the globe. Look for blood in the anterior chamber, lens dislocation, iris disinsertion, blood in the vitreous, retinal detachment, and retained intraocular foreign body (IOFB). A black reflex often indicates the presence of an intraocular hemorrhage. Palpate for discontinuity of the orbital rim and detachment of the medial canthal tendon.
4. Remove nonimpaled conjunctival FBs (using irrigation or a wet cotton-tipped applicator stick) and impaled-lid FBs that can contact the globe.
5. Do not remove impaled conjunctival (intraocular or intraorbital) FBs, but rule out intracranial injuries.
6. Irrigate corneal FBs, and wipe them off the cornea with an applicator stick, if necessary. Apply a broad-spectrum ophthalmic antibiotic ointment and a tight patch.
7. Treat corneal abrasions with a broad-spectrum antibiotic ointment and a tight patch if the patient is not a contact lens wearer. Patients who do wear contact lens have a higher risk of developing a corneal ulcer, so their abrasions should be treated with a broad-spectrum ophthalmic antibiotic ointment or solution and no patching. Do not use corticosteroids.
8. Identify a ruptured, penetrated, or perforated eyeball by edema of the conjunctiva, a shallow or deep anterior chamber, hyphema, decreased ocular motility, decreased visual acuity, or an intraocular hemorrhage (the inside of eye looks black or red). Apply a broad-spectrum ophthalmic antibiotic solution and a Fox or other rigid shield (no patch), and evacuate to a 3rd-echelon ophthalmologist. Apply no pressure to the eye, and ask the patient not to squeeze the lids.
9. Do not apply topical steroids.
10. Do not use ointment on an open eye.
11. Apply moist dressings on eyelid lacerations and medial canthal angle lacerations.
12. Do not attempt enucleation or evisceration (ie, no eye removal) at the 1st or 2nd echelons.
13. Use topical anesthesia *only* for examination purposes. Never give the patient the topical anesthetic for personal use, as self-medication can lead to a serious keratopathy.
14. For chemical burns, provide at least 60 minutes of irrigation and remove any particles from the cornea and conjunctiva, especially the fornices.
15. For white phosphorus burns, identify particles if necessary with 0.5% copper sulfate, and if possible, remove all particles under water.
16. For severe injuries, use tetanus prophylaxis and systemic antibiotics.
17. If intraorbital bleeding causes decreased visual acuity, perform a lateral canthotomy and cantholysis.
18. Tell patients with orbital fractures to refrain from nose blowing, and teach them how to stop sneezing by pressing hard just above the upper lip. If the sneeze cannot be stopped, they should not try to hold it in. Begin systemic antibiotics to cover sinus flora (ie, amoxicillin/clavulanate).
19. Consider repairing lacerations of the eyelid that involve the skin and muscle only without fat prolapse or involvement of the lid margin. Close the eyelid laceration with 6-0 silk.
20. Evacuate casualties with deeper lid lacerations and those involving the margin to a 3rd-echelon ophthalmologist.
21. Look carefully for lacerations of the canaliculi (tear ducts) and evacuate patients with such lacerations to a 3rd-echelon ophthalmologist. Apply a wet dressing on the injured area.
22. Keep orbital soft tissues moist in case of traumatic enucleation/partial exenteration and evacuate to a 3rd-echelon ophthalmologist.
23. Any further decrease in visual acuity after injury demands immediate evacuation to a 3rd-echelon ophthalmologist.
24. Treat laser burns of the cornea with topical ophthalmic antibiotics, patching, and daily examinations.
25. Evacuate casualties with laser burns of the retina to a 3rd-echelon ophthalmologist.
26. After any injury to the eyelids (eg, avulsion, thermal burns), keep the cornea covered. Any corneal exposure requires immediate evacuation to a 3rd-echelon ophthalmologist.

valuable introduction to and overview of this critically important subject. Some specific recommendations are listed in Exhibit 2-1.

The theater Army ophthalmologist should assume responsibility for the continuing education of all eye-care providers in theater. He or she must also work closely with those personnel responsible for aeromedical evacuation to assure that eye casualties are provided necessary in-flight care.

3rd and 4th Echelons: Evacuation to an Ophthalmologist

Pressure exerted on an eye that has been penetrated can extrude intraocular contents through the wound of entry and thereby convert a repairable injury to an irreparable one. Similarly, the administration of ointment to such an eye can result in passage of the ointment into the eye, where it does great damage. Therefore, *only* solutions of ophthalmic medications should be applied to an eye that might be penetrated, and all patients with such injuries must be evacuated wearing a Fox (aluminum) shield or a shield made of some semirigid material (eg, the bottom of a paper cup) over the injured eye. Severe eye injuries must receive an evacuation priority equal to that granted severe extremity injuries and second only to life-threatening injuries, because sight-saving care must rapidly, as well as expertly, be provided. Obviously, medical regulating officers must know at all times which hospitals in theater are prepared to provide care for eye casualties.

At 3rd- and 4th-echelon hospitals (Figure 2-9), the ophthalmologist should be a member of a "head and neck team," composed of a neurosurgeon, otolaryngologist, plastic surgeon, and oral surgeon, as experience in the wars of this century has clearly shown that combat casualty care is thereby optimized.

Definitive, expert, early care will be provided at the 3rd echelon for patients who have sustained an injury to the eye and/or ocular adnexal structures to expedite their return to duty or to save the globe. Watertight closure of the penetrated globe will enable subsequent additional stabilizing surgery to be performed at the 4th echelon. Lacerations of the eyeball, eyelids, and tear ducts will be closed primarily and immediately, utilizing a portable operating microscope. If necessary, the patient will subsequently be evacuated to the 4th echelon, where vitrectomy capability exists. Neurosurgeons and ophthalmologists will work together to decompress the optic nerve as necessary. Various injuries that may be encountered at the 3rd and 4th echelons (Figures 2-10 through 2-12) and sutures that I recommend for their repair are listed in Exhibit 2-2.

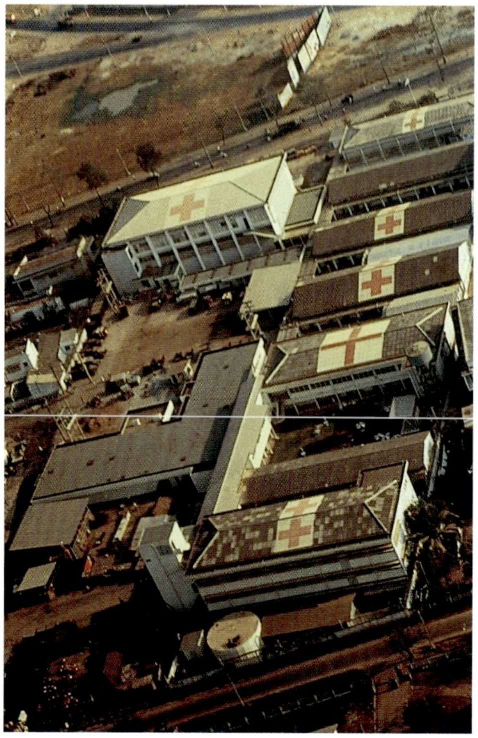

Fig. 2-9. The 3rd Field Hospital in Vietnam. Fourth-echelon hospitals are often in fixed facilities and should have full ophthalmic and head-and-neck capabilities.

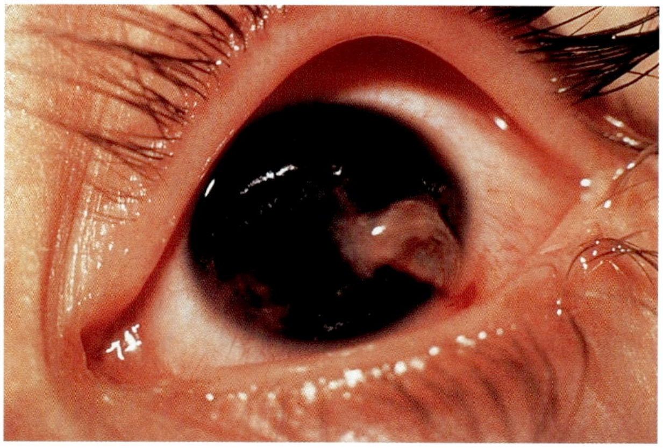

Fig. 2-10. A patient with an open globe with prolapse of uveal tissue needs immediate evacuation to an ophthalmologist for definitive repair of the corneal, scleral, or corneoscleral wound. Photograph: Courtesy of the late Richard M. Leavitt, MD.

a

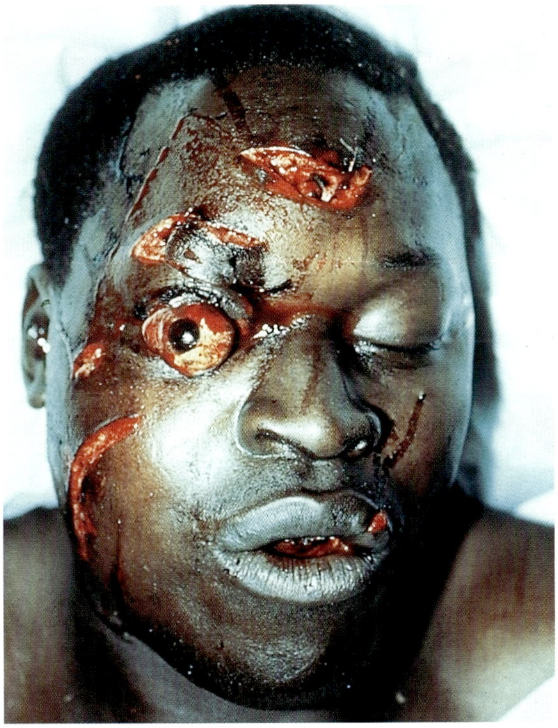

b

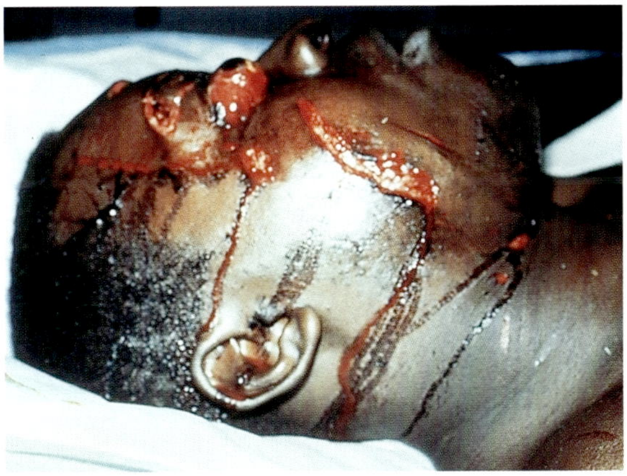

Fig. 2-11. (**a**) The marked proptosis of the eye in this individual is due to a retrobulbar hemorrhage. Without prompt intervention, vision may be permanently lost. (**b**) Also of note is the blood in the mouth and the numerous facial lacerations. Photographs: Courtesy of Blackwell S. Bruner, MD, Potomac, Md.

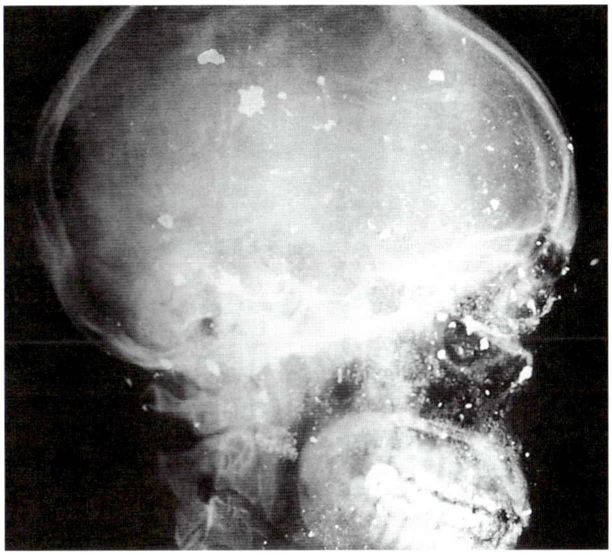

Fig. 2-12. Numerous metallic fragments are seen to involve the cranium and orbit on this lateral skull film (conventional radiograph). Fragmentation injuries commonly injure more than one organ system. Management of these casualties will involve the ophthalmologist for the eye and orbit, the neurosurgeon for the brain, and the otolaryngologist for the airway, sinuses, ears, and nose. Reproduced with permission from Wong TY, Seet B, Ang CL. Eye injuries in twentieth century warfare: A historical perspective. *Surv Ophthalmol*. 1997; 41:433–459.

Ultrasonography is required at the 3rd echelon for the detection and localization of intraocular foreign bodies (IOFBs) and retinal detachments. The portable operating microscope increases the speed of surgery by optimizing the view of the operative field, as well as enabling better surgical results, thereby decreasing ocular morbidity and increasing return to duty. The portable operating microscope can also be employed outside the surgical suite (eg, in the minor/outpatient surgical facility) for minor repairs and suture removal, and it can also be used by other surgeons. The suction/cutter should be available at the 3rd echelon to remove vitreous from the anterior chamber. Irrigation and aspiration of a cataractous lens will be performed only if the lens is ruptured and prolapsed or mixed with vitreous. Otherwise, patients with traumatic cataracts will be evacuated to the 4th echelon.

Surgical repair of eye and adnexal injuries can be performed concurrent with repair of other injuries. CT is necessary for the localization of intraocular and intraorbital foreign bodies (FBs) and for definition of orbital fractures. The CT scanner must be able to provide 1.5-mm cuts and coronal and sagittal reformats.

An eye clinic set is required wherever an ophthalmologist is assigned, as the specialized diagnostic instruments included therein (eg, slitlamp) are mandatory for the care of patients with eye injuries and diseases. The eye clinic should be able to perform minor surgery. Two ophthalmologists (one with anterior segment subspecialty expertise and

EXHIBIT 2-2

RECOMMENDED SUTURES FOR THE REPAIR OF VARIOUS ORBITAL AND ADNEXAL INJURIES

1. Close corneal lacerations with a 10-0 monofilament nylon.
2. Close scleral lacerations with 8-0 nylon, 8-0 silk, or 5-0 Mersilene, as determined by the size and location of the injury.
3. Repair orbital and adnexal soft-tissue lacerations with 4-0 and 6-0 chromic gut.
4. Repair extraocular muscle with 6-0 Vicryl.
5. Repair the medial canthal tendon with 4-0 Mersilene.
6. Close conjunctival lacerations with 6-0 plain gut.
7. Close adnexal skin with 6-0 silk.
8. Repair lid margin with 4-0 or 6-0 black silk suture through the tarsal plate (cut long so that it can be used as a traction suture), and 6-0 black silk suture at the anterior and posterior lid-margin borders.
9. Stent lacerated canaliculi and nasolacrimal duct with silicone tubing or a monocanalicular stent, to be left in place up to 6 months. Close the wound with 6-0 chromic and 6-0 or 8-0 silk sutures.

one with ocular plastic and adnexa subspecialty expertise) are required at the 3rd echelon, where they will be supported by three corpsmen who are trained to assist in ophthalmic surgery.

The ophthalmologists at the 4th echelon not only must be able to handle all the injuries that are usually seen at the 3rd echelon but also able to provide additional subspecialty care. More-extensive ophthalmic surgical procedures to save the globe will be performed at the 4th echelon, where a microsurgical augmentation set and an operating microscope will be located so as to permit vitreoretinal surgery. Required are all diagnostic and therapeutic instruments needed to manage definitively all forms of ophthalmic injury, including IOFB, retinal detachment, and intraocular hemorrhage (including that from laser injury).

Vitreoretinal surgery will generally be performed between 0 and 14 days following an injury; otherwise, fibrous proliferation increases ocular morbidity. Patients requiring vitreoretinal surgery include all those suffering from penetrating eye injuries of the ciliary body and the posterior segment of the eyeball (sclera, choroid, retina). These patients fall into two categories:

1. those without major posterior segment disruption (ie, no major retinal, choroidal, or optic nerve damage) who, after vitrectomy and intraocular lens implant (if necessary), can return to duty within 30 days; one posterior and one anterior chamber–style intraocular lens must be available at this echelon of care; and
2. those whose posterior segments have been significantly disrupted and will require evacuation to CONUS after vitrectomy.

A patient with an IOFB is not to undergo magnetic resonance imaging (MRI) until the FB is shown not to be magnetic (eg, by the magnet-ultrasound test).

Intraorbital, but extraocular, FBs will be left in place unless they are (*a*)large enough to produce a disturbance of eye or optic nerve function, (*b*) composed of vegetable matter or wood, or (*c*) infected. Orbital fractures will be repaired if clinically indicated; few pure blowout fractures of the orbital floor will require surgery.

At the 4th echelon, three ophthalmologists are required: one with vitreoretinal subspecialty expertise, one with anterior segment expertise, and one with ocular plastic and adnexa subspecialty expertise. The ophthalmologists should be supported by five corpsmen trained to assist in the care of ophthalmic patients in the clinic and in surgery. The clinic should be large enough and so equipped that two ophthalmologists can work simultaneously.

It must be kept in mind that surgical ophthalmic patients require evaluation in an outpatient clinic (an "eye lane") before they are returned to duty, and that the ophthalmologists in theater will have many ophthalmic patients (eg, those suffering from infections and inflammations) who require medical care.

One optometrist should be assigned to each 3rd- and 4th-echelon hospital where ophthalmologists are assigned. The optometrist will perform refractions and supervise the optical shop for the region; he or she should be co-located with the ophthalmologists to speed patient care and thereby increase return-to-duty rates.

The benefit of expertly performed ophthalmic surgery at the 3rd and 4th echelons can be totally undone by poor or no care of the eye casualty during aeromedical evacuation to CONUS. The theater Army ophthalmologist must work closely with his or her Air Force counterpart to ensure adequate in-flight care of the eye casualty.

All utilizable ophthalmologists must be identified with a military occupation specialty (MOS) that specifies whether or not the ophthalmologist is a subspecialty expert (eg, 60S9B0, general ophthalmologist; 60S9B1, anterior segment subspecialist; 60S9B2, vitreoretinal expertise). Military ophthalmologists must be prepared, especially if their hospital provides area support, to treat members of allied forces and indigenous peoples—the latter group necessitating an awareness of relevant geographical ophthalmology (eg, the diagnosis and treatment of endemic trachoma). Hygiene is of even more importance, albeit harder to effect, in the combat zone than in the United States. If contact lenses are worn in the combat zone, significant keratopathy can be expected to occur, possibly leading to the loss of an eye. In outpatient facilities, epidemic keratoconjunctivitis and gonococcal conjunctivitis may be encountered. In the operating room (OR), the use of prophylactic antibiotics should be carefully considered.

The vagaries of military medical supply will ensure that military ophthalmologists will have to improvise at times. The ophthalmologist may need to quickly learn to lead and administer an eye service, supervising perhaps an optometrist and several corpsmen, some of whom will be expected to provide optician services.

OPHTHALMIC CARE IN THE PERSIAN GULF WAR

The eye care provided by ophthalmologists during the Persian Gulf War, both its 6-month defensive buildup phase, Operation Desert Shield, and the short (6-wk) offensive phase, Operation Desert Storm, encompassed a broad range of ophthalmic issues and problems in theater, from the combat support hospital (CSH) to the GH. In future conflicts, ophthalmologists will again be charged with the awesome responsibility of preserving the vision of wounded soldiers and civilians. Unfortunately, there are no all-encompassing answers to many of the problems that arose during the Persian Gulf War. Necessity and individual initiative frequently prompted the only pragmatic solutions. Specific ocular injuries encountered during the Persian Gulf War have been described and analyzed elsewhere.[26,27] For the sake of completeness, I (T. H. M.) will briefly comment on these injuries; however, the thrust of this section will be to describe how the theater evolved over time, what problems arose, how attempts were made to deal with these issues, and what lessons were learned.

During the Persian Gulf War, it was my privilege to serve a dual role as both the Theater Ophthalmology Consultant and Deputy Commander for Clinical Services of the mobile 47th CSH. This combination of duties gave me the opportunity to travel to different parts of the theater and interact with many hospitals, both reserve and active duty. The Persian Gulf War evolved as a war of movement, where many medical units (such as my own) moved frequently to provide medical care to a huge army, which moved in a generally northerly direction. The medical mission also gradually shifted as the military strategy changed from the defensive posture of Operation Desert Shield to the offensive one of Operation Desert Storm. In an attempt to convey the changing nature of the medical mission, I will occasionally describe the status of my own unit as the military situation matured and go beyond the scope of a pure ophthalmic discussion. Ophthalmology did not exist in a vacuum during the Persian Gulf War, and any discussion of ophthalmic care must, of necessity, encompass nonophthalmic issues.

Following the invasion of Kuwait in August 1990, the United States responded with the deployment of the 82nd Airborne Division, along with other relatively small Air Force and Navy units. Local Saudi Arabian ophthalmologists provided the initial ophthalmic care for these units. Later, during October and November, as corps-sized combat elements were formed, larger hospitals arrived with surgical subspecialists, including ophthalmologists. The smallest units with ophthalmologists assigned as staff were CSHs. Most of the more than 20 active duty and reserve ophthalmologists in theater throughout operations Desert Shield and Desert Storm were assigned to Army EHs and GHs, as well as to Navy fleet hospitals and hospital ships. Usually, such hospitals had one ophthalmologist each. There were no Air Force ophthalmologists in theater.

I was a staff ophthalmologist at Madigan Army Medical Center (MAMC), Fort Lewis, Washington, at the time of the invasion of Kuwait. Not long after the invasion, I joined the 47th CSH stationed at Fort Lewis, which had been alerted to go to Saudi Arabia. As with nearly all medical units eventually sent to Saudi Arabia, we were by no means completely ready for deployment. Few, if any, medical units had actually inventoried and used their equipment in the field for real surgical cases. Fortunately, our unit had several weeks to break down and examine our equipment. This was indeed fortunate, because some equipment was found to be missing or inadequate. Given the lack of state-of-the-art equipment, particularly in surgical subspecialties, many surgeons "borrowed" equipment from MAMC. This borrowed equipment was to prove invaluable in the treatment of injured and wounded soldiers. (The use of borrowed equipment was very common in active duty medical units deployed to the theater.)

Equipment and Facilities

Because I frequently use the term "state-of-the-art field equipment," it is appropriate to define this term with respect to ophthalmology. With a severe ocular injury, as is frequently observed in war, prompt definitive surgery is absolutely necessary to preserve vision. It is generally accepted that a corneal/scleral laceration, for example, must be sutured with watertight closure within no more than 12 hours of injury. Simultaneously, an anterior vitrectomy and a lensectomy must frequently be performed. These basic procedures help (*a*) prevent hypotony, bacterial contamination, and massive inflammation, and (*b*) preserve the anatomical integrity of the eye, which will improve the success of later ocular surgery, if it is indicated. Any well-trained ophthalmologist can perform these procedures quickly in any field OR with the aid of an OR microscope and a battery-operated vitrectomy unit. Since the mid 1980s, portable OR microscopes (suitcase-sized) and battery-powered vitrectomy units (briefcase-sized) have been available. They are largely designed for ocular surgery in the Third World and have been used under conditions far more crude than those experienced by most military surgeons in a war zone. Thus, for purposes of this discussion, state-of-the-art ophthalmic equipment is defined as

- a portable operating microscope,
- a battery-powered vitrectomy unit,
- appropriate microsurgical instruments,
- appropriate sutures, and
- ophthalmic medications.

Our unit personnel arrived by commercial air in Dhahran, Saudi Arabia, on 11 October 1990. Our hospital equipment, and that of nearly all hospitals of mobile army surgical hospital- (MASH-) size or larger, was transported by ship. We were quickly taken by bus to "Cement City," a heavily guarded, barbed wire–enclosed camp erected within the confines of an old cement factory. It was composed of row after row of large Arab tents. During this time, nearly all incoming units, medical and otherwise, were temporarily billeted in this facility. Early in the deployment, because of the rapid rate of unit arrival, this encampment was overwhelmed with soldiers, the numbers of whom far exceeded this area's capacity for support. The poor sanitary conditions coupled with extreme heat resulted in many diarrhea and heat casualties; numerous soldiers were hospitalized, including some from our unit.

Many hospitals had similar experiences using the Cement City staging area before they moved west into various desert locations. After leaving Cement City, most MASHs and CSHs were established roughly along a north/south line about 100 miles west of Dhahran. This configuration was necessary to support combat divisions, which were spread out in this general area. The larger EH and fleet hospitals were initially constructed near the coast, with three EHs located around Dhahran and a GH and a Navy fleet hospital located in Bahrain. Later, four EHs were located at King Khaleid Medical Center, and several more were located along an east/west line, roughly along Tapline Road from Rafha to near the Persian Gulf coast. There were 21 EHs in theater, and a GH was located in Riyadh. Also, the Navy hospital ships *Mercy* and *Comfort* were present in the Persian Gulf before, during, and after the Persian Gulf War.

Some of the first hospitals constructed in Saudi Arabia, including my own, used Vietnam-era inflatable MUST (medical unit, self-contained, transportable) equipment (ie, the inflatable subsections were latched together to form hospital wards). If left alone, the inflatable sections would leak air, similar to a leaking car tire; to remain functional, the MUST hospitals needed constant reinflation. The first ophthalmic emergency surgical cases performed during Operation Desert Shield were done uneventfully in MUST OR boxes, which are about one-third the size of a standard DEPMEDS (*dep*loyable *med*ical *s*ystem) OR.

Numerous problems became apparent during the hospital-construction phase, and these were to plague medical units for months. Proper supplies and equipment, ophthalmic and otherwise, were almost universally lacking in theater when we arrived. Although many ophthalmologists blamed "the Army," the reasons for this oversight were fourfold:

1. Many ophthalmologists simply never took the initiative to examine their equipment prior to deployment. Thus, even though some PROFIS (*pro*fessional *f*iller *s*ystem) ophthalmologists had been assigned to their hospitals for years, very few had ever performed a hands-on inventory of their equipment.
2. Some ophthalmologists were assigned to units far from their home stations, and for them, equipment inspection was logistically difficult.
3. Some hospital administrators were reluctant to break down equipment for examination by physicians. Many felt that reviewing the equipment list should be enough. However, the equipment list was frequently difficult to interpret and did not necessarily reflect what was actually present.
4. The Table of Organization and Equipment (TO&E) was outdated, and modern equipment and supplies were never part of the plan. This equipment problem was compounded by the fact that many units were undergoing a transition from MUST to DEPMEDS equipment at about the time of the deployment.

For many reasons, therefore, units found themselves without proper equipment. In fact, of more than 20 ophthalmologists in theater, only 1 or 2 at most had operating microscopes on arrival in Saudi Arabia. No vitrectomy units were ever delivered, and very limited supplies of viscoelastics and even basic microsurgery instruments existed in theater.

Thus, the theater MEDSOM (*med*ical *s*upply, *o*ptical and *m*aintenance), which was originally located in Dhahran, was put in the unenviable position of trying to provide medical supplies, ophthalmic and otherwise, to many medical units arriving in theater. Although these dedicated supply personnel did a remarkable job overall, they were never able to supply all medical units with all ophthalmic needs. I might add that the equipment shortfalls were not limited to ophthalmology. For example, some EHs arrived in theater without functioning anesthesia machines, ventilators, proper sutures, and other basic equipment and supplies.

Lack of equipment proved to be an almost insurmountable problem. In late October and early November 1990, it was becoming obvious (for the reasons mentioned above) that surgical units were arriving without even basic ophthalmic equipment. With this in mind, I contacted the Ophthalmology Consultant to the Surgeon General, Colonel Kenyon Kramer, at Walter Reed Army Medical Center, Washington, DC, and we formulated a plan to purchase and ship operating microscopes, slitlamps, and other equipment to Saudi Arabia. Although this equipment acquisition was well coordinated at Walter Reed and the Dhahran MEDSOM, we had no control of the circumstances between these two points, and our plans met with limited success. For example, of the 12 or so operating microscopes purchased and shipped to Saudi Arabia during Operation Desert Shield, I am aware of only 2, including the 1 that I received, that actually arrived at the proper receiving units. Very few of the operating microscopes were ever found—even after the war ended—although numerous attempts were made to track this equipment. Basically, we found that trying to fill such critical gaps in specialty equipment after arriving in theater was hopeless. The result was that ocular casualties were, in general, poorly treated by many hospitals, particularly those nearest where the casualties were generated.

Fortunately, the personnel of one GH and several EHs were actually moved directly into well-equipped, preexisting Saudi Arabian medical centers. Thus, ophthalmologists and other surgical subspecialists from these units inherited relatively high-quality equipment and a modern hospital setting. This arrangement enabled the evacuation system to have several high-quality eye centers in Saudi Arabia, where some severe ocular casualties could be diverted.

At other hospitals, unfortunately, because patients had coexisting wounds that left them unstable for evacuation, ophthalmologists were frequently forced to treat severe ocular injuries with substandard equipment or risk complications as a result of not closing the wounds. For example, suturing corneal lacerations with loupes, inappropriate sutures, and without viscoelastics was commonplace. This resulted in the need for many patients to be resutured on transfer to a hospital with appropriate microsurgical equipment and supplies. There is no question that this lack of proper equipment led to increased ocular morbidity in wounded soldiers. Thus, fewer than a half dozen well-equipped ophthalmologists in Saudi Arabia provided most of the definitive ophthalmic care, which led to some ophthalmologists being overwhelmed with surgical cases.

In addition to equipment needs, ophthalmology supplies such as viscoelastics, silicone tubing, and some antibiotics were difficult to obtain through the overwhelmed medical supply system. Many ophthalmologists found the US mail, coupled with overseas telephone service, to be a viable resupply alternative.

To improve troop morale, the military quickly established civilian-operated satellite telephone banks in Saudi Arabia. These were initially created near the coasts, but by December 1990, divisions in more remote areas also had telephones. This high-priority communication system was of far higher quality than the poor systems used by medical units. In fact, it was easier to contact anyplace in the United States from these telephone banks in Saudi Arabia than to use the military telephones to call an EH that was only 100 miles away. The mail system from the United States was also dependable and well cared for, and it was a major morale booster. Thus, the fastest and most dependable resupply system for small medical items was to call a friend at your parent hospital in the United States and ask him or her to obtain supplies and send them to you via the US mail. This method used two, high-priority, dependable, established systems, and it proved beneficial to physicians and patients; using it and individual initiative could somewhat enhance the supply system.

Frequency and Severity of Eye Injuries

Fortunately, few serious ocular injuries occurred during Operation Desert Shield. Several corneal/scleral lacerations, hyphemas, lid lacerations, and facial fractures were treated, but considering that over half a million troops were present in theater, the number of serious injuries was surprisingly low. I suspect that the no-alcohol policy helped to decrease the incidence of serious accidents, and this was reflected in the low number of ocular injuries. However, corneal abrasions and FBs were extremely common. Several severe sandstorms occurred before Operation Desert Storm, and they produced innumerable soldiers with embedded sand corneal FBs. These injuries were usually painful and incapacitating. Fortunately, several CSHs in the Corps area had slitlamps that were used effectively to remove corneal FBs. This local ability to remove corneal FBs greatly decreased the need for time-consuming medical evacuation to larger hospitals. Frequently, periocular fractures, lid and canalicular lacerations, and corneal/scleral lacerations were also successfully repaired and followed up at CSHs, which greatly lessened the strain on the evacuation system. Finally, contact lens problems related to dust and sand were extremely common early in the deployment, because many soldiers arrived in theater without backup eyeglasses. This situation largely resolved after facilities for making prescription eyeglasses became available in theater.

By the start of the air war in mid January 1991, more than 20 ophthalmologists were in theater. Most were in stationary Army EHs and Navy fleet hospitals, and few had access to state-of-the-art basic ophthalmic field equipment. By various means, however, ophthalmologists were slowly accumulating equipment and supplies that would enable them to provide some form of care to wounded soldiers. Most had acquired slitlamps. The 6 weeks of air war gave ophthalmologists another reprieve in which they cross-leveled equipment and supplies to the best advantage. Although theater ophthalmologists made a concerted effort to share supplies and equipment, the extremely poor theater communication system between hospitals made this difficult.

Simultaneously with the air war, mobile hospitals slowly moved closer to the Iraqi border, roughly in the same area with the divisions they would later support during the ground invasion. For example, by the start of the air war, my unit had moved 150 miles further north and was located about 20 miles south of King Khaleid Medical Center, which was less than 100 miles south of the Iraqi border. During the entire air war, our mobile hospital, as well as most others, was nonfunctional, because all the equipment was packed on trucks in preparation for the invasion of Iraq. Therefore, any serious injury, ocular or otherwise, that occurred during this time was sent directly to the closest EH, bypassing the mobile hospitals. About 3 weeks before the invasion, most mobile hospitals, including my own, moved further north to within about a dozen miles of the Iraqi border. By the time of the invasion, our CSH had been downsized for increased mobility. We went from a 200-bed, partially mobile hospital to a 24- to 30-bed, fully mobile hospital (Figure 2-13). (Note: construction of a 200-bed CSH required

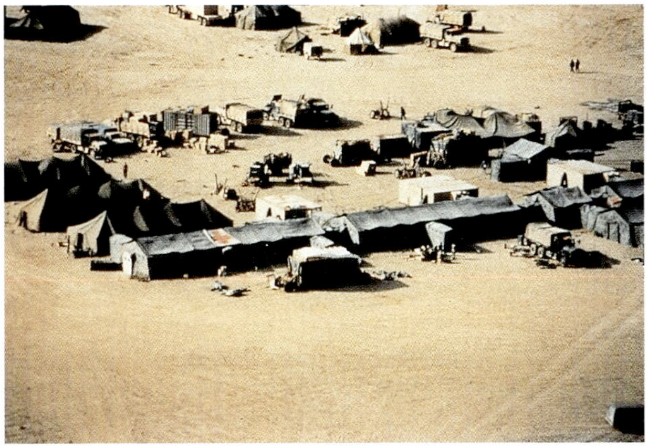

Fig. 2-13. Aerial view of the 47th Combat Support Hospital at Division Support Area 3 in Iraq (24th Infantry Division). Such downsized hospitals were used during the Persian Gulf War to increase mobility.

several days, whereas the small, fully mobile version could be functional in < 6 h.) This change was necessary to keep up with divisions that would soon be advancing fast, deep into Iraq. On the day of the invasion, my unit was incorporated into a huge convoy that entered Iraq in support of the 24th Infantry Division.

During the air war, which began 15 January 1991, ocular casualties continued to be light, for the most part. Most ocular injuries were of the variety that we would expect to see with a large number of young troops, and were related to accidents or athletic injuries. There were two exceptions:

1. Not long into the air war, the Iraqis began to launch SCUD missiles into Saudi Arabia. They were poorly aimed and frequently hit by our Patriot missiles, but the SCUDs occasionally landed in or around the troops or other populated areas and caused numerous injuries, ocular and otherwise. SCUD missile alerts were also a disruptive nuisance to all because they forced soldiers to don their cumbersome chemical protective clothing.
2. The second exception was the Iraqi attack into Kafji, Kuwait, just north of the Saudi Arabian border. This led to an Allied response, largely Marine, which resulted in a small number of serious ocular injuries. Thus, the air war provided a few Allied ocular casualties but nothing that stressed the system.

Medical Evacuation

With the onset of Operation Desert Storm, the medical situation changed drastically and exposed the strengths and weaknesses of the medical care system. All hospitals, from forward surgical teams to GHs, had known for weeks of the plan and timing for the invasion of Iraq and Kuwait. The carefully planned medical evacuation system, heavily dependent on helicopter assets, was well understood by all units (Figure 2-14). The basic medical evacuation plan was (1) to provide lifesaving medical and surgical care to wounded patients at mobile hospitals in Iraq and Kuwait, and then (2) to transport the injured quickly by air to larger, better-equipped hospitals in northern Saudi Arabia for more-definitive care. Because of the long distances traveled into Iraq by Allied forces, however, particularly in the western desert, the evacuation chain was longer and considerably more complex in the Iraqi theater, compared with the less-extended evacuation lines of the Kuwaiti theater.

The chief strength of the plan was the evacuation system itself. The air ambulance assets, largely UH-1 and UH-60 aircraft, were dependable and numerous enough to provide excellent and timely patient transport. For ophthalmologists, the chief weakness of the medical system, as previously discussed, was the lack of appropriate equipment to adequately treat serious ocular injuries, largely at the EH level. Thus, although the movement of patients was well planned and supported, the oph-

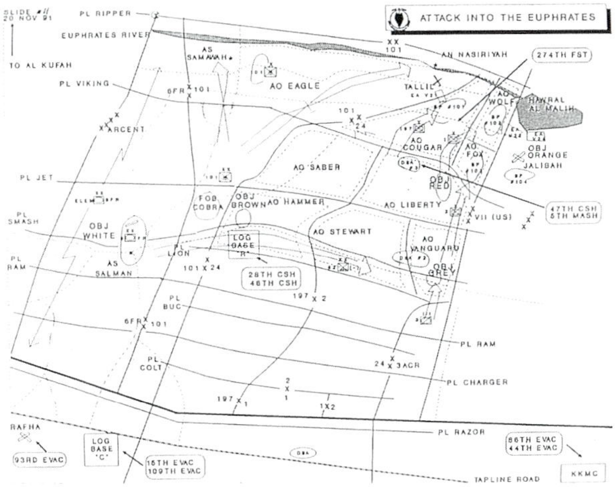

Fig. 2-14. Map showing hospital positions in Iraq and northern Saudi Arabia at the time of the ceasefire in the Persian Gulf War.

thalmic treatment rendered was, in general, substandard.

Insights From the Persian Gulf War

Although detailed descriptions of ocular and ocular adnexal injuries treated during the Persian Gulf War have previously been published,[26,27] four findings should be emphasized:

- Fragmentation injuries from various munitions accounted for 78% of ocular injuries in Operation Desert Storm (Figure 2-15). This approximate percentage has been remarkably consistent in every major war since World War I. Thus, not surprisingly, corneal/scleral lacerations, IOFBs, retinal injury, and traumatic cataract accounted for two thirds of ocular injuries described during Desert Storm. These data suggest that ocular surgeons must have the surgical skill and equipment to treat such injuries—so they can salvage injured eyes.
- Of the nearly 200 serious ocular injuries reported during Operation Desert Storm, 32% occurred in Iraqi troops. The Iraqi medical evacuation and treatment systems were greatly disrupted during the air war before the ground invasion. Thus, many Iraqis who were wounded in the ground war received little or no care before they were treated by advancing Allied medical personnel. In the mobile hospitals in Iraq and Kuwait, where many Iraqis first received care, it was common to see gangrenous, debris-laden, nearly amputated limbs, which had never received even basic first aid. Although no statistics are available, this delay in treatment of injured Iraqi personnel undoubtedly increased ocular morbidity. The most common injury by far in Iraqi soldiers occurred as a result of blast fragmentation from exploding ordnance of an "unknown" variety. Most Iraqis literally had no idea what hit them.
- Among the battle wounded of any nationality during Operation Desert Storm, isolated ocular injuries were rare. Because most ocular injuries resulted from blast fragmentation, the typical wounded soldier had numerous additional nonocular fragmentation wounds. Patients were rarely anesthetized solely to treat an eye wound. Typically, a patient was delivered by helicopter, quickly evaluated in the emergency room by various surgeons, and then, if necessary, taken to the OR. Once anesthesia was achieved, several surgeons would operate simultaneously on the patient to quickly and efficiently treat all the injuries. During mass casualties, OR time was very valuable; the goal was to treat the patient and rapidly turn the room around for the next casualty. Only rarely was time allotted for extensive, time-consuming surgery of any kind. The main ophthalmic goal in a mass casualty situation was to obtain watertight ocular closure. If time was available during the initial surgical procedure, more-complex surgery such as extensive vitrectomy and lensectomy was accomplished. Frequently, such time-consuming procedures were postponed until appropriate operating time was available.
- The Persian Gulf War also demonstrated the occurrence of ocular injuries caused by plastic landmines (Figure 2-16) as well as lasers. Although their mechanisms of injury differ markedly, plastic landmines and lasers have some elements in common: both are relatively inexpensive to produce and easy to use, and their damage potential and lethality will increase with advances in technology. Although the numbers of these injuries were comparatively small during

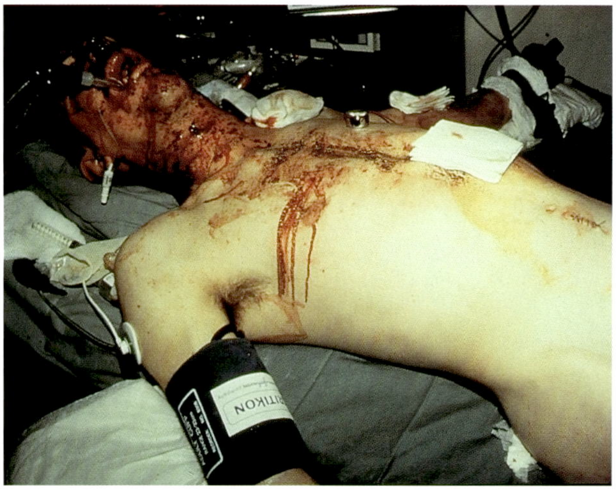

Fig. 2-15. Fragmentation wounds in a young soldier. Note that some degree of protection was offered at the time of injury by the patient's flak vest. This is in contrast to the neck and face areas, which received numerous fragmentation wounds.

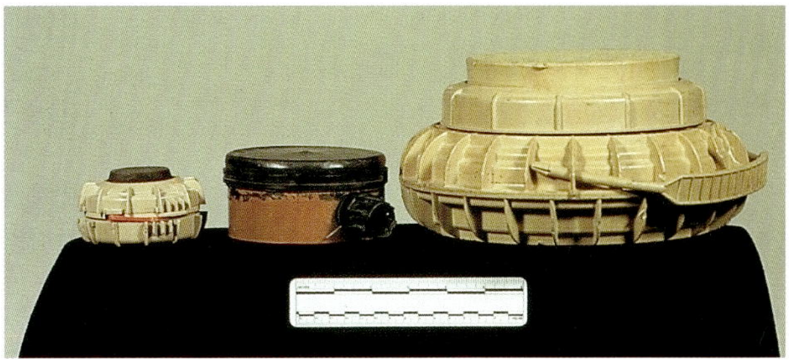

Fig. 2-16. Landmines used by Iraqi forces during the Persian Gulf War. Those on the left and right were made in Italy, and the landmine in the center was manufactured in Russia; all are composed largely of plastic. Reproduced with permission from Mader TH, Aragones JV, Chandler AC, et al. Ocular and ocular adnexal injuries treated by United States military ophthalmologists during Operations Desert Shield and Desert Storm. *Ophthalmology.* 1993;100:1465.

the Persian Gulf War, the potential is huge that such injuries will occur in future conflicts. Unfortunately for the casualties, the localization of plastic FBs and the proper care of laser injuries has been and continues to be problematical.

SUMMARY

Few would contest the proposition that those who stand in the day of battle for us all deserve the best medical care possible. It should, therefore, be the objective of the military ophthalmologist to make the gap between the practice of ophthalmology in the TO and the highest standards in CONUS as small as possible. This is accomplished by

- keeping in mind the principles that underlie such practice in the TO;
- incorporating advances made in civilian ophthalmology into military ophthalmology as soon as possible;
- fighting for the resources required to provide such care;
- educating all who deal with eye-injured casualties;
- putting the best military ophthalmologists in the TO so that they can provide immediate, expert, definitive care to casualties with eye injuries and diseases;
- urging the wearing of eye armor during the conduct of all eye-hazardous activities;
- having a senior ophthalmologist serve as the TO ophthalmology consultant; and
- learning to work with neurosurgeons and head-and-neck surgeons.

The injuries that cannot be prevented should receive the very best care our country is capable of providing, and that care must be provided within the TO. Deferring expert eye care until after the casualty is evacuated from the theater will produce preventable blindness. Denying appropriate eye care to the nontransportable casualty in the TO will do the same.

The Persian Gulf War demonstrated how quickly ocular injuries can be generated in a modern battlefield. The war also exposed the fact that the overall ophthalmic surgical capabilities in theater were suboptimal. It clearly showed the absolute necessity of providing appropriate equipment and training to surgical units during peacetime so that they can be properly prepared for wartime deployment. This conflict may also have given us a preview of new types of ocular injuries to be seen in future wars. Therefore, the Persian Gulf War confirmed the lessons of the past and was perhaps an ominous introduction to the ophthalmic injuries of the future.

REFERENCES

1. Greenwood A. Primary treatment of war injuries of the lids and orbits. *Trans Am Ophthalmol Soc.* 1919;17:105–115.
2. Spaulding SC, Sternberg P. Controversies in the management of posterior segment trauma. *Retina.* 1990;10:S76–S82.
3. La Piana FG, Hornblass A. Military ophthalmology in the Vietnam War. *Doc Ophthalmol.* 1997;93:29–48.
4. La Piana FG, Ward TP. The development of eye armor for the American infantryman. *Ophthal Clin North Am.* 1999;12(3):421–434.
5. Tredici TJ. Management of ophthalmic casualties in Southeast Asia. *Mil Med.* 1968;133:355–362.

6. Aker F, Schroeder DC, Baycar RS. Cause and prevention of maxillofacial war wounds: A historical review. *Mil Med.* 1983;148:921–927.

7. Cotter F, La Piana FG. Eye casualty reduction by eye armor. *Mil Med.* 1991;156:126–128.

8. de Schweinitz GE. Ophthalmology in the United States. In: Ireland MW, The Surgeon General. *Surgery.* Vol 11, Part 2. In: *The Medical Department of the United States Army in the World War.* Washington, DC: Government Printing Office; 1924: 665, 672.

9. Wood CA, ed. *The American Encyclopedia and Dictionary of Ophthalmology*. Vol 18. Chicago, Ill: Cleveland Press: 1921; 13692, 13757.

10. Vail DT. Administrative aspects of ophthalmology in the European Theater of Operations. In: Coates JB, Randolph ME, Canfield N, eds. *Ophthalmology and Otolaryngology*. In: Medical Department, United States Army; Hays SB, The Surgeon General, US Army. *Surgery in World War II.* Washington, DC: Department of the Army, Medical Department, Office of The Surgeon General; 1957: 94.

11. Gunderson T. Personal communication to Martin Wand, MD, Army ophthalmologist, Mediterranean Theater, World War II; 1985.

12. Stone W. Ocular injuries in the Armed Forces. *JAMA.* 1950;142:151–152.

13. King, Edwards. *Recent Advances in Medicine and Surgery*. US Army Medical Service Graduate School, Army Medical Center [now Walter Reed Army Medical Center], Washington, DC: 1954: 477–478, 481.

14. Committee on Trauma, American College of Surgeons. Hospital and prehospital resources for optimal care of the injured patient. *ACS Bull.* 1983;68(10):11–21.

15. Bellamy RF. Contrasts in combat casualty care. *Mil Med.* 1985;150:405–410.

16. Russel SR, Olsen KR, Folk JC. Predictors of scleral rupture and the role of vitrectomy in severe blunt ocular trauma. *Am J Ophthalmol.* 1988;105:253–257.

17. DeJuan E, Sternberg P, Michels RG. Timing of vitrectomy after penetrating ocular injuries. *Ophthalmology.* 1984;91:1072–1074.

18. Randolph ME. Administrative aspects of ophthalmology in Zone of Interior. In: Coates JB, Randolph ME, Canfield N, eds. *Ophthalmology and Otolaryngology*. In: Medical Department, United States Army; Hays SB, The Surgeon General, US Army. *Surgery in World War II.* Washington, DC: Department of the Army, Medical Department, Office of The Surgeon General; 1957: 36.

19. Vail D. Military ophthalmology. *Trans Am Acad Ophthalmol Otolaryngol*. 1950/51; 55:709–715.

20. Carey ME. Learning from traditional combat mortality and morbidity data used in the evaluation of combat medical care. *Mil Med.* 1987;152:6–13.

21. Tressler CS. The incidence of corneal ulcers in soft contact lens wearers among active duty military at Fort Stewart, Georgia. *Mil Med.* 1988;153:247–249.

22. Cohen HB. Colonel, Medical Corps, US Army (Ret). Personal communication, late 1970s–early 1980s.

23. Bowen TE, Bellamy RF, eds. *Emergency War Surgery NATO Handbook*. 2nd rev US ed. Washington, DC: Department of Defense, Government Printing Office; 1988.

24. Committee on Trauma, American College of Surgeons. *Advanced Trauma Life Support Program for Physicians: Instructor Manual.* 5th ed. Chicago, Ill: American College of Surgeons; 1997.

25. Zajtchuk R, Bellamy RF, Jenkins DP, eds. *Combat Casualty Care Guidelines: Operation Desert Storm.* Washington, DC: Department of the Army, Office of The Surgeon General, and Borden Institute; 1991.

26. Heier JS, Enzenauer RW, Wintermeyer SF, Delaney M, La Piana FG. Ocular injuries and diseases at a combat support hospital in support of Operations Desert Shield and Desert Storm. *Arch Ophthalmol.* 1993;111:795–798.

27. Mader TH, Aragones JV, Chandler AC, et al. Ocular and ocular adnexal injuries treated by United States military ophthalmologists during Operations Desert Shield and Desert Storm. *Ophthalmology.* 1993;100:1462–1467.

Chapter 3

OCULAR TRAUMA: HISTORY AND EXAMINATION

MATTHEW J. NUTAITIS, MD*

*Commander, Medical Corps, US Navy; Head, Glaucoma Service, Department of Ophthalmology, National Naval Medical Center, 8901 Wisconsin Avenue, Bethesda, Maryland 20889-5600

INTRODUCTION

Both the soldier fighting on a modern-day battlefield and the civilian residing in a 21st-century city are at risk of ocular trauma. The prevalence of such injury is not trivial. For example, recently gathered data indicate that the rate of ophthalmic injury during military-supported demining missions is 23%.[1] The military and nonmilitary patients who were unlucky enough to be near exploding ordinance, or actually caused the device to explode by tripping the device, or setting the device off as they attempted to remove the explosive ordinance also had a significant rate of nonophthalmic injury and death. It is clear that today's soldiers who survive their time on the battlefield will continue to suffer eye injuries. Additionally, the many other hazards of the modern battlefield—many of which are high- and low-speed particles from fragmentation weapons—cause many injuries to unprotected and partially protected soldiers.[2]

Individuals who sustain eye injuries caused by blunt forces, sharp (ie, penetrating) forces, fragmented projectiles, or a combination thereof can present with a spectrum of ocular problems. There are further indications that if these injuries are not recognized and treated effectively, the outcome for the patient is poor. This fact is exemplified by the spectrum of injuries that were seen during the ophthalmology support trip to Yemen, during which patients injured by land mines were examined.[3] Within 5 years after the civil war between North and South Yemen in 1994, a dichotomy in patient outcomes had become evident. Patients who had sustained minimal or no injury to the ocular structures from land mines had excellent vision. Those who had sustained moderate-to-severe or devastating injuries were uniformly blind.

The ophthalmologist who begins care and the ophthalmologist who finishes the treatment can encounter severe challenges throughout a trauma patient's clinical course. The initial treatment is vitally important, however, because it sets the patient's clinical course and offers a chance for useful vision after injury. This care, of course, begins with the injury itself. This chapter focuses on the steps needed to understand fully the mechanism of injury, discover all the aspects of the eye that have been injured, and set the stage so that the initial repair and follow-on specialty work can yield a successful outcome for the patient. The care of specific problems will be addressed in chapters throughout the book. A concentrated effort to achieve a complete and appropriate history and examination of the traumatized eye follows (Figure 3-1).

Because ocular trauma represents a spectrum of ophthalmic diagnoses, understanding the variety of patients and possible injuries is a requirement for successful treatment of the patient with an ocular injury. In the battlefield or on the city streets, the eye is susceptible to blunt forces, sharp or penetrating forces, and injury by foreign bodies (FBs). The specter of chemical insult looms large over the modern battlefield but is perceived as a smaller threat in the civilian "battlefield." The ophthalmologist and trauma specialist must be prepared to diagnose and treat any of these types of injuries or combinations thereof. The Israeli medical system documented that 11% of their troops' injuries were ocular and adnexal. A significant minority of injuries was multiple,[4–6] notwithstanding protective measures that had been issued but were not in use at the time of the injury.

Before physicians can begin correcting the ocular and adnexal injuries sustained, the patient must be stabilized from an Advanced Trauma Life Support (ATLS) standpoint. In the military during combat, the initial care provided to an injured soldier is unlikely to be rendered by an ophthalmolo-

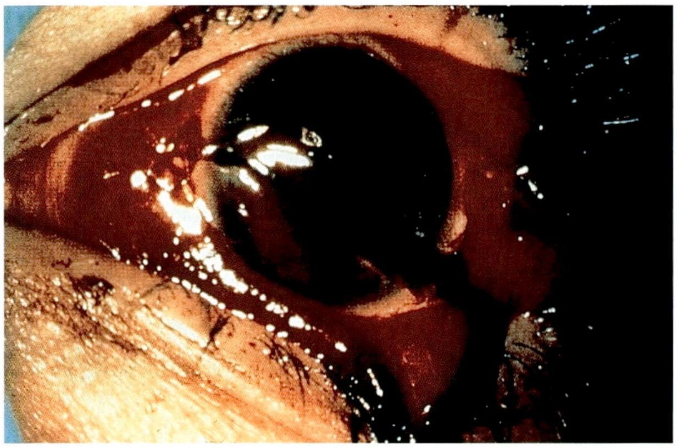

Fig. 3-1. This eye has suffered a typical sharp laceration of the anterior segment structures. The laceration involves limbal structures, the cornea, the trabecular region, lens, and perhaps more posterior structures. The efforts of the initial treating physician and the ophthalmic surgeon in acquiring an appropriate history and physical examination, discovering any occult injuries to the eye, and applying correct and effective diagnostic and surgical techniques can lead to a successful repair of severe eye trauma.

EXHIBIT 3-1

THE FOUR PHASES OF ADVANCED TRAUMA LIFE SUPPORT EVALUATION AND CARE

1. Primary survey: assessment of ABCs (airway, breathing, and circulation)
   A. Airway and cervical spine control
   B. Breathing
   C. Circulation with hemorrhage control
   D. Disability: brief neurologic evaluation
   E. Exposure/environment: completely undress the patient but prevent hypothermia
2. Resuscitation
   A. Oxygenation and ventilation
   B. Shock management-intravenous lines, Ringer's lactate
   C. Management of life-threatening problems identified in primary survey is continued
   D. Monitoring
3. Secondary survey
   A. Head and skull
   B. Maxillofacial
   C. Neck
   D. Chest
   E. Abdomen
   F. Perineum, rectum, vagina
   G. Musculoskeletal
   H. Complete neurological examination
   I. Appropriate roentgenograms, laboratory tests, and special studies
   J. "Tubes and fingers" in every orifice
4. Definitive care

Adapted with permission from Committee on Trauma, American College of Surgeons. *Advanced Trauma Life Support Program for Physicians: Instructor Manual.* 5th ed. Chicago, Ill: American College of Surgeons; 1993: 36–37.

gist; however, stabilization of the patient's airway, and initiation of respiratory and circulatory resuscitation (and their continued support), are in the ophthalmologist's purview. The military surgeon is trained in these abilities, is prepared to carry them out, and should not hesitate to review ATLS treatment algorithms (Exhibit 3-1).[7] Conversely, the civilian emergency room physician must be ready to render aid to trauma patients in accordance with Advanced Cardiac Life Support (ACLS) and ATLS algorithms, but he or she must also be prepared to provide the ATLS care required for the traumatized eye itself. The first physician at the side of a trauma patient should be familiar with the initial steps needed to care for the eye-injured patient as described in these chapters and elsewhere.[8]

We should strive to obtain as complete a history and ocular examination of the patient in the battlefield as we would with any patient seen in a clinical setting. Wartime injuries that include the globe, orbit, and adnexal regions are incapacitating to the soldier,[9] but commanders on the modern battlefield want all soldiers to have minimal time as "walking wounded." The treating ophthalmologist should expect a moderate amount of pressure to treat with success and return the "recovered" soldier to the field commanders in a very short time. Further taxing battlefield medical capabilities, mass casualty scenarios that sometimes occur in

EXHIBIT 3-2

HISTORY AND EXAMINATION SEQUENCE

History
1. Chief complaint
2. Age of patient
3. Details of the traumatic event
4. Review of ocular systems
5. Additional review of systems
6. Past surgical history
7. Past medical history
8. Medication history
9. Allergies

Physical Examination
1. Visual acuity examination
2. Pupil examination
3. Visual field examination
4. Motility examination
5. Intraocular pressure
6. Adnexal examination
7. Anterior segment examination
8. Posterior pole examination

Imaging Studies
1. Ultrasound
2. Plain film radiographs
3. Computed tomography (CT) scan
4. Magnetic resonance imaging (MRI)

combat may preclude doing a complete history and ocular examination, thus forcing the treatment of the injured to move forward with incomplete data.

During conflicts that involve troops and mass casualties, it is important to remember to conduct triage and perform medical maneuvers that allow the most care for the most injured. In the best of all situations, given plenty of time and the appropriate instruments, a detailed ocular history and examination aid in the diagnosis and treatment of military personnel with eye injuries. Exhibit 3-2 can be used to ensure that all significant facets of the patient's history and physical examination are covered in the initial and subsequent interactions with the ocular trauma patient.

HISTORY

Chief Complaint

The chief complaint portion of the history has proven to be a valuable means of eliciting information during any eye examination. This observation is no different for the ocular trauma patient. The amount of time spent on this aspect of the examination depends on the physician and the patient. Most patients, when given the opportunity, can give tremendously useful information toward diagnosing their ocular problems. Obtaining this set of details can be well worth the time spent. Nevertheless, in some instances the acquisition of data toward the chief complaint or for the history in general is not necessary or should not be pursued, at least not immediately.

One scenario in which it is necessary to defer the chief complaint portion of the examination is that of a patient who presents with a chemical injury (for further information, please see Chapter 7, Chemical Injuries of the Eye, in this volume, and *Medical Aspects of Chemical and Biological Warfare,*[10] another volume in the Textbooks of Military Medicine series). The eye must be protected from what could be devastating and vision-affecting damage from an alkali or acid burn. Copious irrigation and removal of any particles are the mainstays of treatment of chemical injuries (Figure 3-2). The issue of an open (ie, perforated or penetrated) globe at this point creates a difficult situation, but the presence of the chemical takes priority over the other injuries and should remain a priority in the treatment plan.

It often happens, especially in warfare, that neither the patient nor witnesses can provide any information that will help elicit the patient's major complaint. A perception or evidence of injury—typically, decreased vision or pain—may be offered, but how the eye was injured may not be known. In this scenario, there is little reason to spend any more

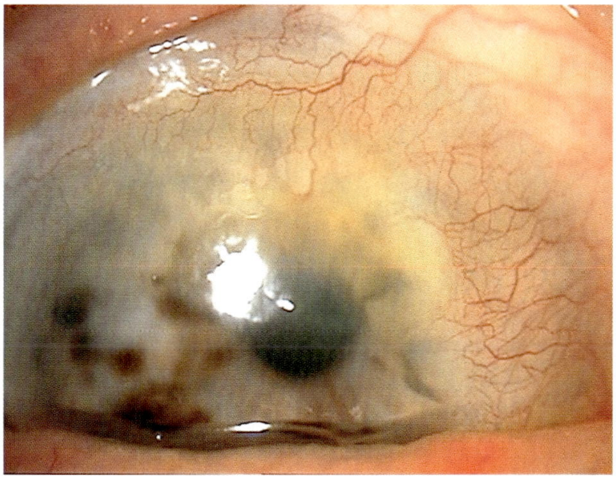

Fig. 3-2. The patient's eye sustained a chemical injury, but early, copious irrigation prevented more serious damage. Note, however, that the anterior segment is damaged. The alkali chemical penetrated the ocular coats and damaged the corneal endothelium. Corneal edema and anterior segment vascularization are the challenges presented to the ophthalmic surgeon by this type of injury.

than the minimum time interviewing the patient, because the likelihood of discovering useful details is quite low. As ophthalmologists we are fortunate, especially when ocular trauma is involved, because we can see the structures and, thereby, gather a wealth of details.

With certain clinical conditions, we can bypass much of the patient's history without jeopardizing the eventual outcome. When the eye is obviously injured, the history may be curtailed to conduct a clinical examination and determine the extent of the injury. Eliminating unnecessary steps and thereby getting the patient treated as soon as possible should be the goal for everyone. Trauma injuries that cross the boundaries separating different classes of injuries challenge the ophthalmologist and decrease the number of successful outcomes. An awareness of this concept and the military ophthalmologist's ability to use the information in the chapters that follow place the ocular trauma patients in the best hands to restore full vision potential.

Age of the Patient

Ocular trauma spans all age categories but does tend to occur more in the younger, more active population[11,12] because these people are participating in activities that put their eyes at risk.[13] Age determination, however, plays only a minor role in the decision to repair ocular trauma. The sequence of events to surgically repair the injured globe does not vary much, whether the patient is 2 or 62 years of age.

Details of the Traumatic Event

During a lull in the action or while waiting for the operating room to be freed up, the examiner can gather details of the event that led to the injury. Additional information about the mechanism of injury may lead to discovery of all the traumatic damage—overt and occult—done to the eye. Minimizing occult damage allows for a more complete primary repair, which, if done early in the course of treatment, can speed the patient's recovery process.

To prompt a full account of the injury, open-ended questions that refer to metal-on-metal events and explosive events are important. This line of questioning allows investigation of possible projectile injury and FB damage that should be included in the initial work-up of the patient. Other mechanisms of injury can also be investigated. The examiner must determine if the patient sustained a true blunt injury or if a sharp injury may have been involved. The examiner knows that the required information has been recovered when it is determined whether a sharp injury occurred and what the weapon of injury was. Was the injury caused by one sharp entry point, or by an explosive or missile injury that caused multiple sharp entries to the globe and the adnexa? To complete the data collection with regard to an FB injury, it is beneficial to determine the type of material, size of the projectiles, shape, metal type and content, and the possibility of contamination (Figure 3-3).

For thermal burns, it is important to gather data about the type of burn, the location of the burn, and the percentage of the total body surface area involved. For electrical injuries, it is beneficial to identify entrance and exit wounds in order to provide lifesaving medical care to the injured fighter.

On the modern battlefield, the physical examination and history need to include an active search for chemical involvement and injury. Identifying the chemical as an acid or base is always important; however, expect the description of the battlefield to be sparse. An additional benefit of identifying the type of chemical injury is that the information can be passed to the field commanders, thus giving them vital data to protect the soldiers who remain in the field. The ability to protect the troops more

a

b

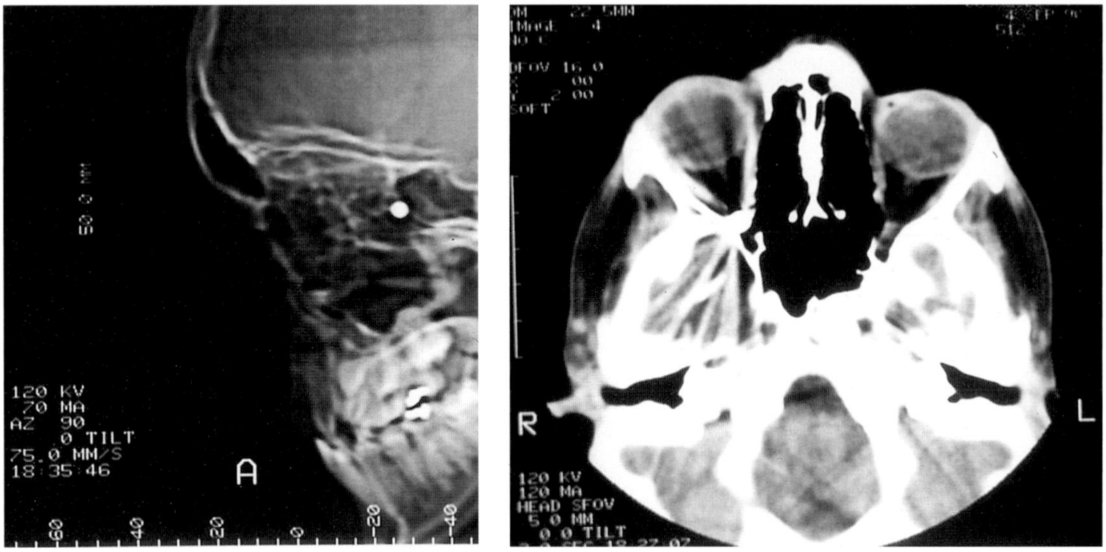

Fig. 3-3. These photographs demonstrate the utility of radiological examination in the ocular trauma patient. The patient history revealed that the injury occurred when a BB gun was discharged at close range during a neighborhood "game." The examination demonstrated a penetrating injury to the anterior segment, but (**a**) the plain scout film and (**b**) the computed tomography scan show the precise location of the foreign body—the critical information needed to plan the ophthalmic care for this patient. The need for radiological examination of the traumatized orbit and globe increases as the history and examination point toward a mechanism of injury that includes multiple, high-velocity foreign bodies—the exact type of environment that exists on the modern battlefield.

effectively is an asset that is well recognized by those in charge of the operational theater.

The final advantage to obtaining carefully documented information about the event is the ability to address any legal issues with solid data. This advantage may not always apply in the operational forces but does exist in nonmilitary health arenas. The armed forces are trending toward a more civilian application of healthcare, so additional well-documented information may be very helpful once the dust settles from the military or civilian event. Issues relevant to the initial level of injury, institution of timely and appropriately addressed surgical and medical care, and a complete treatment of all traumatic damage should have supporting data. This way, any legal scrutiny that may follow can be answered quickly, and care of the patient may be completed.

Review of Ocular Systems

A detailed review of systems for the eye is of next importance. The level of pretrauma vision is an extremely useful piece of data. Also, determination of previously diagnosed problems is key. The presence of glaucomatous optic neuropathy or any optic neuropathy puts the traumatized eye at risk for any pressure elevation experienced. Blunt trauma and postoperative courses are known to be associated with a high incidence of pressure elevations—either short term or chronic. Previous incisional surgery always leaves a weaker area in the ocular coat (Figure 3-4), which reminds us as ophthalmic surgeons to always inspect and be ready to repair these areas of prior surgical injury.

Previous conditions that can affect vision, especially negatively, are useful to uncover. Sometimes knowing the type of eye drops the patient has been using can give some insight into ocular conditions that involve the patient. Also, the need to aggressively repair all eyes with trauma is temporized if the physician knows ahead of time that the visual potential is poor.

Review of Additional Systems

The review of the patient's other systems (Exhibit 3-3) naturally follows the review of ocular systems. Items to be covered and understood are those that put the patient at risk for medical difficulties when surgery is performed, including a history of recent myocardial infarction or recent pulmonary disorders (eg, pneumonia, chronic obstructive pulmonary disease with recent exacerbations, reactive air-

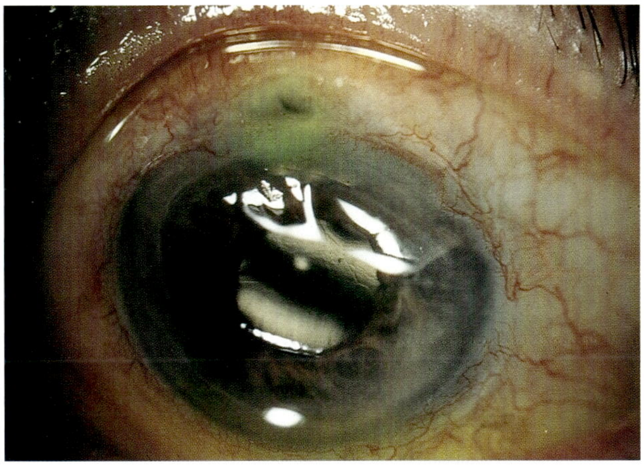

Fig. 3-4. The patient's episode of blunt trauma supports the premise that previous surgical sites never regain the tissue's original tensile strength. They remain areas of possible rupture during traumatic injury. Superiorly in the photograph, the previous cataract incision dehisced and required surgical repair to reinstate the structural integrity of the ocular coats. Other potential weak points in the ocular coats include the limbal region through Schlemm's canal and just posterior to the insertion of the extraocular muscles on the globe. These areas must be inspected before a ruptured globe is ruled out in the case of blunt trauma.

EXHIBIT 3-3

REVIEW OF SYSTEMS LIST

1. Head
2. Eyes
3. Ears
4. Nose
5. Throat
6. Neck
7. Chest
8. Heart
9. Lungs
10. Abdomen
11. Genitalia
12. Musculoskeletal system
13. Extremities
14. Neurological system
15. Skin

way issues). Cancer history with ongoing treatment or the presence of active disease, especially systemic infections, can complicate the care and recovery of the eye. These examples generally do not apply to the active duty military, but prisoners of war or the local civilian population who are offered equivalent treatment may carry some of these concerns to the ophthalmic surgeon. Ultimately, the goals of successful surgery and good vision may be difficult to achieve if these and other preoperative factors are missed or ignored in the time before surgery.

Surgical History

With the completion of the review of systems, information regarding past surgical history should have been discovered. As complete an accounting of previous eye surgeries as possible, in addition to systemic surgeries that the patient has undergone, is needed to allow safe and appropriate surgical care for the patient.

Medical History

A past medical history is developed at this time. The knowledge of the presence of hypertension, diabetes, or cardiovascular disease is important in understanding how the patient may respond to surgery. Time spent evaluating the past medical history, however short, can pay off in the end. For example, discovering a history of aspirin use or a full-blown bleeding diathesis can alter the surgeon's choice of surgical approaches or even the type of repair attempted for the specific injury discovered. The assessment of a patient's risk for having a contagious disease is not out of line today. In the trauma setting, this type of information may not only be unattainable but must be scrutinized for accuracy. The surgeon and other medical care personnel who care for trauma patients are well versed in the need to use universal precautions that protect them from communicable diseases. In a war, the soldiers involved usually have had a certain level of health screening that can detect human immunodeficiency virus, sickle cell trait, or other disorders. Of course, past medical histories for opposing forces or for civilian noncombatant casualties who receive care in the medical system will, to a large extent, be unknown.

Medication History

On the battlefield, most soldiers are fit and free from complex medical disorders. Nevertheless, obtaining a medication history on all trauma patients is wise. The value of this information increases as the patient enters into the category where medications are more commonly used. Medications that put surgical repairs at risk for failure, that put the patient at risk for difficulty with the surgical procedure or the general anesthesia, or that indicate the existence of complicating factors should be identified. Oral and topical steroids, anticoagulant therapy, antineoplastic agents, echothiophate products, and topical or systemic antibiotics tend to fit in those categories. Information about medication to treat systemic diseases—such as diabetes, hypertension, and pulmonary conditions ranging from asthma to pneumonia—are valuable in ensuring better care of trauma patients.

Allergies

If possible, the history portion of the examination needs to include a determination of the medication–allergy profile of the patient. Serious and fatal reactions can occur, and avoidance of known allergens is a wise and useful strategy as patients with ocular trauma are assessed and readied for treatment.

PHYSICAL EXAMINATION

With the history portion of the examination completed in appropriate detail and scope, attention is turned to the examination of the eye. The acquisition of accurate information, using all available examination techniques, allows the ocular surgeon to enter the treatment phase of the injury with knowledge to guide him or her toward appropriate surgery directed at the specific injury. This approach enables the highest success rate in the care of the ocular trauma patient because microsurgery to repair specific, known injuries with no occult injuries equals success for trauma repair.

Visual Acuity

The examination begins, as always, with an assessment of the level of visual acuity. The use of a Snellen visual acuity chart is an objective and familiar technique but is not required. Depending on the setting of initial care, a less formal assessment of visual acuity is acceptable. Assessing the visual acuity level with the "count finger" method is simple, and using the printed letters on an intravenous bag for the trauma patient to read is convenient. Both methods document valuable information for the clinical and surgical course the patient is about to undertake.

Light perception (LP) is an important threshold of vision. Without this level of acuity, initial repair and follow-on procedures may not result in any improvement. However, a patient with no light perception (NLP) should be managed aggressively, since a percentage of these patients will recover some vision.[14] If better vision is detected, repair of the worst injuries can be surprisingly successful.[15] The abilities to perceive light, to see hand movements, and to count fingers at a specific distance are the sequential levels of visual assessment. The ophthalmologist should test for vision in this standard fashion and always remember to test each eye separately. Using the 20/400 E and smaller letters, the Snellen's test type chart provides an accurate and reproducible measurement of the level of vision. The patient should be wearing glasses, if necessary, or the pinhole can be used to get an idea of the best corrected vision. Emphasis is placed on testing the vision early in the patient interaction. As is discussed in subsequent chapters, delay can cause additional clinical factors, such as bleeding and cataract, to depress visual acuity, and the amount of useful information acquired will be adversely affected.

The physician is challenged also to ferret out cases of malingering and secondary gain. These possibilities need to be addressed early in the treatment of the injured eye patient. These patients may take the opportunity to embellish the severity of their injuries or may attempt to fool the examiner into thinking there is "more than meets the eye." If this approach is successful, then the patient may end up with more, rather than appropriate, medical and surgical treatment than the actual condition requires. The accuracy of subjective visual acuity information should be questioned if the healthcare provider suspects a motive of secondary gain or the use of drugs and alcohol, or if the data are not making sense.

Remember that the random Es and Allen figures are to be used if necessary. In the heat of battle or in the mass casualty scenario that war can often produce, a brief but reproducible method should be used and a short time expended to get the best vision estimate. The mass casualty situation also exists in the civilian emergency room and hospitals. We have only to look at the bombing of the Murrah building in Oklahoma City, Oklahoma, in

April 1995 to see a medical system stressed beyond capacity.[16] The 15 seconds it takes to assess monocular visual function is never wasted time.

Pupil

The pupil examination yields a tremendous amount of information in a very short time. The shape and location of the pupil is one of the first and easiest bits of data in the eye examination that yield information about

- the integrity of the globe,
- the presence of blunt and sharp destructive forces in and around the globe, and
- the health and status of the eye with regard to the presence of infection and FBs.

Direct visualization with a simple penlight for illumination is the simplest of techniques and provides a tremendous amount of useful data (Figure 3-5).

The appearance of the pupil (including ovality, irregular borders, missing portions of the pupil border, and blood adhering to the surface or margin of the iris) can indicate that damage has been done to the eye. For example, a peaked pupil usually indicates a globe rupture or laceration in the quadrant that the pupil points toward. On the modern battlefield, high-speed projectiles and explosion-generated particles can be the objects that induce the subtle pupil damage that must be noted if more serious anterior and posterior segment injuries are to be diagnosed at presentation.

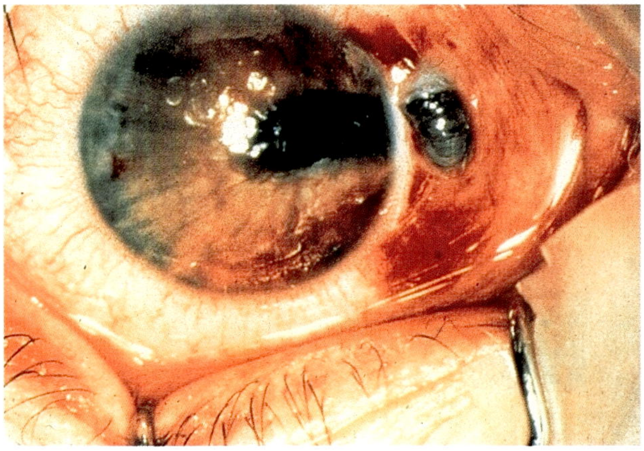

Fig. 3-5. This photograph demonstrates how a pupil examination can add useful information about the amount of damage sustained by the eye during a traumatic event. The shape of the pupil leads to several correct conclusions. The injury is penetrating and is located at the surgical limbus. Note the iris presentation anteriorly on the surface of the sclera, a finding that is also extremely important.

The pupil examination continues with a search for afferent pupillary defect (APD) or Marcus Gunn pupil. The technique of examining each pupil separately and then comparing the pupil's responses to light allows the health and function of the optic nerve to be compared and documented in an objective fashion. The absence of an APD is a powerful (and quick) indication that the intraocular optic nerve, the retroorbital portion of the optic nerve, and the optic canal portion of the optic nerve are relatively intact. That information can be ascertained in as short a time as it takes to check the pupillary reaction to light; this step should never be omitted when a trauma patient is examined.

If the pupil examination reveals a positive APD, we immediately know that there is a severe injury to the optic nerve or retina and posterior pole of the eye. Patients with the combination of NLP and APD tend to have a very poor prognosis. The presence of a relative APD causes concern about the well-being of the optic nerve, and the examiner then must study the eye for potential damage to the areas mentioned previously. Many ways exist to get information about damage or potential damage to the path of the nerve.[17] The detection of an APD on initial examination or subsequent examinations is a strong indication that there is severe damage to the eye or optic nerve.

Visual Field

The next portion of the examination is the determination of the patient's peripheral vision. The ocular trauma patient is at risk for myriad injuries to various portions of the eye. The specific injury determines whether visual field defects will be present. The difficulty in acquiring useful information from this aspect of the physical examination is that many or most of the findings will be nonspecific changes to the visual field. The time that would be spent conducting a more detailed examination to further identify the ocular or adnexal problem is probably best spent moving on to the remainder of the physical examination, ultimately preparing the patient and the eye for treatment and surgical repair of trauma-induced injuries.

Nevertheless, a carefully performed confrontation visual field test can be very useful for injuries that involve the retina, retroorbital spaces, the optic nerve, and the central nervous system. Inferior

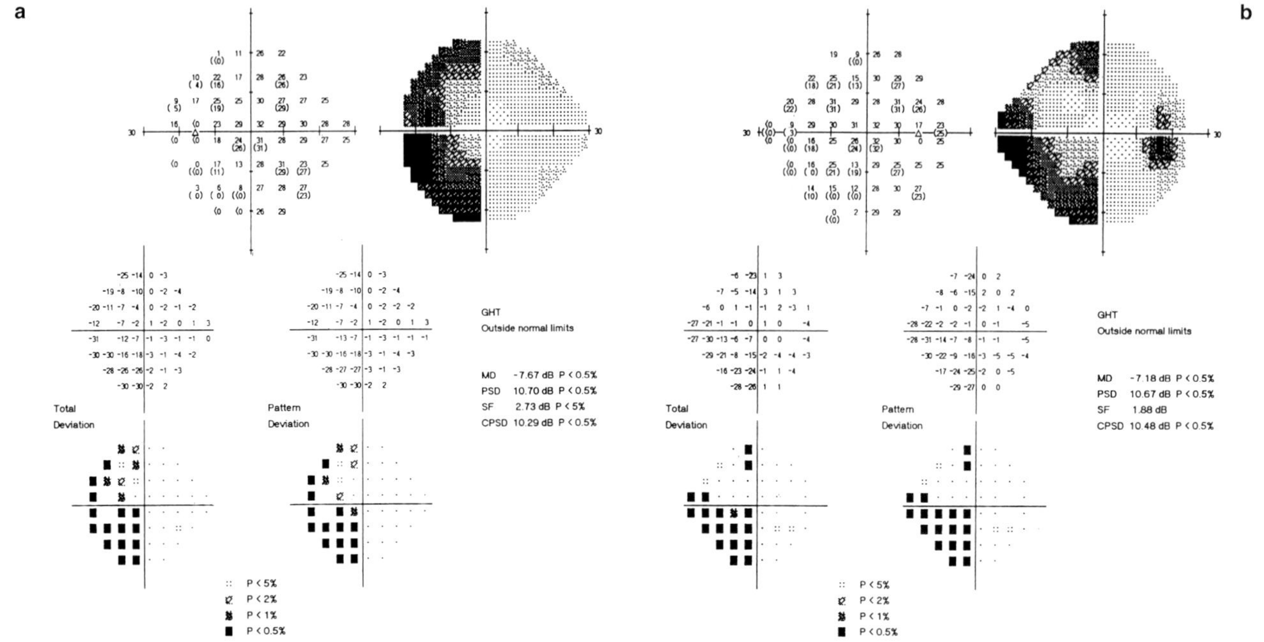

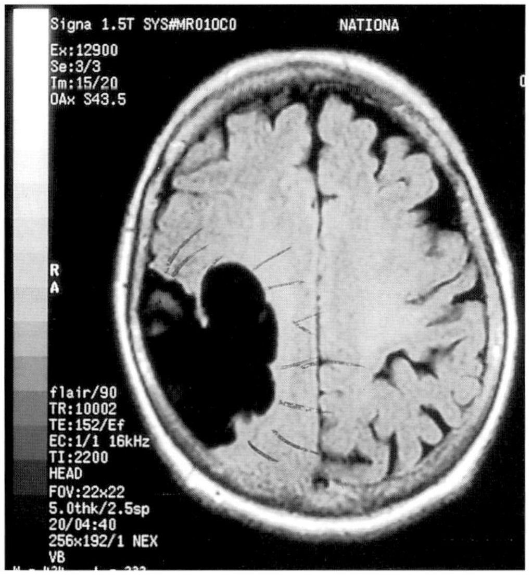

Fig. 3-6. This set of visual fields (**a**, left eye, and **b**, right eye) prompted further examination of this asymptomatic patient. After a magnetic resonance imaging (MRI) examination revealed (**c**) a large tumor of unknown duration in the right hemisphere, the patient underwent a neurosurgical excision of the tumor and the visual fields improved to near-normal.

altitudinal defects can indicate a contusion to the optic nerve in the optic canal or a retinal detachment when vision and the rest of the examination are deceptively "normal." Hemianopsia (Figure 3-6) always requires an evaluation of the posterior portions of the optic nerves and the visual pathways to assess for an injury to this portion of the visual system. However, the astute examiner may be able to gain some of this same information just by recording the quality of visual acuity and whether an APD exists.

In acute settings of trauma, formal or automated field testing is probably unnecessary. Formal visual field testing may be necessary, however, when documenting visual field loss due to traumatic optic neuropathy or a traumatic brain injury. These detailed examinations can usually occur in the weeks following the traumatic injury and need not occupy a priority in the care rendered in the battlefield.

Motility

The evaluation of ocular motility, a portion of the complete routine eye examination, has a purpose in the examination of the traumatized orbit and globe. Foremost, the examination should provide information as to the integrity of the ocular structures. An open globe tends to have decreased motility. However, any injury to the orbit and globe that involves the ocular muscles, motor nerves to those muscles, or origins and insertions of the muscles tends to present with some form of abnormal and decreased motility. Severe injury that leads to muscle and soft-tissue edema also has a certain amount of decreased movement as a presenting finding. Therefore, we can easily understand that although decreased motility can be present in the lacerated or traumatized globe, the clinical finding of abnormal motility does not confirm an open globe.

Several other conditions that decrease motility warrant mention. The examiner must include orbital hemorrhage, orbital wall fractures, and direct injury to the extraocular muscles in the differential diagnosis of a traumatized orbit and a disturbance in the motility of the eye.

Clinical experience helps guide the amount of detail needed to complete the appropriate level of examination. If the anterior segment is grossly unaffected by the individual injury, and if there is concern that periocular structures (muscles) are injured, then time can be spent assessing the motility and developing a differential diagnosis as to the type of injuries that support the clinical appearance of the patient.

The movement of the eye through the cardinal positions of gaze with penlight guidance is standard and easy to complete. If time permits and the patient's other difficulties allow, the assessment for strabismus can be completed at this time with the use of cover-uncover, cross-cover testing and, if available, neutralization of any misalignment with prisms. The quicker estimations of the Krimsky and modified Krimsky tests are also adequate at this level of initial trauma assessment.

As the level of injury and disorganization of the anterior segment increases, the need for detailed and time-consuming motility data decreases. If an open globe or an FB injury is present, then the globe and ancillary structures should be explored in an operating room setting. Direct inspection of the muscles will occur during this phase, and any needed treatment can be planned and completed without causing further delay in critical treatment.

An important observation must be kept in mind with regard to version and duction testing: if the architecture of the wound permits an opening of the ocular coats, then—as the attempt is made to understand the type of motility disturbance present—it is possible that the ocular contents may be extruded. The requirement to understand whether entrapment exists or if a paralytic component is present is not outweighed by the risk to the globe and the possible creation of a worse injury. Forced duction should be considered contraindicated until the eye wall has been confirmed to be intact and the eye can safely undergo more-extensive testing. Only then can the surgeon be confident that the examination itself will not lead to further damage of the eye. This thought process is logical because in a suspected blowout fracture, the repair of the open globe takes precedence over trapped orbital contents.

Adnexa

The time to complete the assessment of the surrounding structures begins as a "work in progress," with direct inspection occurring as the physical examination takes place. Viewing the surrounding soft tissues for signs of penetrating injury, lacerations, and infection while taking a history and completing the steps of the eye examination is a timesaving technique.

Specifically, the margins of the lids are to be examined for laceration. This type of injury may require repair in the operating room under magnification. The surface of the lid must be inspected for any signs of penetrating injury or laceration. If the laceration is superficial and does not involve the lid margin or canaliculi, then a simple closure with loupe magnification is acceptable. The presence of a deep or through-and-through laceration of the lid makes the examination of the globe very important, because the laceration may involve the ocular coats. Once such a laceration is identified, the appropriate steps to repair this injury should be instituted. Extreme caution must be used to ensure that an open globe is detected. Pressure on the globe during further examination or during an oculoplastics repair of a simple lid margin laceration can result in a poor outcome from the ocular trauma, secondary to the expression of ocular contents through the occult globe laceration.

When the injury completely transects the lid structures, a very obvious malfunction of the lid elevators may be present. The clinical examination can reveal specific information about an orbital structure, in this case the levator system. Once this information is known, the surgical plan can include steps to repair the levator damage during the surgical exploration. If the injury is above the tarsal plate in the upper lid, a helpful finding to look for during the examination is orbital fat prolapse. This finding of fat, not lacrimal gland, indicates that the orbital septum has been violated and that damage

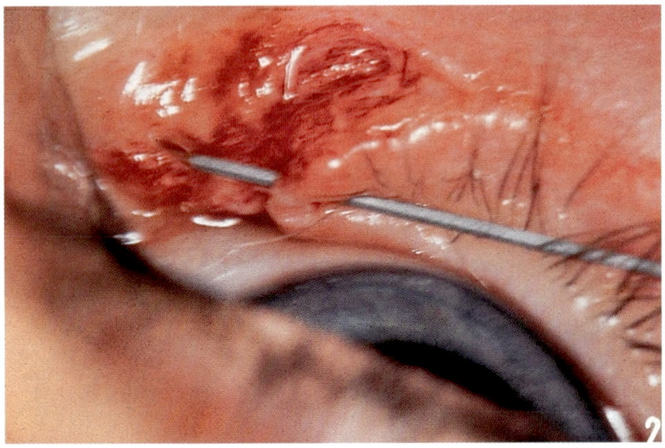

Fig. 3-7. The medial location of the laceration and a high index of suspicion both led to the proper diagnosis of this canalicular laceration and lid margin laceration. Repair under the microscope or with loupes in an operating room setting allows a greater success rate with such lid injuries.

to structures deep in the orbit is possible. Additionally, the orbit has lost an important protective barrier to prevent the spread of infection within the injury site and the orbit. An injury to the canalicular system of the eyelids requires microsurgical repair (Figure 3-7).

Remember to palpate along the orbital rim and the bony structures that make up the orbit, because the detection of a step-off along the frontal, zygomatic, or maxillary portions of the orbital rims is diagnostic of fracture. An inferior floor fracture may entrap orbital soft tissues and require a surgical repair of a floor fracture (Figure 3-8). Testing for numbness of the infraorbital skin and upper teeth is a specific finding of infraorbital nerve damage and indicates a high likelihood that an inferior floor fracture is present. The appearance of more-extreme findings, such as orbital and subcutaneous emphysema, leads the examiner to rule out any traumatic connection that the sinuses may have with the orbit and subcutaneous spaces. These communications tend to arise from fractures of the bony support around the globe or to result from concomitant penetrations of the subcutaneous layers and the sinuses.

Direct inspection can also reveal conjunctival lacerations, which in and of themselves are benign. Once again, if the superficial injury appears deep to the conjunctiva, then surgical exploration of the peribulbar region using a surgical peritomy is required. Further information is best obtained as the examination shifts from inspection, to palpation of the ocular adnexa, to a magnified inspection with

a

b

c

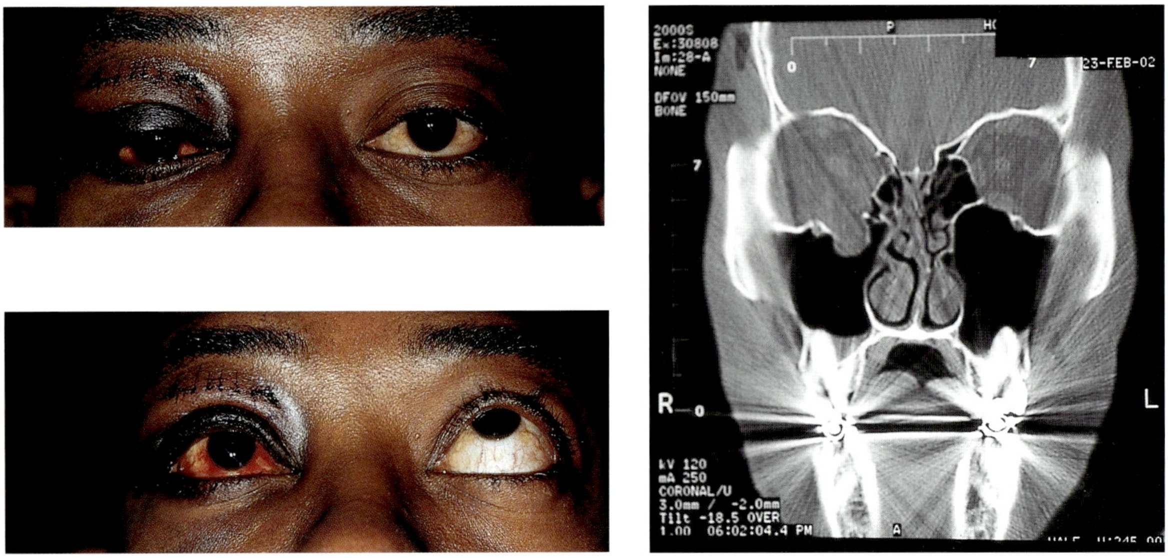

Fig. 3-8. The result of trauma to the orbit and globe can be a fracture of the bony structure of the orbit. After an episode of blunt trauma, this patient suffered (**a**) a superficial upper lid laceration (repaired), upper and lower lid ecchymosis, subconjunctival hemorrhage, 2 mm of enophthalmos, and traumatic mydriasis. (**b**) An inferior floor fracture restricts the movement of the right eye in up-gaze. (**c**) Computed tomography scan evaluation reveals the prolapse of orbital contents through the orbital floor fracture into the maxillary sinus. Surgical intervention was required to restore eye motility. The posterior segment was clear of blunt rupture and commotio retinae.

the slitlamp during the anterior segment portions of the trauma examination.

Anterior Segment

The anterior segment examination is extremely important in patients with ocular trauma. During this portion of the examination, the ophthalmologist has the opportunity to inspect the ocular structures in the anterior portion of the eye with direct and indirect lighting, retroillumination, and magnification. The slitlamp biomicroscope is an important tool for the care of the patient with ocular trauma. If the examining ophthalmologist does not have access to this equipment, then an attempt to provide a light source and magnification is essential. A simple setup of a muscle light and a 20-diopter lens is a crude system that can aid the examiner. However, the use of a small, portable, handheld slitlamp may be the best compromise if the patient cannot get to an examination lane.

Trauma—especially blunt, FB, and penetrating types—leaves clinical signs. We have to become astute at detecting these signs, and that job has become easier with our modern equipment. An orderly sequence of evaluation for the anterior segment helps prevent oversight of any damaged vital structure that should be examined, including the lids and lashes, cornea, conjunctiva, anterior chamber (AC), angle, iris, lens, and anterior vitreous.

The equipment available to the surgeon for examining the anterior segment is vast. In addition to the illuminated magnification system provided by the slitlamp, the use of lid retractors—either a DeMarres or a bent paper clip—will aid in the discovery of damage to the anterior segment. Cotton-tipped applicators, fluorescein strips, local anesthetic to use in regional anesthesia of the lids, and a lid speculum all assist the patient and the ophthalmic surgeon in the completion of the most thorough and safe examination possible.

Direct Inspection

Direct inspection with illumination is the first step in examination of the anterior segment. The lids are examined for lacerations or any evidence of an FB injury. Special attention is given to any areas of swelling and ecchymosis. At this point in the examination, it is still necessary to consider the possibility of projectile injury. The direct examination of the surface of the eye is next. The use of direct, indirect, and retroillumination at the slitlamp are all valuable in assessing and finding damage to the cornea and conjunctiva. A defect in the surface of the conjunctiva or cornea, an area of chemosis or hemorrhage, or a glimpse of a foreign object—all of which can be seen at the slitlamp—lead the physician to the correct diagnosis of ocular injury. Specifically, in the examination of a corneoscleral laceration, the length of the laceration should be noted. The size of the laceration is important in predicting the final outcome for the patient (Figure 3-9).[18]

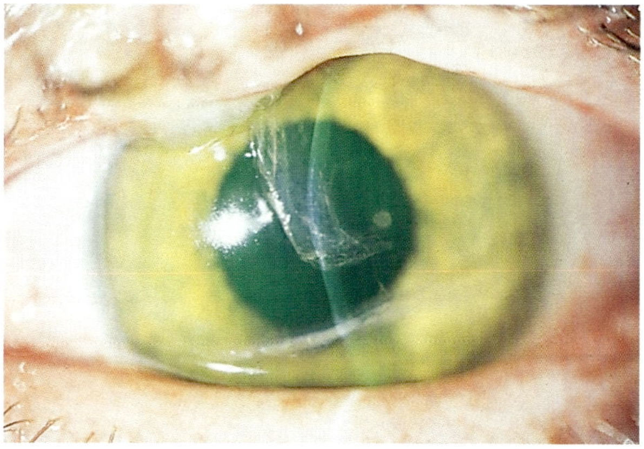

Fig. 3-9. This patient's shelved corneal laceration was first thought by the referring optometrist to be a nonhealing corneal abrasion. Careful slitlamp examination revealed the oblique nature of the laceration and the involvement of Descemet's membrane of the cornea. The use of the slitlamp biomicroscope is an extremely valuable part of the anterior segment examination. A wound leak was not present at the time of the consultant examination.

Penetrating corneal and scleral injuries that are not self-sealing yield additional clinical findings: these wounds will be Seidel-positive. The Seidel test involves the application of a fluorescein dye via a strip of paper, which, when viewed under a cobalt-blue light, reveals a rivulet of diluted dye—the egress of aqueous fluid—casting green fluorescence (Figure 3-10). Using strips of concentrated fluorescein is preferable to using a drop of dye, because the examiner can control the placement of the concentrated fluorescein.

The biomicroscope and the use of fluorescein dye offer another advantage: the differentiation of a corneal abrasion from a corneal ulcer. A break in the epithelium will allow the fluorescein dye to reach the corneal stroma, and the attached molecules will fluoresce. This finding supports the diagnosis of corneal abrasion. If a cellular infiltrate in the stroma (usually appearing white in color) is seen under biomicroscopy, then an infection is also present and the finding is most consistent with a

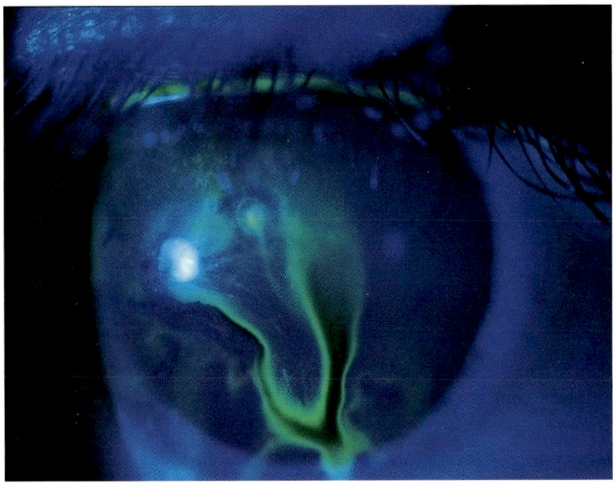

Fig. 3-10. This photograph of a sharp, penetrating corneal injury demonstrates positive findings of a Seidel test: a rivulet of aqueous is seen flowing from the penetration in the layer of concentrated fluorescein. This test is a valuable aid in the determination of anterior segment integrity.

corneal ulcer. The presence of an AC reaction, a history of soft contact lens use, and an absence of trauma to the eye also support the defect's infectious component.

Blunt injury to the eye can produce myriad findings. Globe rupture is the most serious injury and can be diagnosed with a complete examination of the anterior segment. Look for poor vision, a deep or shallow chamber, low intraocular pressure, and media opacities that obscure the view of the fundus.[19] An unusual but known finding of blunt trauma is the presence of concussive endotheliopathy (Figure 3-11). This finding is most common with a blunt FB injury such as a pellet (eg, a BB) that bounces off the cornea. A region of damaged endothelium in the posttrauma phase is present with a corresponding area of corneal edema.[20]

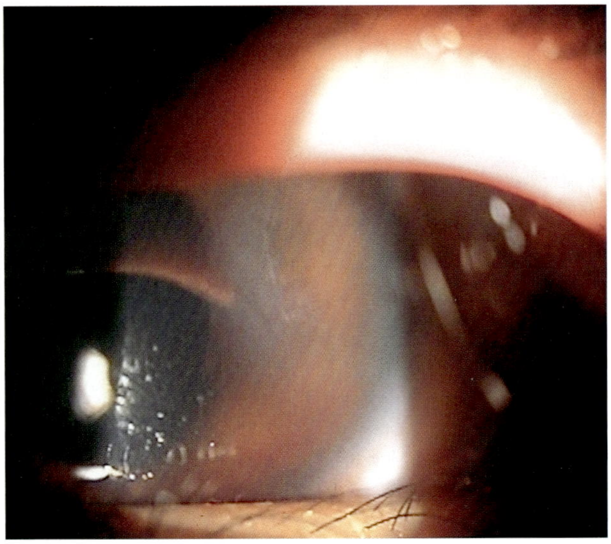

Fig. 3-11. The area of corneal edema seen in this photograph corresponds to the impact area of the BB that caused this blunt injury. Endothelial damage is present in the acute phase of these injuries.

The examination moves past the superficial structures of the eye, and slitlamp viewing of the internal structures allows the detection of further sequelae of ocular trauma. Within the AC—normally a clear, aqueous-filled chamber of the eye—hemorrhage; inflammatory cells; or FBs of metal, glass, or plastic can be seen easily with a careful slitlamp examination. The number, shape, and location of these objects should be noted to ensure removal of all FBs at the time of surgical repair.

Depth of the Anterior Chamber

The depth of the AC is also important. A rupture or laceration of the globe may release fluid from the AC and cause a partial or complete collapse. Some assessment of the chamber angle needs to take place once a blunt injury is suspected, because eyes that have sustained traumatic injury have a 14% incidence of this damage (Figure 3-12).[21] If there is a concern that rupture, laceration, or hyphema has occurred, a gonioscopic evaluation—in which the eye is instrumented with a gonioscopy lens—usually can be delayed. Van Herick's technique allows an initial evaluation of the AC depth for the acutely traumatized eye. A deep AC may indicate a posterior rupture, with increased AC depth due to the prolapse of vitreous from the scleral wound.

Intraocular Pressure

The determination of intraocular pressure (IOP) has questionable value in guiding the examiner toward a specific posttraumatic diagnosis. The differential diagnosis of low pressure after trauma includes rupture or laceration, iritis, retinal detachment, and cyclodialysis cleft. The possible diagnoses for an eye with high IOP after trauma include rupture or laceration, iritis, trabecular damage (contusion or recession), and retinal detachment. There is enough overlap among the clinical data that the examiner should consider IOP measurement only if the data are easily collected and can in no way cause further damage to the eye. There is some

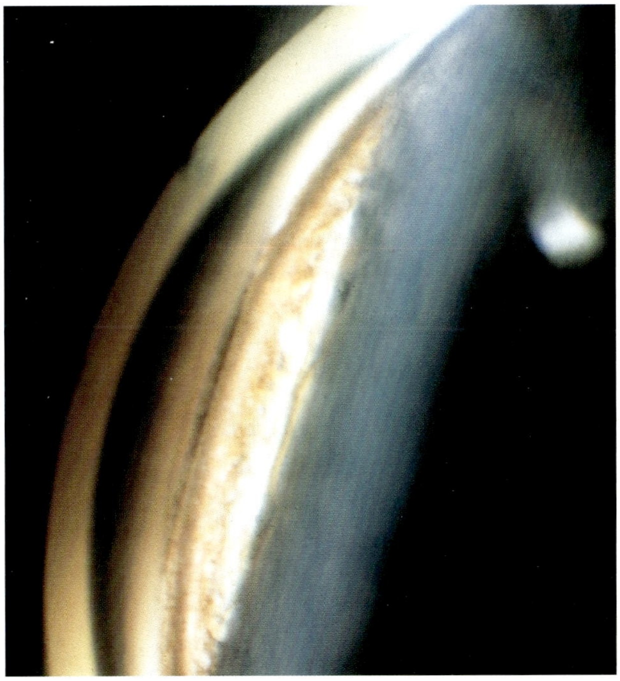

Fig. 3-12. A broad area of angle recession is present in the photograph of this eye after an episode of blunt trauma. This area is asymmetrical with the appearance of the angle in the fellow eye. Because a wide variation exists in the level of insertion of the iris, it is important to examine the fellow eye. A symmetrical posterior insertion seen only unilaterally during an incomplete examination may lead the examiner to an incorrect diagnosis of angle recession.

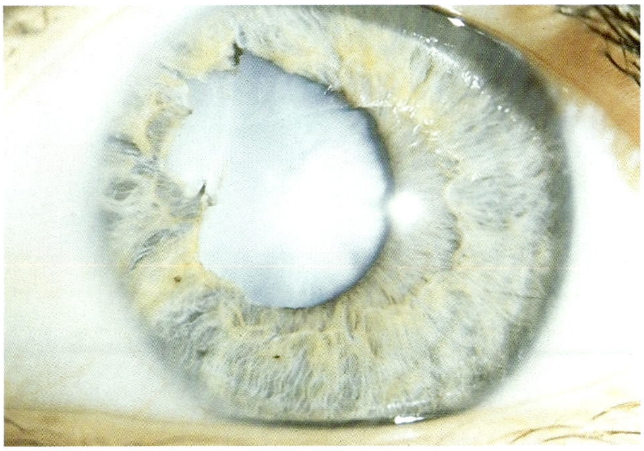

Fig. 3-13. Blunt trauma without rupture of the globe can generate fluid waves in the eye. The movement of the intraocular tissues by these waves can cause the type of iris and anterior segment injuries seen in this photograph. Note the irregular pupil margins secondary to sphincter tears and a developing cataract. This eye's drainage angle is seen in Figure 3-12.

value in knowing if the IOP is at one of the extremes. If there is any concern that the globe is unstable, then the measurement of the pressure of the eye can be postponed.

Iris

The iris may be the structure in the anterior segment that gives the most clinical information as to the damage the eye has sustained. It is a symmetrical, mobile structure. The appearance of the iris is important in all cases of trauma. A peaked pupil indicates that the iris has moved and is trapped or pulled into a defect in the ocular coat. Most likely, the opening is in the cornea or limbal region and is not self-sealing. By plugging the laceration or defect, the iris may have a sealing effect for the wound. Iris sphincter tears and irregularities indicate that the eye has experienced blunt and perhaps sharp trauma (Figure 3-13). The fluid wave generated in the injury is responsible for the traumatic enlargement of the pupil, stretching the pupillary sphincter and causing the tissue to tear.[22] Missing tissue or defects in the iris tissue generally indicate an episode of sharp trauma with possibility of an intraocular FB injury. Thus the iris, by its appearance, is able to lead the eye examination in appropriate directions. Each patient with ocular trauma should have a detailed examination of the iris; any asymmetry noted needs to be explained and understood.

Lens

A critical anterior segment structure to consider when examining a traumatized eye is the lens. This clear tissue lies posterior to the iris and can been seen through the pupil. Simple information about its location, clarity, stability, and the presence of capsular damage is collected in this stage of the eye examination. Lens position is determined primarily by zonular support. A traumatic event that damages zonular fibers (eg, blunt injury, sharp injury, or FB injury from penetration through the zonular fibers) influences the amount of support. Without uniform, 360° support from the fibers, the lens will likely be unstable, have some decentration, and exhibit tremulous movement known as phacodonesis.

The clarity of the lens can be influenced by the traumatic event (Figure 3-14). Focal lens opacities suggest a specific and local injury to the lens. A diffuse decrease in clarity is less specific. One important concept to apply in the examination of the

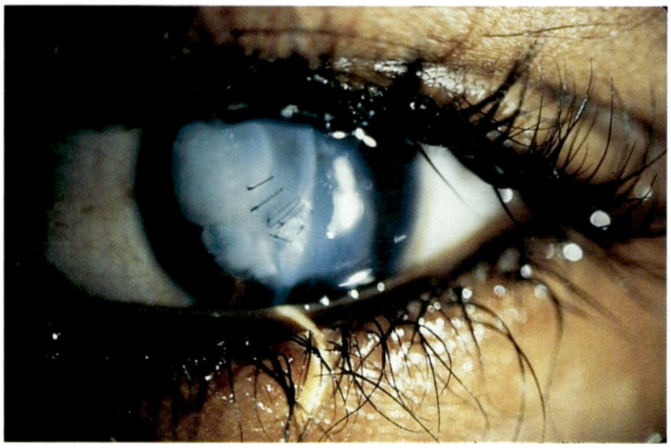

Fig. 3-14. This traumatic cataract developed after a penetrating corneal injury. Such cataracts can progress quickly, prompting the ophthalmic surgeon to examine the back of the eye before the cataract can obscure the view.

trauma patient is to examine the anterior vitreous and posterior pole through the clear media as soon as possible. The posttraumatic eye can undergo changes that inhibit a good examination. Traumatic cataract and intraocular hemorrhage are two excellent examples of traumatic changes that prevent the examiner from completing the routine eye examination.

Anterior Vitreous

The assessment of the anterior vitreous completes this portion of the examination. Taking the opportunity to view this region with the slitlamp allows the precise documentation of foreign objects (location and number); cellular debris, which may indicate early infection; and blood products, which indicate that posterior segment damage may be present. Having the vitreous examination occur at the end of the sequence while the patient is in the slitlamp position accomplishes two important examination goals:

1. The orderly sequence of the examination is maintained, which is important if overlooking any anterior segment structure is to be avoided. Attention must be directed to any disruption of tissues, foreign particles or objects, blood, and signs of infection. All may indicate traumatic injury to the eye, and all require action on the part of the ophthalmologist.
2. The examination can easily shift from the anterior segment to the slitlamp examination of the posterior segment.

Posterior Segment

The examination of the vitreous cavity, retina, choroid, and sclera is best done soon after the injury and with the pupils in a dilated state. A tropicamide (1%) and phenylephrine (2.5%) combination is an acceptable dilating regimen. In a battlefield situation, remember that it is important to document both *on* the patient's forehead and *in* the record that pupil dilation has been achieved pharmacologically. In the confusion of the battlefield, it is critical to maintain an orderly sequence of examination to ensure its completeness. The examination of the posterior segment must include the vitreous cavity; the optic nerve; the retina, including the ora serrata retinae and the pars plana corporis ciliaris; the choroid; and the sclera.

Indirect ophthalmoscopy is the premier examination technique for revealing the myriad findings that can be present in the posterior pole of an injured eye. Knowing this fact and knowing that the usefulness of the indirect examination depends on the clarity of the media, one should realize the importance of completing all the previous examination segments as quickly as possible to ensure accuracy and avoid delay in reaching the posterior pole examination. The development of a traumatic cataract, the accumulation of inflammatory products, the presence of blood, or the disruption of tissues in the visual axis can obscure the view of the back of the eye. Delay can relegate the remainder of the data collection to ancillary tests used to see into eyes with no view or a poor view into the posterior pole. These ancillary tests are extremely useful; nevertheless, they are not a substitute for the indirect ophthalmoscopic examination.

The examination of the posterior segment can begin at the slitlamp when the anterior segment examination is completed. The use of the 78-D or 90-D lens to examine the optic nerve and the surrounding fundus is an excellent examination technique. Close attention should be given to the characteristics of optic nerve health. Signs of pallor, hemorrhage, tissue disruption, and edema are all-important findings and generate concern that the visual system may be damaged at this anterior site.[23] Working methodically from the optic nerve, the presence of FBs and foreign materials will be noted. If found, they should be counted and characterized as to the type of material they are made of, if possible. The macular region is studied for damage that can provide information that helps determine the level of postinjury visual abilities (Figure 3-15). Retinal tears and breaks are searched for as the ex-

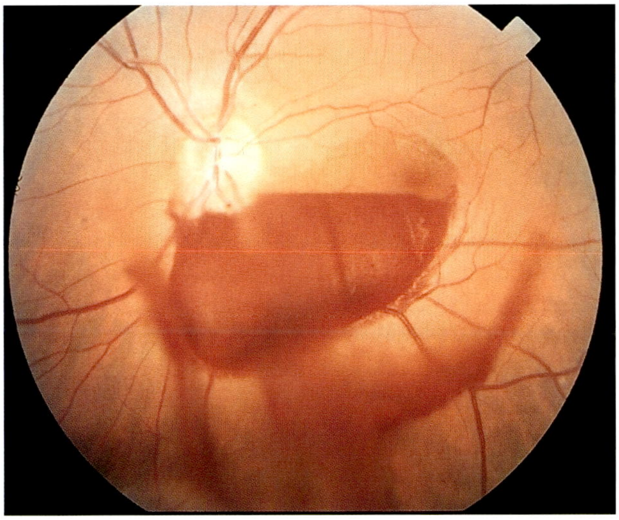

Fig. 3-15. Blunt injury can lead to preretinal hemorrhage with extension into the vitreous cavity, as is seen in this patient. The soldier had noticed decreased vision after carrying a field pack during an extended march. Valsalva's maneuver may have played a role in this particular injury to the posterior pole.

amination continues (Figure 3-16). Subretinal fluid (indicating retinal detachment) and subretinal blood (indicating trauma to the region) are pertinent findings. Inspection of the choroidal and scleral coats is also to be made (Figure 3-17). Retinal detachment and scleral and choroidal rupture, which may be hidden by hemorrhage, are common trauma-related injuries that must be addressed by the ophthalmologist in the hope of recovering the best visual function for the patient.[2,24,25]

Switching to the indirect ophthalmoscope at this point in the examination allows for a more panoramic view, although with less magnification, of the optic disc and the surrounding fundus. The indirect ophthalmoscope is also used to examine the

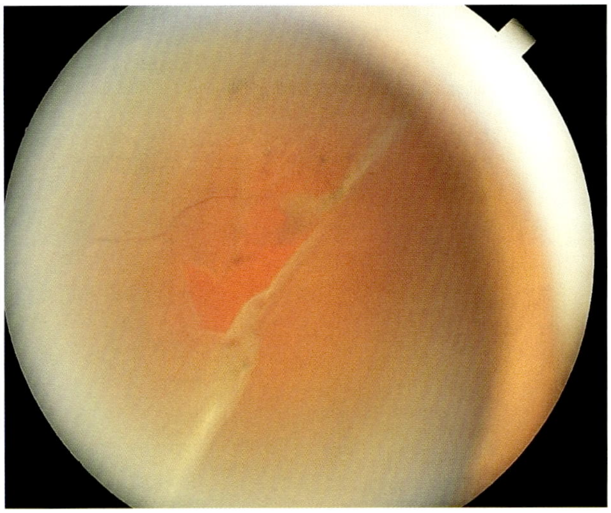

Fig. 3-16. This example of a rhegmatogenous retinal detachment is a reminder that both blunt and sharp injury may produce this type of injury to the retina. Keys to finding retinal injury are to look for injury when the view through the anterior segment allows inspection of the retina and to use available ancillary tests when the view of the posterior pole is poor.

a

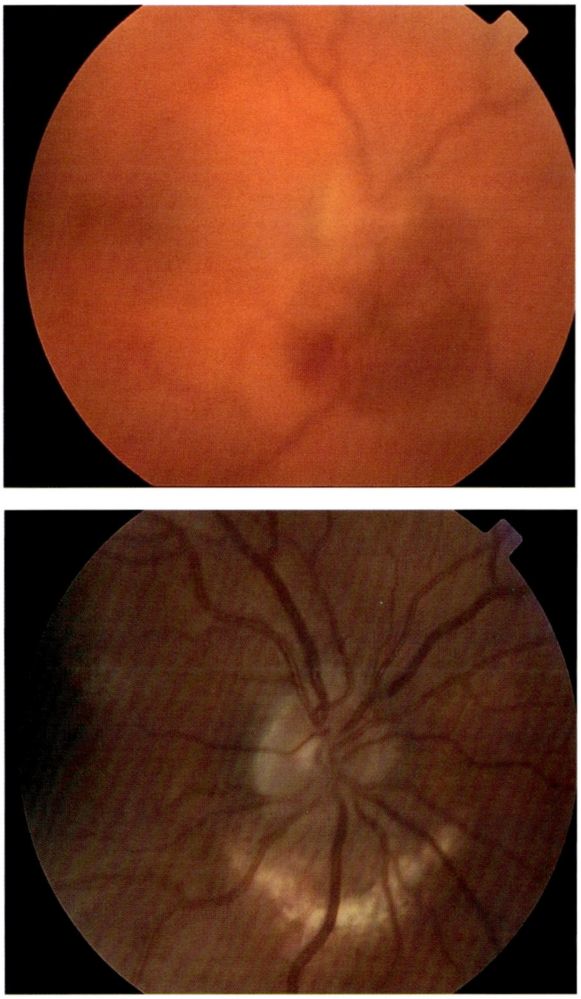

b

Fig. 3-17. Injury to the posterior pole can be extensive. The vitreous cavity can be involved with the collection of blood, the retina can sustain damage, and the choroidal layer can sustain injury. Early in the treatment phase (a) the extent of the injury may not be apparent. If the clinical course permits, serial examinations can reveal additional areas of concern (b) when the choroidal rupture becomes obvious after the vitreous hemorrhage clears.

vitreous, equatorial fundus, peripheral fundus, and vitreous base. Even though complete visualization of the posterior pole allows the most accurate assessment of the injuries to the back of the eye, caution must figure into the decision to use scleral depression. Any possibility of a ruptured ocular coat or an open globe should indicate to the examiner that the scleral depression portion of the examination should be delayed to prevent further damage to the traumatized eye. In the absence of rupture, an alternative technique for viewing the posterior structures is the three-mirror Goldman contact lens, which can provide additional data about the injury.

The evaluation of the injury should include an assessment for surgical repair. How much scar tissue is present? What track did the object take? Which method of removal should be entertained? Is there an associated retinal detachment present with the FB? Is infection present? These issues can be addressed if a view of the injuries is available. Without a good view to the posterior pole, the answers to all these questions become more difficult.

Without a view of the posterior pole structures, the ultrasound B-scan, plain film radiography, CT scan, and MRI technology are brought into use. Chapter 4, Imaging of Ocular and Adnexal Trauma, is devoted to the use of these techniques and a review of the advantages and disadvantages of these examination methods.

PREOPERATIVE PREPARATION

With the ocular and adnexal examinations completed and the ancillary procedures planned, the patient must be readied for the transition in care from data gathering to actual treatment and recovery. This phase's importance should not be underestimated. During the preoperative phase, several aspects of the patient's care are manipulated.

First, the safety of the patient is assessed. The patient should be stabilized and life-threatening surgical and medical conditions treated. The patient is moved expeditiously out of harm's way to an area of the battlefield that allows an initiation of the history and examination portion of the ocular and adnexal examination (and for any of the other body systems that have sustained injury). When attention turns to the ocular injuries, the preoperative phase is used to initiate therapy that can protect the eye from sequelae of the trauma.

Risk of infection is a large concern. The battlefield is a dirty environment where foreign objects achieve high velocities and contribute to ocular and adnexal injuries. The need for preoperative, posttraumatic antibiotic therapy is decided at this time. To best prepare the eye for a successful postoperative course, the use of intravenous antibiotics is recommended for open globe injuries.[8] No ointments or solutions toxic to the retina are recommended until the ocular coats are proven intact. This fact is usually confirmed in the operating room by an ophthalmologist. Medical officers in the field without access to the slitlamp and operating room microscope should not use topical therapy for trauma patients.

One goal worth striving for is to have definitive ophthalmic care occur within 36 hours.[18] An early repair gives the surgeon the opportunity to deal with viable, uninfected tissues. The primary repair then proceeds with greater ease, achieving closed ocular tissues and reapproximated adnexal tissues.

A second goal is the protection of the ocular and adnexal structures from further injury. Metal eye shields are an excellent method of protection. Substitutes are readily made from material at hand, such as the bottom of a paper cup. Preventing further damage to an open globe is the primary concern. The unstable eye is susceptible to injury exacerbation from any external pressure. The patient can cause additional injury by rubbing and squeezing the injured eye. Maneuvers to prevent these actions include chemical or physical restraints, sedation, and anesthetic blocks to decrease lid activity.

The use of pain relief is an important consideration in the ocular trauma patient. Effective analgesic therapy for trauma patients can help stabilize wounds and minimize additional injury during the preoperative phase. Of course, once these medications are administered, the ability to get informed consent from the patient is lost. Again, in the battlefield, the need for consent differs from the requirements of civilian practice. In the care of the injured soldier, the ophthalmologist is entrusted to make the appropriate surgical decisions for the patient.

Valsalva's maneuver can be a huge enemy to the open globe, so antiemetic therapy is important when preparing the patient for both transport and repair of the eye injury. Intramuscular and intravenous routes of administration are recommended. The slow and unpredictable effects of oral medications in trauma patients make this route of administration a less desirable alternative.

SUMMARY

Providing ophthalmic care to patients with ocular trauma in a wartime setting is challenging because of difficulties in accessing both the injured soldier and the equipment necessary for visualizing and diagnosing injuries to the ocular and adnexal structures. Compared with the peacetime civilian arena, these wartime factors make it difficult for military ophthalmologists to care for soldiers with eye trauma and consistently achieve excellent results. Nonetheless, if the sequence of history and examination techniques is followed as presented in this chapter, the chance of overlooking important clinical information is reduced. Adhering to a set sequence reaps even more benefits as the battle intensifies and confusion escalates. The goal to return the injured soldiers to their units and their families as healthy as possible is within reach.

REFERENCES

1. Hagmann J, Marshall, B. *Land Mine Data.* Bethesda, Md: Combat Casualty Research Center; 1999.

2. Mader TM, Aragones JV, Chandler AC, et al. Ocular and ocular adnexal injuries treated by United States military ophthalmologists during Desert Shield and Storm. *Ophthalmology.* 1993;100:1462–1467.

3. Nutaitis MJ. Yemen victim assistance data, September 1999 mission.

4. Heering SL, Shohat T, Heering AS, Seelenfreund M, Lerman Y. Civil unrest and ocular trauma. *Mil Med.* 1992;157:297–298.

5. Belkin M, Treister G, Dotan S. Eye injuries and ocular trauma in the Lebanon war. *Isr J Med Sci.* 1984;20:333–338.

6. Moisseiev J, Belkin M, Bartov E, Treister G. Severe combat injuries in the Lebanon war, 1982. *Isr J Med Sci.* 1984;20:339–344.

7. Committee on Trauma, American College of Surgeons. *Advanced Trauma Life Support Program for Physicians: Instructor Manual.* 5th ed. Chicago, Ill: American College of Surgeons; 1997.

8. Hamill MB. Clinical evaluation. In: Shingleton BJ, Hersh PS, Kenyon KR, eds. *Eye Trauma.* St Louis, Mo: Mosby–Year Book; 1991: 3–24.

9. Hardy RA. Ocular trauma. *Mil Med.* 1996;161:465–468.

10. Sidell FR, Takafuji ET, Franz DR. *Medical Aspects of Chemical and Biological Warfare.* In: Zajtchuk R, Bellamy RF, eds. *Textbook of Military Medicine.* Washington, DC: Department of the Army, Office of The Surgeon General, Borden Institute; 1997.

11. Tielsch JM. Frequency and consequences of ocular trauma. *Ophthalmol Clin North Am.* 1995;8:559–567.

12. Klopfer J, Tielsch JM, Vitale S, See LC, Canner JK. Ocular trauma in the United States. *Arch Ophthalmol.* 1992;110:838–842.

13. Thach AB, Ward TP, Hollifield RD, Dugel PU, Sipperley JO, Marx JL. Ocular injuries from paintball pellets. *Ophthalmology*. 1999;106:533–537.

14. Morris RE, Witherspoon CD, Helm HA, Feist RM, Byrne JB Jr. Eye Injury Registry of Alabama: Demographics and prognosis of severe eye injury [preliminary report]. *South Med J.* 1987;80:810–816.

15. Hutton WL, Fuller DG. Factors influencing final visual results in severely injured eyes. *Am J Ophthalmol.* 1984;97:715–722.

16. Mallonee S, Sharait S, Stennies G, Waxweiler R, Hogan D, Jordan F. Physical injuries and fatalities resulting from the Oklahoma City bombing. *JAMA.* 1996;276:382–387.

17. Klein OG Jr. The initial evaluation in ophthalmic injury. *Otolaryngol Clin North Am.* 1979;12:303–320.

18. Barr CB. Prognostic factors in corneoscleral lacerations. *Arch Ophthalmol.* 1983;101:919–924.

19. Klystra JA, Lamkin JC, Runyan DK. Clinical predictors of scleral rupture after blunt ocular trauma. *Am J Ophthalmol.* 1993;115:530–535.

20. Slingsby JG, Forstot SL. Effect of blunt trauma on the corneal endothelium. *Arch Ophthalmol.* 1981;99: 1041–1043.

21. Salmon JF, Mermoud A, Ivey A, Swanevelder SA, Hoffman M. The detection of post-traumatic angle recession by gonioscopy in a population-based glaucoma survey. *Ophthalmology*. 1994;101:1844–1850.

22. Pieramici DJ, Parver LM. A mechanistic approach to ocular trauma. *Ophthalmol Clin North Am.* 1995;8:569–587.

23. Steinsapir KD, Goldberg RA. Traumatic optic neuropathy. *Surv Ophthalmol.* 1994;38:487–518.

24. Cox MS, Freeman HM. Retinal detachment due to ocular penetration. *Arch Ophthalmol.* 1978;96:1354–1361.

25. Cox MS, Schepens CL, Freeman HM. Retinal detachment due to ocular contusion. *Arch Ophthalmol.* 1966;76: 678–685.

Chapter 4

IMAGING OF OCULAR AND ADNEXAL TRAUMA

JEFFREY P. BLICE, MD*

**Commander, Medical Corps, US Navy, Department of Ophthalmology, National Naval Medical Center, 8901 Wisconsin Avenue, Bethesda, Maryland 20889-5600*

INTRODUCTION

Various imaging modalities exist to aid in the initial and subsequent evaluation of trauma involving the eye and orbit. However, the best imaging modality for the initial evaluation of eye trauma remains indirect ophthalmoscopy. In the first hours after a severe injury, the first examiner can obtain information with a level of detail that no other imaging method can provide. Although the early view may not always be the best one, often the first look into a traumatized eye is the only look.

Standard roentgenography, computed tomography (CT), magnetic resonance imaging (MRI), and ultrasonography all have their strengths and weaknesses. They can be useful adjuncts in the management of globe ruptures, intraocular foreign bodies (IOFBs), and facial and skull fractures.

Before beginning the discussion of available imaging methods, a brief review of orbital anatomy is in order. The orbit is pyramidal in shape, with the base oriented anteriorly and the apex posteriorly. The orbital walls consist of seven bones: the maxilla, zygoma, sphenoid, palatine, ethmoid, lacrimal, and frontal. The roof of the orbit is composed mainly of the frontal bone, with a small contribution from the sphenoid bone. Laterally, the zygoma and greater wing of the sphenoid provide the major component of the wall. Both the lateral and superior walls of the orbit are strong, but the inferior and medial walls have thinner bones and are more likely to be damaged from trauma. Inferiorly, the zygoma and thin roof of the maxilla form the major portion of the floor, and the palatine bone contributes posteriorly. The medial wall is formed from the frontal (superiorly), the sphenoid (posteriorly), the lacrimal (inferiorly and anteriorly), and the thin-walled ethmoid (centrally). The thin walls of the maxilla and ethmoid make these bones particularly susceptible to trauma from compression of the orbital contents or transmitted force applied to the orbital rim.

The optic canal is formed entirely from the lesser wing of the sphenoid. A traumatic injury resulting in dislocated bone fragments from the sphenoid can impinge on the optic nerve, resulting in a neuropathy.

IMAGING MODALITIES

Plain Skull Films

Although largely replaced now by CT scans, plain skull films (ie, roentgenography) can still provide useful information in the evaluation of traumatic injuries. It is likely that CT will not be easily accessible in a deployed medical unit; consequently, plain films of the skull may be the only imaging method available. The occipitofrontal, lateral, occipitooral, and oblique are the standard projections used to evaluate the orbit.

The occipitofrontal view, also called Caldwell's view or the anteroposterior (AP) view, provides a view of the size and shape of the orbit, the orbit floor, zygomaticofrontal suture, and lamina papyracea. The lateral view demonstrates the sella turcica, anterior and posterior clinoids, anterior and posterior walls of the frontal sinus, sphenoid sinus, and nasopharyngeal soft tissues. The occipitooral, or Waters's, view provides the best projection of the maxillary antra and inferior orbital rim. Oblique views are used to assess the shape and diameter of the optic canal, which has a normal range from 4.4 to 6.0 mm in diameter (Table 4-1).[1]

Plain films are relatively inexpensive and almost universally available; soft-tissue definition, however, is poor. Localization of foreign bodies (FBs) is unreliable without more-involved methods of imaging. Specifically, suturing a limbal ring to the eye and repeating AP and lateral views allow a radiologist to chart the position of an FB within the globe.[2] In instances of multiple radiopaque FBs, plain films permit a rapid assessment of the number and shape of the objects.

Computed Tomography

A CT image is a mathematical reconstruction of data obtained from multiple radiographic projections of an object. The basic principle of the CT scan involves an X-ray source and an array of detectors mounted in a gantry. The beam is projected through the object of interest, with the array of detectors measuring the attenuation of the beam. The X-ray source is then moved and the process repeated. The multiple projections are summed and converted to shades of gray, producing the CT image. The patient is then moved the thickness of the image slice, and the process is repeated for the next image.

The relative attenuation of the beam is expressed as Hounsfield units (HU), named in honor of the inventor of CT scanning. Water has a value of 0 HU, air a value of –1,000 HU, and dense bone a value of +1,000 HU (Table 4-2). An object with an HU

TABLE 4-1

APPROPRIATE PLAIN FILM ROENTGENOGRAMS FOR EYE IMAGING

View	Structures Demonstrated
Anteroposterior (AP) (or Caldwell's)	Size and shape of the orbits Superior orbital fissure Lamina papyracea Frontal and ethmoid sinuses Zygomaticofrontal suture
Occcipitooral (or Waters's)	Maxillary antra Orbital roof Inferior orbital rim Zygomatic bone and arch
Lateral	Sella turcica Clinoid processes Clivus Walls of frontal sinus Sphenoid sinus
Oblique (or optic foramen)	Optic foramen Superior orbital fissure Lacrimal fossa Ethmoid air cells

Adapted with permission from Weber AL. Imaging techniques and normal radiographic anatomy. In: Albert DM, ed. *Principles and Practice of Ophthalmology*. Vol 5. Philadelphia, Pa: WB Saunders Company; 1994: 3505.

TABLE 4-2

COMPUTED TOMOGRAPHY ATTENUATION COEFFICIENTS FOR VARIOUS FOREIGN BODIES

Foreign Body	Attenuation Coefficient (HU)*
Air	–1,000
Aluminum	1,150
Bakelite	400
Brick	400
Ceramic	2,000
Chromium	6,000
Copper	1,600
Glass	1,400–2,800
Graphite	260
Iron	3,800–20,600
Lead	11,600
Mica	25
Porcelain	600
Solder	6,500
Stone	500
Water	0
Wood	5

*Hounsfield units

Adapted with permission from Gunenc U, Maden A, Kaynak S, Pirnar T. Magnetic resonance imaging and computed tomography in the detection and localization of intraocular foreign bodies. *Doc Ophthalmol.* 1992;81:371.

value of 0 appears isodense with water, and objects with higher HU values appear brighter—bone, for example. Adjustment of the grayscale window can highlight bony anatomy over soft-tissue anatomy. Modern CT scanners have a fixed array of detectors with a rapidly moving source, permitting decreased scan times and higher spatial resolutions. Relatively new scanners move the patient through the gantry continuously at the rate of one slice thickness per revolution of the X-ray source. This is called a helical or spiral CT; scan time is shortened further, and patient movement artifact is limited.[3–5]

CT scans of the eye and orbit can produce axial or coronal images. The plane of these images and representative slices for an axial and coronal section are demonstrated in Figures 4-1 and 4-2. Slices in the axial plane are usually 1 to 3 mm in thickness when specifically imaging the orbit. Protocols for scanning orbits may vary from institution to institution; if necessary, specify thin sections (1.5 or 3.0 mm) when ordering the study. Axial images provide good cross-sectional anatomical views of the orbit, globe, and skull. Localization of structures in and around the globe is immensely improved over plain films, and the improved view of bony anatomy provides an excellent view of the optic canal.

Coronal images can be reconstructed from the data obtained during an axial scan; however, direct coronal scans offer improved resolution. These sections are usually obtained by placing the patient's neck in a slightly extended position while moving through the gantry. The plane of these images may not be truly coronal but oblique to the true plane. Adjusting the head position can avoid "spray" artifacts from dental work.

Software is now available for reconstruction of three-dimensional images of the entire skull. Although not useful in every case, these images can be useful in the reconstruction of severe orbital trauma.

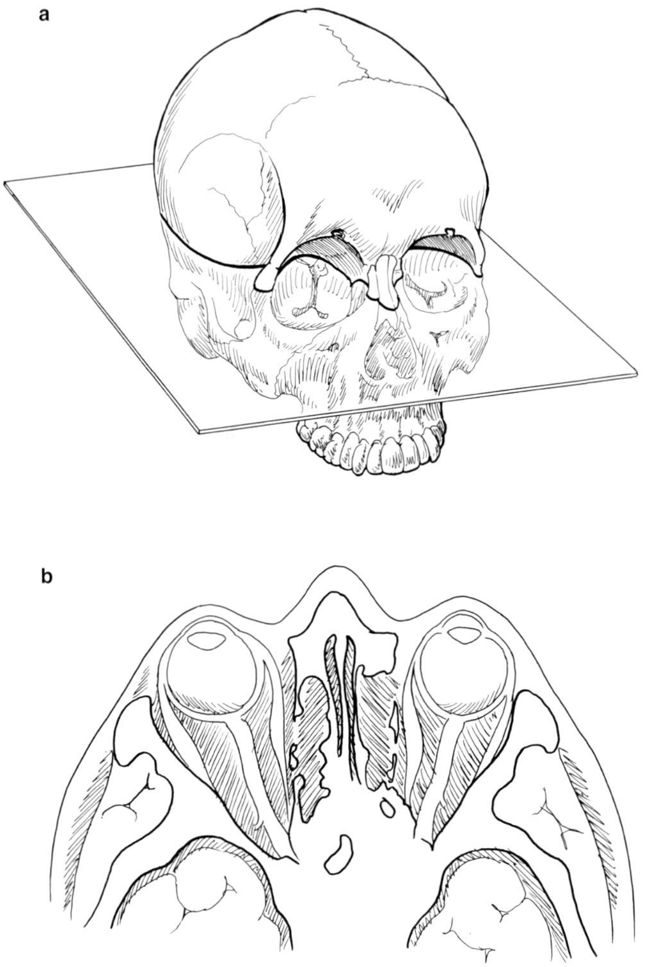

Fig. 4-1. (**a**) A diagram of a skull with the axial plane of the section demonstrated through the midorbit. (**b**) The approximate appearance of a computed tomography section corresponding to the plane of the section in view (a). Fractures of the roof and floor are in the same plane as an axial section and are difficult to detect in these views. Drawings prepared for this textbook by Gary Wind, MD, Uniformed Services University of the Health Sciences, Bethesda, Md.

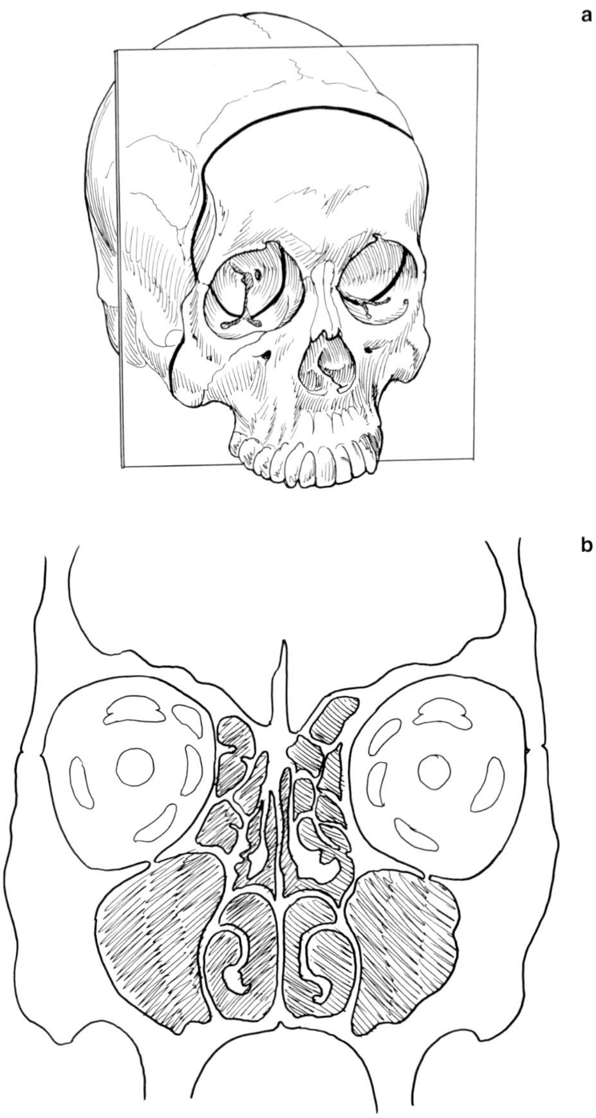

Fig. 4-2. (**a**) A diagram of skull with the coronal plane of a section demonstrated through the midorbit. (**b**) The approximate appearance of a computed tomography section corresponding to the plane of the section in view (a). Fractures through any of the walls of the orbit are more easily seen in these sections. Reconstructed images have suboptimal resolution, so direct coronal sections should be obtained if possible. Drawings prepared for this textbook by Gary Wind, MD, Uniformed Services University of the Health Sciences, Bethesda, Md.

Magnetic Resonance Imaging

A detailed discussion of the theory behind MRI scanning is beyond the scope of this chapter; however, knowledge of the basic principles is useful for understanding the application of this imaging modality in ocular and orbital trauma.

The general principle of MRI is that the nuclei of certain atoms become aligned when placed in a magnetic field. A pulse of radio frequency (RF) energy can be applied to these nuclei, resulting in a shift of the net magnetic vector of 90° or 180°. This process involves the absorption of RF energy. The duration and energy of the pulse affect the hydrogen atoms in human tissue. After the RF pulse is terminated, the nuclei will "relax," or realign

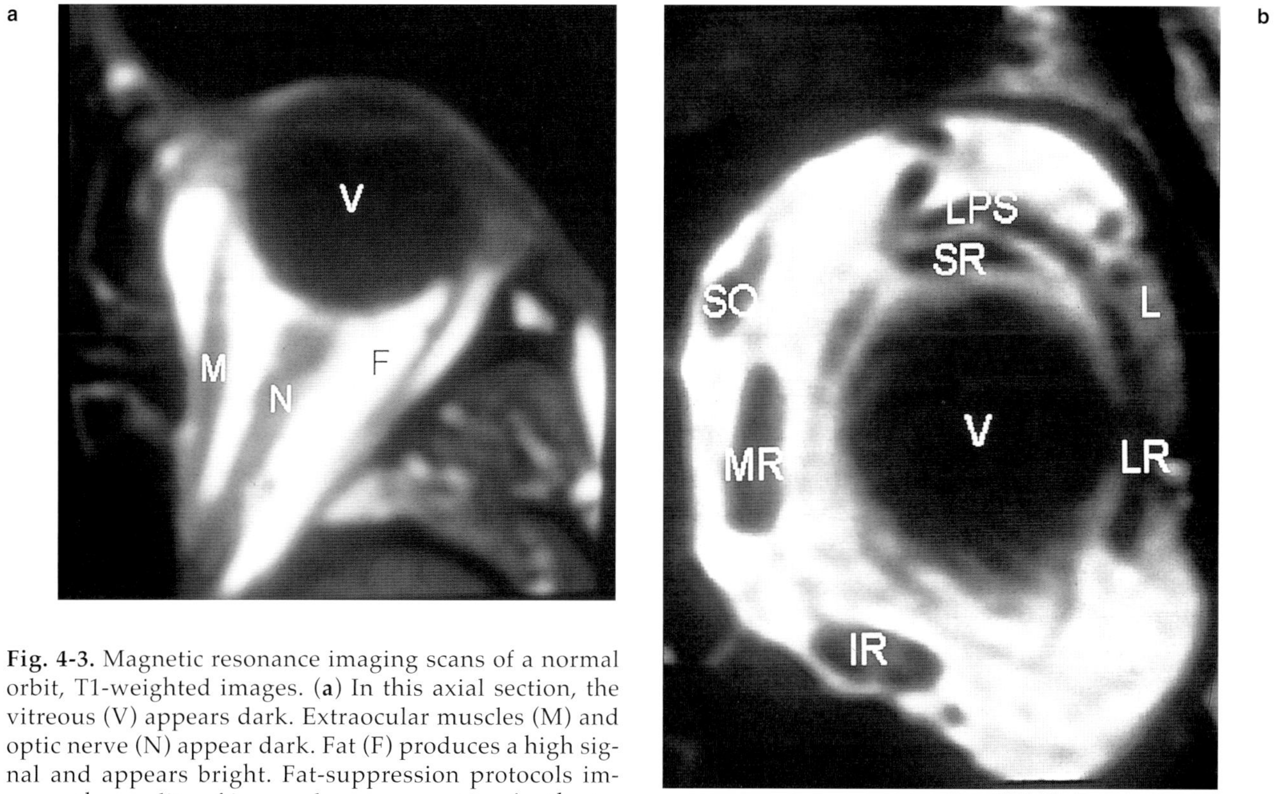

Fig. 4-3. Magnetic resonance imaging scans of a normal orbit, T1-weighted images. (**a**) In this axial section, the vitreous (V) appears dark. Extraocular muscles (M) and optic nerve (N) appear dark. Fat (F) produces a high signal and appears bright. Fat-suppression protocols improve the quality of images by compensating for the increased signal produced by the orbital fat. (**b**) This coronal section provides an excellent view of the vitreous (V) and the lateral rectus (LR), inferior rectus (IR), medial rectus (MR), superior oblique (SO), levator palpebrae superioris (LPS), and superior rectus (SR) muscles. The lacrimal gland (L) can be seen in the lateral orbit; the signal is similar to other soft tissues in the orbit.

themselves with the magnetic field, and they emit RF energy that can be measured with an antenna. This antenna can be intrinsic to the MRI scanner or it can be a surface coil placed over the orbit, which improves image resolution. Gadolinium, a paramagnetic contrast agent, can be given intravenously to enhance vascular anatomy and orbital pathology.

Through manipulation of the various RF pulses and measurements of the resulting emitted energy, different images can be constructed. The most common of these images are the T1-weighted, T2-weighted, and proton density–weighted. The parameters used to produce a T1-weighted image result in a characteristic appearance of ocular structures (Figure 4-3). Vitreous and cerebrospinal fluid appear dark, muscle and nerve appear equally dark with the white matter of the central nervous system, and fat appears very bright. The great contrast between these structures provides the best anatomical detail of the orbit. However, a small orbital lesion may be hidden by the strong signal produced by orbital fat. Melanin and blood appear bright on a T1-weighted image as well; consequently, subretinal hemorrhage and ocular melanomas can be detected on these images.

On T2-weighted images, vitreous and cerebrospinal fluid appear bright, and fat appears dark (Figure 4-4). The scanning times are longer and, consequently, spatial resolution suffers, although tumor infiltration, edema, and demyelination are better demonstrated. Proton density–weighted images reflect the number of MRI-visible protons in a given unit volume. The proton density of the tissues in and around the orbit differs minimally, causing tissue contrast to be relatively low and limiting the usefulness of these images.

Fat-suppression protocols have been developed to decrease the signal intensity of orbital fat, which, in combination with gadolinium, can improve visualization of the optic nerve and enhancing lesions. The views produced with an MRI scan are similar to those produced by CT. There are axial and coronal images, and sagittal images are also produced. Unlike CT, though, the coronal and sagittal images are always reconstructions.

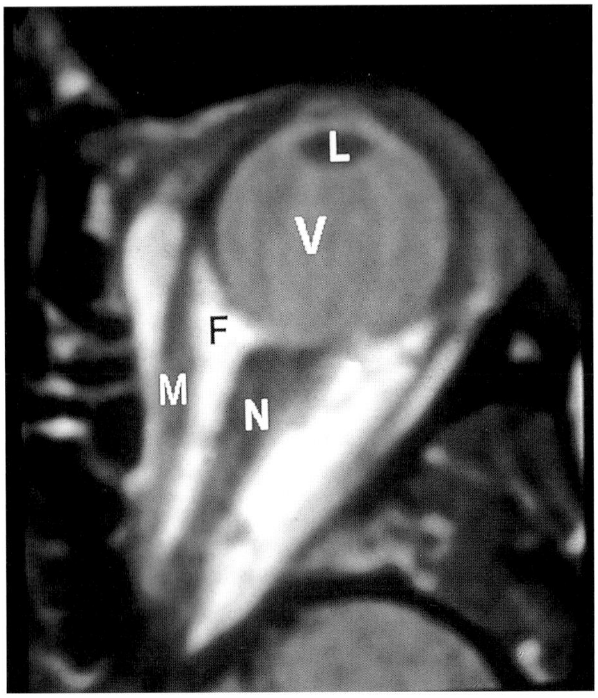

Fig. 4-4. Magnetic resonance imaging scans of a normal orbit, T2-weighted images. The view of the orbit in this axial section is similar to that in Figure 4-3a except that the image is T2-weighted. The vitreous (V) in this case appears relatively bright. The lens (L) produces a low signal and can be seen in the anterior segment. The extraocular muscles (M), optic nerve (N), and fat (F) all appear dark. Bone is poorly demonstrated in all views of the magnetic resonance imaging scan.

Ultrasonography

Ocular ultrasonography is a useful diagnostic tool when media opacities preclude using standard means to view the ocular structures and is especially helpful when used in conjunction with other imaging modalities. Ultrasonography was initially developed in the late 1950s to evaluate intraocular tumors. Over the ensuing decades, improvements in technology have made ultrasonography a routine diagnostic tool.

Ultrasound is defined as sound frequency greater than 20 kHz. Medical applications use ultrasound frequencies in the 2- to 50-MHz range. Lower frequencies provide good penetration of tissue but sacrifice resolution. Higher frequencies provide increased resolution but at the price of tissue penetration. Transducers with a frequency of 7.5 to 12.0 MHz have low penetration, approximately 6 cm at 7.5 MHz with resolution of 0.1 mm at 8 MHz.[6] Higher-frequency transducers operating in the 50-mHz range produce high-resolution images; however, they concentrate on small portions of the anterior segment or anterior structures of the posterior segment. This equipment is relatively expensive and, although useful in certain circumstances, is not readily available at all institutions.[7,8]

The instrument itself consists of a handheld transducer containing a piezoelectric crystal or synthetic ceramic. When an electrical potential is applied across the crystal, the crystal is mechanically deformed, and an ultrasonic pulse is emitted. The echoes produced are received by the transducer and converted back into electrical impulses. These impulses are amplified and converted into a video display.[6] The sound wave produced by the transducer can be reflected, refracted, or absorbed. Different tissues in the eye and orbit have different densities and, therefore, different acoustical impedance. At the anatomical boundaries of these tissues there is a mismatch of acoustical impedance, resulting in reflection and refraction of the sound wave. The intensity of the reflection, or echo, depends on the magnitude of the acoustical impedance mismatch. The intensity of the echo also depends on the angle at which a sound wave reaches an interface: a perpendicular wave is fully reflected, but an oblique wave is only partially reflected. In addition, the shape, size, and regularity of an object can influence the strength of an echo.[9]

The echoes can be displayed in two formats: amplitude (A) or brightness (B) modulation. Amplitude modulation, or A-scan, displays the intensity of the echo as a vertical spike plotted against the echo's time delay, which is equivalent to the distance from the transducer. This mode is useful in measurements of intraocular length for intraocular lens calculations and in diagnosis of intraocular and intraorbital tumors. The usefulness of the A-scan in the evaluation of ocular trauma is limited at best.

Brightness modulation, or B-scan, displays a two-dimensional representation of the eye. The intensity of an echo is proportional to the brightness of a dot on the display. The B-scan is a dynamic examination providing real-time, two-dimensional images of the ocular and orbital structures. Although photographic static images of the B-scan are obtained for a permanent record, the kinetic nature of the study can provide more information than can be documented by a photograph. Therefore, the ability to perform a B-scan can be an invaluable tool in the diagnosis and evaluation of ocular trauma.

Of the imaging modalities discussed, ultrasound is the only one in which the ophthalmologist controls the access to and quality of the study.

SPECIFIC TRAUMATIC INJURIES AND IMAGING

Intraorbital and Intraocular Foreign Bodies

The detection and localization of intraocular and intraorbital FBs are important and potentially difficult tasks in the management of ocular trauma. All the modalities discussed are potentially useful in the detection of FBs and are particularly useful when applied together to obtain a complete picture.

Although almost universally replaced by the CT scan, plain films of the skull, as mentioned earlier, are useful for rapid evaluation of the presence, size, number, and shape of FBs in and around the eye (Figures 4-5 and 4-6). The poor localization of the objects, however, makes the use of other methods necessary. B-scan ultrasonography is a very useful method for determining the presence or absence of FBs that lie within or near the globe.

Ultrasonography can detect an object independent of its radiopacity and can differentiate between intraocular and extraocular objects when they are located near the sclera. Usually, an IOFB will appear as a reflective object either in midvitreous or lying near the retina (Figure 4-7). An example of an extraocular object (a BB) lying next to the medial rectus is shown in Figure 4-8. The ultrasound artifacts of acoustical shadowing (see Figure 4-7) and reverberations (see Figure 4-8) aid in the detection of the FB, and when an object passes through the vitreous, a track can often be seen (Figure 4-9). Air bubbles within the vitreous, which may appear in the globe as a result of trauma, may resemble an FB. Air tends to be more uniform in reflectivity, maintaining its shape and reflectivity from different angles, but the reflection off an FB will only be high from waves that strike perpendicular to its surface.

The use of ultrasound biomicroscopy for the detection and localization of occult FBs was reported in 1999.[10] Ultrasound biomicroscopy is a useful adjunct in the detection and localization of small nonmetallic objects, predominantly in the anterior segment or the anterior, posterior segment (Figure 4-10). Unfortunately, this equipment is not readily available at most facilities.

Although plain films and ultrasonography together may provide enough information to determine the general location of an FB, a CT scan is the standard of care in the evaluation of these injuries. In fact, in cases in which an FB cannot be seen but a high index of suspicion exists, a CT should be obtained to rule out a foreign object.

Without question, CT scanning is useful in de-

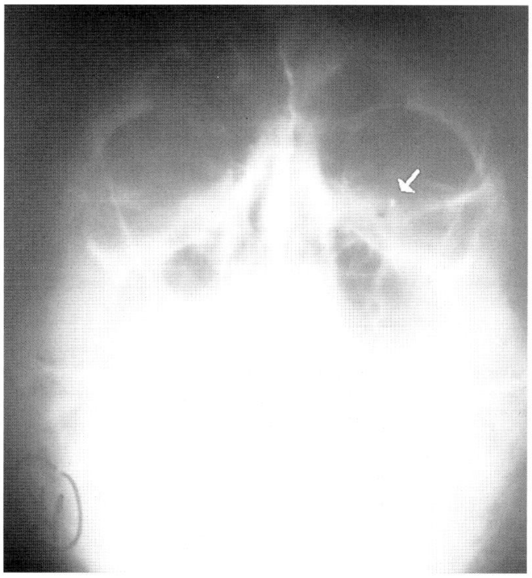

a

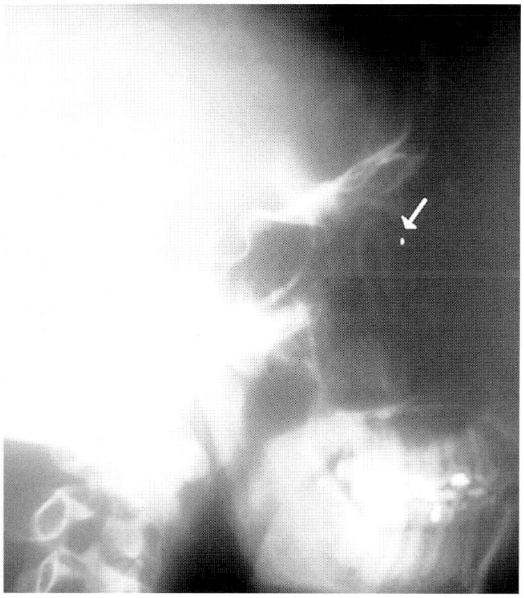

b

Fig. 4-5. (**a**) This is a plain radiograph, occipitooral (Waters's) view, of a patient who was hammering metal on metal and noticed a sudden decrease in vision. On presentation, a self-sealing corneal laceration was present, as well as a developing cataract. The arrow demonstrates a radiopaque foreign body (FB) somewhere in the orbit. (**b**) Lateral plain film of the same patient demonstrates the FB (indicated by arrow) present in the anterior orbit. Although multiple views help localize an FB on plain films, definitive localization of this FB was provided by indirect ophthalmoscopy by the initial examiner. The FB was seen lying nasal to the nerve. Subsequent computed tomography and ultrasonography confirmed an intraocular FB in the vicinity described by the initial exam.

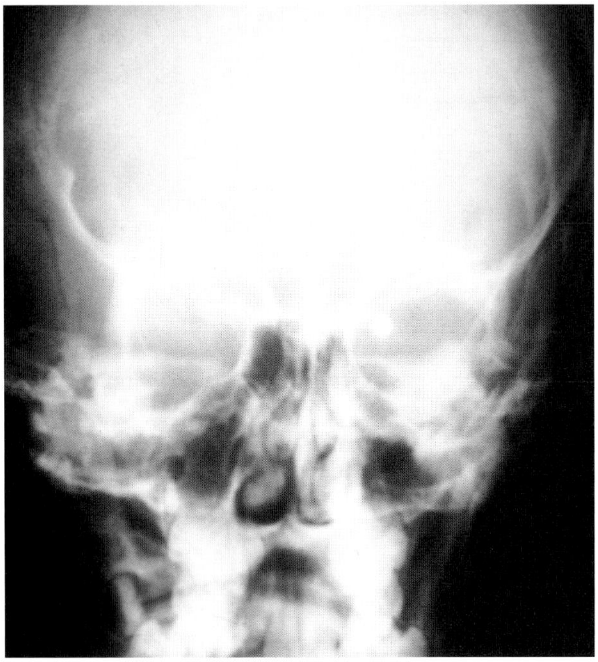

Fig. 4-6. Plain radiograph, occipitofrontal view, reveals a relatively large radiodense object, which can be seen in the orbit. Radiograph: Courtesy of William Benson, MD, Philadelphia, Pa.

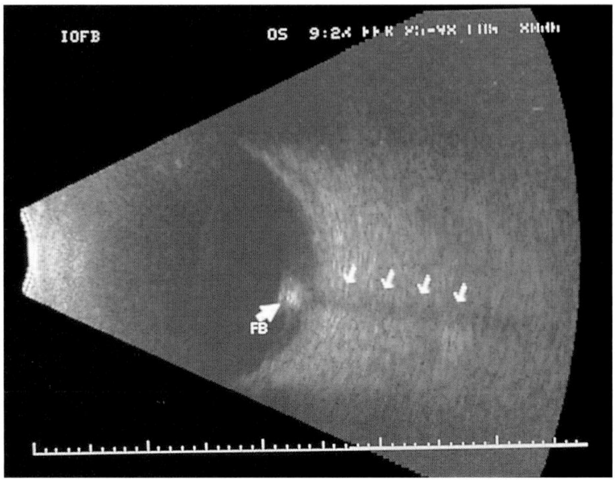

Fig. 4-7. A brightness modulation (B-scan) ultrasound study of an intraocular foreign body (IOFB) reveals a highly reflective FB just anterior to the retina; acoustic shadowing is also seen, as indicated by small arrows. The ultrasound characteristics of an FB depend on the nature and shape of the object. The appearance can also be affected by the angle at which the sound wave strikes the object. When the acoustic wave strikes the object perpendicularly and maximum reflection is obtained, shadowing occurs behind the object. If the angle of incidence is not perpendicular or the surface of the FB is poorly reflective, shadowing may not be seen. Sonogram: Courtesy of Elizabeth L. Affel, MS, RDMS, Philadelphia, Pa.

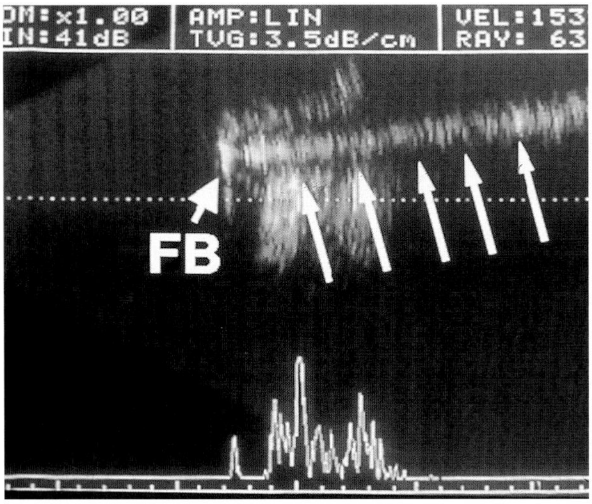

Fig. 4-8. A patient was shot in the eye with a BB gun; however, no clinical evidence of a ruptured globe was found. A brightness modulation (B-scan) ultrasound examination revealed a highly reflective foreign body (FB) with multiple reverberations, indicated by small arrows. The reverberations seen here are classic for a BB pellet. Although other foreign bodies produce reverberations, the spherical shape of this object produces this unique appearance. The B-scan does not demonstrate a vitreous cavity because the object is lying outside the globe near the medial rectus muscle. This position was confirmed on exploration of the orbit and removal of the object.

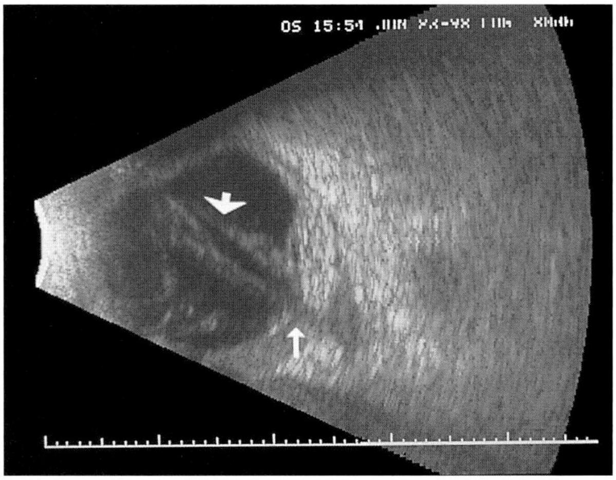

Fig. 4-9. A brightness modulation (B-scan) ultrasound examination of patient with a posterior rupture of the globe. When a foreign body passes through the vitreous cavity, an apparent track through the vitreous can be seen, as demonstrated by the short arrow. In this case, the object passed through the posterior sclera at a point indicated by the longer arrow. The B-scan does not demonstrate the foreign body directly but does provide useful information about the status of the intraocular structures in a circumstance in which the view is likely to be poor. Sonogram: Courtesy of Elizabeth L. Affel, MS, RDMS, Philadelphia, Pa.

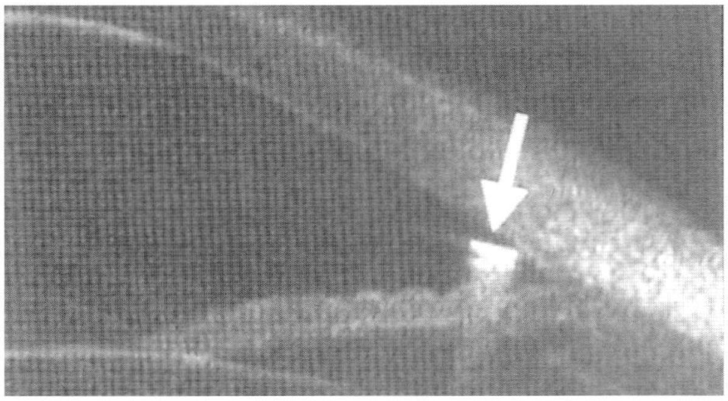

Fig. 4-10. Ultrasound biomicroscopy revealing an occult foreign body. Although ultrasound biomicroscopy requires specialized equipment, the exquisite detail of anterior segment structures makes it an excellent tool for detecting small, otherwise poorly visualized foreign objects. Reproduced from Deramo VA, Shah GK, Baumal CR, Fineman MS, Correa Zm, Benson WE. Ultrasound biomicroscopy as a tool for detecting and localizing occult foreign bodies after ocular trauma. *Ophthalmology.* 1999;106:303.

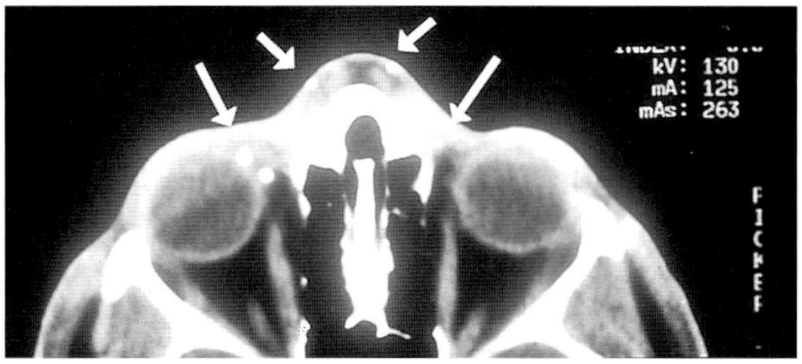

Fig. 4-11. A patient involved in ordnance disposal was injured by an explosion and presented with multiple facial lacerations and visual symptoms in the right eye. This computed tomography scan, axial section, through the orbit reveals multiple radiodense objects in the superficial tissues of the face and within the orbits bilaterally. Note the two objects lying outside the medial aspect of the left globe.

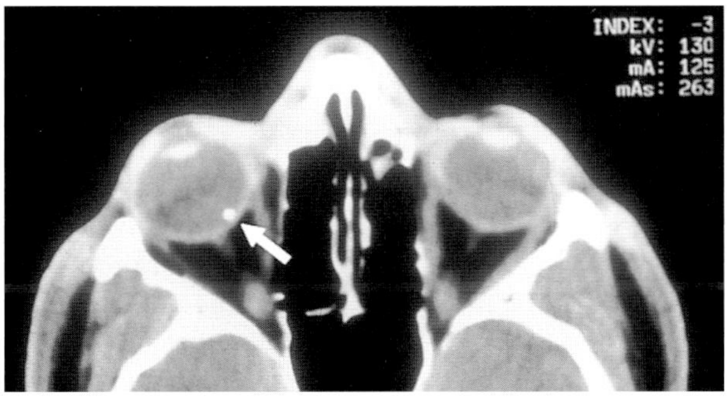

Fig. 4-12. Another computed tomography scan, axial section, from the same patient as in Figure 4-9, at the level of midglobe. The lens is clearly visible on both sides. A single radiodense object, indicated by the arrow, is seen within the globe. The object appears to be located adjacent to the nerve on the nasal retina. The position of the object was confirmed by indirect ophthalmoscopy to be one disc diameter nasal to the optic disc.

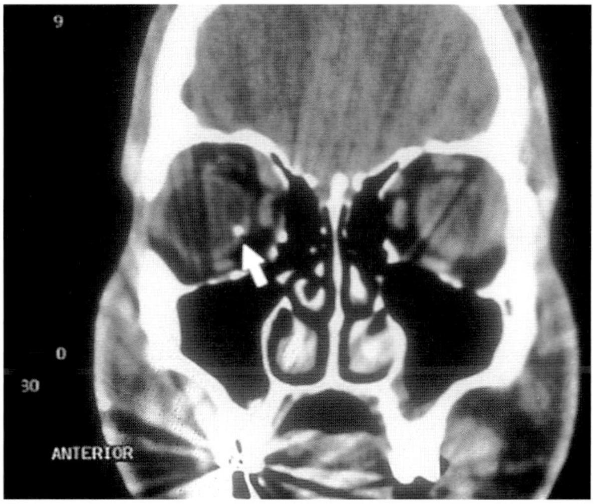

Fig. 4-13. This computed tomography scan, direct coronal section, of the same patient whose plain films are seen in Figure 4-5, demonstrates the same radiodense foreign body (FB), indicated by an arrow, in the globe on the nasal aspect. The combination of the coronal and axial sections provided an accurate determination of the position of the FB. Surgical removal of the FB was required; a metallic FB was located on the nasal retina. Spray artifact from dental work also can be seen.

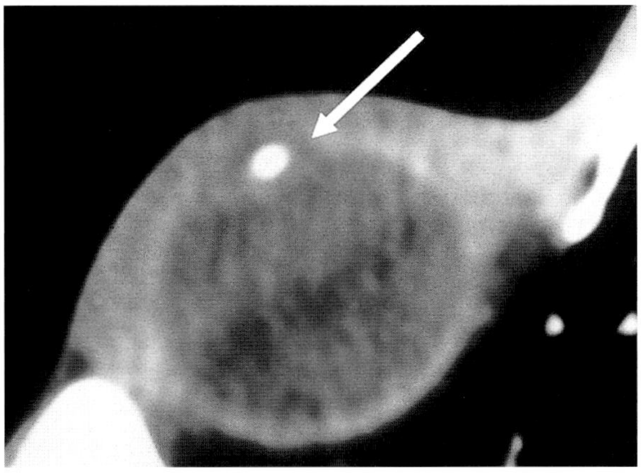

Fig. 4-14. While training on the rifle range, this patient noticed a sudden pain in his eye after a shell casing was discharged from a nearby rifle and struck the concrete beside him. Anterior segment examination revealed an area of fibrin in the inferior angle, but no foreign body could be confirmed. The computed tomography enlarged view of axial section seen here demonstrated a single, radiodense foreign body in the anterior segment, indicated by the arrow. On exploration, a small limbal laceration was noted and a 1-mm piece of mineral material was located in the anterior chamber.

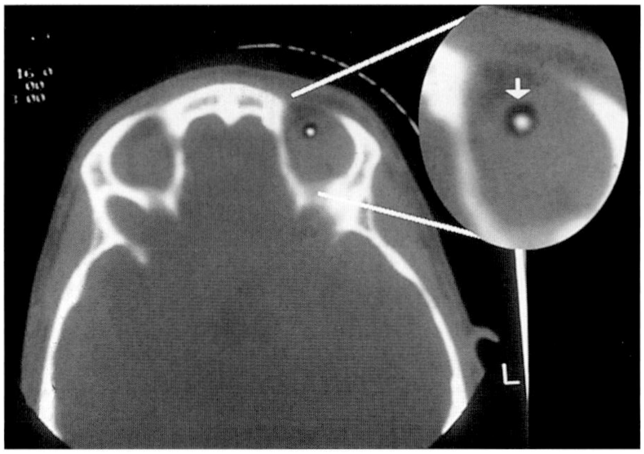

Fig. 4-15. A computed tomography scan, axial section, with enlargement of orbit (inset) of a patient in whom a pencil had passed through the eyelid and into the orbit and brain. The relative radiopacity of the graphite is clearly seen, as well as the relative radiolucency of the surrounding wood. This demonstrates how a wooden foreign body within the orbit may escape detection; a magnetic resonance imaging scan might well provide more information in cases like this. Computed tomography scan: Courtesy of Allen Thach, MD, Phoenix, Ariz.

tecting FBs made of glass, metal, or mineral (Figures 4-11 to 4-14). Lead, iron, solder, and chromium have relatively high attenuation coefficients; glass and stone have lower coefficients but still appear relatively bright. Wood is almost isodense with water and may be difficult to distinguish from the surrounding soft tissue (Figure 4-15). The size and volume of these objects are also factors in their detection.[11,12] Steel objects with a volume as small as 0.048 mm^3 are detectable by CT scan, although steel objects with a volume greater than 0.06 mm^3 were detected with a greater sensitivity in one experimental model.[4]

Helical or spiral CT scans present some benefits over conventional CT scanning, and the ability to detect steel IOFBs seems equivalent to that of conventional CT.[4] Scan times for the entire orbital volume can be as fast as 18 seconds, which will minimize motion artifact and reduce radiation exposure. Furthermore, unlike conventional CT, high-resolution coronal and sagittal images can be reconstructed from the axial scans, further limiting radiation exposure. Total exposure may be approximately one fourth that required for a conventional CT.[5] Helical CT may be ideal for patients with limited ability to cooperate or limited ability to position for conventional coronal CT scans.

Although excellent for the detection of high-density materials, CT is poor for organic matter of comparable size.[13,14] MRI has been suggested[15] as a reliable method to detect nonmetallic FBs (glass, plastic, or mineral), but the detection of organic matter may be much less reliable. A retrospective study[16] concluded that identification of foreign material in the orbit was possible in only about 50% of cases with the use of CT and MRI.

The potential danger of MRI in the face of a ferromagnetic FB in or outside the globe is clearly recognized. An intraocular magnetic object can move and grossly deform the globe[17] or move through the orbit, potentially causing a blinding injury.[18] A CT scan or plain film to exclude an iron or steel FB is a prerequisite for an MRI in the setting of an intraorbital or intraocular FB.

Orbital Fractures

Fractures of the orbital bones can result from direct trauma to the facial bones or compression of the orbital soft tissues, resulting in a blowout fracture of the orbit. Plain films of the skull are still used in emergency departments to screen for these fractures, and usually the telltale sign of an air–fluid level in the maxillary sinus prompts further radiographic evaluation. The definitive evaluation of bony anatomy provided by the CT scan is an integral part of the management of these injuries.

When an orbital fracture is suspected, a CT scan with both axial and direct coronal sections should be obtained. A section 1.5 mm to 3.0 mm in thickness is the usual protocol; very thin sections require a longer scan time, straining the resources of the radiologist, and the extra information obtained may not alter the management of the injury. The recent development of the helical CT may provide imaging options in patients with limited ability to cooperate or position for direct coronal sections. Three-dimensional reconstruction, which requires the manipulation of digital images with special software, may also be useful in the management of complex orbital fractures. Although three-dimensional imaging may not be useful to the general ophthalmologist, an orbital surgeon faced with a difficult reconstruction may find the information valuable. When considering these more-complex imaging options, we should consult a radiologist early in the process to ensure that the desired result is obtained most efficiently.

Fractures of the orbital walls are most easily seen on coronal sections. Irregularities in the contours of the medial or inferior orbital walls, as well as

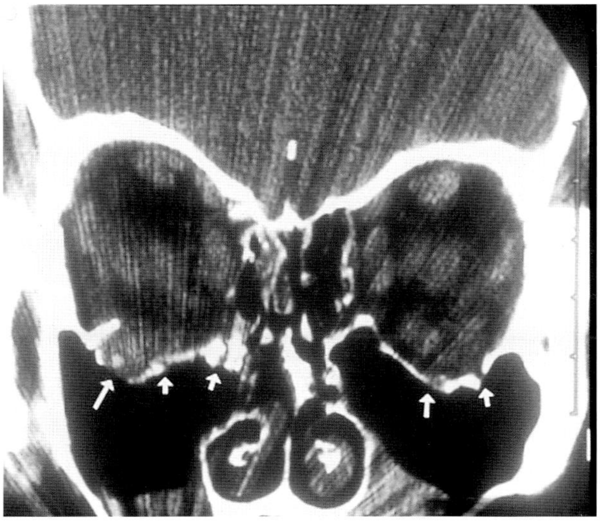

Fig. 4-16. The patient is a young woman who was involved in a serious automobile accident, which resulted in multiple facial fractures. The arrows on this computed tomography scan, coronal view, demonstrate bilateral, commuted orbital floor fractures. Other fractures involving the ethmoid sinuses also can be seen. Note how spray artifact from dental work affects the overall quality of the image.

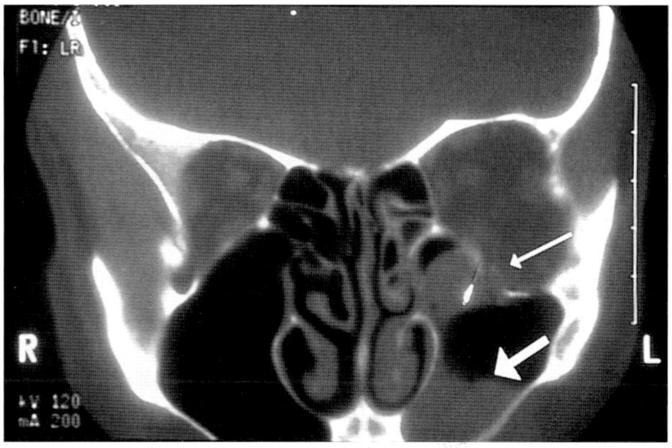

Fig. 4-17. This computed tomography scan, coronal view, is of a patient who sustained a direct blow to the face. The grayscale window is adjusted to highlight bone. The longer arrow demonstrates a fracture of the orbital floor, left orbit. Hemorrhage into the maxillary sinus causes opacification of the maxillary sinus and an air–fluid level, demonstrated by the shorter arrow.

opacification of the ethmoidal or maxillary sinuses, are the usual findings in blowout fractures of the orbit (Figures 4-16 and 4-17). Prolapse of orbital contents into the maxillary sinus or intraorbital emphysema may also be seen. Because entrapment of the inferior rectus is often at issue in these injuries, careful examination of sections through the muscle cone is required. An area of prolapsed orbital fat or hemorrhage into the sinus mucosa must be differentiated from a truly entrapped rectus muscle (Figure 4-18). Fractures of the lateral and superior orbital rims are less common but can impinge on the intraorbital contents (Figure 4-19).

Following the fracture from the point of initial detection and summing the thicknesses of the sections involved until the end of the fracture can yield an estimate of the size of the fracture. The involvement of neurovascular structures can also be assessed by examination of the infraorbital canal. A depression of the bony canal or groove will often correlate with infraorbital hypesthesia (Figure 4-20).

The optic nerve is subject to trauma from bony fragments impinging on it at or near the optic canal. Axial CT images can provide high-resolution images of the bony anatomy surrounding the nerve. If optic nerve damage is suspected, the possibility

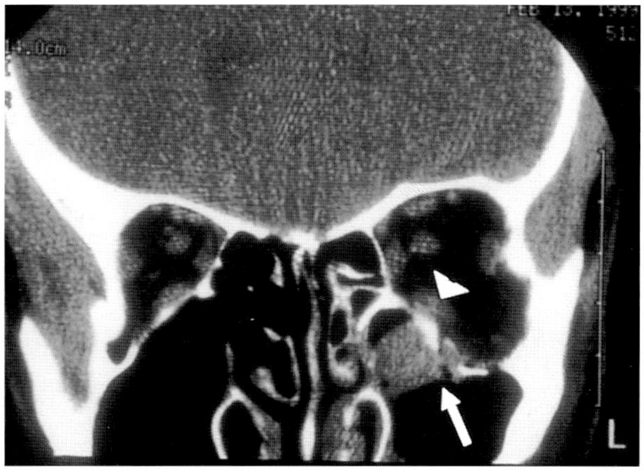

Fig. 4-18. The patient sustained head and facial trauma from a fall down a staircase. This computed tomography scan, coronal view, reveals an orbital floor fracture in the left orbit. The grayscale is adjusted to highlight the view of orbital soft tissues. A short arrow points directly to the inferior rectus muscle, which does not appear to be trapped in the fracture site; a mass of tissue is seen protruding at the fracture site (long arrow). On close examination, the mass appears inferior to the nondisplaced bone fragment; most likely, it represents a hemorrhage into the mucosa of the maxillary sinus, not a herniation of orbital fat. These findings are consistent with the unimpaired ocular motility of the patient.

a b

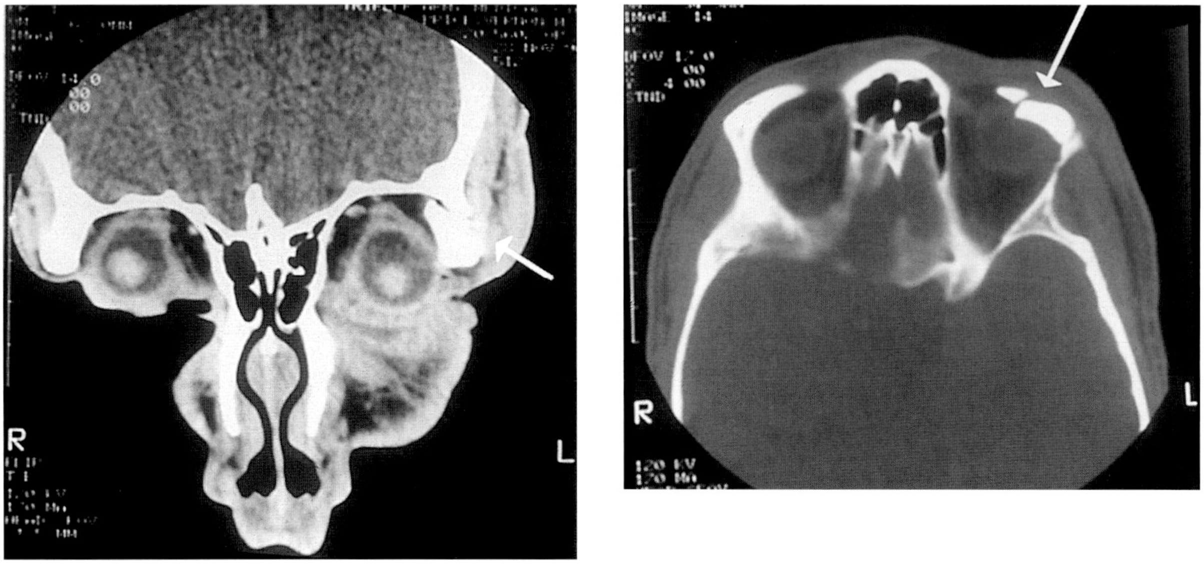

Fig. 4-19. (**a**) This computed tomography scan, coronal section, demonstrates an orbital fracture involving the zygomatic-frontal suture (arrow) with displacement of the bone fracture into the orbit. Associated soft-tissue swelling is also visible on the lateral aspect of the skull. The patient was unable to elevate the globe. (**b**) This computed tomography scan, axial section, of the same patient demonstrates bony fragments (indicated by arrow) impinging on the globe and interfering with supraduction. Computed tomography scans: Courtesy of Allen Thach, MD, Phoenix, Ariz.

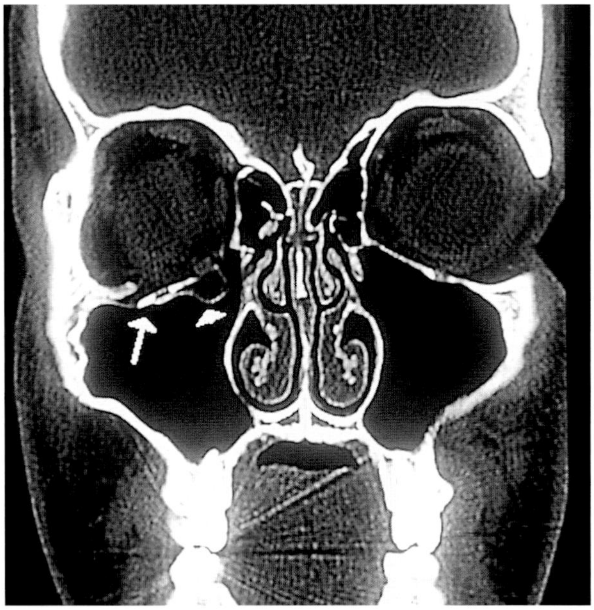

Fig. 4-20. The patient sustained sports injury to the right orbit 6 months before this computed tomography study, coronal view, was done. The long arrow indicates a fracture of the right orbital floor involving the infraorbital canal. The depression of the canal is consistent with the infraorbital hypesthesia seen in these fractures. The absence of an air–fluid level and a clear picture of the displaced sinus mucosa (arrowhead) suggest that the injury is not acute.

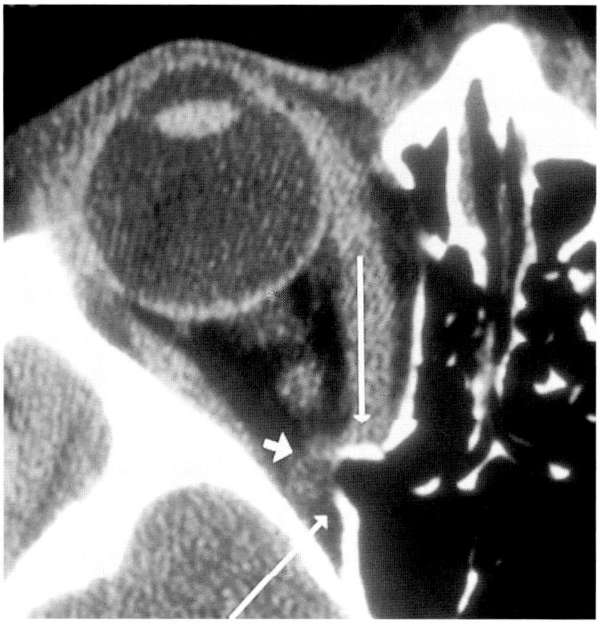

Fig. 4-21. A computed tomography scan, axial view, of a patient with multiple skull fractures and no light perception following a motor vehicle accident. Fragments of the sphenoid bone (long arrows) can be seen impinging on the optic nerve (short arrow). The axial section through the optic canal can provide valuable information when a traumatic injury from a bone fragment is suspected.

should be brought to the attention of the radiologist before the study is obtained to ensure adequate imaging of the nerve and surrounding bone. Early detection of bone fragments impinging on the nerve can provide an opportunity for treatment by decompression, or at least early detection can provide useful information to guide the treatment of the traumatized eye and aid in the formulation of a realistic prognosis (Figure 4-21). In any case, when visual loss seems out of proportion to findings on ophthalmoscopy, the possibility of traumatic optic neuropathy must be considered.

Blunt Ocular Trauma

The value of radiographic evaluation of the globe with CT is limited except in those incidents in which a nebulous history cannot exclude the presence of an FB. Although a CT scan may confirm a deformed globe in cases of occult ruptures, the findings on a CT scan are unlikely to precipitate or prevent an exploration of a bluntly traumatized eye. An eye that is suspected to have an occult rupture on clinical examination should be explored with or without supporting radiographic evidence.

Although MRI is of limited use in the general evaluation of ocular trauma, in specific instances it can be helpful. The exceptional images of orbital soft tissues provided by MRI can aid in the evaluation of trauma to the extraocular muscles. Figure 4-22 demonstrates a case involving blunt ocular trauma with an inability to infraduct the eye. CT was not able to demonstrate the injury to the inferior rectus muscle.

Ultrasonography, on the other hand, can be an invaluable tool in the evaluation of a bluntly traumatized eye with a poor or absent view of the posterior segment. Although extreme care must be exercised to avoid any pressure on the eye with a suspected rupture, an ultrasound examination can be performed to confirm a globe rupture and assess the status of the retina (see Figure 4-9). For a patient with a ruptured globe, B-scan is often the only source of information to guide postoperative care.

A dislocated lens or lens fragment, vitreous detachments, retinal tears, retinal detachments, and choroidal detachments are all complications of blunt ocular trauma that can be diagnosed by ultrasonography (Figures 4-23 to 4-26). CT and MRI are capable of imaging some, if not all, of the aforementioned entities; however, ultrasonography is a more economical and practical method for diagnosis and follow-up examinations. Because the quality of the examination is

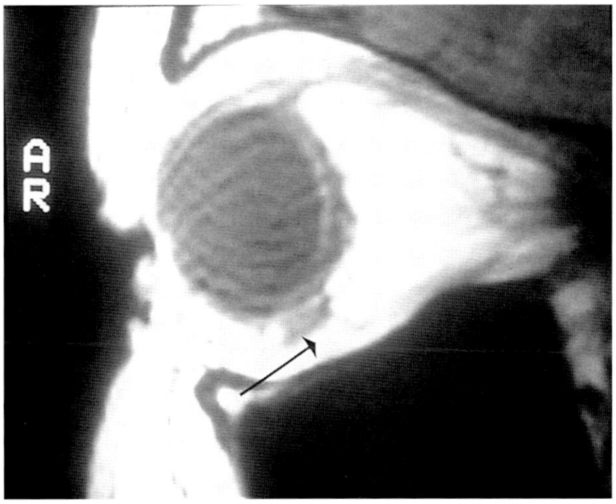

Fig. 4-22. A sagittal magnetic resonance imaging scan of an orbit, T1-weighted. This patient fell on a metal pipe, subsequently losing the ability to infraduct the eye. A computed tomography scan was not helpful in the evaluation of the problem; the magnetic resonance imaging scan, however, demonstrated a discontinuity in the inferior rectus muscle. Magnetic resonance imaging provides excellent images of the orbital soft tissues, especially the extraocular muscles; the arrow highlights the discontinuity in the inferior rectus. Adapted from Ward TP, Thach AB, Madigan WP, Berland JE. Magnetic resonance imaging in posttraumatic strabismus. *J Pediatr Ophthalmol Strabismus.* 1997;34:132.

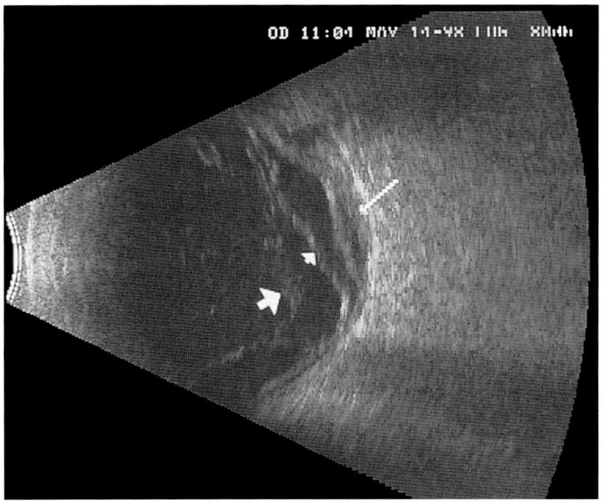

Fig. 4-23. High-quality ultrasound can provide information about the anatomical status of the intraocular structures when no view is possible. This brightness modulation (B-scan) ultrasound study demonstrates a posterior vitreous detachment (large arrow), a retinal detachment (smaller arrow), and a choroidal detachment (long arrow). Sonogram: Courtesy of Elizabeth L. Affel, MS, RDMS, Philadelphia, Pa.

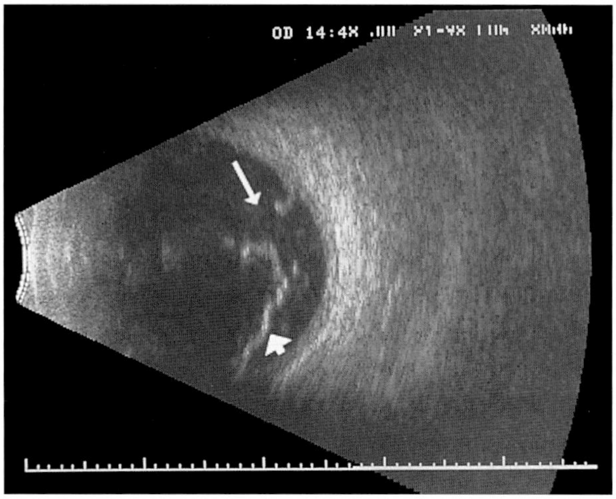

Fig. 4-24. In the hands of a skilled examiner, a high-quality ultrasound can demonstrate details usually only detectable on ophthalmoscopy. This brightness modulation (B-scan) ultrasound study demonstrates a retinal detachment, indicated by the small arrow, and the cause, a retinal tear demonstrated by the larger arrow. Sonogram: Courtesy of Elizabeth L. Affel, MS, RDMS, Philadelphia, Pa.

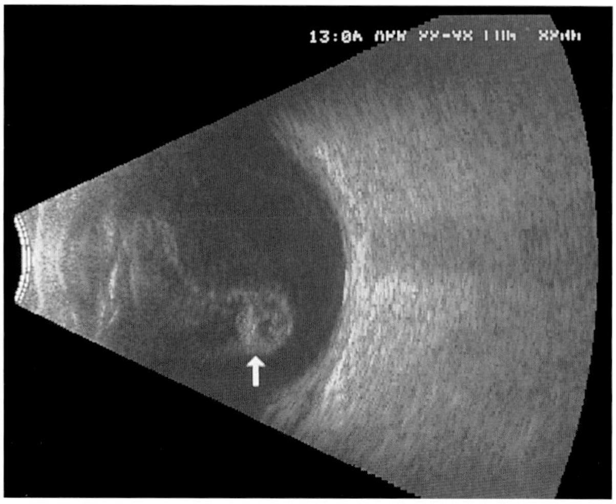

Fig. 4-25. A lens dislocated into the posterior segment (arrow) can easily be detected by brightness modulation (B-scan) ultrasonography. Sonogram: Courtesy of Elizabeth L. Affel, MS, RDMS, Philadelphia, Pa.

a

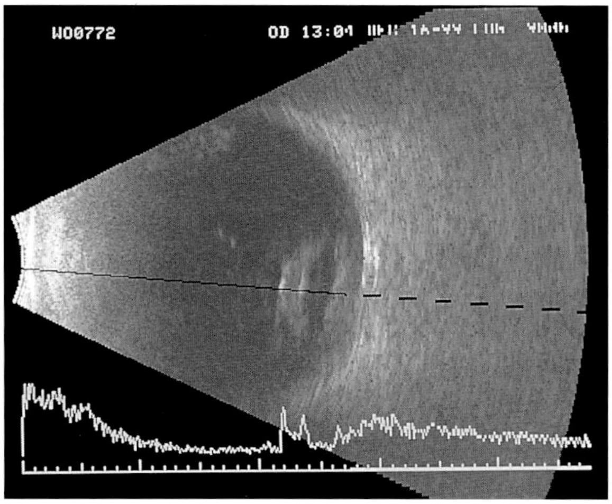

b

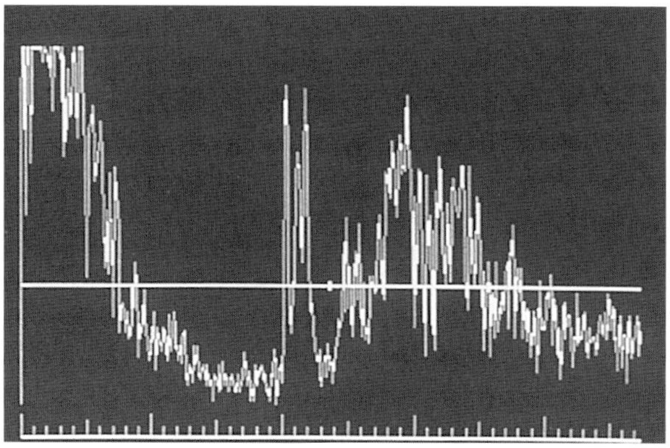

c

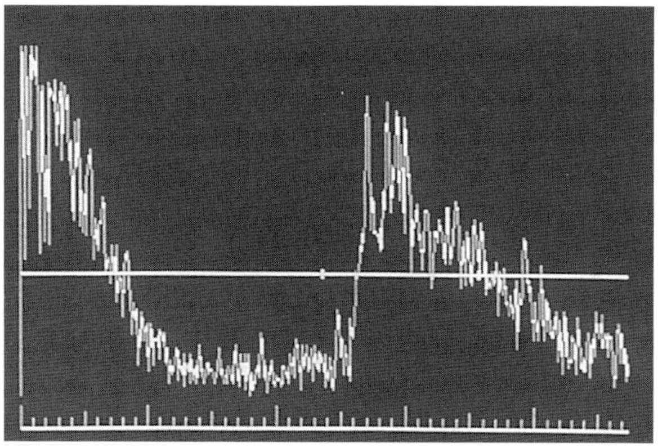

Fig. 4-26. (**a**) A brightness modulation (B-scan) ultrasound study of a patient with a remote history of ocular trauma. The dislocated native lens can be seen resting on the surface of the retina. (**b**) An amplitude modulation (A-scan) ultrasound study of the same patient demonstrates a peak at the position of the anterior surface of the dislocated lens. (**c**) An A-scan ultrasound study of a normal eye, in which echoes are plotted against time, reflecting the distance of the target from the probe. An absence of echoes is noted through the vitreous cavity until a sharp peak generated by the surface of the retina is encountered. In the hands of most ophthalmologists, for the detection and analysis of foreign bodies, the usefulness of A-scan ultrasonography is limited.

dependent on the skill of the examiner, a basic level of competence with the ultrasound examination of the eye should be the goal of every ophthalmologist who manages traumatized eyes.

SUMMARY

Plain film radiography, CT, MRI, and ultrasonography are all methods used to image the ocular and adnexal structures in the evaluation of trauma. Although CT is the best and standard method of evaluating the orbital fractures and aids in the detection of orbital and ocular FBs, both MRI and ultrasonography play supporting roles. In instances of blunt trauma to the globe, however, the roles are reversed: ultrasonography becomes much more important as a diagnostic tool, and radiographic evaluation and MRI play minor roles in the detection and management of the ocular pathology.

REFERENCES

1. Weber AL. Imaging techniques and normal radiographic anatomy. In: Albert DM, ed. *Principles and Practice of Ophthalmology*. Vol 5. Philadelphia, Pa: WB Saunders Company; 1994: 3505–3510.
2. Moseley L. The orbit and eye. In: Sutton D, ed. *A Textbook of Radiology and Imaging*. Vol 2. London, England: Churchill Livingstone; 1993: 1287–1309.
3. Wiesen EJ, Miraldi F. Imaging principles in computed tomography. In: Haaga JR, ed. *Computed Tomography and Magnetic Resonance Imaging of the Whole Body*. Vol 1. St. Louis, Mo: Mosby; 1994: 3–25.
4. Chacko JG, Figueroa RE, Johnson MH, Marcus DM, Brooks SE. Detection and localization of steel intraocular foreign bodies using computed tomography: A comparison of helical and conventional axial scanning. *Ophthalmology*. 1997;104:319–323.
5. Lakits A, Prokesch R, Scholda C, Bankier A, Weninger F, Imhof H. Multiplanar imaging in the preoperative assessment of metallic intraocular foreign bodies: Helical computed tomography versus conventional computed tomography. *Ophthalmology*. 1998;105:1679–1685.
6. Berges O. Orbital ultrasonography: Principles and technique. In: Newton TH, ed. *Radiology of the Eye and Orbit*. New York, NY: Raven Press; 1990: 6.1–6.20.
7. Pavlin C, Harasiewicz K, Sherar M, Foster I F. Clinical use of ultrasound biomicroscopy. *Ophthalmology*. 1991;98:287–295.
8. Pavlin C, Sherar M, Foster F. Subsurface ultrasound microscopic imaging of the intact eye. *Ophthalmology*. 1990;97:244–250.
9. Kramer M, Hart L, Miller JW. Ultrasonography in the management of penetrating ocular trauma [review]. *Int Ophthalmol Clin*. 1995 Winter;35(1):181–192.
10. Deramo VA, Shah GK, Baumal CR, Fineman MS, Correa ZM, Benson WE. Ultrasound biomicroscopy as a tool for detecting and localizing occult foreign bodies after ocular trauma. *Ophthalmology*. 1999;106:301–305.
11. Gunenc U, Maden A, Kaynak S, Pirnar T. Magnetic resonance imaging and computed tomography in the detection and localization of intraocular foreign bodies. *Doc Ophthalmol*. 1992;81:369–378.
12. Kadir S, Aronow S, Davis KR. The use of computerized tomography in the detection of intraorbital foreign bodies. *Comput Tomogr*. 1977;1:151–156.
13. Grove AS Jr. Computed tomography in the management of orbital trauma. *Ophthalmology*. 1982;89:433–440.
14. Zinreich SJ, Miller NR, Aguayo JB, Quinn C, Hadfield R, Rosenbaum A. Computed tomographic three-dimensional localization and compositional evaluation of intraocular and orbital foreign bodies. *Arch Ophthalmol*. 1986;104:1477–1482.

15. LoBue TD, Deutsch TA, Lobick J, Turner DA. Detection and localization of nonmetallic intraocular foreign bodies by magnetic resonance imaging. *Arch Ophthalmol.* 1988;106:260–261.

16 Nasr AM, Barret GH, Fleming JC, Al-Hussain HM, Karcioglu ZA. Penetrating orbital injury with organic foreign bodies. *Ophthalmology.* 1999;106:523–532.

17. Williamson TH, Smith FW, Forrester JV. Magnetic resonance imaging of intraocular foreign bodies. *Br J Ophthalmol.* 1989;73:555–558.

18. Kulshrestha M, Mission G. Magnetic resonance imaging and the dangers of orbital foreign bodies. *Br J Ophthalmol.* 1995;79:1149.

Chapter 5

ANESTHETIC CARE OF THE TRAUMATIZED EYE

ANDREW S. EISEMAN, MD*; AND DANIEL J. JANIK, MD†

*Lieutenant Colonel, Medical Corps, US Army; Chief, Oculoplastics and Orbit Service, Walter Reed Army Medical Center, Washington, DC 20307-5001

†Lieutenant Colonel, US Air Force (Ret); Associate Professor of Anesthesiology and Associate Medical Director of Operating Room Services, University of Colorado Health Sciences Center, Denver, Colorado 80162; formerly, Anesthesia Service, Walter Reed Army Medical Center, Washington, DC

INTRODUCTION

Ocular injuries account for a significant percentage of combat injuries, even though the eyes account for only 0.27% of the body's total surface area, 0.54% of the body's total frontal silhouette, and 4% of the surface area of the face.[1] The incidence of ocular injury in combat is 20 to 50 times greater than that expected by its surface area alone.[2] This differential is largely the result of the increased exposure of the head and eyes during combat and the ease with which the eye can be injured by such seemingly innocuous mechanisms as windblown foreign bodies. Many of these foreign bodies would be easily stopped by the skin or clothing elsewhere but can incapacitate a soldier if they strike the eye.

The medical literature has shown that the rate of ocular injuries during combat has steadily increased since the American Civil War.[3–8] Ocular injuries accounted for 0.57% of casualties during the American Civil War, 2% of casualties during World War I and World War II, and nearly 3% during the Korean War. The Israeli experience from 1967 until 1982 showed rates that started at 5.6% during the 1967 Arab–Israeli Six-Day War and increased to 6.8% during the war in Lebanon. This parallels the US experience during the Vietnam War, in which 5% to 9% of the casualties were ocular. Finally, in the Persian Gulf War (1991/92), ocular injuries accounted for up to 13% of all war injuries. These rates indicate the need for a significant number of well-trained medical personnel who are experienced with the complexities of the care of the injured eye. This includes not only modern ophthalmic surgical techniques but also the subtleties and intricacies of providing adequate anesthesia.

Interested readers may find additional information on anesthesia for eye trauma in another volume in the Textbooks of Military Medicine series, *Anesthesia and Perioperative Care of the Combat Casualty,* particularly Chapter 17, Eye Injuries.[9]

PREOPERATIVE ASSESSMENT

The preoperative assessment of the patient injured in combat must first identify and treat any life-threatening condition. The algorithms published for Advanced Cardiac Life Support and Advanced Trauma Life Support are extremely effective in identifying and treating such conditions in a systematic way. This is especially important in a patient who has multisystem trauma, a common occurrence on today's battlefield. Patients with ocular trauma often have midfacial trauma as well. Such trauma can significantly complicate airway management and may require early intervention by an anesthesiologist or an otolaryngologist for definitive airway control. A cribriform plate injury with cerebrospinal fluid leak must also be considered when ocular and midface trauma are present. Nasotracheal intubation and the placement of nasogastric tubes should be avoided in patients with cribriform plate injury to prevent inadvertent intracranial placement.

Once the initial ABCs of airway, breathing, and circulation have been stabilized, a more definitive examination of the eye and ocular adnexa can be performed. If the patient has other life-threatening injuries, the ophthalmologist may be able to perform only a cursory examination, with the main goal of determining whether an open (ie, penetrating) globe injury is present or suspected. The most important ocular consideration before the induction of anesthesia is the integrity of the eye. If an ocular examination cannot be performed before life-threatening injuries must be managed, the injured eye should be presumed to have an open globe injury. A metal protective shield should be placed so that no pressure is exerted on the eye, and anesthesia should be induced to minimize the risk of extrusion of the intraocular contents.

The importance of a careful preanesthetic evaluation cannot be overemphasized. The importance of the integrity of the eye has already been discussed; other important considerations include the presence of preexisting disease, prior anesthesia and surgery, current medications used chronically or given in the posttrauma time frame, drug allergies, and physical examination. Most patients who sustain injury in combat are young and otherwise healthy without underlying disease; however, cardiovascular and pulmonary dysfunction can occur with multisystem trauma or exposure to chemical or biological warfare agents.

A common anesthetic problem in acute trauma is a full stomach. Combat-injured patients should all be treated as if they have full stomachs. In the setting of ocular trauma in which an open globe is verified or suspected, mechanical gastric emptying with nasogastric or orogastric tubes should be avoided because placement of the tubes may evoke coughing and vomiting, which could result in expulsion of the intraocular contents. Neutralization of gastric acid should be undertaken in all patients to minimize the risk of aspiration pneumonitis. Sodium citrate 0.3 molar (30–40 mL, administered orally) given 30 minutes before induction can raise the gastric contents' pH but at the expense of a small increase in gastric volume. Cimetidine (300 mg, orally, or 150 mg, intramuscularly) or ranitidine (150 mg, orally, or 50 mg, intramuscularly) given 90 minutes before induction can also provide some protection. Additionally, these agents do not appear to affect the intraocular pressure (IOP) of the closed eye.[10] Metoclopramide (10 mg, intravenously) may reduce the volume of the stomach contents by promoting gastric emptying. However, preliminary data demonstrate this drug's tendency to raise IOP[11]; it should, therefore, be used with caution in open globe injuries.

TOPICAL ANESTHESIA

Topical anesthesia is commonly used during routine ophthalmic examinations and procedures. It allows a more complete examination, especially when corneal epithelial defects are present or when such procedures as lacrimal probing and irrigation, nasal examination, and forced duction testing are used to obtain more detailed information concerning the anatomy or physiology of the injured area. To add to patient comfort, topical anesthesia is also useful before facial preparation. If an open globe is suspected and topical anesthetic is required, care should be taken to minimize the amount used and to ensure that the drops are sterile.

Several topical anesthetic agents are available for use during ophthalmic examinations and procedures (Table 5-1). Proparacaine is an ester preparation available in 0.5% solution. It is quickly absorbed through the corneal epithelium because of its high lipid solubility and thus causes less discomfort than a more hydrophilic solution such as lidocaine.[12] Long-term use can result in corneal epithelial toxicity and delayed corneal healing. Local-

TABLE 5-1

COMMONLY USED TOPICAL AND LOCAL ANESTHETICS IN OPHTHALMIC SURGERY

Kind of Agent	Concentration	Max. Dose	Onset	Duration	Comments
Topical:					
Proparacaine	0.5%	—	Seconds	10–20 min	Any topical anesthetic can cause superficial punctate keratitis[1]
Tetracaine	0.5%	—	Seconds	10–20 min	
Lidocaine	1%–4%	—	Seconds	10–20 min	
Regional:					
Lidocaine	1%–2%	500 mg[1]	4–6 min	40–60 min	Least painful on injection[2]
Mepivacaine	1%–2%	500 mg[1]	3–5 min	2–3 h	Duration of action greater without epinephrine[3]
Bupivacaine	0.25%–0.75%	23 mL of 0.75% solution[2]	5–11 min	3–12 h	Most painful on injection[2]
Adjuvant:					
Epinephrine	1:100,000 to 1:200,000	—	—	—	Increases duration of action of all except mepivacaine[3]
Hyaluronidase	150 U per vial	Standard dose is 150 U/10 mL of local	—	—	Can decrease duration of action of local[2]
Sodium Bicarbonate	8.4% (1 meq/mL)	Standard dose is 1 mL in 10 mL of local	—	—	Can decrease pain on injection[2]

1. Medical Economics Data. *Physicians' Desk Reference for Ophthalmology*. 22nd ed. Montvale, NJ: Medical Economics Co; 1994: 9.
2. Bilyk JR, Sutula FC. Anesthesia for ophthalmic plastic surgery. In: Stewart WB, ed. *Surgery of the Eyelid, Orbit, and Lacrimal System*. Vol 1. San Francisco, Calif: American Academy of Ophthalmology; 1993: 33.
3. Everett WG, Vey EK, Finlay JW. Duration of oculomotor akinesia of injectable anesthetics. *Trans Am Acad Ophthalmol*. 1961;65:308.

ized allergic reactions have also been reported; if a reaction occurs, tetracaine, another ester preparation in 0.5% solution, can be substituted.[13] However, tetracaine is more toxic to the epithelium and has significantly more systemic toxicity. Fatalities with excessive topical use have been reported.[14]

Cocaine is another ester derivative that not only provides excellent topical anesthesia but also causes vasoconstriction by preventing the reuptake of norepinephrine.[15] This added property of cocaine makes it an excellent agent when examination or manipulation of the nasal mucosa is required. Before lacrimal drainage surgery, the nasal cavity is usually packed with neurosurgical cottonoids soaked in 4% cocaine solution. Care must be taken to place the cottonoids directly against the nasal mucosa and in the location of the anterior middle meatus where the nasal mucosa will be opened. Cocaine is toxic to the corneal and conjunctival epithelium, and its use in the eye is usually limited to detecting the sympathetic dysfunction of Horner's syndrome. A drop or two of the 2% solution can confirm the diagnosis of Horner's syndrome when less dilation is noted on the affected side. When cocaine is used, the vital signs must be monitored closely because hypertension, tachycardia, and ventricular dysrhythmias can occur. Concomitant use of other systemic agents, such as monoamine oxidase inhibitors and tricyclic antidepressants, can potentiate this effect and require extra vigilance.[16] Additionally, because cocaine is detoxified by plasma and liver cholinesterases, persons with cholinesterase deficiencies are at risk for sudden death from the use of cocaine.[17]

Lidocaine is an amide preparation that recently has been used more frequently as a topical anesthetic agent. In the past it was used mostly as a local injectable anesthetic agent. However, the 4% solution used topically can provide enough anesthesia to perform cataract surgery or allow for a much more comfortable examination. It is particularly helpful when performing forced duction testing and when probing and irrigating the nasolacrimal system. A pledget can be fashioned from the tip of a cotton-tipped applicator and soaked in a 2% or 4% lidocaine solution. It can then be placed either over the muscle insertion or over the lacrimal punctum for several minutes before the procedure is performed.

EMLA Cream (an emulsion of lidocaine 2.5% and prilocaine 2.5%, mfg by AstraZeneca LP, Wilmington, Del) is a topical agent that may be an alternative to local anesthesia of the skin. It is not suitable for use in the eye but can be used in the periocular region if care is taken to avoid contact with the ocular surface. EMLA Cream is particularly useful for providing anesthesia before venipuncture. It can also be used for superficial surgical procedures, such as removal of superficial foreign bodies or laser skin resurfacing, but anesthesia can only be achieved to a depth of approximately 5 mm. EMLA Cream has a relatively long onset of action and should be applied 1 hour before the planned procedure.[17]

LOCAL ANESTHESIA

All local anesthetics inhibit sodium ion influx across neuronal cell membranes and produce a blockade of the nerve impulse. However, not all neuronal functions are affected by local anesthetics in equal fashion. The rates of blockade of the components of a peripheral nerve occur at different speeds with loss of sympathetic function first, followed by a pin-prick sensation, touch, temperature, and finally motor function. The reason for this differential blockade is not totally clear but may have to do with small or nonmyelinated fibers being affected more quickly than large or myelinated fibers.[17]

Local anesthetics are benzoic acid derivatives and can be separated into two different groups on the basis of whether there is an amide or ester link between the lipophilic head and the hydrophilic tail.[17] Amides and esters differ in several respects. Amides are metabolized in the liver, whereas esters require a plasma pseudocholinesterase for breakdown. Amides cause fewer allergic reactions than esters do, but are more toxic.[15] Allergic cross-reactions between the ester and amide groups do not occur, so if an individual is allergic to one group of agents, it may be possible that the other group can be used safely. Commonly used agents that are members of the ester group are tetracaine, cocaine, and procaine. The amide group includes lidocaine, mepivacaine, and bupivacaine.

Specific Local Anesthetic Agents

Lidocaine is the most commonly used local anesthetic agent and is available in 1% and 2% solutions (see Table 5-1). It produces the least pain on injection and has a rapid onset of action and a moderate duration of action.[18] Mepivacaine is available in 1%, 2%, and 3% solutions and, like lidocaine, has a rapid onset of action and moderate duration. Unlike lidocaine, however, it has no topical activity.[19] Bupivacaine is a more potent agent and is more toxic, probably because of its increased lipid solubility. It is available in 0.5% and 0.75% solutions and has a delayed onset of action and longer duration of action. One of the shorter-acting agents can be combined with bupivacaine to facilitate rapid onset of action and prolonged duration. This is commonly done when performing retrobulbar blocks, when postoperative analgesia is necessary, or when a longer procedure is anticipated.

Adjuvant Agents

Several adjuvant agents (see Table 5-1) can be added to any of the local anesthetics. One commonly added agent is epinephrine, which has several beneficial effects, including

- prolonging the duration of anesthesia,
- minimizing the peak level of local anesthetic in the blood,
- increasing the intensity of the blockade, and
- reducing surgical bleeding.

Epinephrine concentrations from 1:100,000 to 1:400,000 are available. One study[20] showed that decreasing the concentration from 1:200,000 to 1:400,000 caused the same vasoconstrictive result locally. Using lower concentrations might minimize the potential for systemic toxicity, including tachycardia, hypertension, and dysrhythmia. Epinephrine should be used cautiously in patients with unstable angina, malignant dysrhythmias, uncontrolled hypertension, or hyperthyroidism, and in patients taking monoamine oxidase inhibitors and tricyclic antidepressants, which can enhance the effects of catecholamines. To prevent tissue necrosis, epinephrine should also be used with caution in areas with poor collateral blood flow.

Hyaluronidase is another adjuvant often added to local anesthetics. Hyaluronic acid inhibits the diffusion of foreign substances in interstitial spaces. Hyaluronidase, on the other hand, depolymerizes hyaluronic acid and facilitates the spread of local anesthetics,[17] which can hasten their onset of action. However, hyaluronidase significantly shortens the duration of action and may cause diffusion of the anesthetic agent into undesirable locations. If a local anesthetic agent with hyaluronidase is used in the upper lid, the drug may diffuse into the levator muscle, paralyzing it and making intraoperative adjustment of lid height difficult. If hyaluronidase is used, 150 units (U) can be added to 10 mL of local anesthetic.

Sodium bicarbonate can also be added to local anesthetics to raise the pH and increase the concentration of nonionized free base. In theory, these actions increase the rate of diffusion and speed the onset of action.[17] Raising the pH has also been shown to decrease the pain of injection when 1 mL of 1 mEq/mL sodium bicarbonate solution is added to 10 mL of local anesthetic, for a final concentration of 0.1 mEq/mL.[21]

Adverse Reactions to Local Anesthetic Agents

Local anesthetic agents present a continuum of toxic effects as systemic blood concentrations increase. The earliest signs of toxicity may include numbness of the tongue, lightheadedness, visual disturbances, and muscle twitching. Further progression results in central nervous system (CNS) signs such as unconsciousness, convulsions, and coma. Finally, the cardiovascular system collapses, with respiratory arrest and refractory dysrhythmias.

Treatment of local anesthetic toxicity is mainly supportive, with the immediate administration of oxygen and the use of an agent to stop seizure activity. The first item recommended is succinylcholine to facilitate ventilation. Then, either a barbiturate or benzodiazepine can be given, as tolerated by the cardiovascular system, to reduce CNS metabolic demands. To treat cardiovascular effects, high-dose epinephrine may be needed to support the heart rate and blood pressure. Atropine may be needed to treat bradycardia, and ventricular dysrhythmias should be treated with an agent like bretylium tosylate instead of lidocaine.[17]

The best treatment for toxic reactions is prevention. The toxic dose of the agent being used must be known. For 2% lidocaine without epinephrine, the maximum recommended dose is 15 mL, and for 2% lidocaine with epinephrine, it is 25 mL. The maximum recommended dose of 0.75% bupivacaine is 23 mL.[12] Other preventive measures include using meticulous technique to avoid intravascular administration and assessing for individual risk factors (eg, liver failure, pseudocholinesterase deficiencies) that could slow the metabolism of the agent.

TECHNIQUES FOR ANESTHETIZING THE OCULAR ADNEXA

Several techniques are available to adequately anesthetize the ocular adnexa after injury. These techniques are usually a combination of subcutaneous regional infiltration, field block, and nerve block. When any of these techniques are used, we must remember that a sharp needle tip is close to the globe. It is advisable to place a plastic globe protector over the eye when possible to reduce the risk of inadvertent penetration. A globe protector also decreases the discomfort often reported from the bright operating room lights.

Subcutaneous Regional Infiltration

Subcutaneous regional infiltration is easily administered because it requires the least amount of knowledge of neuroanatomy. When this method is used, the surgeon must remember that the motor and sensory nerves run deep to the orbicularis muscle; therefore, the anesthetic must be injected in this plane. Injection in this plane also facilitates surgical dissection, because hydraulic dissection has already occurred.

Field and Nerve Blocks

Successful administration of field and nerve blocks requires much more detailed understanding of the neuroanatomy of the ocular adnexa. A field block is defined as infiltration of anesthetic into tissue to block neural transmission and provide anesthesia to distal tissue. Nerve blocks, in contrast, involve the injection of anesthesia directly around a nerve to provide anesthesia to an area supplied by that nerve. These two techniques often meld into one in the ocular adnexa because the nerves are often in close proximity to each other and because there is significant redundancy of sensory innervation.[12]

Neuroanatomy for Ocular Adnexal Blocks

The sensory nerve supply to the ocular adnexa is provided by the first two branches of the trigeminal nerve (Figure 5-1). The first branch, known as the ophthalmic division, enters the orbit via the superior orbital fissure and has three branches: the

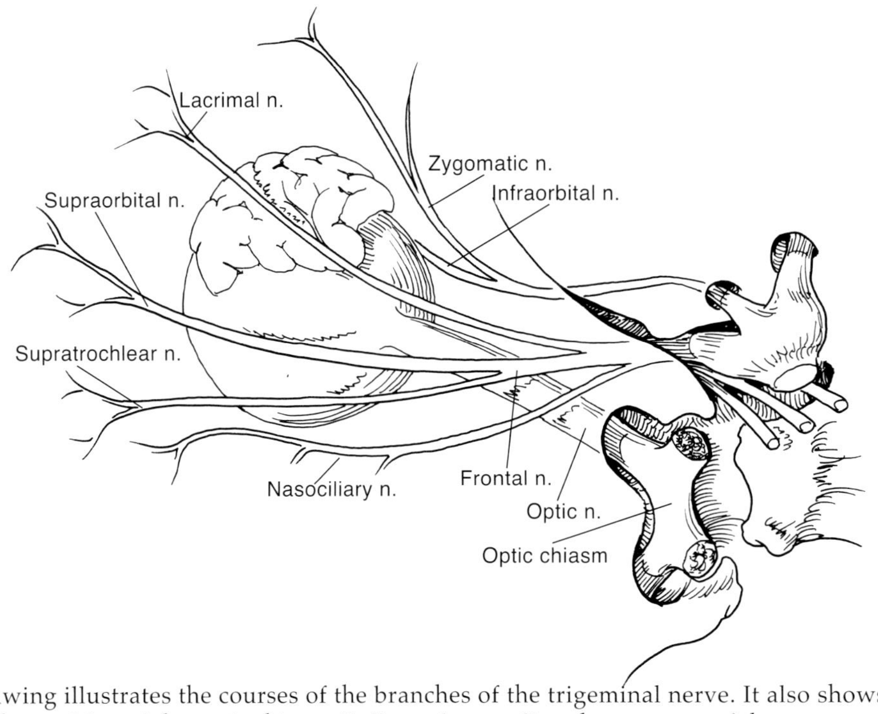

Fig. 5-1. This drawing illustrates the courses of the branches of the trigeminal nerve. It also shows the course of the optic nerve and the position of the optic chiasm. Fully understanding the anatomy of the sensory supply to the orbit and orbital adnexa will allow the development of a standardized approach to local anesthetic and infiltrative blocks. Drawing prepared for this textbook by Gary Wind, MD, Uniformed Services University of the Health Sciences, Bethesda, Md.

lacrimal, the frontal, and the nasociliary.[22] The lacrimal nerve supplies sensation to the lacrimal gland and to the skin of the lid and periorbital region superolaterally. The frontal nerve runs forward in the roof of the orbit just under the periorbita. It divides into the supraorbital and supratrochlear nerves, which supply sensation to the skin and deeper tissues of the lid and periorbital regions in the superonasal and frontal areas. The nasociliary nerve gives off sensory fibers to the ciliary ganglion and then passes above the optic nerve, where long ciliary nerves branch to the globe. It continues forward superiorly and nasally in close proximity to the ophthalmic artery, dividing into the anterior ethmoidal nerve, the posterior ethmoidal nerve (often not present), and the infratrochlear nerve. The ethmoidal nerves supply sensation to the nasal mucosa. The infratrochlear nerve supplies sensation to the side and tip of the nose and the lacrimal sac and canaliculi.[22]

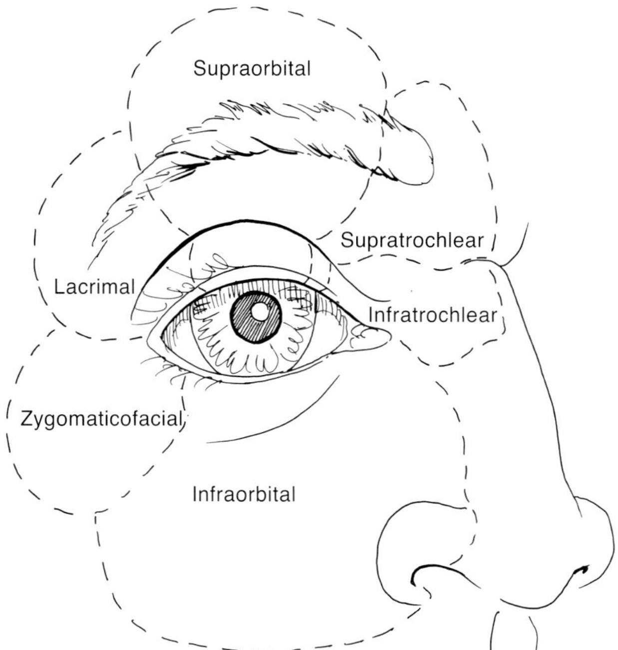

Fig. 5-2. This drawing illustrates the occular adnexal sensory innervation. Each sensory nerve is responsible for providing sensation to a certain area (seen above), although there is some overlap in innervation. An understanding of this nerve supply is the basis for the local anesthetic techniques and nerve blocks utilized. Drawing prepared for this textbook by Gary Wind, MD, Uniformed Services University of the Health Sciences, Bethesda, Md.

The maxillary nerve is the second division of the trigeminal nerve and courses forward through the foramen rotundum. The zygomatic nerve is a branch that subdivides into the zygomaticofacial and zygomaticotemporal nerves.[22] These sensory branches exit through foramina in the lateral wall of the orbit and supply sensation to the skin of the lateral orbit. The infraorbital nerve is the terminal branch; it runs along the orbital floor, supplying sensation to skin of the lower lid, the upper lip, and some teeth (Figure 5-2).

Fully understanding the anatomical relationships of these nerves as they exit the orbit allows for successful anesthetic infiltration. Four of the nerves are palpable as they leave the orbit: the supraorbital, the infraorbital, the supratrochlear, and the infratrochlear.[23] The supraorbital foramen is usually located 2.7 cm lateral to the midline of the glabella, and the supratrochlear and infratrochlear nerves are 1.7 cm lateral to the midline. The infraorbital nerve exits approximately 1 cm below the inferior orbital rim in a vertical line drawn from the supraorbital notch.[23] To effectively block these nerves' sensory distribution, a few milliliters of local anesthetic can be infiltrated around their points of exit from the orbit. When injecting the local anesthetic, anesthesia providers should always aspirate before injecting to minimize the risk of an intravascular injection, because these nerves also run with blood vessels (Figure 5-3).

The motor nerve supply to the eyelids and ocular adnexa is from the seventh cranial nerve—the facial nerve—which exits the stylomastoid foramen behind the ramus of the jaw and then courses through the parotid gland. It divides into five branches: temporal, zygomatic, buccal, mandibular, and cervical. The temporal and zygomatic branches innervate the orbicularis muscle of the upper and lower lid respectively, allowing for full lid closure. Blocking lid closure can allow complete examination in a patient with excessive blepharospasm and can facilitate safer surgery by minimizing squeezing, which can increase IOP.[24]

Block Techniques for the Seventh Nerve Supply

Several techniques can be used to block the seventh cranial nerve supply to the orbicularis muscle (Figure 5-4). The modified van Lint method is performed by placing a needle approximately 1 cm lateral to the lateral orbital rim. The needle is directed in the suborbicularis plane, and anesthetic agent is injected perpendicularly to the skull above the pe-

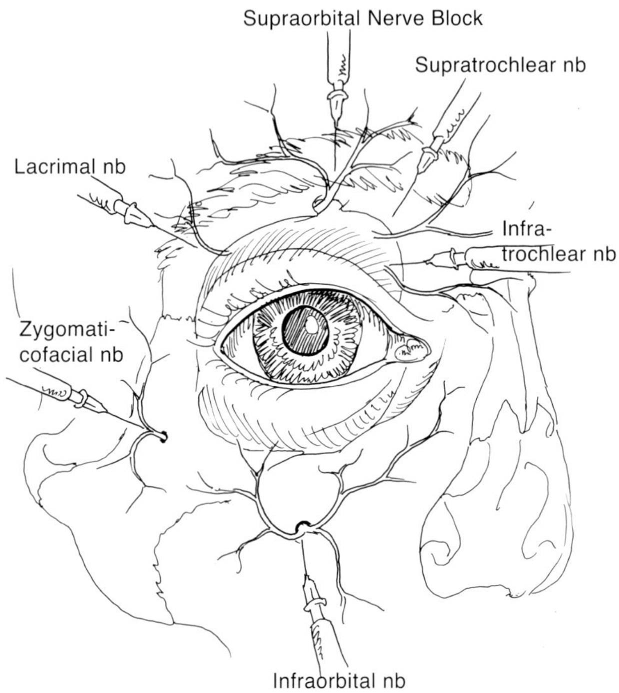

Fig. 5-3. This drawing illustrates the locations that would be used to administer the various ocular adnexal nerve blocks. When administering the blocks it is important to remember that each nerve is also accompanied by vasculature. To avoid intravascular injections of local anesthetic, one should pull back on the syringe before injection to ensure that blood return does not occur and that the needle is not within a blood vessel. Drawing prepared for this textbook by Gary Wind, MD, Uniformed Services University of the Health Sciences, Bethesda, Md.

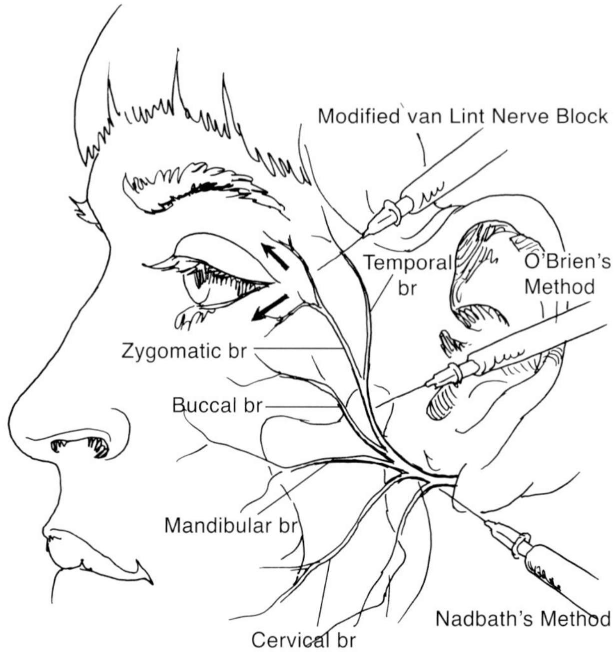

Fig. 5-4. The drawing illustrates both (1) the course of the branches of the seventh cranial nerve, which provides the motor function for the face and for eyelid closure, and (2) the location of the various seventh nerve blocks. The modified van Lint block is the most distal nerve block and causes only eyelid closure weakness. O'Brien's method and Nadbath's method are more proximal and cause increaced facial weakness in addition to eyelid weakness. Drawing prepared for this textbook by Gary Wind, MD, Uniformed Services University of the Health Sciences, Bethesda, Md.

riosteum. The needle is then directed in a cephalad and caudad direction while more anesthetic is injected to block the terminal branches of the seventh nerve and avoid blocking other facial muscles. The disadvantages of this method include pain on injection and the possibility of bruising and swelling of the eyelids.

O'Brien's method involves injecting local anesthetic agent just anterior to the tragus of the ear, below the posterior portion of the zygomatic process, and directly over the condyloid process of the mandible. A short needle is used; it goes straight inward until the bony condyloid process is felt, usually 1 cm deep. Two to six milliliters of local anesthetic is injected.[25] The disadvantage of this block is that an incomplete block or a failed block is possible because of variations in the course of the branches of the seventh nerve.

The Nadbath method results in complete hemifacial akinesia because the injection is given over the main trunk of the seventh nerve. The needle is inserted behind the posterior border of the ramus of the mandible in front of the mastoid process. Having the patient open his or her mouth widely can help identify this space. A short needle is advanced in an anterocephalad direction. Three to five milliliters of local anesthetic is injected.[25] Potential complications of this block include hoarseness, dysphagia, pooling of secretions, laryngospasm, respiratory distress, and agitation. These effects are believed to be due to the close proximity of other cranial nerves, including the vagus and glossopharyngeal nerves.[24] This block is usually not needed in the setting of ocular trauma management because paralysis of the lower facial muscles is usually not necessary.

Retrobulbar Block

The retrobulbar block has been used successfully for more than 80 years in intraocular surgery. It can effectively cause globe akinesia and anesthesia by

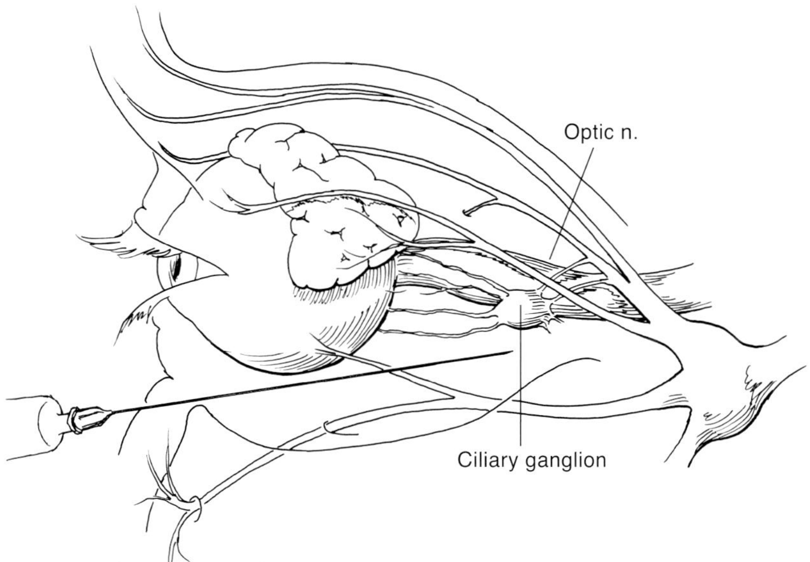

Fig. 5-5. This drawing illustrates the course of the retrobulbar needle during a retrobulbar block. It also illustrates the final position of the needle within the intraconal space. This block will effectively paralyze all the extraocular muscles that receive their nerve supply from within the intraconal space. The only muscle spared is the superior oblique muscle, as it receives its nerve supply from outside the intraconal space. Care must be taken while performing this block not to damage the eye or the optic nerve. Drawing prepared for this textbook by Gary Wind, MD, Uniformed Services University of the Health Sciences, Bethesda, Md.

blocking the sensory and motor nerve supply of the intraconal space. However, in the trauma setting it must *only* be used when there is assurance that the globe is not ruptured. If such a block is performed in the setting of an open globe, the pressure used to inject the anesthetic into the orbit can cause extrusion of the intraocular contents.

The retrobulbar block is performed by inserting a 25- or 27-gauge, 1.5-in. needle through the skin of the lower lid directly above the orbital floor at the border of the lateral limbus. The needle is advanced until it has passed the equator of the globe, then it is directed upward and medially to place the tip within the muscle cone (Figure 5-5). Approximately 4 mL of local anesthetic is injected. A 50/50 mixture of 2% lidocaine without epinephrine and 0.75% bupivacaine is commonly used. Often 15 to 20 U of hyaluronidase per milliliter of local anesthetic is added to facilitate diffusion of the local.

The classic Atkinson method called for the patient to look upward and medially while the block was being given. This method has fallen out of favor because several studies have shown that such an eye position places the optic nerve closer to the path of the needle.[25] Most ophthalmologists now have the patient look straight ahead.

Several complications have been reported after retrobulbar anesthesia. Although rare, serious complications, including blindness and death, have occurred. This method should be used only if there is no risk of an open globe injury. If an open globe is even suspected, then general anesthesia should be used. The complications of retrobulbar anesthesia include direct injection of anesthesia into the sheath of the optic nerve, causing blindness from anesthetic toxicity or direct trauma to the nerve. Direct injection into the optic nerve sheath can also cause brainstem anesthesia with respiratory collapse if the anesthetic agent travels to the CNS. Retrobulbar hemorrhages have also been reported that can lead to an orbital compartment syndrome with increased IOP and optic nerve compression. Finally, globe perforation has been reported with resultant retinal detachment and blindness from anesthetic toxicity to the retina.[24]

Several techniques—including peribulbar and parabulbar anesthesia—have been developed since the mid to late 1970s to minimize such complications. In peribulbar anesthesia, an injection is given below the globe in a fashion similar to the technique for retrobulbar anesthesia, except that the needle is not directed upward and inward and more anesthetic agent is injected. This injection is sometimes supplemented with another injection above the globe and below the supraorbital notch. Parabulbar anesthesia is given in the sub-Tenon's fascia plane with a blunt cannula. Unfortunately, complication rates have not diminished significantly, and these alternative blocks do not provide the same level of akinesia as the retrobulbar block does.

MONITORED ANESTHESIA CARE

Monitored anesthesia care (MAC) involves the use of intravenous sedation and analgesia with noninvasive monitoring during a surgical case also involving local anesthetics. MAC has several advantages over straight local anesthesia and general anesthesia. Two major advantages over local anesthesia are the following[26]:

1. MAC's ability to reduce the anxiety of the patient by providing some amnesia and by providing for noninvasive monitoring, which allows the surgeons to concentrate solely on the task at hand while the anesthesiologist delivers the sedation and monitors vital signs; and
2. conversion to general anesthesia is readily available if needed.

The major advantages of MAC over general anesthesia are the following[26]:

1. it is less stressful to the normal body physiology and
2. recovery time is shorter.

Ideally, MAC is used when the patient has had nothing to eat for at least 6 hours. In the trauma setting, a full stomach is assumed so the same techniques described in the preoperative management section to minimize gastric contents should be used if MAC is to be employed.

The most common sedatives used for MAC (Exhibit 5-1) include benzodiazepines (eg, midazolam), narcotics (eg, fentanyl), and other agents (eg, propofol). Benzodiazepines act primarily on the CNS and produce sedation, retrograde amnesia, anxiolysis, and muscle relaxation. These drugs are metabolized in the liver and must be used with care in patients with underlying liver disease. Hypotension and respiratory depression may occur, especially when benzodiazepines are used in combination with narcotics.[27] Midazolam is a widely used benzodiazepine because of its short half-life and because it produces little irritation at the injection site. When administered intravenously, sedation occurs within 3 to 5 minutes. Its peak sedation is seen in about 30 minutes and lasts for approximately 2 hours. It is usually given in small doses starting at 1 mg because the respiratory depressant effects may not manifest immediately.[28] Flumazenil, a newly available benzodiazepine antagonist, can be used to reverse the sedation and respiratory depression caused by agents like midazolam. The recommended dose is 0.2 mg/min, intravenously, with a maximum dose of 3 mg within an hour.[12] After administration of flumazenil, patients should be monitored for at least 2 hours because of the risk of resedation.

Often, a benzodiazepine is given in conjunction with a narcotic such as fentanyl. The main effect sought with the narcotic is analgesia. Narcotics, however, also cause respiratory depression and decreased gastrointestinal motility and nausea. Vital signs must be closely monitored when narcotics are used with or without other agents. Fentanyl is short-acting, with onset of action within 2 minutes. If respiratory depression occurs, assisted ventilation may be required with naloxone. Naloxone is an effective opioid antagonist that is routinely used in doses of 0.1 to 0.2 mg, intravenously, to reverse opioid-induced sedation and respiratory depression.[12] Naloxone can produce its own cardiovascular side effects,

EXHIBIT 5-1

RECOMMENDED DOSAGES OF SELECTED SEDATIVES AND ANALGESICS

Oral
- Diazepam 0.2 mg/kg
- Lorazepam 1–4 mg
- Midazolam 0.3–0.8 mg/kg

Intramuscular
- Diazepam 0.2 mg/kg
- Midazolam 0.07–0.30 mg/kg
- Methohexital 8–10 mg/kg
- Meperidine 1–2 mg/kg
- Morphine Sulfate 0.1–0.2 mg/kg

Intravenous
- Fentanyl 0.5–2.0 µg/kg
- Meperidine 0.5–1.5 mg/kg
- Morphine sulfate 0.05–0.10 mg/kg
- Methohexital 50–1,000 µg/kg load, 15–50 µg/kg/min infusion
- Midazolam 50–100 µg/kg load, 0.6–2.0 µg/kg/min infusion
- Propofol 250–1,000 µg/kg load, 25–75 µg/kg/min infusion

including hypertension, hypotension, acute pulmonary edema, and dysrhythmia. Additionally, patients must be monitored for resedation.

A newer, short-acting sedative–hypnotic that has been found to be extremely useful for MAC is propofol. After injection, hypnosis is usually induced with only one pass through the CNS and takes effect within 2 minutes. Patients are usually wide awake several minutes after a single bolus is given.[28] Propofol can also be given as a continuous drip to maintain sedation throughout a procedure. The usual dosage for MAC is a slow infusion of 0.5 mg/kg over 3 to 5 minutes followed by 1.5 to 4.5 mg/kg/h if continued sedation is desired. The major adverse side effects of propofol include respiratory depression and hypotension. Vital signs must be monitored closely during its use, and ventilatory support should be immediately available.

GENERAL ANESTHESIA

General endotracheal anesthesia is commonly used to provide adequate and safe anesthesia for a patient with multisystem trauma. It is also the only technique available for patients with open globe injuries or presumed globe rupture. The objectives in a patient with an open globe injury include overall patient safety, maintenance of decreased extraocular muscle tone, avoidance of elevation of intraocular volume, and avoidance of external pressure on the eye.[10] As has been discussed above, all trauma patients must be treated as full-stomach encounters and should be pretreated as outlined.

Induction of Anesthesia

The induction of anesthesia, the most critical period of anesthetic management, is encountered after pretreatment. A rapid-sequence induction technique is usually chosen to minimize the risk of aspiration. Nevertheless, each step must be evaluated for its effect on ocular pressure to minimize the risk of extruding the intraocular contents. Several basic techniques are widely accepted to minimize risk during such inductions. The debate continues, however, over the selection and use of neuromuscular blocking agents for facilitating intubation. Widely accepted techniques include the following[29]:

- preoxygenation with care to avoid pressure on the eye from the face mask,
- cricoid pressure during intubation to prevent regurgitation,
- establishment of a deep enough level of anesthesia prior to laryngoscopy to prevent coughing and sudden increases in arterial blood pressure, and
- controlled ventilation after intubation to avoid hypercapnia-associated increases in IOP.

Which neuromuscular blocking agent should be used during induction? The controversy centers mostly on the transient increase in IOP noted with the use of depolarizing agents such as succinylcholine. This effect is due to the initial contraction of the extraocular muscles, which can increase IOP about 8 mm Hg.[10] More-recent clinical studies have challenged the aversion to using depolarizing agents in open globes.[30] Two major disadvantages should be kept in mind when using a very fast-acting agent such as succinylcholine[10]:

1. If a nondepolarizing agent, with its delayed onset, is used, then coughing and straining may occur if intubation is attempted before complete blockade is achieved.
2. Conversely, if enough time is left to ensure complete blockade, then the airway is left unprotected in a situation in which the casualty may well have a full stomach.

Many techniques have been developed to overcome these inherent problems. The techniques include[29]

1. using large doses of nondepolarizing agent to hasten onset,
2. using a priming dose of nondepolarizing agent followed by a larger dose, and
3. pretreatment with a nondepolarizing agent followed by a barbiturate–succinylcholine sequence.

All three techniques have met with variable results, and globe rupture should no longer be considered an absolute contraindication to the use of succinylcholine. The specific muscle relaxant and technique to be used should be decided by the anesthesiologist on a case-by-case basis.

Maintaining Anesthesia

Once the induction is complete, maintenance of adequate anesthesia becomes the next priority. Extraocular muscle tone must be kept to a minimum to keep IOP low, and straining and bucking that can increase choroidal congestion must be minimized by deep anesthesia. Deep anesthesia can usually be achieved with an inhalational agent, narcotics, or muscle relaxants titrated to an appropriate response on the neuromuscular function monitor.[29]

Inhalational Agents

Several inhalational agents are available, including the halogenated hydrocarbons (sevoflurane, desflurane, halothane, enflurane, and isoflurane) and nitrous oxide. Often, nitrous oxide is combined with one of the other agents to decrease their relative concentrations and minimize side effects.[10] Each has its own advantages and disadvantages; the choice of which agent to use is best left to the anesthesiologist. Other factors that must be continually assessed during anesthesia maintenance are the effects of the anesthetic agents and other adjuvant medications on IOP.

Inhalational anesthetics all cause dose-related decreases in IOP.[31] The exact mechanisms are unknown, but possible etiologies include depression of a CNS control center, reduction of aqueous humor production, enhancement of aqueous humor outflow, and relaxation of the extraocular muscles.[31]

There is, however, one situation in which nitrous oxide must be used with caution. To facilitate retinal detachment repair, an intraocular gas bubble may be injected as a tamponade for retinal tears. Agents used include sulfur hexafloride and octafluoropropane. These agents are relatively insoluble and slowly increase in size over several days. Nitrous oxide can also fill the vitreous cavity intraoperatively. Nevertheless, its solubility coefficient allows for a more rapid increase in volume and a more rapid liberation from the vitreous. This phenomenon presents two possible problems if nitrous oxide is used concomitantly with one of the other agents:

1. an inadequate fill of the tamponading agent, because the nitrous oxide fills some of the space in the vitreous cavity; when the nitrous oxide is then liberated postoperatively, an inadequate tamponade can result; and
2. an intraoperative rise in IOP, which results from the rapid expansion of the nitrous oxide bubble filling the vitreous cavity, in addition to the other agent used.

To prevent these problems, it is recommended that if nitrous oxide is used, it should be turned off at least 15 minutes before the gas is injected into the eye. Furthermore, if a reoperation is required after intraocular gas injection, then nitrous oxide should be avoided for 5 days after an injection of air and for 10 days following the injection of sulfur hexafluoride.[32]

Anesthetics and Intraocular Pressure

Other agents influence IOP, too. The CNS depressants (eg, barbiturates, neuroleptics, opioids, tranquilizers, hypnotics, propofol) all seem to lower IOP. Ketamine, on the other hand, appears to be able to increase the pressure; one study,[31] using indentation tonometry, showed a rise in pressure, although subsequent studies have not always corroborated this finding. Nonetheless, ketamine should be used with caution if an open globe is present or suspected because of its possible role in increasing pressure and because it has also been shown to induce nystagmus and blepharospasm.[31]

Hypertonic solutions (eg, mannitol, dextran, urea, sorbitol), when administered intravenously, all increase plasma oncotic pressure and, thereby, decrease IOP. These agents may produce acute intravascular volume overload, which can place a heavy workload on the heart and kidneys. Hypertension, prolonged diuresis, and dilution of plasma sodium may result. Acetazolamide is a carbonic anhydrase inhibitor; its administration interferes with the sodium pump. The resultant decrease in aqueous humor formation leads to decreased IOP. Its action is not limited to the eye, and systemic effects include loss of sodium, potassium, and water secondary to renal tubular effects. Such electrolyte imbalances can then increase the risk of cardiac dysrhythmias during general anesthesia.[31]

Medications are not the only factors that influence IOP. Ventilatory status and temperature can also affect the pressure within the eye. Hyperventilation decreases IOP, whereas asphyxia, increased levels of carbon dioxide, and hypoventilation have all been shown to increase IOP.[31] Hypothermia decreases IOP secondary to decreased aqueous humor formation from vasoconstriction and the subsequent decrease in ocular blood flow.[31]

Ramifications of Ophthalmic Interventions for Anesthesia Care

The preceding discussion illustrates how actions taken by anesthesia providers can alter the work environment of the ophthalmologist by influencing IOP. The reverse can also be true when surgical maneuvers or medications given by the ophthalmologist force changes in the anesthetic care provided. One common occurrence is the initiation of the oculocardiac reflex, which is triggered by pressure on the globe or manipulation of the extraocular muscles. This can lead to bradycardia or other serious dysrhythmias, including junctional rhythm, atrioventricular blockade, premature ventricular contractions, ventricular tachycardia, and asystole. This reflex has its afferent limb along the trigeminal nerve and its efferent limb along the vagus nerve. The reflex may appear with the use of any anesthetic technique; however, it is more prevalent with hypoxemia, hypercarbia, and inappropriate anesthetic depth.[31]

Retrobulbar blocks may decrease the incidence of the oculocardiac reflex; however, the administration of the block itself will occasionally *cause* the reflex.[33] If ocular manipulation causes bradycardia or another dysrhythmia, the first step is to have the surgeon stop the surgical maneuver. The patient's anesthetic depth and ventilatory status are then evaluated. The heart rate will usually return to normal within 20 seconds after these measures are instituted. Repeated manipulation of the eye has been shown to decrease the recurrence of the reflex secondary to fatigue of the reflex arc at the level of the cardioinhibitory center.[33] If, however, the initial dysrhythmia was significant or if the reflex continues to recur, the treatment of choice is intravenous atropine. Additionally, careful monitoring of the intraoperative electrocardiogram must be maintained throughout the surgical case.

Several medications that the ophthalmologist administers have the potential for undesirable systemic effects and deleterious anesthetic implications. Topical ophthalmic preparations can be significantly absorbed through the conjunctiva or nasal mucosa after drainage through the nasolacrimal duct. To minimize this, patients can be instructed to occlude the nasolacrimal sac with pressure on the inner canthus of the eye after the administration of a drop. The anesthesiologist must continually monitor for undesirable effects and potential drug interactions.

Acetylcholine is a medication commonly used intraocularly to produce miosis after the lens is removed. The local use of this drug may occasionally result in bradycardia, increased salivation, increased bronchial secretions, bronchospasm, and hypotension. If these occur and require treatment, they can be reversed with intravenous atropine.[31] Echothiophate is a long-acting anticholinesterase and is used to treat chronic glaucoma. When used for more than 1 month, it can decrease plasma pseudocholinesterase activity by 95%, and its effects can last for 4 to 6 weeks even after cessation of the drug.[31] Both succinylcholine and ester local anesthetics are metabolized by plasma pseudocholinesterases, so if either of these is used, ophthalmologists should expect a longer-than-normal duration of action. This phenomenon can lead to prolonged apnea even with usual doses of succinylcholine.

Phenylephrine is commonly used to dilate the pupil. It has α-adrenergic effects that can cause hypertension, headache, tachycardia, and myocardial ischemia. These side effects are rare if the 2.5% solution is used, but they occur more commonly when the 10% solution is used. Caution should be used in the elderly and those with preexisting coronary artery disease to avoid problems. The topical β-blockers are medications commonly used to treat patients with glaucoma. They are contraindicated in patients who have obstructive pulmonary disease, congestive heart failure, preexisting bradycardia, and greater than first-degree heart block.

Cocaine, which was discussed earlier as a topical anesthetic, must be used with care during general anesthesia. Acetazolamide and mannitol, discussed earlier in regard to their being administered by the anesthesiologist, are also frequently used by ophthalmologists to lower IOP. If they are given intraoperatively, the same precautions that were discussed previously must be used to avoid problems.

Anesthetic Emergence

The importance of the anesthetic induction has already been discussed. Another important stage in the care of the traumatized eye is the anesthetic emergence. During emergence, the patient's IOP is likely to increase. Although the adverse consequences of this stage on the repaired eye are less important than for the open globe, coughing, straining, and vomiting during this stage can cause intraocular or orbital bleeding that can jeopardize the results of the surgery. Lidocaine (1.5 mg/kg, intravenously) may attenuate these responses to emergence and extubation.[10]

Shivering after anesthesia can increase IOP and should be treated by warming the patient.[34] Another method for reducing shivering is to administer a small dose of meperidine or hydroxyzine. Methods to minimize postoperative nausea and vomiting are discussed later in this chapter. During transportation to the recovery room, patients should be kept in a head-up position to facilitate venous drainage from the eye and the orbit. Postoperative hypertension may develop in some patients, owing to anxiety, pain, or urinary retention, and should be treated promptly to prevent straining and elevated eye pressure. Finally, patients who are either blind or bilaterally patched may need psychological support from the recovery room staff and physicians involved in the case.

ANESTHESIA COMPLICATIONS

Major risks of general anesthesia include cardiovascular collapse, allergic or anaphylactic reactions, and malignant hyperthermia. The first two can also occur after the administration of local anesthesia or during MAC. Luckily, such complications are rare, especially if an adequate preoperative assessment is performed. There are also a number of ocular complications from general anesthesia, including corneal abrasions, hemorrhagic retinopathy, retinal ischemia, and periocular nerve compression. Each is discussed here, with an emphasis on prevention.

Allergic Reactions

Allergic reactions may occur from any of the anesthetic agents discussed so far. For local anesthetics, such reactions are typically characterized by pruritus, urticaria, and edema at the site of the injection. Coughing and wheezing may also be present, but if the cardiovascular system is maintained, the reaction can usually be treated with either oral or intramuscular diphenhydramine. The oral dose for an adult is 50 mg, and the intramuscular dose for an adult is 10 to 50 mg, depending on the severity of the reaction. Patients treated in this manner should be observed for at least 6 hours to ensure that their status does not worsen.[12]

If the allergic symptoms occur with cardiovascular collapse, the reaction is considered to be anaphylaxis and requires immediate care. Treatment includes immediate cessation of the drug, volume expansion with intravenous normal saline, and intramuscular or intravenous epinephrine. Oxygen and intravenous aminophylline are administered to reduce the effects of bronchospasm.[12] Dysrhythmias are possible; their treatment is guided by the standards found in Advanced Cardiac Life Support protocols.[35]

Malignant Hyperthermia

A rare defect in muscle metabolism, malignant hyperthermia results in more generation of heat than the body can dissipate. It is inherited in an autosomal-dominant fashion with incomplete penetrance.[36] During the preoperative assessment, questions regarding family history of death under anesthesia should be raised. If a history exists and the cause is unclear, the clinician should be alerted to the possibility of malignant hyperthermia as the cause. Malignant hyperthermia is more common in children, in the Midwest, and in patients with a history of strabismus. It is incited most commonly by a combination of the use of succinylcholine and halogenated anesthetics.[36] Amide local anesthetic agents are usually safe in this setting.

Malignant hyperthermia is best managed by anticipation and prevention. Its earliest signs may be subtle and include tachycardia, darkening of the blood on the operative field, and masseter muscle rigidity. This can be followed by sweating, increased temperature, dramatic oxygen consumption, increased carbon dioxide production, muscle rigidity, cardiac dysrhythmias, unstable blood pressure, and death.[36] Treatment consists of immediate cessation of the agent presumed to be causing the problem and the administration of 100% oxygen. The patient may need to be cooled by gastric or rectal lavage with ice or ice water. Electrolyte imbalance, especially acidosis, is treated as needed. Intravenous dantrolene (2–10 mg/kg) is administered to stabilize calcium outflow from the sarcoplasmic reticulum, and procainamide is given to stabilize cardiac dysrhythmias.[12] If the preoperative assessment uncovers a possibility of malignant hyperthermia, then screening tests, including resting serum creatinine phosphokinase and muscle biopsy, can be ordered. Because these tests sometimes produce false positives or negatives, it is extremely important to carefully observe the patient during all phases of anesthesia.

Ocular Complications of Anesthesia

One of the most common ophthalmic complications of anesthesia is corneal abrasion. This can occur from direct trauma to the cornea from the anesthesia mask or surgical drapes, or can be the result of chemical injury from the surgical skin preparation solution. Prevention is the best management. The eyes should be closed during skin preparation. During the surgical procedure, the eye not being operated on should be taped closed with or without a bland petroleum-based ophthalmic ointment being applied. If a patient awakens from general anesthesia complaining of pain, tearing, foreign body sensation, or photophobia, a corneal abrasion should be suspected. If confirmed on examination, prophylactic antibiotic ointment should be applied until healing has occurred.

Hemorrhagic retinopathy can occur in otherwise healthy patients during turbulent emergence from anesthesia or if protracted vomiting occurs after anesthesia.[37] It is commonly called Valsalva retinopathy and is related to increased intrathoracic pressure that is transmitted to the ocular vasculature, leading to intraocular bleeding. The bleeding is usually from the venous side and is found in front of the retina beneath the internal limiting membrane. Visual loss is noted if the hemorrhage is in front of the macula or if the hemorrhage breaks through the internal limiting membrane and causes a vitreous hemorrhage. Luckily, most of these hemorrhages are self-limiting and resolve completely in several weeks. Intervention is rarely required unless a vitreous hemorrhage does not clear, and a vitrectomy is needed.

Retinal ischemia and infarction also may result from direct ocular trauma secondary to pressure on the globe. The pressure can be from an ill-fitting anesthesia mask or from excessive force on the globe during surgical manipulation. Care must also be taken if the patient is positioned prone to make sure that external pressure is not being placed on the eye. External pressure on the eye is even more dangerous if systemic hypotension is present.[37] Finally, retinal infarction can occur from emboli during cardiac or vascular surgery. Such emboli can also lead to optic nerve damage as well.

Periorbital nerve compression is most likely secondary to poor positioning of the patient in the prone or jackknife position or excessive pressure from the face mask. Care must be taken to prevent excessive pressure on the orbital rims and to ensure adequate padding. The supraorbital, supratrochlear, and infraorbital nerves are at risk for this complication, which can lead to postoperative numbness and swelling. These symptoms usually resolve without intervention, but several weeks may be needed for full recovery.

POSTOPERATIVE PAIN AND NAUSEA MANAGEMENT

The goal of postoperative analgesia is to maximize pain control while minimizing the side effects of the analgesic agent. The most common side effects of analgesia are sedation, nausea, and vomiting. Most ophthalmic procedures do not lead to significant amounts of pain. However, in the patient with multisystem trauma, severe pain may be caused by the repair of injuries in other areas than the head and neck region. For these areas, the use of strong narcotics (intravenous or intramuscular) may be necessary. If surgery of only the head and neck is performed, often acetaminophen alone or acetaminophen combined with an oral narcotic is enough.

Ice-Cold Compresses

One easy postoperative pain control method that is often overlooked is the liberal use of ice. Cold (ice) compresses not only decrease pain, they also minimize bleeding and swelling by causing vasoconstriction, which prevents the egress of transudate.[12] Packs of crushed ice are better than ice cubes because crushed ice conforms better to the shape of the body. Ice-cold compresses should be used for 10 minutes four times a day for the first 48 to 72 hours.

Narcotics

Narcotics are commonly used analgesics and can be used orally, intramuscularly, or intravenously, depending on the severity of the pain. Oral opioids have a slower onset of action but provide longer pain relief. In addition to their analgesic properties, however, opioids have several other effects that ophthalmologists should keep in mind, including decreased gastrointestinal motility, respiratory depression, orthostatic hypotension, pupillary miosis, nausea, and vomiting.[12]

Commonly used narcotics include morphine, meperidine, codeine, and oxycodone. Morphine is usually reserved for severe pain when it is used either intramuscularly or intravenously. The usual dose is 2 to 10 mg every 4 to 6 hours as needed. Meperidine is also usually reserved for severe pain and can be given in doses of 50 to 100 mg, intramuscularly, every 4 to 6 hours as needed. If the pain is moderate, oral doses of codeine or oxycodone can

TABLE 5-2

ANTIEMETICS FOR NAUSEA AND VOMITING AFTER OPHTHALMIC SURGERY

Antiemetic	Dose (mg)	Duration (h)	Drug Category and Side Effects
Metoclopramide	10	1–2	Dopamine antagonist Extrapyramidal reactions Abdominal cramping
Droperidol	0.625–2.500	3–6	Dopamine antagonist Extrapyramidal reactions Sedation Dysphoria
Ondansetron	1–8 (4)	4	5-HT3 antagonist Headache Dizziness Muscle pains
Dolasetron	12.5	8	5-HT3 antagonist ECG interval changes (PR, QRS) Headache Dizziness Muscle pain
Prochlorperazine	5–10	3–4	Phenothiazine Extrapyramidal reactions Neuroleptic malignant syndrome Sedation Hypotension
Perphenazine	1–5	6–24	Phenothiazine Extrapyramidal reactions Neuroleptic malignant syndrome Sedation Hypotension
Promethazine	12.5–50.0	4–6	Phenothiazine Extrapyramidal reactions Neuroleptic malignant syndrome Sedation (less so) Hypotension
Chlorpromazine	12.5–50.0, administered *slowly*	2–4	Phenothiazine Hypotension Sedation Extrapyramidal reactions Neuroleptic malignant syndrome

Sources: (1) Davidson JK, Eckhardt WF, Perese DA. *Clinical Anesthesia Procedures of the Massachusetts General Hospital,* 4th ed. Boston, Mass: Little, Brown; 1993. (2) Miller RD. *Anesthesia.* 4th ed. New York, NY: Churchill Livingstone; 1994. (3) Medical Economics Data. *Physicians' Desk Reference.* Montvale, NY: Medical Economics Co; 1998.

be used, usually in combination with acetaminophen. The effectiveness of codeine and acetaminophen combined is greater than if each agent were used alone.[12] The usual dose of codeine is 30 to 60 mg every 4 to 6 hours, and the usual dose of oxycodone is 5 to 10 mg every 4 to 6 hours as needed. If the pain is mild, acetaminophen alone may be all that is needed. The usual dose of acetaminophen is 325 to 650 mg, orally, every 4 to 6 hours as needed.

Antinausea and Antiemetic Agents

Postoperative nausea and vomiting can be caused by several different factors. One cause is the oculogastric reflex, whereby ocular manipulation, especially of the extraocular muscles, causes nausea and vomiting. This reflex is especially common after surgery for strabismus. Other causes of nausea and vomiting are the use of preoperative or intraoperative narcotics or their use in the postoperative period for analgesia. The detrimental effects of vomiting on IOP have already been discussed. For these reasons, the use of prophylactic antiemetics is important (Table 5-2). Metoclopramide is an H_1 (histamine) receptor and dopamine antagonist and can help, intraoperatively and postoperatively, decrease the incidence of nausea and vomiting. In addition to its antiemetic effect, metoclopramide also increases the tone of the lower esophageal sphincter and speeds gastric emptying, minimizing the risk of aspiration. The disadvantages of using metoclopramide include its side effect of dystonia, which occurs in 2% of the patients receiving it intravenously.[12] Drowsiness and anxiety can also occur. Metoclopramide is not available as a suppository, and, when used orally, it is less predictable and less effective secondary to metabolism in the liver before it becomes available systemically. Trimethobenzamide is another benzamide antiemetic in the same family as metoclopramide. It is available in suppository form, which is the major difference between it and metoclopramide.

Dopaminergic antagonists of the phenothiazine group include prochlorperazine and promethazine. Both are effective agents to manage postoperative nausea and vomiting. Neither drug increases the tone of the lower esophageal sphincter; thus, they do not influence the risk of aspiration.[12] Both agents have fairly high rates of dystonic reactions, however, and can cause hypotension if used parenterally. They can also cause pupillary dilation and should be used with care in patients with narrow-angle glaucoma.[12]

Droperidol is a butyrophenone with neuroleptic properties. It is an active antagonist at the dopamine receptor and is very useful in preventing nausea and vomiting, even in small doses. Droperidol may result in dyskinesia, restlessness, dysphoria, and hypotension.[38] To limit theses side effects, the lowest effective doses should be used, especially when the goal is prophylaxis.

Ondansetron selectively blocks serotonin receptors with little or no effect on dopamine receptors.[39] It is an effective antiemetic in the postoperative period. It is very expensive and, therefore, is not recommended for routine prophylaxis. Ondansetron is usually reserved for patients with a history of postoperative nausea and vomiting and for those undergoing procedures that often cause nausea and vomiting. Side effects other than pain on intravenous injection are rare, and the drug does not appear to cause sedation, extrapyramidal signs, or respiratory depression.[39]

SUMMARY

Ocular injuries account for a significant and growing percentage of combat injuries. To effectively care for these injuries, highly skilled eye surgery teams, well-versed in the most modern microsurgical techniques, are required. Anesthesia providers must be comfortable with the subtleties of administering anesthesia for ocular trauma, especially when an open globe is suspected or confirmed. The first step to providing such care is a thorough preoperative assessment. If there are ocular injuries that require anesthesia for further evaluation or definitive care, the optimal method must be chosen for the particular situation. The anesthetic choices include topical, local, MAC, and general endotracheal anesthesia.

Topical anesthesia is commonly used during the complete ophthalmic evaluation to determine IOPs, examine the nasolacrimal system and the nose, and perform forced duction testing. Commonly used topical agents include amide agents (eg, lidocaine) and ester agents (eg, proparacaine, tetracaine, and cocaine).

Local anesthesia is often used to repair ocular adnexal injuries, as well as soft-tissue facial injuries. Lidocaine and bupivacaine are amide local anesthetics that are often used in combination because the lidocaine has a quicker onset of action and the bupivacaine has a longer duration of action. Several adjuvant agents can be added to these local anesthetics to enhance their effectiveness. Epinephrine reduces bleeding and lengthens the duration of the neural blockade, but it can cause hypertension and tachycardia and must be used with caution in patients susceptible to these side effects.

There are several techniques available to adequately anesthetize the ocular adnexa. These techniques are usually a combination of subcutaneous regional infiltration, field block, and nerve block. Regional infiltration is the easiest of the techniques because it requires the least knowledge of the neuroanatomy of the ocular adnexa; field and nerve blocks, on the other hand, require a detailed understanding. Successful anesthesia can be achieved with blocks of the supraorbital, supratrochlear, infratrochlear, infraorbital, and lacrimal nerves.

In cases where more than local anesthesia is required, MAC can be used. MAC involves the use of intravenous sedation and analgesia with noninvasive monitoring in combination with local anesthetics. The most commonly used sedatives for MAC include benzodiazepines, narcotics, and propofol.

If a patient has multisystem trauma or if an open globe injury is present or suspected, general endotracheal anesthesia is usually required. Controversy exists about which neuromuscular blocking agents should be used during induction. Succinylcholine reportedly increases IOP and could cause extrusion of the intraocular contents, but it is not absolutely contraindicated. The decision to use succinylcholine must be made by the anesthesiologist on a case-by-case basis. Once induction is complete, extraocular muscle tone, straining, and bucking must be kept to a minimum as anesthesia is maintained, usually with one of the inhalational halogenated hydrocarbons and nitrous oxide.

During maintenance anesthesia, the effects of the anesthetic agents and other adjuvant medications on IOP must be continually assessed. All inhalational anesthetics cause dose-related decreases in IOP. One must also be vigilant for the oculocardiac reflex. It is usually the result of extraocular muscle manipulation and can result in bradycardia or asystole. To block or reverse the reflex, intravenous atropine should be used.

Emergence from anesthesia must also be handled smoothly to prevent uncontrolled increases in IOP. Intravenous lidocaine can be helpful to prevent coughing and straining during extubation. Keeping the patient warm can minimize shivering, which has also been shown to increase IOP.

There are several major risks of general anesthesia. Allergic reactions range from mild symptoms to full-blown anaphylaxis. Treatment includes cessation of use of the inciting agent, volume expansion, and the administration of oxygen and intravenous epinephrine. Malignant hyperthermia is another major risk. Its early presentation can be subtle and may include tachycardia and darkening of the blood on the surgical field. This phase can be followed by elevated body temperature, unstable blood pressure, and death. Treatment consists of immediate cessation of the inciting agent, the administration of oxygen and intravenous dantrolene, and correction of electrolyte imbalances.

General anesthesia can cause ophthalmic complications, as well. Corneal abrasions can occur from the anesthesia mask or from the surgical preparation solution. Hemorrhagic retinopathy can be the result of a turbulent emergence or postoperative vomiting. Retinal ischemia can result from external pressure on the globe. Finally, periorbital nerve compression can result from poor patient positioning or excessive pressure from the anesthesia mask.

Postoperative pain and nausea management is the final stage in successful anesthesia care. The goal is to maximize pain control while minimizing side effects. Commonly used narcotic analgesics include morphine, meperidine, codeine, and oxycodone. These agents may be administered orally, intramuscularly, or intravenously.

The oculogastric reflex can lead to vomiting, especially after extraocular muscle manipulation. Prophylactic antiemetics minimize the risk of vomiting, which can elevate IOP. Metoclopramide, a widely used antiemetic, increases the tone of the lower esophageal sphincter and speeds gastric emptying.

When ocular trauma is identified on the battlefield, the eye care team must be ready to act. Ophthalmologists and anesthesiologists must be willing to work together to optimize the care provided. Only through attention to detail and adherence to the techniques described in this chapter can risk to the injured eye be minimized before, during, and after the repair.

REFERENCES

1. Wong TY, Seet B, Ang CL. Eye injuries in twentieth century warfare: A historical perspective. *Surv Ophthalmol*. 1997;41:433–459.

2. Treister G. Ocular casualties in the Six-Day War. *Am J Ophthalmol*. 1969;68:669–673.

3. Steindorf K. Die kriegschirurgie des schorganz. *Berlin Klin Wochenschr.* 1914;51:1787–1789.

4. Stone W. Ocular injuries in the armed forces. *JAMA.* 1950;142:151–152.

5. Reister FA. *Medical Statistics in World War II.* Washington, DC: Office of The Surgeon General; 1975: 330–331; 387–389.

6. Reister FA. *Battle Casualties and Medical Statistics, US Army Experience in the Korean War*. Washington, DC: Office of The Surgeon General; 1973: 48.

7. Belkin M, Treister G, Doton S. Eye injuries and ocular protection in the Lebanon War, 1982. *Isr J Med Sci.* 1984;20:333–338.

8. Hornblass A. Eye injuries in the military. *Int Ophthalmol Clin*. 1981;21:121–138.

9. Zajtchuk R, Grande CM, eds. *Anesthesia and Perioperative Care of the Combat Casualty.* In: Zajtchuk R, Bellamy RF, eds. *Textbook of Military Medicine*. Washington, DC: Department of the Army, Office of The Surgeon General, Borden Institute; 1995.

10. Capan LM, Mankikar D, Eisenberg WM. Anesthetic management of ocular injuries. In: Capan LM, Miller SM, Turndorf H, eds. *Trauma Anesthesia and Intensive Care*. Philadelphia, Pa: JB Lippincott Company; 1991: 372–384.

11. Parris WCV, Kambam JR, Flanagan JFK, Elliott J. The effects of metoclopramide on intraocular pressure. *Anesth Analg*. 1987;66:S135.

12. Bilyk JR, Sutula FC. Anesthesia for ophthalmic plastic surgery. In: Stewart WB, ed. *Surgery of the Eyelid, Orbit, and Lacrimal System.* Vol 1. San Francisco, Calif: American Academy of Ophthalmology; 1993: 26–57.

13. Bruce RA. Local anesthetics. In: Bruce RA, McGoldrick KE, Oppengeimer P, eds. *Anesthesia for Ophthalmology*. Birmingham, Ala: Aesculapius Publishing Co; 1982: 27–33.

14. Bennett RG. Anesthesia. In: Bennett RG, ed. *Fundamentals of Cutaneous Surgery*. St Louis, Mo: Mosby; 1988: 194–239.

15. Ritchie JM, Greene NM. Local anesthetics. In: Gilman AG, Rall TW, Neis AS, Taylor P, eds. *Goodman and Gilman's The Pharmacological Basis of Therapeutics*. 8th ed. New York, NY: Pergamon Press; 1990: 311–331.

16. Libonati MM. General anesthesia. In: Tasman WE, Jaeger EA, eds. *Duane's Clinical Ophthalmology*. Vol 5. Philadelphia, Pa: JB Lippincott Co; 1991; Chap 12.

17. Carpenter RL, Mackey DC. Local anesthetics. In: Barash PG, Cullen BF, Stoelting RK, eds. *Clinical Anesthesia.* 3rd ed. Philadelphia, Pa: Lippincott-Raven; 1997: 413–440.

18. Morris RW, Whish DKM. A controlled trial of pain on skin infiltration with local anesthetics. *Anaesth Intensive Care*. 1984;12:113–114.

19. McCracken JS. Major ambulatory surgery of the ophthalmic patient. *Surg Clin North Am*. 1987;67:881–889.

20. Dolsky RL, Fetzek J, Anderson R. Evaluation of blood loss during lipo-suction surgery. *American Journal of Cosmetic Surgery.* 1987;4:257–261.

21. McKay W, Morris R, Mushlin P. Sodium bicarbonate attenuates pain on skin infiltration with lidocaine, with or without epinephrine. *Anesth Analg*. 1987;66:572–574.

22. Sullivan JH, Beard C. Anatomy of the eyelid, orbit, and lacrimal system. In: Stewart WB, ed. *Surgery of the Eyelid, Orbit, and Lacrimal System.* Vol 1. San Francisco, Calif: American Academy of Ophthalmology; 1993: 84–99.

23. Bruce RA. Regional anesthetic techniques. In: Bruce RA, McGoldrick KE, Oppengeimer P, eds. *Anesthesia for Ophthalmology*. Birmingham, Ala: Aesculapius Publishing Co; 1982: 34–47.

24. Zahl K. Selection of techniques for regional blockade of the eye and adnexa. In: McGoldrick KE, ed. *Anesthesia for Ophthalmic and Otolaryngologic Surgery*. Philadelphia, Pa: WB Saunders Co; 1992: 235–247.

25. Greenbaum S. Anesthesia for cataract surgery. In: Greenbaum S, ed. *Ocular Anesthesia.* Philadelphia, Pa: WB Saunders Co; 1997: 1–56.

26. Wilson RP. Local anesthesia in ophthalmology. In: Tasman WE, Jaeger EA, eds. *Duane's Clinical Ophthalmology*. Vol 6. Philadelphia, Pa: JB Lippincott Co; 1991; Chap 2.

27. Bailey PL, Pace NL, Ashburn MA, Moll JWB, East KA, Stanley TH. Frequent hypoxemia and apnea after sedation with midazolam and fentanyl. *Anesthesiology*. 1990;73:826–830.

28. Biesman BS, Hornblass A. Anesthesia for oculoplastic surgery. In: Greenbaum S, ed. *Ocular Anesthesia*. Philadelphia, Pa: WB Saunders Co; 1997: 195–209.

29. McGoldrick KE. Anesthetics and intraocular pressure: Management of penetrating eye injuries. In: McGoldrick KE, ed. *Anesthesia for Ophthalmic and Otolaryngologic Surgery*. Philadelphia, Pa: WB Saunders Co; 1992: 183–189.

30. Libonati MM, Leahy JJ, Ellison N. Use of succinylcholine in open eye injury. *Anesthesiology*. 1985;62:637–640.

31. McGoldrick KE. Anesthesia and the eye. In: Barash PG, Cullen BF, Stoetling RK, eds. *Clinical Anesthesia*. 3rd ed. Philadelphia, Pa: Lippincott-Raven; 1997: 911–928.

32. McGoldrick KE. Anesthetic ramifications of ophthalmic drugs. In: McGoldrick KE, ed. *Anesthesia for Ophthalmic and Otolaryngologic Surgery*. Philadelphia, Pa: WB Saunders Co; 1992: 227–234.

33. Moonie GT, Rees DI, Elton D. Oculocardiac reflex during strabismus surgery. *Can Anaesth Soc J*. 1964;11:621.

34. Mahajan RP, Grover VK, Sharma SL, Singh H. Intraocular pressure changes during muscular hyperactivity after general anesthesia. *Anesthesiology*. 1987;66:419.

35. Cummins RO, ed. *Advanced Cardiac Life Support*. Dallas, Tex: American Heart Association; 1997: Chaps 1–17.

36. Ingraham HJ, Donnenfeld ED. Anesthesia for corneal surgery. In: Greenbaum S, ed. *Ocular Anesthesia*. Philadelphia, Pa: WB Saunders Co; 1997: 57–89.

37. McGoldrick KE. Ophthalmologic and systemic complications of surgery and anesthesia. In: McGoldrick KE, ed. *Anesthesia for Ophthalmic and Otolaryngologic Surgery*. Philadelphia, Pa: WB Saunders Co; 1997: 272–290.

38. Ostman PL, White PF. Outpatient anesthesia. In: Miller RD, ed. *Anesthesia*. 4th ed. New York, NY: Churchill Livingstone; 1994: 2213–2246.

39. Morgan GE, Maged SM. *Clinical Anesthesiology*. 2nd ed. Stamford, Conn: Appleton and Lange; 1996: 204.

Chapter 6

OCULAR TRAUMA SCALES

DARRYL J. AINBINDER, MD*; ROBERT A. MAZZOLI, MD†; WILLIAM R. RAYMOND IV, MD‡; ELIZABETH A. HANSEN, MD§; AND E. GLENN SANFORD, MD¥

*Lieutenant Colonel, Medical Corps, US Army; Director, Ophthalmic Oncology and Pathology; Staff, Ophthalmic Plastic, Reconstructive, and Orbital Surgery, Madigan Army Medical Center, Tacoma, Washington 98431-5000

†Colonel, Medical Corps, US Army; Chief and Chairman of Ophthalmology; Director, Ophthalmic Plastic, Reconstructive, and Orbital Surgery, Madigan Army Medical Center, Tacoma, Washington 98431-5000; Clinical Associate Professor of Surgery (Ophthalmology), Uniformed Services University of the Health Sciences, 4301 Jones Bridge Road, Bethesda, Maryland 20814-4799

‡Colonel, Medical Corps, US Army; Director, Pediatric Ophthalmology and Strabismus, Madigan Army Medical Center, Tacoma, Washington 98431-5000; Clinical Assistant Professor of Surgery (Ophthalmology), Uniformed Services University of the Health Sciences, 4301 Jones Bridge Road, Bethesda, Maryland 20814-4799

§Colonel, Medical Corps, US Army; Director, Comprehensive Ophthalmology, Madigan Army Medical Center, Tacoma, Washington 98431-5000; Clinical Assistant Professor of Surgery (Ophthalmology), Uniformed Services University of the Health Sciences, 4301 Jones Bridge Road, Bethesda, Maryland 20814-4799

¥Major, Medical Corps, US Army; Chief, Department of Ophthalmology, Blanchfield Army Community Hospital, Fort Campbell, Kentucky 42223-1498

INTRODUCTION

It is essential that we implement lessons learned from experienced military surgeons to improve surgical support for the injured soldier. Within this arena, ocular trauma scales may not appear to be as critical as, say, a discussion of the modern surgical approaches to treating an injury. However, trauma scales are a vital aspect of effective triage and focused readiness training. Trauma scales strengthen our readiness to restore soldiers with eye and orbital injuries by providing a triage framework for facilitating timely, accurate diagnoses and appropriate treatment. Trauma scales have also had a historical role of improving our ability to match injury patterns with the appropriate urgency of surgical support. We have realized the benefit of the Advanced Trauma Life Support (ATLS) system for soldiers with multiple trauma[1]; we must seek the same benefit to restore soldiers with sight-threatening injuries. Unit commanders can use the same database to recognize and prevent common injury patterns through the broad use of protective eye armor.

RATIONALE FOR USING TRAUMA SCALES

Efficient triage, initial stabilization, coordinated evacuation, and strong surgical team care are all vital elements of combat surgical support. An effective trauma scale can benefit each link in the chain. The Glasgow Coma Scale was introduced in 1974 as an evaluation tool for patients with severe head injuries.[2] This simple tool, with its index categories that include eye opening and verbal and motor evaluation, filled the need for a system that defined severe head trauma. The Glasgow Coma Scale provided a common language, and improved triage communication.

As with head trauma, prompt identification of severe ocular and orbital injuries is critical for reducing soldier morbidity and conserving military fighting strength. Because ocular and orbital injuries are frequently unrecognized or are obscured by other wounds, an effective triage tool is necessary so that sight-threatening injuries will not be overlooked. To rapidly identify soldiers with potentially vision-threatening wounds and to achieve broad use by field medics and other triage personnel, the ocular trauma scale must be simple and require little more than a penlight and a trained triage soldier.

The newly developed Madigan Eye and Orbit Trauma Scale (MEOTS)[3] achieves these objectives (Figure 6-1); the trauma index categories include vision, eyeball structure, proptosis, pupils, and motility. Although MEOTS has been applied effectively in a peacetime emergency room setting, its true value will not be completely validated until it has been used and evaluated in battlefield conditions.

Proper use of trauma scales requires a reference of common ocular trauma terms to clearly define the most common injury patterns. Significant works have provided a basic understanding of such terms as penetrating globe injuries, perforating injuries, and traumatic optic neuropathy. A standardized classification of ocular trauma is as important to military medicine as it is to the international ophthalmic community. The international classification presented in 1996 provided a simple anatomical scheme, which defined basic ocular injury patterns. The globe is consistently used as the tissue of reference, adding clarity to such terms as "penetration" or "perforation" (Table 6-1).[4] Under this system, a fragmentation injury with a corneal entrance wound and no exit wound would be identified as a penetrating ocular injury with a retained intraocular foreign body (IOFB). This system provides an effective classification for surgeons and command to review ocular injury patterns. The international Ocular Trauma Classification is useful for multivariate analyses of ocular injuries. However it does not provide a rapid numerical triage value for use on the battlefield, which is the main advantage of the MEOTS.

Ocular structures are at great risk in the modern battlefield. Severe ocular injuries represent 9% to 14% of total severe battlefield injuries. High-velocity, fragment injuries predominate, representing 78% of the serious ocular and adnexal injuries during the Persian Gulf War. But reported injuries greatly underestimate the number of soldiers who sustain corneal abrasions and superficial corneal foreign bodies (FBs).[5–7] Understanding the most common injury patterns is the first step toward implementing effective triage and, more important, encouraging command interest in injury prevention with eye armor.[8]

Ocular trauma scales and ocular trauma registries depend on lessons learned from previous conflicts to make clear progress toward improved readiness. These lessons have taught us that soldiers

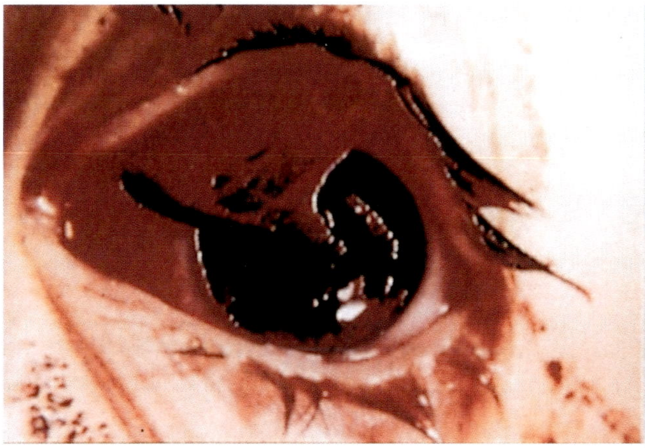

MADIGAN EYE & ORBIT TRAUMA SCALE

Index	Points	Standards
Vision:		
Small Print: 20/40	3	
Large Print: 20/100	2	
Count Fingers:	1	Urgent Referral
Less than CF:	0	Urgent Referral
Eyeball Structure:		
Eyeball structurally intact:	3	
Possible Violation eye, Low suspicion:	2	
Possible Violation eye, High suspicion:	1	Shield, Surg. Support*
Gross Violation of eye:	0	Shield, Surg. Support**

*Apply Fox shield and Seek Urgent Ophthalmic Surgical Support. Increase suspicion with lid laceration, distortion of pupil, alteration in ocular chamber depth, clinical history at risk for penetrating or blunt injury.
**Adult patients consider Cipro PO or IV, Prepare for surgery.

Index	Points	Standards
Proptosis: "Bulging"		
No displacement of eye	2	
Proptosis ≤ 3 mm	1	CT
Gross Proptosis > 3 mm, orbit Tense	0	Urgent, Steroid, CT**

**Lateral canthotomy, it a relative afferent pupil defect (APD) is present. High dose IV Steroids to reduce compression of optic nerve. Ophthalmic surgical support.

Index	Points	Standards
Pupils: Consider Neurosurgical & Ocular Trauma		
Equal, Reactive, No APD*	2	
Unequal or Possible APD	1	
Dilated pupil, Definite APD	0	Urgent, See proptosis

*(APD) Afferent Pupillary Defect (swinging light test)

Index	Points	Standards
Motility:		
No subjective or objective problem	2	
Double vision, or restriction	1	CT
Eyeball barely moves, "Frozen"	0	Urgent, CT, see proptosis

Overall Score: MAX 12

Patients with a total score ≤ 6 require urgent treatment to maintain sight. An initial score > 6 does not exclude a blinding injury. See Urgent referral guidelines listed above. *, ** All previous surgical support standards still apply.

Fig. 6-1. The Madigan Eye and Orbit Trauma Scale (MEOTS) was developed at Madigan Army Medical Center, Tacoma, Washington. The five categories on which the scale is based are Vision, Eyeball Structure, Proptosis, Pupils, and Motility (in red, above); each category has at least three criteria, for which "points" are assigned during an examination for trauma of the eye and orbit. The maximum overall score—the total points scored above—is the cumulative from all categories. Scores of 7 and above do not exclude a blinding injury; SCORES OF 6 AND LOWER REQUIRE URGENT TREATMENT.

should wear polycarbonate ballistic protective eyewear to prevent most injuries. Moreover, soldiers with sight-threatening injuries must be identified in the triage process so they can receive timely surgical care. Senior, experienced ophthalmologists with field operating surgical equipment should be positioned with head trauma teams so they can repair injuries that, if delayed, would have little potential for retained sight. These concepts are not new, reflecting the afteraction reviews of numerous ophthalmologists with experience spanning the years from the Vietnam War to the Persian Gulf War.[6,7,9]

Ocular trauma scales and trauma registries have many functions, including

- defining injury patterns,
- facilitating effective triage,
- improving surgical readiness,
- predicting visual prognosis, and
- serving as a critical command briefing element on the military perspective of ocular trauma.

Away from the battlefield, ocular trauma scales have prognostic counseling applications. Visual

TABLE 6-1

DEFINITIONS OF OCULAR TRAUMATOLOGY TERMS

Term	Definition	Comments
Eyewall	Sclera and cornea	Technically, the wall of the eye has three tunics (coats) posterior to the limbus; therefore, for clinical purposes, it is best to restrict the term "eyewall" to the rigid structures of the sclera and cornea.
Closed-globe injury	Eyewall does not have a full-thickness wound	Either there is no corneal or scleral wound at all (contusion) or it is only of partial thickness (lamellar laceration). Rarely, a contusion and a lamellar laceration coexist.*
Open-globe injury	Full-thickness wound of the eyewall	The cornea, the sclera, or both sustained a through-and-through injury. Depending on the inciting object's characteristics and the injury's circumstances, ruptures and lacerations are distinguished. The choroid and the retina may be intact, prolapsed, or damaged.
Rupture	Full-thickness wound of the eyewall, caused by a blunt object; the impact results in momentary increase of the intraocular pressure and an inside-out injury mechanism	The eye is a ball filled with incompressible liquid; a blunt object with sufficient momentum creates energy transfer over a large surface area, greatly increasing intraocular pressure. The eyewall gives way at its weakest point, which may or may not be at the impact site. The actual wound is produced by an inside-out force; consequently, tissue herniation is very frequent and can be substantial.
Laceration	Full-thickness wound of the eyewall, usually caused by a sharp object; the wound occurs at the impact site by an outside-in mechanism	Further classification is based on whether an exit wound or an intraocular foreign body is also present. Occasionally, an object may create a posterior exit wound while remaining, at least partially, intraocular.
Penetrating injury	Single laceration of the eyewall, usually caused by a sharp object.	No exit wound has occurred. If more than one entrance wound is present, each must have been caused by a different agent.
Intraocular foreign body (IOFB) injury	Retained foreign object causing entrance laceration	Technically, an IOFB is a penetrating injury, but it is grouped separately because of the different clinical implications (treatment modality, timing, endophthalmitis rate, etc).
Perforating injury	Two full-thickness lacerations (entrance + exit) of the eyewall, usually caused by a sharp object or missile	The two wounds must have been caused by the same agent.

*The injury is so atypical that characterization is very difficult; the clinician should use his or her best judgment based on the information provided here.

Reproduced with permission from Kuhn F, Morris R, Witherspoon CD, Heimann K, Jeffers JB, Treister G. A standardized classification of ocular trauma. *Ophthalmology*. 1996;103:241.

outcomes and enucleation rates depend on the nature and extent of the injury as well as on the availability of surgical support. These factors are important to ensure command distribution of assets to areas where they will have the greatest impact. Soldiers with nonfatal, multitraumatic injuries often have salvageable, but injured, eyes.[7] Retaining soldiers with useful vision requires forward placement of experienced surgeons and effective combat surgical support.[6,9]

WARTIME OCULAR INJURY PATTERNS

A comprehensive military perspective requires the compilation of trauma data from multiple sources. The international classification system (see Table 6-1) was an important step toward the development of a common ocular trauma language; however, the terminology for traumatic optic neuropathy and orbital injuries was not included. Chemical injuries, burns, laser injuries, and extensive craniofacial trauma are all of great importance to military ophthalmologists but are excluded from many civilian trauma classification systems.[10,11] Small, high-velocity fragment injuries predominate in nonfatal ocular trauma in wartime, and these injuries are also excluded from many civilian trauma series.[4,11–13]

A wartime injury pattern base must be established to set the stage for effective use of ocular trauma scales. The first step is to acknowledge the injury patterns observed by military ophthalmologists in previous conflicts.[5–7,9] The second step is to reflect this body of experience in a simplified trauma scale that can be used as an effective triage and readiness training tool. On the battlefield, medics must rapidly identify the most severe ocular injuries in a sea of soldiers who have corneal FBs.

Sustaining the force requires the capacity to treat common, minor injuries that would otherwise degrade a soldier's ability to fight. Ocular trauma scales must enable the separation at triage of corneal abrasions and superficial FBs from penetrating fragmentation injuries. Corneal FBs requiring slitlamp removal were extremely common during the Persian Gulf War.[7] During the 1967 Arab–Israeli Six-Day War, 46% of the total Israeli injured sustained corneal injuries from FBs, mostly from sand and rock missiles associated with blast injuries. These minor corneal injuries degraded the ability of injured Israeli soldiers to fight or to assist in their own evacuation off the battlefield. Although temporary, corneal FBs are not minor when they degrade a soldier's ability to fight. Many can be prevented by simply using protective eye armor. Polycarbonate eyewear can also prevent most serious eye injuries resulting from small, high-velocity fragments.[5]

High-velocity fragments are the principal cause of severe eye injuries in modern combat.[6,7,14] Small, high-velocity fragments that might be stopped easily by heavy clothing and skin can penetrate the eye with devastating results.[9] Of the 35 enucleations performed during the Persian Gulf War, 94% were the result of fragmenting munitions. Several authors have reported on the incidence and clinical presentation of fragmentation injuries from shells, grenades, and mines. Fragmentation wounds caused more than 80% of ocular injuries during World Wars I and II, 72% during the Korean War, 78% during the 1967 Arab–Israeli Six-Day War, and 78% during the Persian Gulf War.[7,14] In nonlethal trauma, most high-velocity fragments are quite small. This was true of the military ophthalmology experience in the Vietnam War, where most of the fragments that were removed from the eye and adnexal structures had a mass less than 100 mg (Figure 6-2).[6] In the Persian Gulf War, 40% of corneal scleral lacerations from blast fragments were less than 10 mm in length, caused by proportionately small fragments.[7]

In addition to the high percentage of fragment injuries, wartime ophthalmic wounds have several distinguishing characteristics. These injuries are typically multiple, often presenting with adnexal, bilateral ocular, and concurrent orbital injury patterns. The injury patterns are complex, contaminated, and severe.[5,6,9] Frequently, secondary missiles from gravel and organic material cause more damage than the primary missile.[9] Unlike civilian case series, military trauma scales have no exclusion criteria for complex wounds, burns, or chemi-

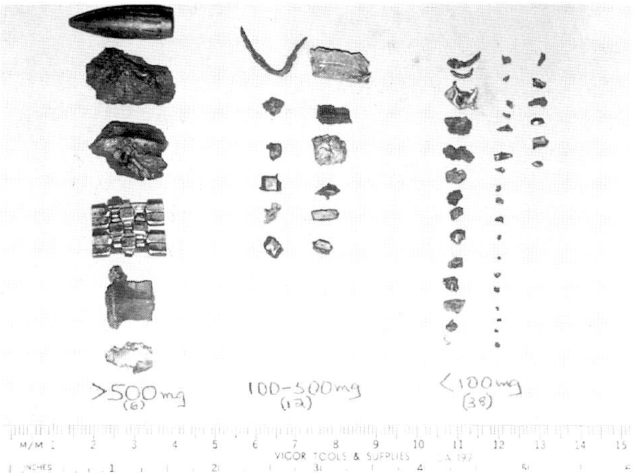

Fig. 6-2. These foreign bodies (FBs) were removed from the eye, orbital, and adnexal soft tissue of soldiers and Marines at the US Naval Hospital, Da Nang, Vietnam, 1968–1969, by Drs. Sponaugle and Mackinley. Note that more than twice as many small (< 100 mg) FBs were removed than medium (100–500 mg) and large (> 500 mg) FBs *combined*. Photograph: Courtesy of Francis G. LaPiana, Colonel, Medical Corps, US Army (Ret), Washington, DC.

cal injury patterns.[3,4]

Vesicant agents, such as mustard gas, remain a constant medical threat and have significant ocular morbidity. These persistent, rapidly absorbed, oil-droplet agents have a latent period followed by mucosal activation, making the eye an especially vulnerable target. Six to 12 hours after exposure, soldiers may present with ocular, skin, gastrointestinal, and pulmonary symptoms. The corneal epithelium is particularly vulnerable, and the result is pain, photophobia, tearing, and reduced vision.[15]

Military ophthalmologists have provided a thorough accounting of wartime injury patterns[5–7,9]; their experience provides the basis for future triage and readiness training. When we implement an ocular trauma triage and readiness training module, we must continue to ask the question, "Will it work on the battlefield?"

TRIAGE APPLICATIONS OF OCULAR TRAUMA SCALES

Battlefield triage presents a unique challenge for field medics and triage personnel. Wartime experience, combined with combat-oriented triage training, will improve our readiness to restore soldiers with ocular injuries. MEOTS is a triage training module that uses simple observational categories and a penlight to identify soldiers with sight-threatening injuries[3] (see Figure 6-1). A soldier with basic medic skills can be trained to perform ocular triage using MEOTS. Sight-threatening injuries are recognized by their overall pattern. For example, a retrobulbar hematoma is recognized by decrease in vision, proptosis, abnormal pupils with an afferent pupillary defect (APD), and reduced motility (Figure 6-3). An open globe is recognized by an overall low trauma score, a clinical history of risk for penetrating or blunt trauma, and by evidence of violation of the globe (Figure 6-4). Recognition of sight-threatening injuries triggers urgent intervention. For example, identification of an open globe activates both the application of a Fox shield and urgent ophthalmic surgical support (Figure 6-5). It is

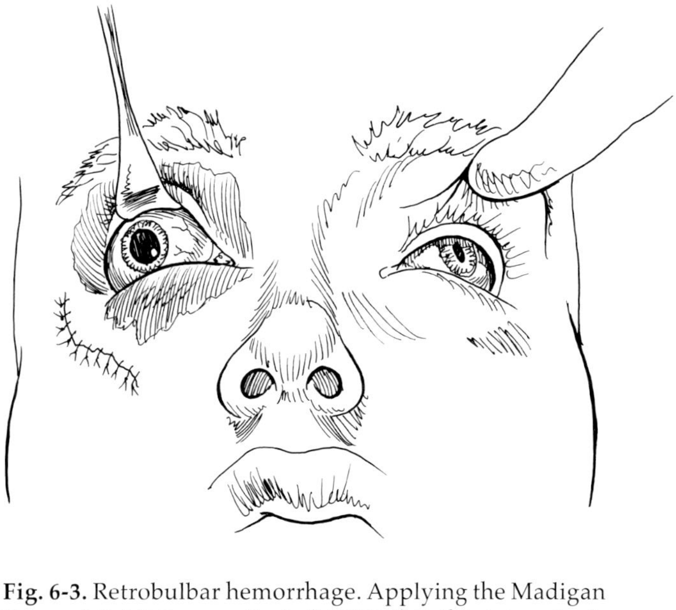

Fig. 6-3. Retrobulbar hemorrhage. Applying the Madigan Eye and Orbit Trauma Scale (MEOTS) to this injured soldier facilitates prompt recognition and treatment for of a retrobulbar hemorrhage. Urgent action is triggered by recognition of: vision reduced to Count Fingers, a firm proptotic orbit with evidence of facial trauma, unequal pupils with a definite afferent pupillary defect, and a frozen globe. A lateral canthotomy/cantholysis, cold compresses, elevation of the head, high-dose steroids, and ophthalmic surgical support restored this soldier to normal function. MEOTS score: total 4 of 12. Drawing prepared for this textbook by Gary Wind, MD, Uniformed Services University of the Health Sciences, Bethesda, Md.

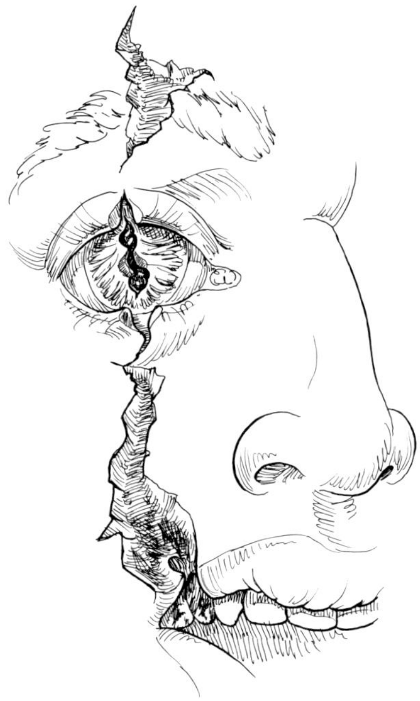

Fig. 6-4 Extensive facial trauma with a corneal-scleral laceration. Gross violation of the globe is recognized by: vision of bare light perception, contiguous lacerations and fractures with gross violation of the eye, no view of a pupil, and an eye that does not move normally. The soldier requires a Fox shield, oral or intravenous ciprofloxacin, and immediate ophthalmic surgical support. MEOTS score: total 1 of 12. Drawing prepared for this textbook by Gary Wind, MD, Uniformed Services University of the Health Sciences, Bethesda, Md.

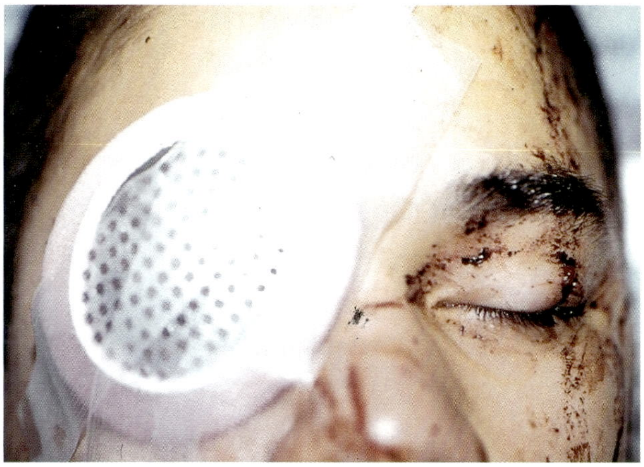

Fig. 6-5. Fox shield for an open globe. The injured soldier receives an immediate protective shield for gross violation of the right eye caused by glass fragments, and careful examination of the left eye. Urgent ophthalmic surgical support is required.

vital that we provide our triage personnel with focused training and basic equipment to yield the benefits of improved surgical readiness.

The training module for MEOTS follows a simple, commonsense approach for each index category. The act of measuring *visual acuity* is the most critical starting point. Medics are trained to use the small print and large print on a 4 in. x 4 in. gauze dressing, the count fingers method, and a penlight to determine levels of visual acuity. The overall score and injury pattern dictate the need for urgent intervention and referral. Critical points on individual indices, such as vision less than or equal to count fingers, require urgent referral.

During the MEOTS training module, medics are given multiple examples of an open globe. They are trained to recognize an open globe based on a mechanism of injury and *eyeball structure* criteria, including the following:

- adjacent lid lacerations,
- loss of normal eye anatomy,
- distortion of the pupil, and
- alterations in ocular chamber depth.

Medics are trained to recognize *proptosis* by observing the injured soldier's face from above and noting a relative proptosis in the frontal view. Medics are trained to gently palpate the orbit if absolutely no signs of an open globe are present. A firm, proptotic orbit prompts immediate reassessment of pupils, vision, and motility to exclude a blinding orbital hemorrhage.

The *pupil* examination involves a large dose of common sense. A dilated pupil in a comatose patient with head trauma is considered to be evidence of brain injury until proven otherwise. The swinging flashlight test is used to assess for a relative APD. A definite APD is a critical finding for evidence of an orbital hemorrhage or optic nerve injury.

The *motility* examination is based on both the subjective complaint of double vision and the objective evidence of restricted movement. A "frozen globe," with severely limited motility, prompts an urgent assessment of the orbit. Multiple examples of open globes and severe, sight-threatening orbital injuries are presented during MEOTS training to strengthen overall pattern recognition and reinforce the need for immediate intervention.

Improved Readiness

Ocular trauma is an important battlefield injury because of its frequent occurrence and its effect on a soldier's capacity to fight. Although the eye constitutes only 0.1% of the frontal body surface, it is extremely vulnerable to small fragments that on other parts of the body would have minimal effect. Ocular injuries are common, representing more than 9% of all battle injuries in the Vietnam War and 12% to 17% of battle injuries in World War II.[6] Ocular wounds are associated with landmine injuries and the increasing range of explosives.[11] Ocular trauma increases with a static battlefront, as soldiers must take to trenches and foxholes where the body is protected while the head and eyes are exposed for observation and fire. Battlefield eye injuries are severe. In World War II and the Vietnam War, 50% of ocular penetrating injuries resulted in enucleation.[6] The need for ocular trauma readiness is clear.

The primary goal for military ophthalmologists is to improve readiness through prevention and expert surgical management of eye and orbital injuries in soldiers. Ocular trauma scores can help achieve this goal by providing tools for both the command and unit levels of training. The collective body of ocular trauma score literature is most notable for its diversity. The focus and intended application are equally diverse for each system.

Several trauma scales provide excellent prognostic and research applications, including those from the United States Eye Injury Registry[10] and the Ocular Trauma Classification Group.[11] Ocular trauma scales of this caliber provide valuable command data regarding probable visual outcomes based on the soldier's mechanism of injury, initial vision, and a panel of prognostic factors. The data are based on an initial examination and operative findings from the first surgical repair. The readiness applications of these types of trauma scales are more global, providing probabilities of visual outcomes at 6 months and a database for trauma research. Trauma scales of this nature could be used to assess the visual outcomes of ocular trauma following an entire conflict.

Most ocular trauma scales include surgical findings in their assessment. Such data are of little use in a battalion aid station. Readiness training for medics and triage personnel requires a battlefield focus of sustaining the fighting force and instilling confidence in our ability to restore injured soldiers. The MEOTS trauma scale is designed for use in the field with acutely injured soldiers. This scale provides a readiness-training tool designed to identify and initiate care for soldiers with immediate, sight-threatening injuries. Restoration of the injured soldier requires effective triage, prompt first line of care, timely evacuation, and strong forward surgical support.

A hands-on active training environment is created through the use of multiple gross clinical examples, a plastic skull, Fox shields, field surgical instruments, and an experienced instructor. Figures 6-6 through 6-19 show a cross-section of the injury patterns and treatment modalities. Out of respect for severely injured soldiers and their families, some wartime images are limited to presentations in small-group settings.

A laminated trauma scale card serves as a pocket reference and training aid (see Figure 6-1). This trauma scale and the 45-minute training module help medics and triage personnel to decide rapidly which ocular injury to evacuate first, and why. It also helps the triage personnel to determine the urgency status of a given injury and to provide first-line care. Treatment examples include Fox shields and ophthalmic surgical support for open globes, lateral canthotomy for orbital injuries with optic nerve compression, and irrigation of chemical injuries (see Figures 6-5, 6-12, 6-13, and 6-14).

The MEOTS training module has gained support at many national and international meetings. The most vigorous reception, however, has been at the military unit level of instruction. The training module has been well received by multiple units, including medics of the 2/75 Ranger battalion, forward surgical teams, combat support hospitals, emergency department personnel, and members of several facial trauma teams. This decentralized training module is best suited for direct unit instruction

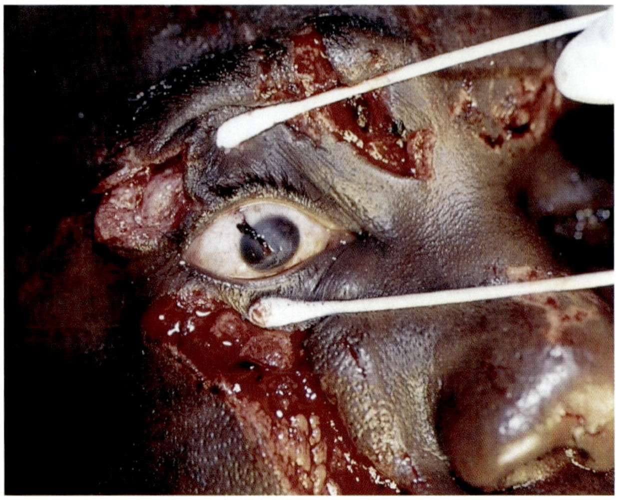

Fig. 6-6. Recognition of an open globe in a soldier with multiple trauma. Airway and breathing are always prime concerns in the primary survey of a multiply injured soldier, such as this one with multiple facial fractures and an open globe. The Madigan Eye and Orbit Trauma Scale (MEOTS) is a useful triage tool to be applied during the secondary survey for serious injuries.
The soldier's eyelids were swollen shut, yet serious eye injuries were anticipated, considering the deep lacerations and fractures above and below the eye. The eyelids were carefully retracted to obtain a patient vision and inspect the eye. MEOTS examination demonstrated the following: Vision: bare light perception (MEOTS 0); Eyeball Structure: gross violation (MEOTS 0); Proptosis: < 3 mm (MEOTS 1); Pupil: grossly abnormal (MEOTS 0); Motility: barely moved (MEOTS 0). Under the care of a cohesive Facial Trauma Team, this soldier returned to duty with an intact eye, normal face, and useful vision. MEOTS score: total 1 of 12.

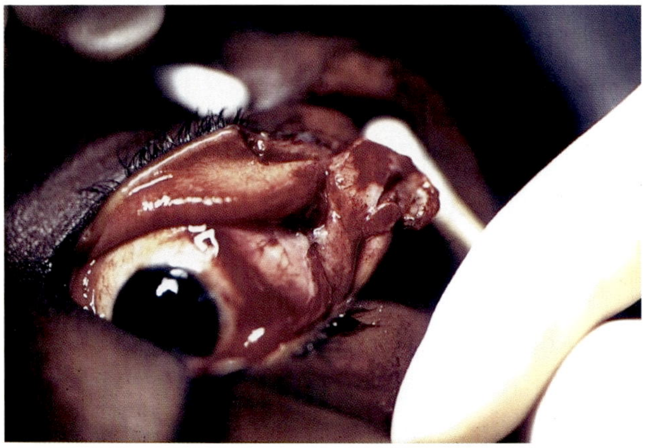

Fig. 6-7. Extensive laceration of the eyelid prompts examination of the eye to exclude injury. A complex, full-thickness injury of the eyelid raises great concern for the underlying globe. In this case, the eye was intact. Ophthalmic surgical support was required to "clear" the eye and repair the eyelid. Repair of the eyelid could be delayed until all soldiers with open globes are repaired. MEOTS score: total 11 of 12.

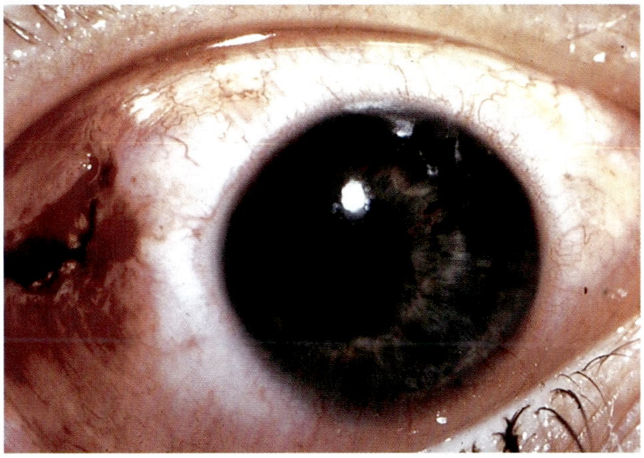

Fig. 6-8. Open globe with a scleral wound. This soldier's open globe is readily identified by its Madigan Eye and Orbit Trauma Scale (MEOTS) findings of Vision: Count Fingers (MEOTS 1); Eyeball Structure: gross violation as evident by the scleral wound, alteration in ocular chamber depth, distortion of the pupil, blood inside the eye, and a history of penetrating injury (MEOTS 0); Proptosis: no (MEOTS 2); Pupils: abnormal with possible afferent pupillary defect (MEOTS 1); Motility: abnormal (MEOTS 1). Immediate action was required on identification of the open globe. MEOTS score: total 5 of 12. Photograph: Courtesy of Francis G. LaPiana, MD, Colonel, Medical Corps, US Army (Ret), Washington, DC.

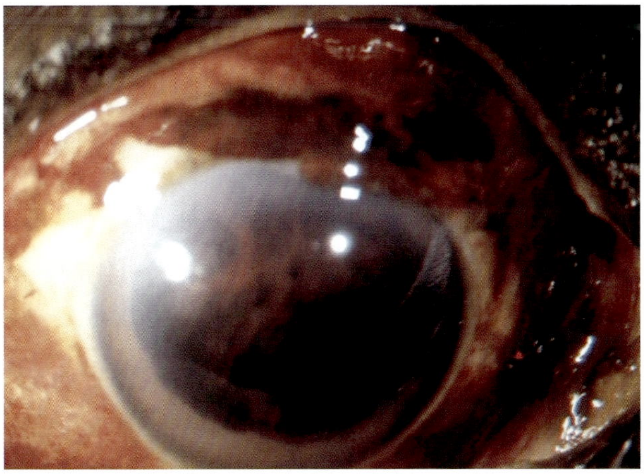

Fig. 6-9. Open globe with critically abnormal findings in all categories. Some very serious injuries are difficult to recognize; however, critical findings in all categories of the Madigan Eye and Orbit Trauma Scale (MEOTS) help identify the serious nature of this injury. A ruptured globe with prolapsed uvea and no view of a pupil results in critical deficits in the categories of Vision (MEOTS 0); Eyeball Structure (MEOTS 1); Proptosis (MEOTS 1); Pupils (MEOTS 0); and Motility (MEOTS 1). Medics evaluating this soldier *must* apply a Fox shield and seek urgent ophthalmic surgical support. MEOTS score: total 3 of 12.

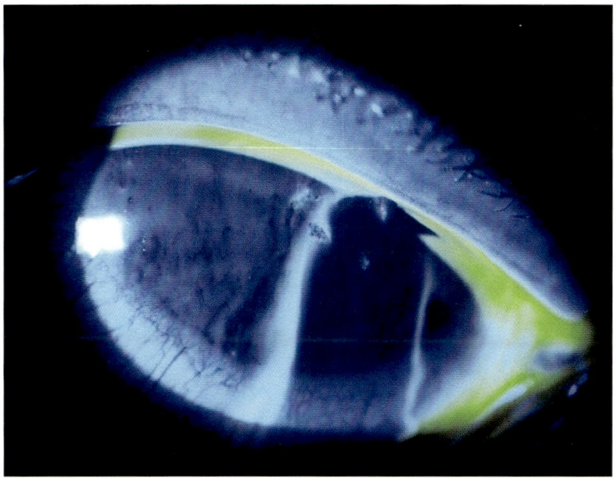

Fig. 6-10. Penetrating wound with leakage of aqueous fluid. A history of a penetrating injury leads to prompt assessment of this penetrating wound, application of a Fox shield, and urgent ophthalmic surgical support. Field units should consider giving 1.5 g oral ciprofloxacin as a loading dose for all open globe injuries to reduce the risk of serious infection. MEOTS score: total 6 of 12.

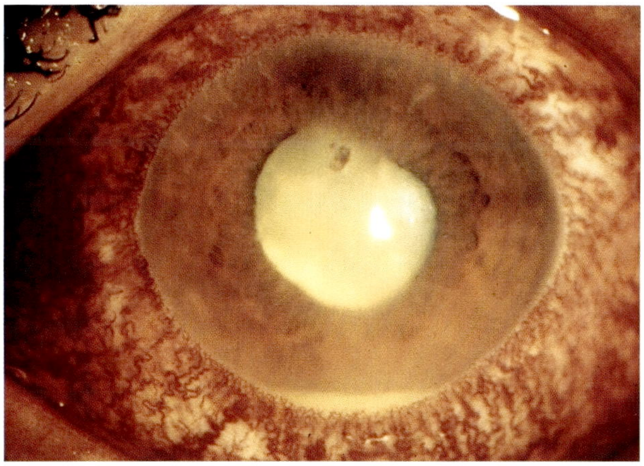

Fig. 6-11. Endophthalmitis following a penetrating wound from a wire. A history of a penetrating injury is critical. The soldier with a corneal wound can develop an eye full of pus in less than 24 hours. The findings of endophthalmitis include Vision: light perception (MEOTS 0); Eyeball Structure: severe pain; a hot, red eye; and a corneal wound with pus layered in the anterior chamber (MEOTS 0); Pupil: no view through the pupil, which is adherent to a traumatic white cataract (MEOTS 0). An inflammatory infiltrate is probably filling the posterior segment of the eye, as well. Medics in a field unit should give a loading dose of 1.5 g oral ciprofloxacin, apply a Fox shield, and immediately evacuate this soldier to a unit with ophthalmic surgical support. MEOTS score: total 3 of 12. Photograph: Courtesy of Thadeus Krolicki, MD, Wausau, Wisc.

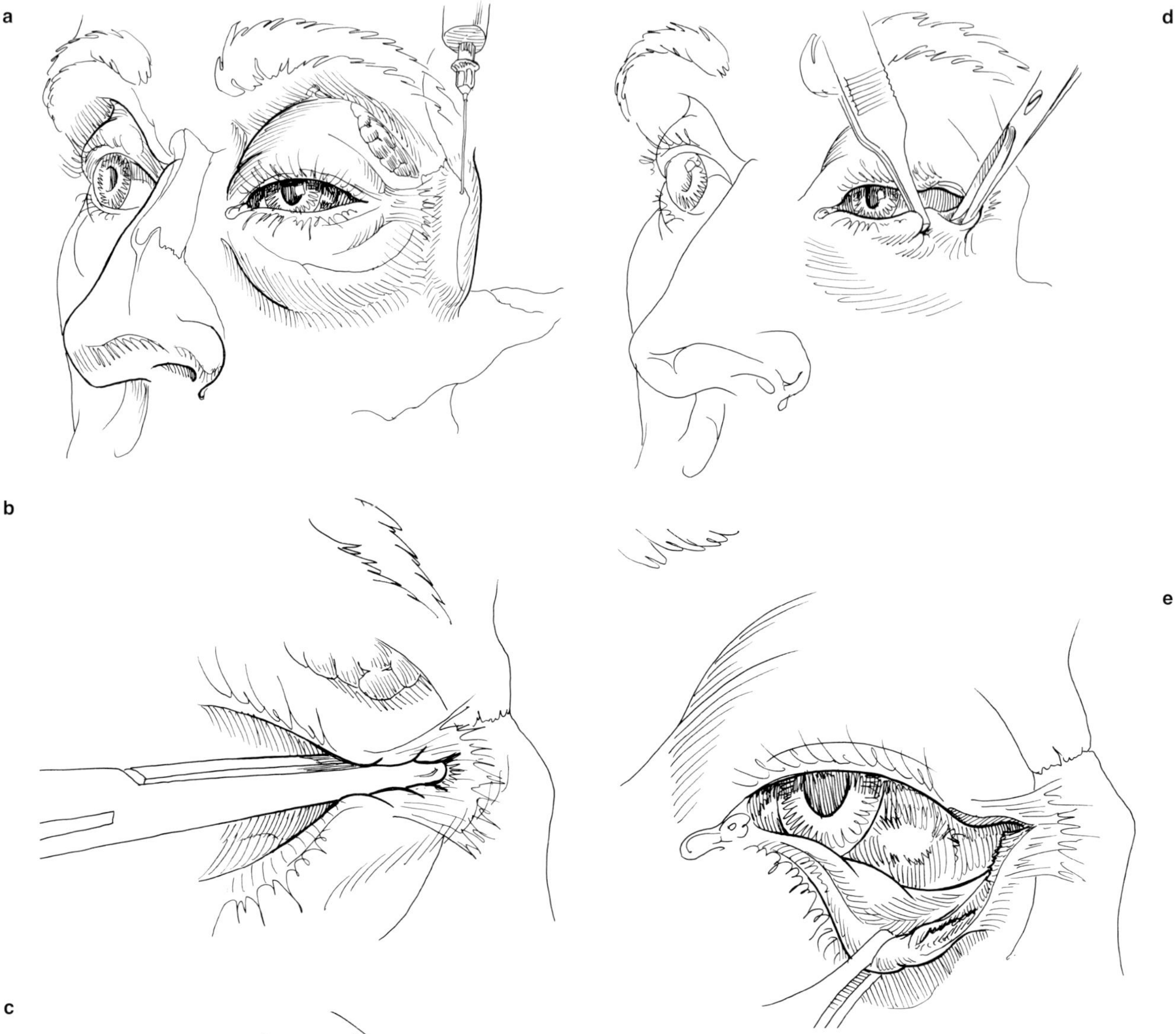

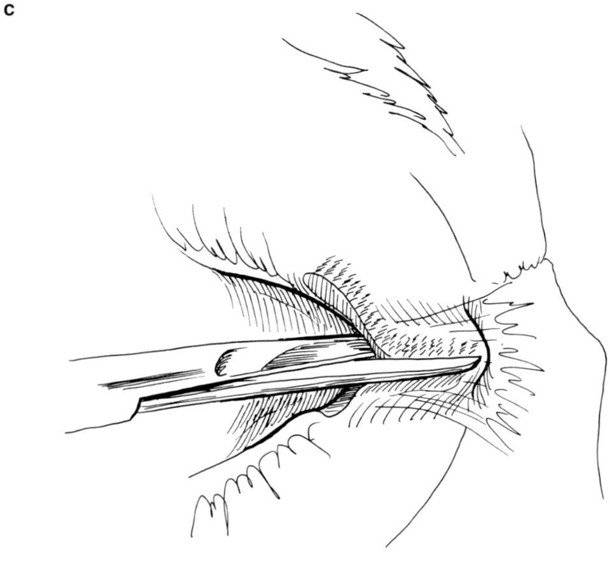

Fig. 6-12. Lateral canthotomy and inferior cantholysis are indicated for casualties presenting with serious orbital hemorrhage. These soldiers present with a history of trauma, decreased vision, firm proptosis, an abnormal pupil, and decreased motility. *Do not perform such procedures if the eyeball structure has been violated. If the eye is sliced open, apply a Fox shield for protection and seek immediate ophthalmic surgical support.* If the eyeball is intact, check the Madigan Eye and Orbit Trauma Score (MEOTS) categories: Vision, Eyeball Structure, Proptosis, Pupils, and Motility. Cut the lower lid if the orbit is swollen hard and is squeezing on an intact eyeball. The procedure is as follows:

a

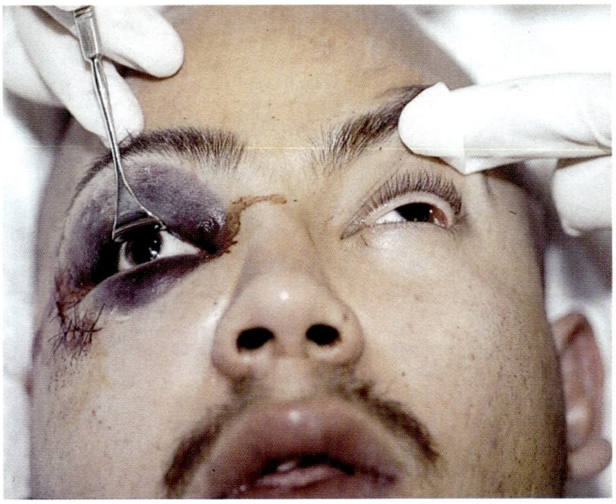

b

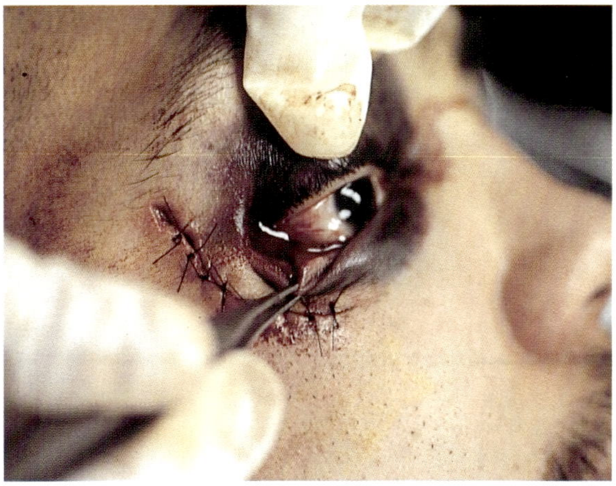

Fig. 6-13. (**a**) Orbital hemorrhage following blunt trauma with a crowbar, in an alert soldier with no neck pain. An orbital hemorrhage is identified by the Madigan Eye and Orbit Trauma Scale (MEOTS) criteria of Vision: reduced to large print (MEOTS 2); Eyeball Structure: appears intact (MEOTS 3); Proptosis: firm (MEOTS 0) Pupil: dilated, poorly responsive right pupil with consideration of both orbital and potential neurosurgical causes (MEOTS 0); Motility: frozen right eye (MEOTS 0). (**b**) The result of a lateral canthotomy and cantholysis. A lateral canthotomy was performed, releasing the blinding pressure of a firm, swollen orbit. One week later, the Head and Facial Trauma Team returned the soldier to duty; he had regained completely normal function. MEOTS score: total 5 of 12.

Fig. 6-12. *continued*

(**a**) Step 1: Injection. Inject 3 mL of 2% lidocaine with epinephrine 1:100,000 in a single, slow, vertical injection. Inject lateral to the orbital rim, with the needle pass at a depth just beneath the skin. Apply gentle pressure for 2 minutes over the injection site and away from the eye.

(**b**) Step 2: Horizontal clamp. Clamp the lateral canthal tendon with a thin hemostat in a straight horizontal position, pulling away from the swollen eye.

(**c**) Step 3: Horizontal cut. Using scissors, make a 1-cm horizontal incision of the lateral canthal tendon in the middle of the crush mark.

(**d**) Step 4: With scissors parallel to the face and tips pointing toward the chin, cut the lower eyelid. Grasp the lateral lower lid with a large-toothed forceps, pulling the eyelid away from the face. This pulls the inferior crus (band) of the lateral canthal tendon tight as a rope so it can be easily cut loose from the orbital rim. You can "strum" this band with closed scissors to feel what needs to be cut. Use a pair of blunt-tipped scissors to cut the inferior crus. Keep the scissors parallel (flat) to the face with tips pointed toward the chin. Place the inner blade just anterior to the conjunctiva and the outer blade just deep to the skin. The eyelid should pull freely away from the face, releasing pressure on the globe. Cut residual lateral attachments of the lower eyelid if it does not move freely. (Remember, you can feel the residual attachment bands best when you grab the eyelid with forceps and pull toward the ceiling, making the bands tight and easy to cut.) Do not be concerned about cutting half a centimeter of conjunctiva or skin, just keep the scissors out of the eyeball and orbital fat.

(**e**) Step 5: Success. The lower eyelid has been cut, relieving orbital compression. Compression of vital vascular structures in the orbit has been reduced by releasing the restraining belt of the lower eyelid. As the edema and hemorrhage resolve, the eyeball will recede back into the orbital space. If the intact cornea is exposed, apply hourly copious erythromycin ophthalmic ointment or ophthalmic lubricant ointment to prevent devastating corneal desiccation and infection. Relieving orbital pressure must be followed by lubricating protection of the cornea and urgent ophthalmic surgical support. Do NOT apply absorbent gauze dressings over an exposed cornea. Drawings prepared for this textbook by Gary Wind, MD, Uniformed Services University of the Health Sciences, Bethesda, Md.

a

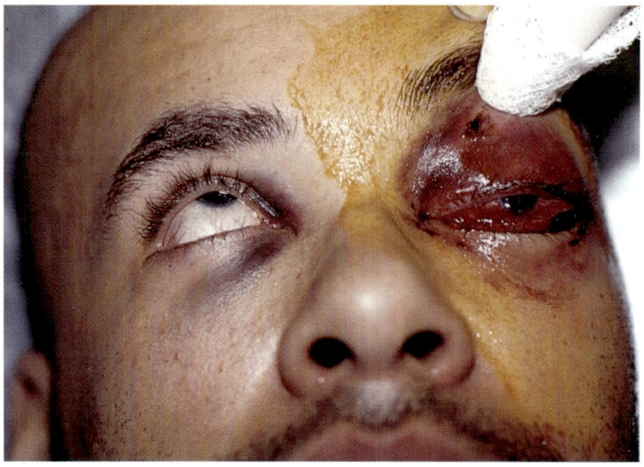

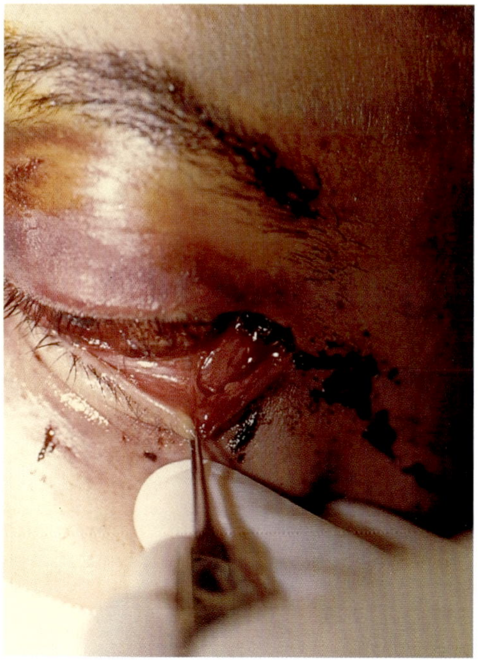

b

Fig. 6-14. (**a**) Orbital hemorrhage from a punch resulting in complete blindness. The severity of injury from optic nerve compression within a swollen orbit was not appreciated on initial presentation with Count Fingers vision under very swollen eyelids. Twelve hours after initial presentation, the soldier was urgently referred when he could no longer detect light in his left eye. The Madigan Eye and Orbit Trauma Scale (MEOTS) findings included Vision: No Light Perception (MEOTS 0); Eyeball Structure: intact (MEOTS 3); Proptosis: > 3 mm and rock hard (MEOTS 0); Pupil: dilated with a definite afferent pupillary defect (MEOTS 0); Motility: frozen (MEOTS 0). (**b**) Postlateral canthotomy and cantholysis. The soldier's vision remained at no light pereption (NLP) despite immediate action including canthotomy / cantholysis, 2.5 g intravenous methylprednisolone, and surgical decompression of the orbit. MEOTS score: total 3 of 12.

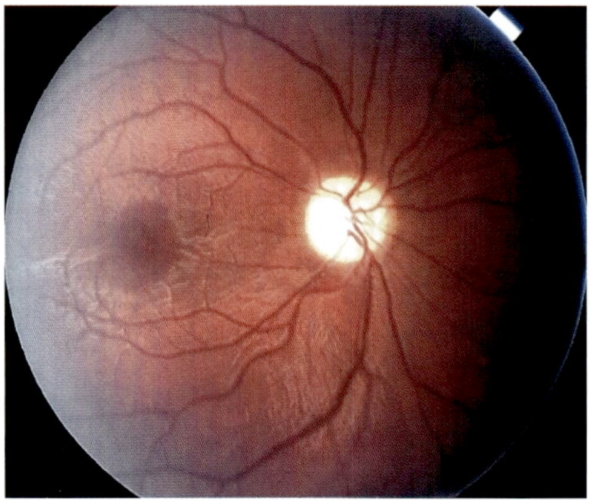

Fig. 6-15. Appearance of a blind optic nerve head 6 months after orbital compression. Gross pallor of the optic nerve head is a delayed finding when the optic nerve loses its blood supply in a rock-hard, traumatized orbit.

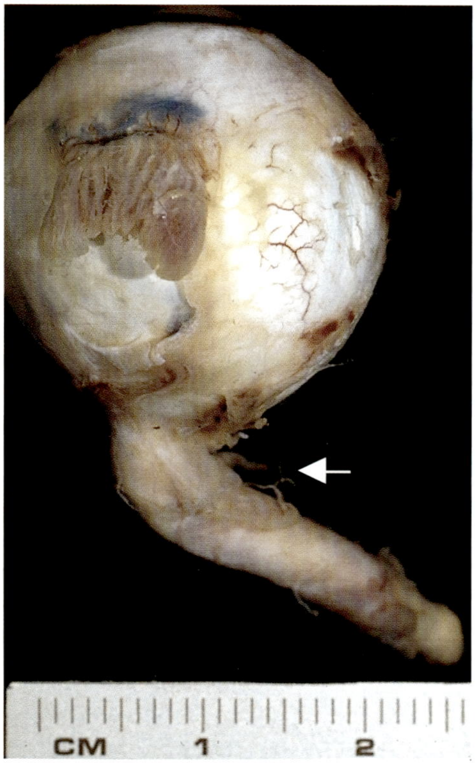

Fig. 6-16. Traumatic enucleation of the eye and extensive optic nerve segment. The delicate multiple penetrating blood vessels to the orbital section of the optic nerve (arrow) are at risk of compression in the setting of a firm orbital hemorrhage. This pathology specimen resulted from blunt trauma with extrusion of the globe and amputation of the optic nerve from the orbital apex. The specimen shows a clear view of the small blood vessels that nourish the orbital segment of the optic nerve.

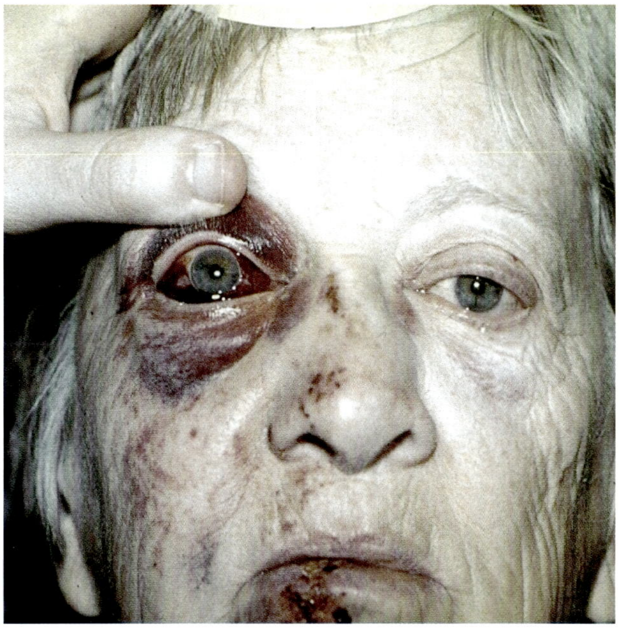

Fig. 6-17. This 70-year-old woman fell; as a result, she had a superior globe displacement caused by an inferior orbital hemorrhage. The patient had a normal vision and pupillary examination with less than 3 mm of proptosis, which was managed medically with modest oral steroids. A lateral canthotomy was not required. MEOTS score: total 10 of 12.

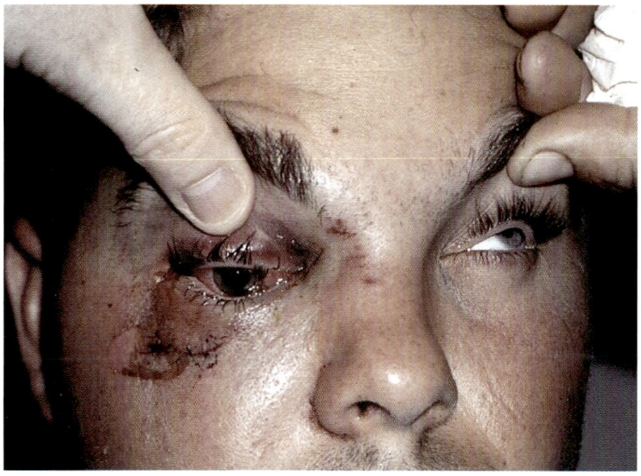

Fig. 6-18. Severe orbital hemorrhage associated with a zygomatic-maxillary complex fracture, requiring emergent treatment. This patient developed progressive orbital hemorrhage from blunt trauma complicated by vomiting and ingestion of alcohol and aspirin. The Madigan Eye and Orbit Trauma Scale (MEOTS) findings included Vision: reduced to Count Fingers (MEOTS 1); Eyeball Structure: intact (MEOTS 3); Proptosis: gross (MEOTS 0); Pupil: dilated with definite afferent pupillary defect (MEOTS 0); Motility: frozen (MEOTS 0). This patient received an emergent canthotomy/cantholysis plus high-dose intravenous (IV) steroids. Decadron (dexamethasone; mfg by Merck & Co, West Point, Pa) was administered IV, with a loading dose of 0.5 mg/kg (35 mg), followed by 10 mg IV every 8 hours for six doses, followed by an oral taper of prednisone. Surgical repair of the displaced fracture was performed without complication 1 week after the injury. The patient regained normal function. MEOTS score: total 4 of 12.

a

b

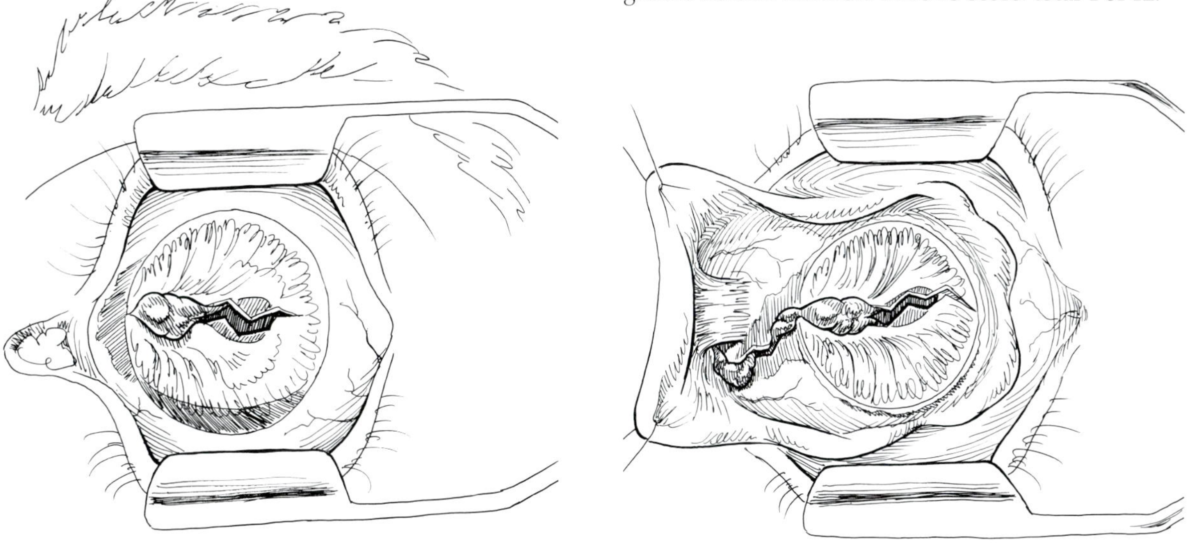

Fig. 6-19. For corneoscleral lacerations, the extent of injury is a critical predictive factor of visual outcome. (**a**) Following wound exploration the laceration was 11 mm in length. (**b**) In a different patient, after wound exploration the laceration was 21 mm in length, with a far worse prognosis.[1] (1) Grossman MD, Roberts DM, Barr CC. Ophthalmic aspects of orbital injury. *Clin Plast Surg*. 1992;19:71–85. Drawings prepared for this textbook by Gary Wind, MD, Uniformed Services University of the Health Sciences, Bethesda, Md.

in the aid station training room of any field or emergency trauma unit.

Prognostic Applications of Ocular Trauma Scales

Predicting visual outcomes is a major feature of a number of civilian and military ocular trauma scores. Numerous studies have shown that initial vision, extent of initial damage, and mechanism of injury are most predictive of ocular trauma outcome (Table 6-2; also see Figure 6-19). Although these concepts are valid, we must be vigilant in distinguishing between a civilian database and a battlefield environment. Many of these scales are not designed for battlefield use. The mechanism and extent of injuries are often restricted to subsets of mechanical globe injuries. IOFBs, complex contaminated injuries, burns, and chemical and craniofacial trauma are often not included.[11,12,16–18] In an excellent study regarding prognostic factors of corneoscleral lacerations, Barr[16] found the overall early (< 10 d) enucleation rate was 17%. This database of corneoscleral lacerations excluded injuries from retained IOFBs, globe perforation, burns or chemical injuries, and blunt trauma. Wartime experience has no such exclusion criteria; therefore, it is difficult to compare such studies to the enucleation rates following disruption of the globe during the Vietnam War (50%)[6,9] or the Persian Gulf War (18%).[7] These wartime enucleation rates represent the surgical outcomes of a very different group of wounds and battlefield circumstances.[6,7,9] However, keeping in mind the differences that exist in wartime, the prognostic applications of ocular trauma scales are worthy of examination.

The Ocular Trauma Score (OTS) developed by May and colleagues[10] is a product of the United States Eye Injury Registry and the Hungarian Eye Injury Registry. This group evaluated more than 2,000 mechanical injuries to the globe over a 10-year period. Initial vision was the most important predictor of final visual outcome. Probability of visual outcome at 6 months was further refined by adding the following predictive factors: globe rupture, endophthalmitis, perforating injury, retinal detachment, and the presence of an APD.

Next on the list of important predictors of final visual outcome, according to several major studies,[11,16–20] is the extent of injury (see Table 6-2). In a major study[13] of prognostic factors in corneoscleral lacerations, poor initial vision and extent of trauma, including the length of the corneoscleral laceration, were predictive of outcome. In this study, the enucleation rate was 4% for lacerations less than 9 mm in length and 68% for more-extensive lacerations (13–32 mm long) (see Figure 6-19).

Defining the posterior extent of injury is a major contribution of the Ocular Trauma Classification Group's classification of mechanical ocular injuries.[11] Patients were divided into two injury groups: those with open globe injuries and those with closed. The predictive factors supported by the study are the type of injury, initial vision, presence of an APD, and zone of injury.

In open globe injuries, the zones of injury are classified as I: corneal-limbal wounds; II: corneal scleral wounds less than 5 mm posterior to the limbus; and III: wounds extending more than 5 mm posterior from the limbus. Numerous studies[12,16,17,19,21–23] have identified the adverse relationship of posterior uveal prolapse; vitreous hemorrhage; and extrusion of intraocular contents with longer, more posterior wounds. A major contribution of the Ocular Trauma Classification Group study was this concept of posterior zone (III) wounds.

Mechanism of injury is another critical predictive factor, in addition to initial vision and extent of trauma. De Juan and colleagues[17,19] showed that blunt trauma and perforating injuries have significantly worse outcomes than injuries from sharp objects or penetrating missiles. However, military ophthalmologists must keep in mind that there is a great difference between the mechanism of an injury encountered in a civilian industrial setting and one encountered in a wartime environment. This difference is most evident with fragmentation wounds. Battlefield fragmentation wounds are not like metallic chips from hammers and chisels. If we consider only nonfatal injuries, then ocular fragmentation wounds from munitions tend to be caused by multiple, high-velocity, contaminated missiles (see Figure 6-2). Mechanism of injury is *the* critical prognostic factor that is most likely to be different in a battlefield versus a civilian database.

Command Perspective of Ocular Trauma Scales

Ocular trauma scales and trauma registries are critical elements of an effective command brief on ocular trauma. Only at the command level can we convert lessons learned by individual surgical units into broad, effective action. The critical message is that ocular trauma that degrades a soldier's ability to fight is a common battlefield event. The most vital command aspects of ocular trauma are prevention and ophthalmic surgical readiness.

TABLE 6-2

PROGNOSTIC FACTORS OF VISUAL OUTCOME

Study	Prognostic Factors of Visual Outcome	Comments
Ocular Trauma Score[1]	Initial visual acuity Globe rupture Endophthalmitis Perforating injury Retinal detachment Afferent pupillary defect (APD)	Initial vision is the most important predictor of final visual outcome. Cases limited to mechanical, nonburn eye injuries.
Prognostic Factors in Corneoscleral Lacerations[2]	Initial visual acuity Amount of hyphema Presence of posterior uveal prolapse or vitreous hemorrhage Length of laceration Extent of lens damage	Enucleation rate was 4% for lacerations < 9 mm and 68% for lacerations of 13 to 32 mm. Excluded from the study were all patients with retained intraocular foreign body (IOFB) or perforating globe injuries.
Penetrating Ocular Injuries: Types of Injuries and Visual Results[3]	Initial visual acuity Presence of an APD Type of injury Location and extent of penetrating wound Type of lens damage Presence and severity of vitreous hemorrhage Type of IOFB	This study emphasizes that the prognosis after penetrating injury is strongly influenced by the nature of the injury and the extent of initial damage. Blunt trauma has a less favorable outcome compared with sharp lacerations or missile injuries.
Multivariate Analysis of Prognostic Factors in Penetrating Ocular Injuries[4]	Initial visual acuity Mechanism of injury: blunt, sharp, or missile Length and location of laceration Laceration limited to the cornea Laceration anterior to the rectus muscle insertion Expulsion of the lens Posterior scleral laceration Severe vitreous hemorrhage Presence of an APD BB pellet IOFB	Initial vision and extent of injury are the most critical predictive factors of visual outcome. 12 eyes had BB pellet IOFB injuries. None of these patients achieved a final visual acuity of 20/800 or better.
Factors Influencing Final Visual Results in Severely Injured Eyes[5]	Visual-evoked potential Initial visual function Extent of injury	Study relies on visual-evoked potential as a gauge of central visual function in severely injured eyes. Damage to either the macula or optic nerve causes reduction in amplitude of the visual-evoked potential.

Studies and sources cited:

1. Kuhn FP, MD. Professor of Ophthalmology, University of Alabama at Birmingham, Birmingham, Alabama. Personal communication, Jan 2001; and May DR, Kuhn FP, Morris RE, et al. The epidemiology of serious eye injuries from the United States Eye Injury Registry. *Graefes Arch Clin Exp Ophthalmol.* 2000;238(2):153–157.
2. Barr CC. Prognostic factors in corneoscleral lacerations. *Arch Ophthalmol.* 1983;101:919–924.
3. de Juan E Jr, Sternberg P Jr, Michael RG. Penetrating ocular injuries: Types of injuries and visual results. *Ophthalmology.* 1983;90:1318–1322.
4. Sternberg P Jr, de Juan E Jr, Michels RG, Auer C. Multivariate analysis of prognostic factors in penetrating ocular injuries. *Am J Ophthalmol.* 1984;98:467–472.
5. Hutton WL. Factors influencing final visual results in severely injured eyes. *Am J Ophthalmol.* 1984;97:715–722.

The military need for protective eye armor is clear and well established.[6,7,9] Small fragments that might be stopped by the battle dress uniform and the skin may, even from a great distance, penetrate the eye.[5] Polycarbonate eye armor could prevent many of the small-fragment injuries and countless corneal FBs that degrade a soldier's ability to fight.[5–9,24]

The second critical command brief message is that ophthalmologists are required members of an effective head trauma team. Soldiers with craniofacial injuries frequently suffer occult, severe ocular trauma.[9] Combat eye injuries are rarely limited to the globe. In the 1967 Arab–Israeli Six-Day War, 72% of the ocular injuries had associated wounds, most commonly to the head and neck.[14] In his personal account of Vietnam War injuries, Hornblass[9] stressed the importance of including senior ophthalmologists in forward-positioned head-and-neck trauma teams. La Piana and Mader strongly support this concept (see Chapter 2, Lessons Learned), based on their experiences in the Vietnam War and the Persian Gulf War. These experienced leaders remind us that military ophthalmologists must work aggressively within the chain of command to obtain adequate resources, equipment, and experienced personnel to restore injured soldiers with ocular and orbital injuries.

SUMMARY

Ocular trauma scales in various forms are a vital aspect of effective triage and wartime readiness training. Trauma scales provide a triage and training framework that strengthens our ability to restore soldiers with eye and orbital injuries. Recognition of common injury patterns facilitates command input for prevention and combat health-support planning. Small, high-velocity fragments from munitions caused 78% of the serious ocular and ocular adnexal injuries during the Persian Gulf War; military command structure must be informed of such injury patterns to initiate protective eye armor measures.

Trauma scales and eye injury registries support critical efforts to obtain the equipment and trained personnel necessary to restore soldiers with sight-threatening injuries. In 1974, it would have been easy to overlook the value of a head trauma scale that evaluated such basic elements as eye opening and verbal and motor responses. Yet the Glasgow Coma Scale has provided the critical function of defining severe head trauma, providing a common language, and improving triage communication. We must seek the same benefit for soldiers with eye and orbital injuries. MEOTS, a triage training module developed at Madigan Army Medical Center, Tacoma, Washington, provides for recognition of immediate vision-threatening injuries and triggers urgent intervention, coordinated evacuation, and surgical support—all of which should make MEOTS a valuable tool on the battlefield. The use of MEOTS and other trauma scales improves triage, initial stabilization, coordinated evacuation, and utilization of surgical teams. MEOTS strengthens each link in the treatment chain and thus improves our capacity to provide effective ophthalmic combat surgical support.

REFERENCES

1. American College of Surgeons, Committee on Trauma. *Advanced Trauma Life Support Program*. 5th ed. Chicago, Ill: American College of Surgeons; 1997.
2. Rush C, interviewer. The history of the Glasgow Coma Scale: An interview with Professor Bryan Jennett. *International Journal of Trauma Nursing*. 1997;3:114–118.
3. Ainbinder DA, Sanford EG, Raymond WR IV, et al. Madigan Eye and Orbit Trauma Scale. Presented at the Annual Meeting of the American Academy of Ophthalmology; October 1999; Orlando, Fla.
4. Kuhn F, Morris R, Witherspoon CD, Heimann K, Jeffers JB, Treister G. A standardized classification of ocular trauma. *Ophthalmology*. 1996;103:240–243.
5. Bellows JG. Observations on 300 consecutive cases of ocular war injuries. *Am J Ophthalmol*. 1947;30:309–323.
6. La Piana FG, Hornblass A. Military ophthalmology in the Vietnam War. *Doc Ophthalmol*. 1997;93:29–48.
7. Mader TH, Aragones JV, Chandler AC, et al. Ocular and ocular adnexal injuries treated by United States military ophthalmologists during Operations Desert Shield and Desert Storm. *Ophthalmology*. 1993;100:1462–1467.

8. Simmons ST, Krohel GB, Hay PB. Prevention of ocular gunshot injuries using polycarbonate lenses. *Ophthalmology*. 1984;91:977–983.

9. Hornblass A. Eye injuries in the military. *Int Ophthalmol Clin*. 1981;21(4):121–138.

10. May DR, Kuhn FP, Morris RE, et al. The epidemiology of serious eye injuries from the United States Eye Injury Registry. *Graefes Arch Clin Exp Ophthalmol*. 2000 Feb;238(2):153–157.

11. Pieramici DJ, Sternberg P Jr, Aaberg TM, et al, and The Ocular Trauma Classification Group. Perspective: A system for classifying mechanical injuries of the eye (globe). *Am J Ophthalmol*. 1997;123:820–831.

12. Hardy RA. Ocular trauma: Battlefield injuries. *Mil Med*. 1996;161:465–468.

13. Grossman MD, Roberts DM, Barr CC. Ophthalmic aspects of orbital injury. *Clin Plast Surg*. 1992;19:71–85.

14. Treister G. Ocular casualties in the Six-Day War. *Am J Ophthalmol*. 1969;68:669–675.

15. Solberg Y, Alcalay M, Belkin M. Ocular injury by mustard gas. *Surv Ophthalmol*. 1997;41:461–466.

16. Barr CC. Prognostic factors in corneoscleral lacerations. *Arch Ophthalmol*. 1983;101:919–924.

17. de Juan E Jr, Sternberg P Jr, Michael RG. Penetrating ocular injuries: Types of injuries and visual results. *Ophthalmology*. 1983;90:1318–1322.

18. Hutton WL. Factors influencing final visual results in severely injured eyes. *Am J Ophthalmol*. 1984;97:715–722.

19. Sternberg P Jr, de Juan E Jr, Michels RG, Auer C. Multivariate analysis of prognostic factors in penetrating ocular injuries. *Am J Ophthalmol*. 1984;98:467–472.

20. Guerrissi JO. Maxillofacial injuries scale. *J Craniofac Surg*. 1996;7:130–132.

21. Davidson PC, Sternberg P Jr. Management of posterior segment ocular trauma. *Curr Opin Ophthalmol*. 1991; 2:337–343.

22. de Souza S, Howcroft MJ. Management of posterior segment intraocular foreign bodies: 14 years' experience. *Can J Ophthalmol*. 1999;34:23–29.

23. Klein BE, Karlson TA, Rose J. An anatomic index for the severity of ocular injuries. *Eur J Ophthalmol*. 1993;3:57–60.

24. Varr WF III, Cook RA. Shotgun eye injuries: Ocular risk and eye protection efficacy. *Ophthalmology*. 1992;99:867–872.

Chapter 7

CHEMICAL INJURIES OF THE EYE

EDWARD W. TRUDO, JR, MD*; AND WILLIAM RIMM, MD†

*Lieutenant Colonel, Medical Corps, US Army Reserve; Azar Eye Institute, 31519 Winter Place Parkway, Suite 1, Salisbury, Maryland 21804, and Assistant Professor of Surgery (Ophthalmology), Uniformed Services University of the Health Sciences, 4301 Jones Bridge Road, Bethesda, Maryland 20814-4799; formerly, Director, Corneal and External Disease, Walter Reed Army Medical Center, Washington, DC 20307-5001

†Colonel, Medical Corps, US Army; Ophthalmology Service, Walter Reed Army Medical Center, Washington, DC 20307-5001

INTRODUCTION

Military forces face possible chemical injury caused not only by hazards of the battlefield but also by occupational hazards in the military's industrial base. Therefore, an understanding of the physiological damage and the treatment of chemical eye injuries is required for both the battlefield and the peacetime environment.[1] Occupational hazards come in the form of common chemicals that can injure the eye, including acids (eg, automobile battery acid, refrigerants, vinegar) and alkalis (eg, drain cleaners, fertilizers, building supplies). Military forces run the risk of being exposed to offensive chemical weapons that pose specific ocular risks. The principles of treatment are similar, however, whether the injury occurred as the result of chemical weaponry or of occupational hazards.

Chemical injuries of the eye are true emergencies requiring prompt recognition and treatment. Rapid dilution of the chemical agent is the immediate treatment necessary to reduce tissue damage and preserve vision. The extent of ocular injury is proportional to the departure of the corrosive substance from the neutrality of pH 7.4, the time that it remains in contact with the eye, and the quantity requiring neutralization.

Other factors must be considered when treating patients with injuries caused by chemical warfare agents. Ocular chemical injuries can cause immediate loss of vision, combat ineffectiveness, and even permanent blindness. Some effects are more subtle: the mere *threat* of chemical agents on the battlefield reduces unit morale and efficiency. Medical personnel who discern that injuries might be the result of chemical agents may be in a position to alert field command to the possible use of chemical warfare on the battlefield. In addition, medical personnel must be aware of specific antidotes for treating systemic and ocular effects stemming from exposure to chemical warfare agents.

Three other volumes in the *Textbooks of Military Medicine* series contain additional information on chemical injuries to the eye, which interested readers can peruse: *Occupational Health: The Soldier and the Industrial Base*[2]; *Military Dermatology,* particularly Chapter 5, Cutaneous Reactions to Nuclear, Biological, and Chemical Warfare[3]; and *Medical Aspects of Chemical and Biological Warfare*.[4]

INJURIES OF THE EYE CAUSED BY COMMON CHEMICALS

Chemical Agents

Chemical agents with the potential to cause ocular injury are often found in the home, at work within the military's industrial base, on the training field, and on the battlefield. Industrial and household cleaners often contain acidic or alkaline products in sufficient concentrations to cause eye and skin injury. Building materials, such as mortar and plaster, and automobile batteries are the most common sources of household chemical eye injuries today. Any of these agents can significantly damage human tissue after contact (Table 7-1).

Some common examples of acid-containing products are automobile batteries (sulfuric acid), refrigerants, and vinegar (acetic acid). Common alkali products include drain cleaners, fertilizers, refrigerants, and building supplies. Another household chemical injury can occur when an individual mixes cleaning agents and unknowingly liberates chlorine gas. This event can precipitate acute respiratory distress syndrome from chlorine gas inhalation and also cause ocular surface damage.

Peacetime training exposes military personnel to additional chemical hazards. Tear gas is often an element of training scenarios. The term *tear gas* refers to several different agents that can cause lacrimation. Ordinary tear gas (2-chloro-1-phenylethanone, also called CN and Mace) is used in riot control and civilian police activity. The most common military tear gas is 2-chlorobenzalmalonitrile (CS). In addition to its lacrimatory effect, tear gas produces a mild chemical keratitis, which is usually self-limited.[5] In its most concentrated form, tear gas has the potential to rapidly cause significant damage to the ocular surface.

In military field-training exercises, weapon and grenade simulators, flares, and other incendiary devices also are ocular hazards. These training devices may cause thermal injury in addition to chemical injury from the magnesium hydroxide contained in them.[6] Also, the projectile and explosive nature of these devices poses a risk of penetrating or perforating foreign bodies in addition to their toxic effects. Open globe injury must always be suspected.

Acids and Alkalis

The normal pH of the human eye is approximately pH 7.4. Acids (considered here as substances

TABLE 7-1

COMMON SOURCES OF CHEMICAL INJURY

Chemical	Example
Acids	
Sulfuric acid	Battery acid Industrial cleaner
Acetic acid	Vinegar Glacial acetic acid
Hydrochloric acid	Chemistry laboratories Muriatic acid (cleaner)
Sulfurous acid	Bleach Refrigerant Fruit and vegetable preservative
Hydrofluoric acid	Glass polishing and etching Gasoline alkylation Silicone production
Alkalis	
Ammonia	Fertilizer Refrigerant Cleaning agent
Lye	Drain cleaner
Lime	Plaster Mortar Cement Whitewash
Potassium hydroxide	Caustic potash
Magnesium hydroxide	Sparklers Incendiary devices

with lower-than-normal pH values) precipitate tissue proteins, creating a barrier to further ocular penetration. The corneal epithelium offers some protection against weaker acids. Very weak acids may cause only temporary loss of the corneal epithelium with minimal damage to the deeper structures.

Sulfuric acid is the most common cause of chemical ocular injury, usually the result of the explosion of a car battery.[7,8] Sulfuric acid has a great potential for permanent ocular damage; it reacts with the water present in the preocular tear film, producing heat sufficient to cauterize the corneal and conjunctival epithelium. Hydrochloric acid is commonly found in school and college chemistry laboratories. Fortunately, it has poor ocular penetration in its usual laboratory concentration. Acidic refrigerants contain oils, which make removal and decontamination difficult and prolong contact with the body. Hydrofluoric acid and heavy metal acids are exceptions to the penetration rules of acidic agents. They penetrate quite rapidly and destroy the corneal endothelium. Most of the ocular damage is the direct result of fluoride ion toxicity. Although acids usually do not penetrate the eye to cause the deeper destruction associated with alkali injuries, their injury of the ocular surface tissues results in corneal vascularization, scarring, and reduced vision.

Alkalis (bases) are agents with a pH in the higher-than-normal physiological range. In contrast to acids, alkaline agents rapidly penetrate the cornea, reacting with the cellular lipids to form soaps. Alkaline agents essentially dissolve the cell membranes; they continue destroying tissues much longer than acids do, permanently damaging ocular tissues and entering the anterior chamber in as short a time as 5 seconds. Alkaline substances continue their destruction of tissues within the eye for up to several days. Alkalis also dehydrate cells and destroy enzymatic and structural proteins. The most severe effects occur in the pH range 11.0 to 11.5. Penetration rates differ by the type of base; ammonium hydroxide is one of the fastest penetrating bases, followed by sodium hydroxide, potassium hydroxide, and calcium hydroxide.

Thermal Injury

In addition to the damage created by the pH of chemical agents, associated thermal injury is also encountered. When the face and eyes are exposed to pure water at its boiling point, the normal cells

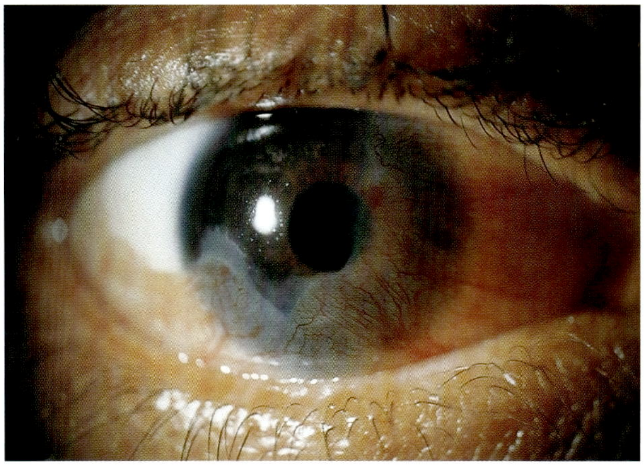

Fig. 7-1. Localized corneal scarring as a response to limbal stem cell thermal damage from pure water at the boiling point.

that populate the cornea (limbal stem cells) are destroyed, resulting in altered corneal surface healing. Scarring and opacification ensue (Figure 7-1). Chemical munitions are often delivered at a high temperature generated by explosions, or they may generate heat due to exothermic chemical reactions. For these reasons, the extent of injury from a chemical agent may have additional thermal damage not evident when the casualty presents to medical personnel.[8]

OCULAR RESPONSE TO CHEMICAL INJURY

Each ocular structure responds uniquely to a chemical insult. The conjunctival tissues are cauterized. The corneal epithelium sloughs; the corneal stroma swells and opacifies; endothelial cells die and are replaced by neighboring cells that stretch to cover the resultant empty space. The angle structures scar, resulting in increased intraocular pressure (IOP). Cataracts form as a result of insult to the lens.[9–12]

Weak acids and alkalis in the eye cause similar injurious effects, including injection, chemosis, mild corneal clouding, and edema with minimal visible inflammation. In severe acid burns, however, the cornea and conjunctiva rapidly turn white and opaque. Nitric and chromic acids turn tissue yellow-brown. An initially deepithelialized cornea with clear stroma may belie the severity of the burn. The most severe acid burns produce corneal anesthesia, limbal pallor, and uveitis. Severe alkali burns can result in corneal melting and perforation within 2 to 4 weeks.[13]

The extent of injury to the limbal area is critical in determining the severity and prognosis of chemical burns. The ocular reparative response to chemical injuries involves reepithelialization and vascularization. If the perilimbal blood supply is damaged, sterile necrosis of the peripheral cornea can ensue. Injury to deep structures at the limbus can destroy the normal source (stem cells) for reepithelialization.

CLINICAL COURSE OF CHEMICAL OCULAR INJURY

According to McCulley,[14] the clinical course of ocular chemical injury can be divided into the following four phases: immediate, acute, early reparative, and late reparative.

Immediate Phase

The immediate phase begins the moment a chemical agent comes in contact with the ocular surface. The major determinants of prognosis are based on the initial clinical examination, although predictors of ocular recovery after chemical injury have proven to be more accurate if the evaluation is made 24 to 48 hours after the injury. Animal models demonstrate that the pH of the involved substance, its concentration, and the length of time the substance is in contact with the tissue are the major determinants of the depth of penetration and damage to deeper ocular structures.[15]

Because these factors are often unknown to the presenting physician and may not be recoverable from the patient's history, classification schemes and prognostic data have been based on examination findings. The clinical utility of classification schemes is to better predict which patients will respond to conventional medical therapy and which will require extensive treatment or are at risk for loss of the eye. In a military scenario, this classification of chemical injury is useful during triage for assigning patients for therapy on-site versus immediate evacuation. The most common classification schemes of ocular chemical injury are those by Ralph (Exhibit 7-1),[16] Hughes (Table 7-2),[17,18] and Thoft (Table 7-3).[19] The key elements for determining the extent of chemical ocular injury and prognosis are

- the total area of the corneal epithelial defect;
- the area of the conjunctival epithelial defect;
- the number of clock hours or degrees of limbal blanching (ischemia);
- the area and degree of density of corneal opacification;
- evidence of increased IOP on presentation, especially if resistant to treatment; and
- any loss of lens clarity.

The last two elements imply deeper effects of the chemical agent and damage to the inner ocular structures.

Acute Phase

The first 7 days after chemical eye injury constitute the acute phase of recovery. During this time, the tissues rid themselves of contaminants while reestablishing the superficial protective layer of the corneal epithelium. *Reepithelialization is the most crucial factor in ultimate visual recovery; therefore, the first*

EXHIBIT 7-1
RALPH'S CLASSIFICATION OF OCULAR CHEMICAL INJURY

Clinical Finding	Prognosis Code (Total score determines prognosis)
Perilimbal hyperemia	0
Chemosis	1
Spotty perilimbal ischemia	1
Clouded epithelium	1
Spotty denudation of epithelium	1
Up to 50% loss of epithelium	2
Mild stromal haze (iris detail visible)	2
Vertically oval fixed pupil (long posterior ciliaries)	2
Iridocyclitis	2
Perilimbal ischemia < $\frac{1}{3}$ of circumference	2
Complete epithelial loss	3
Moderate stromal haze (iris details barely visible)	3
Perilimbal ischemia $\frac{1}{3}$ to $\frac{1}{2}$ of circumference	3
Sustained intraocular pressure during the first 23 h	3
Severe stromal haze (no iris details visible)	4
Perilimbal ischemia > $\frac{1}{2}$ of circumference	4

Total Score (from above)	Category of Injury	Prognosis
0–3	Insignificant injury	Rapid recovery expected without permanent sequelae
4–6	Mild injury	Rapid reepithelialization and clearing of stromal haze Return to baseline acuity in 1–2 wk
7–9	Moderately severe burn	Complete reepithelialization takes 1–3 wk Persistent haze may reduce visual acuity Stable pannus of 1–2 mm is common Perforation not expected
10–12	Severe burn	Slow reepithelialization and frequent pannus Furrow from collagenolytic activity in advance of pannus is common Perforation very possible Final visual acuity is low because of pannus and stromal haze
≥ 13	Worse cases	Inflammation quiets only after months Dense pannus Perforation is common Vascularized corneal scar, cataract, and secondary glaucoma often ensue in those who retain the globe

Adapted with permission from Ralph RA. Chemical burns of the eye. In: Duane TD, Jaeger EA, eds. *Clinical Ophthalmology*. Vol 4. Philadelphia, Pa: Harper & Row; 1987: 4, 6.

TABLE 7-2

HUGHES'S CLASSIFICATION OF OCULAR CHEMICAL INJURY

Category of Injury	Clinical Finding
Mild	Erosion of corneal epithelium Faint haziness of cornea No ischemic necrosis of conjunctiva or sclera
Moderately severe	Corneal opacity blurs iris detail Mild ischemic necrosis of conjunctiva or sclera
Very severe	Blurring of pupillary outline Significant ischemic necrosis of conjunctiva or sclera

Source: Ralph RA. Chemical burns of the eye. In: Duane TD, Jaeger EA, eds. *Clinical Ophthalmology*. Vol 4. Philadelphia, Pa: Harper & Row; 1987: 4.

important therapeutic consideration is prompt, unhindered reepithelialization. In severe eye injury, reepithelialization may determine whether the globe is retained. The epithelium serves as a protective barrier against the enzymes in tears that lead to corneal thinning and progression to perforation. It also modulates stromal regeneration and repair. Exposed stromal surfaces are a target for tear-borne enzymes of destruction and modulators that promote the release of stromal collagenases.[13,20]

Significant inflammatory mechanisms begin to evolve on the ocular surface and inside the eye. *Control of ocular inflammation is the second important therapeutic consideration during this period.* If severe, ocular inflammation can impair reepithelialization. Corticosteroid drops are the standard therapy during this period. In addition to promoting rapid reepithelialization and controlling inflammation, medical officers should also pay special attention to corneal clarity, IOP, degree of intraocular inflammation, and development of lens opacification. An acute rise in IOP may be due to the shrinkage of ocular collagen. After the acute rise abates, a more sustained increased IOP is the result of the elaboration of prostaglandins.[12]

Early Reparative Phase

The healing period from 8 to 20 days after the injury constitutes the early reparative phase. This is the transition period of ocular healing, in which the immediate regeneration of ocular surface epithelium and acute inflammatory events give way to chronic inflammation, stromal repair, and scarring. The most important treatment goal remains the establishment of an intact epithelium. If the corneal epithelium did not fully heal during the acute phase, then the physician must aggressively treat the patient to minimize the risk of corneal thinning and perforation.

TABLE 7-3

THOFT'S CLASSIFICATION OF OCULAR CHEMICAL INJURY

Category of Injury	Clinical Findings	Prognosis
Grade I	Corneal epithelial damage No ischemia	Good
Grade II	Cornea hazy, but iris detail seen Ischemia less than ⅓ of limbus	Good
Grade III	Total loss of corneal epithelium Stromal haze blurs iris detail Ischemia of ⅓ to ½ of limbus	Guarded
Grade IV	Cornea opaque, obscuring view of iris or pupil Ischemia more than ½ of limbus	Poor

Sources: (1) Roper-Hall MJ. Thermal and chemical burns. *Trans Ophthalmol Soc UK*. 1965;85:631. (2) Thoft RA. Chemical and thermal injury. *Int Ophthalmol Clin*. 1979;19(2):243–256. (3) Parrish CM, Chandler JW. Corneal trauma. In: Kaufman HE, Barron BA, McDonald MB, eds. *The Cornea*. 2nd ed. Boston, Mass: Butterworth-Heinemann; 1998: 642.

Ocular inflammation must also be controlled during this stage because inflammation can continue to inhibit epithelial migration over the corneal defects.[21] High-dose corticosteroids are usually required for the first 10 days of treatment, tapering at 14 days if an epithelial defect persists. The use of corticosteroids for more than 21 days in an eye without an intact epithelium risks collagenolysis and perforation.[22]

Late Reparative Phase

Three weeks after a chemical injury occurs, the healing process begins the late reparative phase. Application of ocular lubricants and tear substitutes must be continued to ensure a healthy epithelium. Chemical agents can cause loss of corneal sensation, decreasing the blink reflex and reducing the production of tears. Destruction of the associated mucin and lipid-producing cells also leads to an inadequate corneal tear film. Severe injury can lead to pannus formation during this time. Persistent corneal epithelial defects or recurring epithelial breakdown can be surgically managed by tarsorrhaphy.

PATIENT TREATMENT AND EVALUATION

Immediate Action

At first glance, this section appears to be erroneously titled. However, in any known or even *suspected* chemical injury of the eye, immediate treatment with irrigation precedes patient evaluation. Prompt recognition and immediate treatment of a chemical injury are the most important aspects in the preservation of vision because only then can reepithelialization be optimized. In a wartime scenario, maintaining a high degree of suspicion that a chemical attack is imminent or has occurred is also important to ensure that proper protective measures are taken and that medical resources are preserved. Observing isolation and decontamination regimens and recognizing the type of agent involved may support intelligence gathering in the combat zone and preserve the lives of the evacuation and medical teams.

Immediately on suspecting a chemical injury, medical personnel should begin treatment. The most readily available nontoxic liquid is used to flush the area of the face, eyes, and any other areas of contact. Tap water is usually the most readily available, but using iced tea, milk, or any neutral liquid is better than delaying treatment. Research indicates that attempts to chemically neutralize the original agent (eg, using a dilute acidic solution such as vinegar to neutralize an alkali injury) are contraindicated because they may cause even more damage. The exception is the use of prepared neutralization kits, specific for the known chemical agent encountered.

Medical treatment begins by irrigating with 2 L of normal saline or lactated Ringer's solution over 20 to 30 minutes. Because of its flexibility, an intravenous line attached to the bottle is a useful means of delivering the irrigation fluid. These injuries are painful and result in blepharospasm and squeezing of the eyelids. These responses to pain often oblige medical personnel to hold the patient's eyelids open with a speculum or bent paperclips while the diluting solution is delivered to the globe (Figure 7-2). Because the pain is severe, topical anesthetics are helpful in maintaining patient cooperation. (It is essential that irrigating fluid be kept from running into the patient's ears to preclude any chemical agent from contacting the tympanic membrane; eg, the eardrums of casualties of a blast may be perforated). After irrigation is completed, the pH of the eye is measured with pH paper or a urine dipstick (for ease of use, the strip is cut to expose the pH plate at the edge of the strip).

After sufficient irrigation, the eyes and ocular adnexa are inspected for particulate matter. Evert-

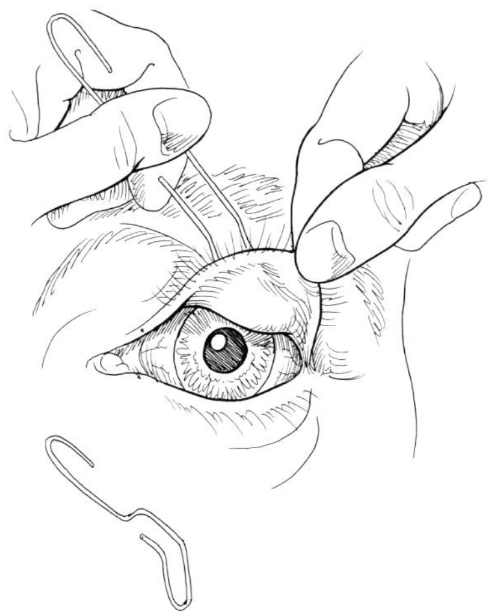

Fig. 7-2. Eyelid eversion using a bent paper clip. Drawing prepared for this textbook by Gary Wind, MD, Uniformed Services University of the Health Sciences, Bethesda, Md.

ing both the upper and lower eyelids is mandatory to search for retained particles trapped in the conjunctival fornix or embedded in the tissues themselves. Five minutes after the end of irrigation, the pH is again measured. If the pH is nearly normal, irrigation is temporarily suspended, particulate matter removed, and the examination portion begun. If the pH is not normal, irrigation is again performed with an additional 2 L of fluid. If the observed pH does not match the initial incident history, the patient and others should be questioned again.

Patient Examination

Once a normal pH level is attained and the patient's eye remains neutralized, a full ophthalmological examination is performed. Visual acuity measurements are taken for each eye independently. If a Snellen chart is not available, recording the ability of the patient to read newspaper headlines of "x" inches in height at a distance of "y" feet away is helpful.

Pupil examination is performed, noting any irregular shape or sluggish response to light. An irregular response may indicate iris ischemia due to chemical coagulation of the blood vessels in the iris or in the ciliary vessels. The external examination consists of the facial skin, eyelids, lashes, and lacrimal apparatus. Look for areas of lid burn, which can cause incomplete globe coverage, and for residual chemical particulate matter.

Ask the patient to look at an object straight in the line of view as the examiner looks at the eyelid position. Then the examiner should talk to the patient about other subjects while observing for a more relaxed lid position as well as blink reflex excursion and frequency. The patient is then asked to look up and down while the examiner observes the upper and lower eyelid position over the globe during the motion. Finally, the patient is asked to squeeze his or her eyelids tightly and then relax. It is also important for the physician and the assisting staff to observe the eyelid position and exposure of the globe while the patient is sleeping. Corneal or conjunctival exposure can lead to epithelial breakdown, infection, and corneal melting, and is a risk factor for loss of the eye.

Attention is then directed to the globe itself. A penlight, or preferably a slitlamp, examination is performed to detect epithelial loss, corneal opacification, and limbal ischemia. First, shine a light onto the corneal surface and observe the luster of the epithelium. Injured epithelial cells lack their typical reflective luster, resulting in an irregular corneal light reflex from the ocular surface. Note any gray or white areas of stromal opacification by observing whether iris detail or pupillary border is apparent when looking through the cornea. Limbal ischemia is measured by the number of clock hours of blood vessel loss of the conjunctival tissues where it nears the peripheral edge of the cornea.

Once the previous examination details are noted, a fluorescein strip may be wetted and placed on the ocular surface to delineate the extent of corneal epithelial loss (see also Chapter 3, Ocular Trauma: History and Examination). IOP is measured with one of the many instruments for this purpose or simply by comparing the tactile IOP of an intact globe by gently placing the fingertips on the closed eyelids. To facilitate evaluation of the posterior segment of the eye, eye drops (tropicamide or cyclopentolate) are instilled to achieve pupillary dilation. Cycloplegic eye drops also help control pain by effectively "splinting" pupillary reaction and reducing the pain associated with pupil constriction in bright light. Pupil dilatory drops also enhance the outflow of aqueous from the eye, helping to control IOP. The use of phenylephrine is not recommended, because its vasoconstrictive properties may lead to an increased risk of ocular ischemia.

A summary of evaluation and treatment is provided for rapid reference (Exhibit 7-2).

Acute Phase Treatment

Once the emergency treatment and evaluation are completed, the challenging task of healing the chemically injured eye begins. The major treatment goals that are important throughout the healing phases are (*a*) the reestablishment and maintenance of an intact and healthy corneal epithelium, (*b*) control of the balance between collagen synthesis and collagenolysis, and (*c*) minimizing the adverse sequelae that often follow a chemical injury. This triad of care for casualties with ocular chemical injuries takes place in the acute (urgent) phase of treatment.

The top priority in the acute phase is the reestablishment of an intact corneal epithelium. Without an intact epithelium, the risks of corneal thinning and perforation (melt), infection, and other complications that follow a chemical injury are significantly higher. The source for healthy epithelial cells is the rim of corneal epithelial stem cells that lie near the limbus.[23] A severe ocular chemical injury may permanently damage all stem cells. The corneal surface is therefore lacking in progenitor epithelial cells, and the surface is replaced with

EXHIBIT 7-2

CHEMICAL INJURY: EVALUATION AND TREATMENT SUMMARY

A. History

1. Suspected or known chemical contact
2. Possible wartime/lethal chemical agent
    a. Observe mission-oriented protective posture (MOPP) gear or self-protection
    b. Sound chemical alarm

B. Initiate Treatment

1. Irrigation
    a. 1–2 L normal saline or lactated Ringer's solution (30 min)
    b. Intravenous tubing
    c. Speculum
    d. Topical anesthetic
2. Inspection
    a. Remove particulate matter
    b. Pull down lower eyelid, inspect fornix
    c. Evert upper eyelid, inspect fornix
3. Indicator test: test pH at end of irrigation and 5 min after completion of irrigation
    a. If pH = 7: Stop irrigation
        Begin examination (see below)
        Recheck pH after 20 more min elapse
        Debride devitalized tissue
        Initiate medical therapy
    b. If pH < 7 or > 7: Restart irrigation with another 2 L
    c. If pH matches history (eg, low pH for acid injury), continue therapy
    d. If pH does not match history, obtain more details of injury while continuing treatment
4. Examination
    a. Visual acuity
        DISTANCE: Right Left
        NEAR: Right Left
    b. Pupils
        SHAPE: Round/Irregular
        REACTION: Fast/Sluggish
    c. External examination
        (1) Facial skin
        (2) Eyelid skin
        (3) Lashes
            (a) Loss
            (b) Eversion
            (c) Inversion
    d. Slitlamp or pen light examination
        (1) Conjunctiva
            (a) Number of clock hours of limbal ischemia
            (b) Areas of fluorescein staining

(**Exhibit 7-2** *continues*)

Exhibit 7-2 *continued*

(2) Cornea
- (a) Epithelium: Fluorescein staining/cell loss
- (b) Stroma
  - (i) Tissue loss
  - (ii) Thickening
  - (iii) Opacity
    - Haze, but iris detail visible
    - Haze blurs iris detail
    - Haze obscures view of iris or pupil
- (c) Descemet's: Folds

(3) Anterior chamber
- (a) Depth
- (b) Foreign body
- (c) Red blood cells layered
- (d) White blood cells layered
- (e) Inflammation

C. Additional Information

1. Intraocular pressure:	Low	Normal	High*
2. Lens:	Clear		Clouded*

*Elevated intraocular pressure or loss of lens clarity suggests significant intraocular penetration

slower-growing conjunctival epithelial cells and fibrosed and vascularized tissue.[24] In less-severe injury, corneal epithelial stem cells that survive a chemical injury act as progenitor cells for epithelial cell division and subsequent migration of the cells to cover the epithelial surface.[25] Promotion of a healthy microenvironment for these processes is the mainstay of therapy.

The preocular tear film is normally rich in moisture, lipids, mucus, and mineral cofactors. Treatment is usually aimed at replacing the aqueous portion of the tear film with preservative-free artificial tears, ointments, and antibiotics that are relatively nontoxic to the epithelium. If the eye is significantly damaged or eyelid closure is not sufficient to maintain a healthy tear surface, prevention of tear evaporation is aided by eyelid closure with a patch, eyelid taping, or tarsorrhaphy. Again, control of inflammation is important because significant inflammation immediately after a chemical injury inhibits reepithelialization. Corticosteroids should be used if there is no evidence of coexisting infection.

The second priority in the acute phase of healing after a chemical injury is maintaining a positive balance between collagen synthesis and collagenase activity. This balance is necessary for achieving the removal of damaged collagen tissue while rebuilding the stroma proper. Recent studies of chemical eye injuries[26–28] have indicated the importance of the stroma and epithelial interactions in the modulation of corneal wound healing, and thus the achievement of an intact epithelium is vital. These same studies have also shown that treatment with citrate and ascorbate eye drops with oral supplementation of ascorbate (vitamin C) can enhance collagen synthesis.

Limiting adverse sequelae is the third goal in the triad of care for the ocular chemical injury. Reducing the risk of infection is accomplished with an antibiotic that presents little toxicity to the epithelial cells. Control of IOP by suppression of aqueous production is often effective. Oral and intravenous medication may be preferred in the acute setting to minimize the amount of drops administered to the eye. Control of pain should never be taken lightly, as chemical injuries are often severely painful. Long-acting cycloplegics help in pain management, because they prevent the repeated movement of the pupillary muscles. Again, oral, intramuscular, and intravenous pain control are preferred.

Limitation of conjunctival scarring can be one of

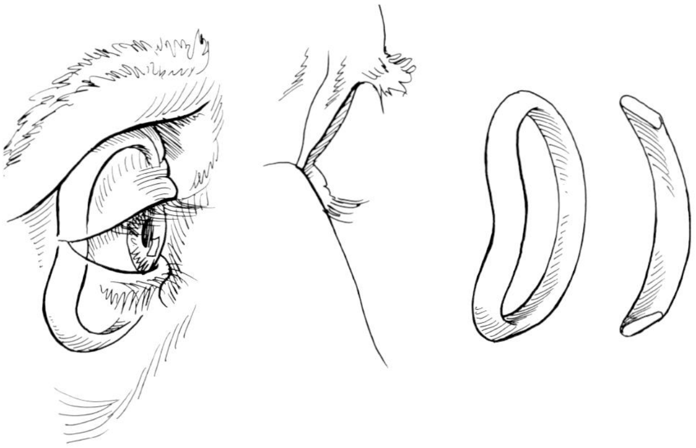

Fig. 7-3. A plastic symblepharon ring surrounds the globe and maintains the conjunctival fornices. Drawing prepared for this textbook by Gary Wind, MD, Uniformed Services University of the Health Sciences, Bethesda, Md.

the most challenging tasks for the physician. Prevention or breaking of formed symblepharon requires almost daily diligence. A symblepharon ring (conformer) is often helpful in these situations (Figure 7-3).

Early Reparative Phase Treatment

An intact epithelium should have already been achieved by the third phase of therapy. If it has not been, aggressive therapy is instituted by the use of lubrication, punctal plugs, punctal occlusion with cautery, bandage contact lens, or tarsorrhaphy. If the epithelium is not intact, corticosteroids are prescribed in a tapering dosage to be discontinued by the 14th day after injury. If significant inflammation remains, progestational steroids (eg, medroxyprogesterone) may be substituted or added to the regimen.[29,30] Ascorbate and citrate are continued. Antiglaucoma therapy is continued as required. If the epithelium is not intact, antibiotics are maintained. Examination for the formation of symblepharon is continued.

Late Reparative Phase Treatment

The patient whose injured eye has not achieved an intact epithelium by the 21st day, is at significant risk of permanent vision loss. Furthermore, long-term reduction in the amount of tear and mucus production, decreased corneal sensation, and the risk of sight-threatening infection place the patient at risk for loss of the globe. Aggressive surgical intervention is usually required in eyes that have not epithelialized within 3 weeks. Progressive thinning is treated as required with tissue glue, lamellar keratoplasty, patch graft, or pericardial tissue graft.

Rehabilitative Phase

After the eye has stabilized, most surgeons prefer to wait months to years to consider rehabilitative surgery. Limbal stem cell transplantation has shown remarkable promise in rehabilitating ocular chemical injuries that have resisted treatment or were considered too great for rehabilitation.[24,31–34] Limbal stem cells can be donated from the patient's uninjured fellow eye, a blood relative, or a postmortem globe. All have shown promise in reestablishing a healthy ocular surface prior to further reconstructive surgery. Once a healthy surface is achieved, penetrating keratoplasty or a keratoprosthesis may be considered.[35]

INJURIES OF THE EYE CAUSED BY CHEMICAL WARFARE AGENTS

The earliest military use of chemical weapons included the burning of sulfur and other choking agents to "smoke out" an enemy holding in a defensive position. Chemical weapons were later used as defensive tools. Burning oils and other noxious agents were poured from cauldrons high atop castle towers onto attackers below to repel their assault.

Modern chemical weapons were used in the attempt to break the stalemate that had developed in the trench warfare of World War I. German forces discharged chlorine gas, allowing the prevailing wind to sweep it over the British and French soldiers entrenched in Belgium in April 1915. The wartime element of surprise effectively devastated the unsuspecting soldiers, who were not wearing protective equipment, and the toxic gas killed and injured unknown numbers because of its effect on the respiratory system. Sulfur mustard was first used in warfare at Ypres, Belgium, in 1917 by German forces.[36,37] By the war's end, both sides were using choking agents (eg, phosgene) and vesicants (eg, mustard) as modern weapons of the era.[38]

The images of chemical casualties from World War I and political issues were part of the reasons that chemical agents were not used in World War II. Despite active research in chemical agents, military use of chemical weapons declined for a time. During a phase of the Vietnam War (primarily in the late 1960s), chemical defoliants such as Agent Orange were sprayed to destroy the thick jungle

a

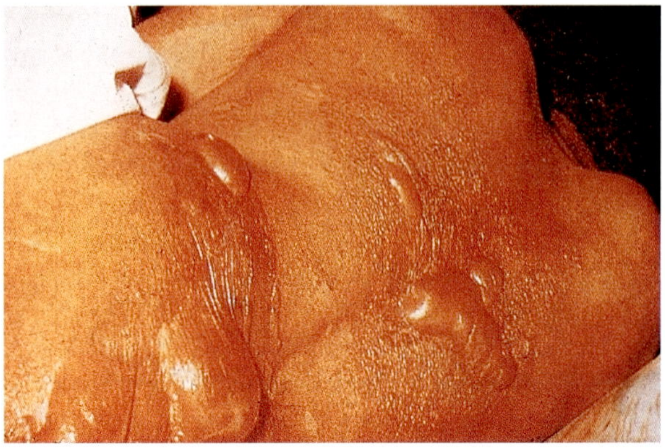

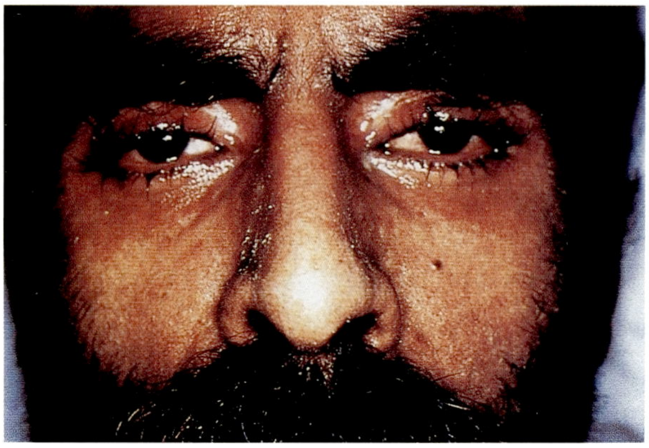

b

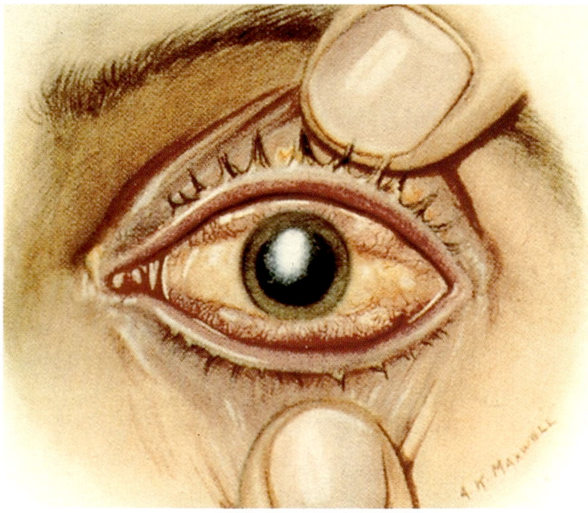

c

Fig. 7-4. (**a**) Although the vesicular effects of mustard agent on the skin of the casualty's back are impressive (the casualty's head is seen in the upper right of this photograph), (**b**) the eyes are significantly more sensitive to mustard's effects; the eye involvement seen here is relatively severe even though the skin is only minimally affected. (**c**) In 1918, the British prepared for the American Expeditionary Force a series of color drawings and descriptions of injuries by chemical warfare agents. This drawing depicts a severely burned eye in the acute stage after exposure to mustard vapor. A portion of the original description follows:

> [Severely burned eyes] may be recognized by certain characteristic features ... . Whenever a dead white band crosses the exposed area of the conjunctiva, while the parts of this membrane covered by the upper and lower lids are red and oedematous, serious injury from the burning is likely to have occurred.
>
> In the case illustrated, the caustic effect of the vapour is seen chiefly in the interpalpebral aperture. On each side of the cornea there is a dead white band due to coagulative oedema, which compresses the vessels, impairs the circulation, and thus acts as a menace to the nutrition of the cornea. The swelling in the region of this white band is slight, while the protected conjunctiva above and below it is greatly swollen and injected and may even bulge between the lids.
>
> The exposed portion of the cornea is grey and hazy; it has lost its lustre, and when viewed with a bright light and a magnifying glass it shows a blurred "window reflex" and a typical "orange skinned" surface. The haze gradually faces off above in the region of the protected part of the cornea where the surface is bright and smooth. The pupil is at first contracted as a result of irritation and congestion. In this drawing it is shown as artificially dilated by atropine ointment, which should always be used early in severe cases or where there is much pain and blepharospasm.

Photograph b: Courtesy of Dr Luis Requena, Universidad Autónoma de Madrid, Spain. Reproduced from Bennion SD, David-Jabar K. Cutaneous reactions to nuclear, biological, and chemical warfare. In: James WD, ed. *Military Dermatology*. In: Zajtchuk R, Bellamy RF, eds. *Textbook of Military Medicine*. Washington, DC: Department of the Army, Office of The Surgeon General, Borden Institute; 1994: 95. Drawing c: Reproduced from *An Atlas of Gas Poisoning*. 1918: Plate 11A. Handout provided by the American Red Cross to the American Expeditionary Force. In: Joy RJT. Historical aspects of medical defense against chemical warfare. In: Sidell FR, Takafuji ET, Franz DR, eds. *Medical Aspects of Chemical and Biological Warfare*. In: Zajtchuk R, Bellamy RF, eds. *Textbook of Military Medicine*. Washington, DC: Department of the Army, Office of The Surgeon General, Borden Institute, 1997: 99.

plants and thereby deny the enemy concealment. Whether antipersonnel chemical agents were used during the Vietnam War continues to be debated.

A sharp rise has been seen in the distribution and use of chemical weapons in events around the world. Chemical injuries have increased both on and off the battlefield in recent decades. For example, as many as 45,000 casualties may have occurred when Iraq employed mustard agent during its war (1982–1988) with Iran[39,40]; Iraq also deployed vesicants in its suppression of the 1988 rebellion in Kurdistan (Figure 7-4).

Military-strength chemical injuries have also occurred outside the classically defined boundaries of warfare. In the United States, highly toxic agents, both industrial and weapons grade, are commonly transported throughout the country. A significant industrial toxic chemical spill from a tanker truck in the Washington, DC, area required almost 24 hours for HAZMAT (hazardous material) team operations to completely decontaminate a major highway and the surrounding residential area.

In addition to the immediate effects, chemical injuries produce long-term problems with reduced vision, as well as employment and rehabilitation issues.[41] One patient who was exposed to mustard agent during the 1988 attack in Iraq presented 10 years later with delayed mustard gas keratopathy.[42] This and the recent examples above are just a few of the readiness issues for chemical injury that the military physician must be prepared to identify and treat whether in combat or everyday life.

Chemical munitions currently available include blister agents (vesicants), nerve agents, irritants, and blood agents (Tables 7-4 and 7-5). These agents can affect different organ systems, producing temporary incapacitation, temporary illness, permanent disability, or even death. The eyes can be very sensitive to many chemical agents (Table 7-6); permanent damage to the eye with loss of vision may occur.

Blister Agents

The major agent in the vesicant, or blister agent, class is sulfur mustard. During World War I, there were as many as 400,000 chemical casualties, but fewer than 3% died of their chemical wounds.[43] Of the casualties of mustard agent, 86% had ocular involvement, and many had skin involvement, especially in warm, moist areas such as the scrotum, buttocks, axillae, neck, face, and areas that were

TABLE 7-4

CHEMICAL AGENTS

US Army Code	Name of Agent
Vesicants	
H	Sulfur mustard, munitions grade (30% impurities)
HD	Distilled sulfur mustard
HN	Nitrogen mustard (once used in chemotherapy)
L	Lewisite (an arsenical)
Nerve Agents	
GA	Tabun
GB	Sarin
GD	Soman
VX	*o*-Ethyl *S*-[2-(diisopropylamino)ethyl] methylphosphonothiolate
Irritants (Tear Gas)	
CN	2-Chloro-1-phenylethanone (also known as Mace)
CS	2-Chlorobenzalmalononitrile
Vomiting Gas	
DM	Adamsite
Other Agents	
CG	Phosgene (alveolar toxicity)
AC	Hydrogen cyanide
CK	Cyanogen chloride
BZ	3-Quinuclidinyl benzilate (anticholinergic agent with psychoactive properties)

TABLE 7-5

MILITARY CHEMICAL AGENTS OF OPHTHALMOLOGICAL INTEREST

Military Designation	Agent	Onset of Symptoms	Odor at Higher Concentrations
H	Sulfur mustard $S(CH_2\text{–}CH_2\text{–}Cl)_2$	4–12 h	Garlic or mustard
HN*	Nitrogen mustard $N(CH_2\text{–}CH_2\text{–}CL)_3$	1–6 h	Fishy
L	Lewisite $ClCH{=}CH\text{–}As\text{–}Cl_2$	Immediate	Geranium
CX	Phosgene oxime $CCl_2{=}NOH$	Immediate	Low concentrations: newly mown hay; higher concentrations: acrid, pungent, disagreeable

*Although HN has previously been used only as a chemotherapeutic agent, it might be used as a weapon in the future.

TABLE 7-6

OCULAR EFFECTS OF CATEGORIES OF CHEMICAL WARFARE AGENTS

Category of Agent	Ocular Effects
Vesicants (Blister Agents)	Conjunctivitis Irritation blepharospasm Photophobia Corneal clouding and vascularization Inflammation Symblepharon Lid burns Corneal perforation
Nerve Agents	Miosis Pain Dimming of vision Ocular pain
Mycotoxins	Tearing Pain/burning Decreased vision Conjunctivitis Keratitis
Riot Control Agents	Burning/irritation Conjunctival injection/conjunctivitis Lacrimation Blepharospasm Photophobia Keratitis
Phosgene	Pain Keratitis Conjunctivitis
Cyanide	Irritation Difficulty focusing (late mydriasis)

constricted by clothing, such as the waist.[43] The British reported many thousands of eye casualties, with 75% mildly affected (2 wk on average before casualties were returned to duty); 15% were intermediate (incapacitated, 4–6 wk); and 10% were severe (their ocular injuries remained active for 4–6 mo before stabilizing). Fifty-one soldiers were blinded, and 180 were given vision-related pensions.[43] On the other hand, the Americans reported 1,500 chemical casualties, with 15% recovering in 10 to 14 days and 80% recovering in 5 to 8 weeks. They also reported cases of panophthalmitis.[44,45]

The apparent discrepancy between the British and American experience in World War I is hard to explain. The important fact remains that most patients recovered without significant damage but were incapacitated for a long time. The symptoms of photophobia, grittiness, pain, and blepharospasm effectively immobilized those affected. Keep in mind that 10% to 20% of those evacuated from the front during World War I for ocular injuries were suffering a combat reaction (gas hysteria) and either did not sustain a physical injury or demonstrated symptoms far in excess of their injuries. Today, our troops are better trained and equipped to deal with the chemical threat, and medical therapy for these types of exposures has been improved.

Between 75% and 90% of vesicant casualties can be anticipated to have ocular involvement,[44,46] with symptoms usually peaking 6 to 12 hours after exposure. Of these, 90% should have no significant corneal involvement.[47,48] They may present with a gritty sensation, conjunctivitis, chemosis, lid edema, blepharospasm, photophobia, blurred vision, tearing, and exudates.[39,48] The 10% with corneal involvement may additionally demonstrate corneal edema, keratitis, ocular pain or headache, temporary blindness, tissue necrosis, iridocyclitis, glaucoma, vascularization, delayed keratopathy, and rarely ulceration or perforation.[39,49–52]

Mechanisms of Injury

The vesicants are alkylating agents that have a pronounced intracellular effect, especially on replication of deoxyribonucleic acid (DNA).[53] Irreversible histological changes occur within 10 minutes, and these changes become pronounced at 30 minutes. Additionally, the arsenical Lewisite liberates hydrochloric acid. The acid lowers the pH of the eye to 1.3, which causes superficial opacities, but arsine oxide is its main toxin.

Lewisite, developed in the United States at the end of World War I but never used, was nevertheless extensively studied in World War II, revealing the following facts[50,54]:

- the corneal surface is free of toxins within 2 to 4 minutes,
- toxins are in the stroma within 2 minutes,
- toxins are in the anterior chamber within 1.5 minutes,
- the anterior chamber is free of toxins within 30 minutes, and
- some stromal toxins are present for 1 to 26 hours.

Research with mustard agent shows similar penetration, with the eye being free of toxins within 15 minutes.[50] The delay in symptoms with mustard thus makes timely decontamination difficult. Early detection and prevention of injury become critical.

Signs and Symptoms

Exposure to minute quantities (0.001 mg/L) of mustard agent for periods up to 1 hour does not affect the skin or the respiratory tract significantly. Yet, within 4 to 12 hours, lacrimation occurs, and a sandy sensation in the eyes becomes manifest. The conjunctivae and lids become swollen and edematous. Exposure to increased concentrations shortens the latent period, causes more damage with corneal involvement, and prolongs recovery to 2 to 6 weeks. Hot, humid weather increases the rapidity of action but also decreases the persistence of the agent.

The skin shows erythema similar to a sunburn after a latent period, and then large, thin-walled bullae usually form. Irritating these affected areas (eg, by scrubbing during decontamination), can promote vesicle formation in casualties who might not have developed them otherwise. The fluid in these vesicles is not contaminated and may safely be drained when necessary. These lesions behave much like second-degree burns and heal in several weeks, depending on the area affected.

Respiratory tract effects begin with hoarseness and a persistent cough that can progress to bronchopneumonia; these effects usually do not reach maximum severity for several days. This delay should prompt us to carefully observe those with ocular or facial burns for subsequent signs of pulmonary damage.

Working with casualties of mustard agent puts medical personnel at risk. Exhibit 7-3 lists some properties of mustard that healthcare personnel must keep in mind while aiding casualties who have

EXHIBIT 7-3

FACTS TO KEEP IN MIND WHEN WORKING WITH CASUALTIES OF MUSTARD AGENT

1. Mustard agent sensitizes, and reexposure to it—even to a small amount—may cause a more severe reaction.
2. Mustard agent is toxic in concentrations so slight that it may not be detected by its odor.
3. Contact with mustard agent is initially painless. Casualties may be produced hours or days after contaminated areas were exposed. (Lewisite, in contrast, causes immediate symptoms.)
4. Mustard-contaminated clothing, weapons, and the like may produce severe lesions for some time after the initial exposure. Contact with persons who were injured and with clothing unrecognized as contaminated with mustard has accounted for many secondary casualties among medical personnel.
5. Mustard agent is easily soluble in organic solvents and lipids but poorly soluble in water. Therefore, it can easily penetrate clothing and shoes and be absorbed into the skin. Decontaminate with water because organic solvents may actually promote its absorption.
6. Vaporized mustard agent is denser than air.
7. Mustard agent is persistent and is used to deny terrain to the enemy. This persistency varies from weeks in a cold climate to days in hot weather.
8. Mustard can be combined with other chemical agents such as Lewisite, phosgene, or nerve agents to enhance the toxicity. Keep this in mind if you are treating apparent nerve-agent casualties to avoid contaminating yourself and others.
9. Mustard agents can be delivered by airplane sprays, bombs, artillery and mortar shells, and by missiles. Mustard's boiling point is 220°C, and thefore to be effective, it must be atomized or vaporized by the munition.
10. Mustard agent that is not vaporized can contaminate the area as a contact poison with a long persistence and can serve as an inhalational poison as it evaporates.
11. Mustard agent can be destroyed by chlorination, but only dilute chlorine preparations should be used because of the great heat and sometimes flame that are generated by the chemical reaction. Decontaminating solutions are toxic to the eyes and should not be used.

Source: Blewett WK. *Defense Against Mustard: A P2NBC2 Review and Analysis.* Aberdeen, Md: Aberdeen Proving Ground, Physical Protection Directorate; 1992. Chemical Research and Development Engineering Command Technical Report 3270.

been exposed to mustard agent. Wounds per se are unlikely to be sources of mustard contamination of medical personnel, given the rapid fixation of mustard by tissues.

Treatment

There is no specific treatment used for mustard injuries; the treatment described above for alkali injuries should prove beneficial in dealing with such casualties. If decontamination is not performed within the first 5 minutes or certainly within the first 15 minutes, however, it is probably inconsequential to the outcome of the ocular injuries. The delay in the onset of symptoms probably precludes effective decontamination of the eyes, but decontamination of the casualty's clothing, skin, and hair can help prevent recurring exposure and secondary casualties. When a casualty with an injury caused by mustard agent arrives at a 3rd- or 4th-echelon medical treatment facility with an ophthalmology service, medical personnel may find it necessary to use a standing operating procedure (SOP) for mustard injuries of the eye (Exhibit 7-4).

However, a specific treatment for Lewisite injuries is available. British anti-Lewisite (BAL), which is dimercaprol, is extremely effective against Lewisite but *only* if administered topically within 2 to 10 minutes after exposure. Treatment for as long as an hour after exposure may have some benefit in an otherwise destructive lesion. Subsequent treatment of injuries caused by Lewisite and other vesicants should also follow the recommendations given for the treatment of alkali injuries.

Several publications advocate using topical anesthetics for the eye to relieve pain. However, these

EXHIBIT 7-4

EXAMPLE[*] ORDER SHEET FOR A PATIENT WITH OCULAR MUSTARD INJURIES

ADMIT:

Dx: Chemical ocular injury. *WARNING! MUSTARD EXPOSURE DECONTAMINATED*

COND:

VITALS:

ALLERGIES:

ACTIVITY: Restricted to room/bed (to minimize the risks of contaminating others and of infection)

MEDS (*examples only*):

Polytrim ophthalmic solution: one drop 5 times daily
Ilotycin or bacitracin *ophthalmic* ointment: 3 times daily and at bedtime
Prednisolone phosphate: one drop to affected eye every 2 hours while awake
Vitamin C: 2 g by mouth, 4 times daily
10% ascorbate: one drop to the affected eye
10% citrate: one drop to the affected eye every 2 hours while awake
Homatropine 2%: one drop to the affected eye 3 times daily
Timoptic 0.5%: one drop to affected eye twice daily
Neptazane 50 mg: one by mouth, 3 times daily

[*]The listed medications are for a patient with ocular injuries from exposure to mustard agent, who has no contraindications or allergies that would preclude their use. This example is *only* a guide.

anesthetics *should be avoided* except as needed for periodic examinations, as they can have serious deleterious effects on the eye if used frequently. The use of systemic analgesics would be appropriate as needed.

Nerve Agents

The nerve agents are organophosphates that bind cholinesterase. Tabun (GA), sarin (GB), and soman (GD) are essentially volatile, nonpersistent agents used for their immediate effect, but they can be combined with a thickener for more persistence. They are clear, colorless, and odorless—except for tabun, which is said to have a slightly fruity odor. In March 1995, a terrorist attack with sarin in the Tokyo, Japan, subway system injured many civilians, 12 of whom died. Another nerve agent, *o*-ethyl *S*-[2-(diisopropylamino)ethyl] methylphosphonothiolate (VX; no common name), is oily with little volatility except in high temperatures and is used as a persistent agent.

These agents are mentioned here in the discussion of ocular injuries because they can cause miosis of the pupils, blurred vision, dimmed vision, and ocular pain. Atropine (as much as 20 to 100 mg may be needed in severe intoxication) and pralidoxime chloride (2-PAM Cl), which can remove the agent from sites on the enzyme acetylcholinesterase only if the nerve agent is not "fixed" on the enzyme molecule, are used to counter the effects of these nerve agents. Atropine is given as long as signs of intoxication are present and is usually titrated by minimizing nasal, bronchial, and salivary secretions. The miosis or pupil size should not be used as an index of atropinization.

Mycotoxins

Trichothecene mycotoxins—the most memorable example is the infamous "yellow rain" from the Vietnam War era—are produced by certain strains of *Fusarium* fungi. They seem to inhibit synthesis of proteins. Symptoms appear from 1 hour (pulmonary route) to 24 hours (cutaneous route) after exposure and include vomiting, weakness, hypotension, and burns in exposed areas including the cornea.[55] Microgram quantities can cause irreversible corneal injury. Victims have complained of tearing, eye pain, conjunctivitis, a burning sensation, and blurred vision.[56,57]

SUMMARY

Despite advances in treatment for chemical injury, knowledge of risks and prevention remain the best ways to avoid the often-long therapeutic course for recovery of vision. When a patient with a chemical ocular injury presents to the treating physician, early recognition and prompt treatment remain the standards to minimize ocular tissue damage and provide hope for preservation of vision.

Military chemical agents are usually not part of the daily training environment of civilian physicians, but chemical warfare agents remain a real threat on the battlefield. Knowledge of battlefield chemical munitions, their characteristics, and expected treatment is important for patient care as well as protection of medical personnel.

Chemical ocular injuries—whether they happen on the battlefield, in the military industrial base, or at home—will occur. When they do, knowledgeable physicians can minimize tissue destruction and enhance healing throughout all phases of treatment.

REFERENCES

1. Bowen TE, Bellamy RF, eds. *Emergency War Surgery NATO Handbook.* 2nd rev US ed. Washington, DC: Department of Defense, Government Printing Office; 1988.

2. Deeter DP, Gaydos JC, eds. *Occupational Health: The Soldier and the Industrial Base.* In: Zajtchuk R, Bellamy RF, eds. *Textbook of Military Medicine.* Washington, DC: Department of the Army, Office of The Surgeon General, and Borden Institute; 1993.

3. James WD, ed. *Military Dermatology.* In: Zajtchuk R, Bellamy RF, eds. *Textbook of Military Medicine.* Washington, DC: Department of the Army, Office of The Surgeon General, and Borden Institute; 1994. Also available at www.armymedicine.army.mil/history/borden/default.htm.

4. Sidell FR, Takafuji ET, Franz DR, eds. *Medical Aspects of Chemical and Biological Warfare.* In: Zajtchuk R, Bellamy RF, eds. *Textbook of Military Medicine.* Washington, DC: Washington, DC: Department of the Army, Office of The Surgeon General, and Borden Institute; 1997. Also available at www.armymedicine.army.mil/history/borden/default.htm.

5. Laibson PR, Oconor J. Explosive tear gas injuries of the eye. *Trans Am Acad Ophthalmol Otolaryngol.* 1970:74:811–819.

6. Harris LH, Cohn K, Galin MA. Alkali injury from fireworks. *Ann Ophthalmol.* 1971;3:849–851.

7. Minatoya HY. Eye injuries from exploding car batteries. *Arch Ophthalmol.* 1978;96:477–481.

8. Wagoner MD. Chemical injuries of the eye: Current concepts in pathophysiology and therapy. *Surv Ophthalmol.* 1997;41:275–313.

9. Pfister RR. The effects of chemical injury on the ocular surface. *Ophthalmology.* 1983;90:601–609.

10. Matsuda H, Smelser GK. Epithelium and stroma in alkali-burned corneas. *Arch Ophthalmol.* 1973;89:396–401.

11. Matsuda H, Smelser GK. Endothelial cells in alkali-burned corneas: Ultrastructural alterations. *Arch Ophthalmol.* 1973;89:402–409.

12. Paterson CA, Pfister RR. Intraocular pressure changes after alkali burns. *Arch Ophthalmol.* 1974;91:211–218.

13. Kenyon KR. Inflammatory mechanisms in corneal ulceration. *Trans Am Ophthalmol Soc.* 1985;83:610–663.

14. McCulley JP. Chemical injuries. In: *The Cornea: Scientific Foundation and Clinical Practice.* Smolin G, Thoft RA, eds. Boston, Mass: Little, Brown & Co; 1987: 527–542.

15. Pfister RR. Chemical corneal burns. *Int Ophthalmol Clin.* 1984;24:157–168.

16. Ralph RA. Chemical burns of the eye. In: Duane TD, Jaeger EA, eds. *Clinical Ophthalmology.* Vol 4. Philadelphia, Pa: Harper & Row; 1987: 1–10.

17. Hughes WF Jr. Alkali burns of the eye, I: Review of the literature and summary of present knowledge. *Arch Ophthalmol.* 1946;35:423–449.

18. Hughes WF Jr. Alkali burns of the eye, II: Clinical and pathologic course. *Arch Ophthalmol.* 1946;36:189–214.

19. Roper-Hall MJ. Thermal and chemical burns. *Trans Ophthalmol Soc UK.* 1965;85:631.

20. Kenyon KR, Berman MB, Rose J, Gage J. Prevention of stromal ulceration in the alkali-burned rabbit cornea by glued-on contact lens: Evidence for the role of polymorphonuclear leukocytes in collagen degradation. *Invest Ophthalmol Vis Sci.* 1979;18:570–587.

21. Wagoner MD, Kenyon KR, Gipson IK. Polymorphonuclear neutrophils delay corneal epithelial wound healing in vitro. *Invest Ophthalmol Vis Sci.* 1984;25:1217–1220.

22. Donshik PC, Berman MB, Dohlman CH, Gage J, Rose J. The effect of topical corticosteroids on corneal ulceration in alkali-burned corneas. *Arch Ophthalmol.* 1978;96:2117–2120.

23. Pfister RR. Stem cell disease. *CLAO J.* 1993;20:64–72.

24. Huang AJW, Tseng SCG. Corneal epithelial wound healing in absence of limbal epithelium. *Invest Ophthalmol Vis Sci.* 1991;32:96–105.

25. Chen JJ, Tseng SCG. Corneal epithelial wound healing in partial limbal deficiency. *Invest Ophthalmol Vis Sci.* 1990;31:1301–1314.

26. Pfister RR, Paterson CA, Hayes SA. Topical ascorbate decreases the incidence of corneal ulceration after experimental alkali burns. *Invest Ophthalmol Vis Sci.* 1978;17:1019–1024.

27. Pfister RR, Nicolaro ML, Paterson CA. Sodium citrate reduces the incidence of corneal ulceration and perforation in extreme alkali-burned eyes: Acetylcysteine and ascorbate have no favorable effect. *Invest Ophthalmol Vis Sci.* 1981;18:486–490.

28. Pfister RR, Haddox J, Barr D. The combined effect of citrate/ascorbate treatment in alkali-injured rabbit eye. *Cornea.* 1991;10:100–104.

29. Lass JH, Campbell KC, Rose J. Medroxyprednisone on corneal ulceration: Its effects after alkali burns on rabbits. *Arch Ophthalmol.* 1981;99:673–676.

30. Newsome DA, Gross JA. Prevention by medroxyprogesterone of perforation of the alkali burned rabbit cornea: Inhibition of collagenolytic activity. *Invest Ophthalmol Vis Sci.* 1977;16:21–31.

31. Thoft RA. Conjunctival transplantation as an alternative to keratoplasty. *Ophthalmology.* 1979;86:1084–1092.

32. Herman WK, Doughman DJ, Lindstrom RL. Conjunctival autograft transplantation for unilateral ocular surface disease. *Ophthalmology.* 1983;90:1121–1126.

33. Weise RA, Mannis MJ, Vastine DW. Conjunctival transplantation: Autologous and homologous grafts. *Arch Ophthalmol*. 1985;103:1736–1740.

34. Kenyon KR, Tseng SCG. Limbal autograft transplantation for ocular surface disorders. *Ophthalmology*. 1989;96:709–722.

35. Dohlman CH, Schneider HA, Doane MG. Prosthokeratoplasty. *Am J Ophthalmol*. 1974;77:694–700.

36. Prentiss AM. *Chemicals in War: A Treatise on Chemical War*. New York, NY: McGraw-Hill; 1937.

37. Heller CE. *Chemical Warfare in World War I: The American Experience, 1917–1918*. Fort Leavenworth, Kan: US Army Command and General Staff College, Combat Studies Institute; 1984. Leavenworth Papers 10.

38. National Research Council, Division of Medical Sciences, Committee on Treatment of Gas Casualties. *Fasciculus on Chemical Warfare Medicine: Eye*. Vol 1. Washington, DC: NRC; 1945.

39. Lashkari K, Lashkari MH, Kim AJ, Crane WG, Jalkh AE. Combat-related eye trauma: A review of 5320 cases. *Int Ophthalmol Clin*. 1995;35:193–203.

40. Carus WS. *Chemical Weapons in the Middle East*. Washington, DC: Washington Institute for Near East Policy; 1988. Research Memorandum 9.

41. The Johns Hopkins University Press. *Studies on the Physiologic, Biochemistry, and Cytopathology of the Cornea in Relation to Injury by Mustard Gas and Allied Toxic Agents*. Baltimore, Md: The Johns Hopkins University Press; 1948: 82(2): n.p.

42. Pleyer U, Sherif Z, Baatz H, Hartman C. Delayed mustard gas keratopathy: Clinical findings and confocal microscopy. *Am J Ophthalmol*. 1999;128:506–507.

43. Duke-Elder J, MacFaul PA. Chemical injuries. In: *Non-Mechanical Injuries*. Part 2. In: *Injuries*. Vol 14. In: Duke-Elder J, ed. *System of Ophthalmology*. St Louis, Mo: CV Mosby; 1972: 1112–1153.

44. Gilchrist HL. *A Comparative Study of WWI Casualties from Gas and Other Weapons*. Edgewood, Md: US Chemical Warfare School; 1928: 1–51.

45. Combat Casualty Care Office. *Medical Management of Chemical Casualties Handbook*. Aberdeen Proving Ground, Md: Combat Casualty Care Office, US Army Medical Research Institute of Chemical Defense; 1994.

46. Hughes WF Jr. Mustard gas injuries to the eyes. *Arch Ophthalmol*. 1942;27:582–609.

47. Greenmeaux P. Ocular lesions following the action of lacrymatory gases [abstract]. *Br J Ophthalmol*. 1917;1:512.

48. Teulieres M, Valois G. The action of asphyxiating or lacrymatory gases on the visual apparatus [abstract]. *Br J Ophthalmol*. 1917;1:512–513.

49. Mann I, Pullinger BD. Experiments on effect of ascorbic acid in mustard gas burns of the eye. *Br J Ophthalmol*. 1940;24:444–451.

50. Cordes FC. Nonsurgical aspects of ocular war injuries. *Am J Ophthalmol*. 1943;26:1062–1071.

51. Davis WT. Military ophthalmology. *Am J Ophthalmol*. 1944;27:26–44.

52. Zagora E. *Specific Protein Denaturants and Selective Enzyme Inhibitors in Eye Injuries*. Springfield, Ill: Charles C Thomas; 1970: 308–309.

53. Papirmeister B, Feister AJ, Robinson SI, Ford RD. *Medical Defense Against Mustard Gas: Toxic Mechanisms and Pharmacologic Implications*. Boca Raton, Fla: CRC Press; 1991.

54. Wiener M. The treatment of recent injuries to the eye and adnexa. *Trans Am Acad Ophthalmol Otolaryngol*. 1944; 49:425–433.

55. Wannemacher RW Jr, Bunner DL, Neufeld HA. Toxicity of trichothecenes and other related mycotoxins in laboratory animals. In: Smith JE; Henderson RS, eds. *Mycotoxins and Animal Foods*. Boca Raton, Fla: CRC Press; 1991: 499–552.

56. Haig AM Jr. *Chemical Warfare in Southeast Asia and Afghanistan. Report to the Congress.* Washington, DC: US Government Printing Office; 22 March 1982.

57. Watson SA, Mirocha CJ, Hayes AW. Analysis for trichothecenes in samples from Southeast Asia associated with "yellow rain." *Fundam Appl Toxicol*. 1984;4:400–417.

Chapter 8

BLUNT TRAUMA AND NONPENETRATING INJURIES OF THE ANTERIOR SEGMENT

GLENN C. COCKERHAM, MD*

**Colonel, US Air Force (Ret); Cornea Service, Allegheny General Hospital, 420 East North Avenue, Suite 116, Pittsburgh, Pennsylvania 15212; formerly, Chief, Ophthalmology Service, Malcolm Grow Air Force Medical Center, Andrews Air Force Base, Maryland*

INTRODUCTION

The anterior segment of the eye consists of the conjunctiva, cornea, anterior chamber, trabecular meshwork, iris, and crystalline lens. Despite the surrounding facial bones, which protect the orbital contents from lateral or tangential blows, the anterior segment is vulnerable to direct trauma. Blunt ocular trauma may occur on the battlefield from missile injury, concussive effects from high explosives, and physical blows. It may also occur in industrial accidents, sports injuries, domestic assault, violent crime, motor vehicle accidents, fireworks, and in other military and civilian settings.

The numerous sequelae of blunt anterior segment trauma (Exhibit 8-1) can cause transient or permanent visual loss and disability. These injuries may be associated with globe rupture and damage to the orbital bones; eyelids and ocular adnexa; and posterior ocular structures, including the retina, choroid, and optic nerve.

EXHIBIT 8-1

SEQUELAE OF ANTERIOR SEGMENT TRAUMA

- Conjunctiva
  - Conjunctival abrasion
  - Foreign body
  - Conjunctival laceration
  - Subconjunctival hemorrhage
- Cornea
  - Abrasion
  - Foreign body
  - Traumatic keratopathy
  - Corneal laceration/rupture
  - Ultraviolet radiation injury
- Iris
  - Traumatic iritis
  - Traumatic mydriasis
  - Iridodialysis
  - Traumatic hyphema
- Ciliary Body
  - Cyclodialysis
  - Angle recession
- Lens
  - Subluxation/Dislocation
  - Traumatic cataract
- Traumatic Glaucoma

Incidence of Ocular Trauma

From World War II to the Persian Gulf War, ocular injuries have accounted for 2% to 13% of wartime injuries.[1] Ocular injuries are also seen frequently in civilian trauma. Of 727 patients with maxillofacial trauma evaluated in a large urban hospital, 90 (1.24%) patients had a serious eye injury, including hyphema in 38 (0.52%) patients.[2] Of 6,254 eye admissions at a large, metropolitan eye hospital, 7.5% of the patients were admitted with ocular trauma; hyphema was the most common injury, present in 25% of the ocular trauma cases.[3] Severe injury (defined as hyphema, open globe, intraocular foreign body [IOFB], or orbital/facial fracture) was present in 5% of 3,184 patients with ocular trauma who were evaluated in an urban tertiary care hospital over a 6-month period.[4]

Prevention of Injuries

A polycarbonate protective lens will stop small-caliber gunshot, low-velocity projectiles (eg, blast shrapnel), and windblown dust and sand. It affords some protection against a direct blow to the eye. In the Arab–Israeli Yom Kippur War (6–24 October 1973), combatants who wore protective lenses sustained fewer ocular injuries than those who did not wear them.[1] Military ophthalmologists must emphasize that soldiers in the theater of operations must continuously wear their protective eyewear.

CONJUNCTIVA

The conjunctiva is a smooth, thin, transparent mucus membrane that covers the globe and lines the posterior eyelid surfaces. It consists of nonkeratinizing, stratified, columnar epithelium and an underlying stroma composed of connective tissue with blood vessels and lymphatic vessels. The portion overlying the eye—the bulbar conjunctiva—is loosely attached to the underlying episclera and sclera, whereas the portion lining the eyelids—the palpebral conjunctiva—is more firmly attached.

Blunt trauma may damage the conjunctival layer by means of scrapes and tears to the conjunctiva itself, and by allowing blood to pool in and trapped air to enter the subconjunctival layers.

Conjunctival Abrasions and Lacerations

Conjunctival abrasions and lacerations are caused by a direct or shearing force, such as may be applied by a fist, finger, or other object. The patient can usually recall the time and type of injury. Symptoms of a conjunctival abrasion include a foreign body (FB) sensation and discomfort. Localized redness is noted at the area of injury. Subconjunctival hemorrhage is possible. Fluorescein staining reveals a discontinuity in the conjunctival surface.

Treatment consists of the use of a broad-spectrum ophthalmic ointment (eg, bacitracin or erythromycin) several times per day in the affected eye. Physicians can reassure their patients by telling them that conjunctival abrasions typically heal within several days.

Patients with conjunctival lacerations may present with the same history and symptoms as those with conjunctival abrasion. Inspection with anesthetic eyedrops reveals a full-thickness tear in the conjunctival epithelium, possibly with hemorrhage. A thorough examination, including dilation, is necessary to exclude an associated globe injury in that area or a retained FB. Small lacerations do not require closure and may be managed with antibiotic ointment and, if the patient is uncomfortable, application of a pressure patch for 1 or 2 days. Larger lacerations, usually more than 1 cm long, should be closed with an absorbable suture, such as 7-0 or 8-0 polyglactin (Vicryl, mfg by Johnson & Johnson, Summerville, NJ), on either a tapered or a spatulated needle. Tenon's fascia should be excluded from the wound to avoid an unsightly scar.[5]

Subconjunctival Hemorrhage and Emphysema

The subepithelial connective tissue underneath the bulbar conjunctiva, known as the lamina or substantia propria, contains numerous blood vessels derived from the anterior ciliary artery. These vessels are mobile and are vulnerable to rupture or tear in blunt trauma (Figure 8-1). Consequently, subconjunctival hemorrhage is common. Isolated subconjunctival hemorrhages require no specific therapy and will resorb within several weeks.

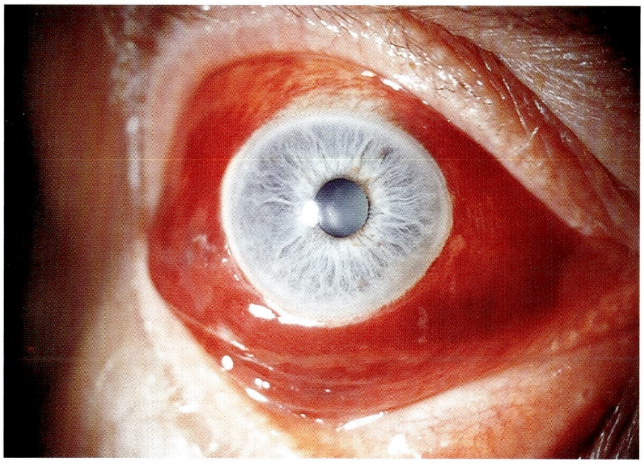

Fig. 8-1. In this patient with subconjunctival hemorrhage, diffuse hemorrhage can be observed underneath the conjunctiva following blunt trauma. There was no evidence of globe rupture.

Subconjunctival emphysema is loculated air in the lamina propria and is distinguished by a cystic appearance of the conjunctiva and by crepitus on palpation. These findings signify fracture of the periorbital sinuses with leakage of free air under the conjunctiva. Most commonly, the orbital fracture involves the lamina papyracea of the ethmoid sinus or the orbital floor overlying the maxillary sinus.[5]

The presence of subconjunctival hemorrhage, edema, or air may be associated with other eye injuries. Conjunctival edema, or chemosis, may accompany blunt trauma of the anterior segment. Specifically, localized hemorrhagic chemosis may overlie the site of a globe rupture. A complete ocular examination with imaging of the orbital bones is indicated in these cases.

CORNEA

The cornea is a specialized, transparent area of the outer coat of the eye. Its anterior location and aspheric conic shape make it susceptible to trauma. The cornea is most thin centrally, where it averages 0.52 mm in thickness, and increases to 0.65 mm peripherally.[6] Superficially, it consists of nonkeratinizing stratified squamous epithelium. The stroma, which constitutes 90% of the corneal thickness, consists of avascular collagen. Underlying the stroma is a thick basement membrane known as Descemet's membrane. Nonreplicating endothelial cells line Descemet's membrane and are responsible for maintaining corneal clarity by removing water from the corneal stroma.

Abrasion

Blunt or sharp trauma may disrupt the surface epithelium, producing a corneal abrasion. Because of the rich innervation by the corneal nerves, such injuries are very symptomatic and are accompanied by tearing, pain, photophobia, and protective closure of the eyelids. The visual acuity is usually decreased, from both the abrasion and profuse tearing. Topical anesthetic drops may be necessary for adequate anterior segment examination. Fluorescein, a dye applied either as a 2% solution or with a paper strip wetted with a sterile solution, will stain areas of epithelial discontinuity. Use of a cobalt filter with the slitlamp or of a hand-held Wood's ultraviolet (UV) lamp stimulates a green fluorescence by fluorescein and facilitates the diagnosis. Magnification of the cornea may be obtained with a slitlamp, a Wood's lamp, or a direct ophthalmoscope set at high-plus diopters (black).

Traumatic corneal abrasions have traditionally been treated with an antibiotic ointment, a mild cycloplegic agent, and a pressure patch. Patched patients require daily examinations to determine if the abrasion has healed and to verify that there is no corneal infection. Pressure patching has disadvantages, including occlusion of vision in the injured eye, discomfort, and an increased risk of infection, especially in contact lens-associated corneal abrasions.[7] Small- to moderate-sized traumatic abrasions have been shown[8] to heal faster with less discomfort, compared with pressure patching, if treated only with a broad-spectrum antibiotic (polymyxin [Polysporin Ophthalmic Ointment, mfg by Burroughs Wellcome Co, Research Triangle Park, NC] or erythromycin) and a mild cycloplegic (1% tropicamide). Topical nonsteroidal drops (0.5% ketorolac tromethamine) used four times daily for 3 days in conjunction with the no-pressure patch regimen described above can reduce the pain associated with traumatic corneal abrasion.[9] However, institution of topical nonsteroidal drops requires medical supervision and discontinuation after 3 days, as prolonged use may cause persistent epithelial defects.

A traumatic corneal abrasion may also be treated successfully with a bandage contact lens, topical antibiotic drops instilled four times daily, and topical nonsteroidal drops also instilled four times daily, which allow quicker visual rehabilitation.[10] For active duty soldiers, the increased risk of corneal infection and the expense associated with use of a bandage contact lens and nonsteroidal eyedrops must be weighed against the possible benefit of a quicker return to duty.

Uncomplicated, small corneal abrasions usually heal within a day or two. Superficial abrasions involving the epithelium heal without scarring, although corneal irregularity may impair vision for days to weeks. If a corneal wound breaches the underlying Bowman's layer and involves the stroma, scarring is usual. Topical anesthetics are *never* prescribed for pain management of corneal disorders, because their continued use may cause persistent epithelial defects and stromal scarring.

Corneal abrasions breach a protective layer of the eye and may become secondarily infected with bacterial, fungal, or parasitic agents. A white or gray infiltrate, best seen under magnification, is an indicator of corneal infection. Contact lenses are a predisposing factor for bacterial infection, especially Gram-negative bacteria such as *Pseudomonas* species. Inoculation of a corneal abrasion with vegetable matter is a risk factor for fungal infection. If microbiological laboratory support is available, diagnostic scraping with topical anesthesia and either a platinum spatula or a surgical blade is indicated. Appropriate studies include microscopic examination with Gram's or Giemsa stains, as well as microbial culture on solid media, such as blood agar, chocolate agar, and Sabouraud's agar (fungal). Until the results of the cultures are available, the initial treatment can be based on the results of the Gram's stain.

Fortified topical antibiotics should be used for infiltrates that (1) are associated with contact lens wear and (2) involve the visual axis or (3) are unresponsive to antibiotic monotherapy. Commonly used regimens include fortified cefazolin or vancomycin for coverage against Gram-positive bacteria and fortified gentamycin or tobramycin for coverage of Gram-negative organisms. Monotherapy with a single, broad-spectrum, fluoroquinolone antibiotic (eg, ciprofloxacin or ofloxacin) can be used for small or peripheral infiltrates or ulcers. However, fluoroquinolone antibiotics may not eradicate some Gram-positive bacteria, including *Staphylococcus* and *Streptococcus* species.

Patients with corneal infiltrates or ulcers should be followed closely. As previously noted, pressure patching of abrasions or ulcers associated with contact lens use is contraindicated. Topical steroids should not be used in the initial management of corneal infections.

Traumatic Keratopathy

Concussive force may directly damage endothelial cells with sector corneal edema. Damaged endothelial cells may regain function, or undamaged adjacent cells may slide over and cover the injured area, leading to eventual clearing.[11] Sufficient concussive force may cause a single or multiple breaks in Descemet's membrane and severe corneal edema due to acute hydrops.[5] Endothelial cells will slide over the gap and eventually regenerate a new basement membrane. However, a tear in the original Descemet's membrane will remain visible, owing to scrolling or curling of the edges.

Corneal edema will often clear in weeks to months. The efficacy of topical steroids in the treatment of traumatic corneal edema remains unproven. Persistent sector edema, especially if localized inferiorly, can indicate an IOFB in the chamber angle. Gonioscopy is necessary to rule out this possibility.

Corneal Foreign Bodies

Foreign objects in the cornea may occur in a variety of industrial or military settings. The mechanism of injury is an important clue to possible occult ocular damage. High-velocity FBs (eg, particles generated by a blast, power tools, or metal striking metal) can lodge within any level of the cornea or even penetrate the ocular coat and locate anywhere within the eye. The presence of a conjunctival or corneal FB should prompt a thorough examination of the entire external area, including eversion of the upper and lower eyelids.

Like corneal abrasions, corneal FBs may be very painful, with blurred vision, photophobia, and tearing. Slitlamp examination will reveal single or multiple imbedded FBs at any level of the cornea. Superficial objects may be irrigated or removed with a moistened sterile swab under topical anesthesia. Deeper objects may be removed with a spud or a sterile hypodermic needle (22-gauge or smaller) mounted on a tuberculin syringe. This is best done at the slitlamp with firm support for the hand or wrist. A rust ring, common with iron FBs, may be removed with a hypodermic needle, dental burr, or spud. Residual rust may be left in the cornea, especially if the object was located away from the central cornea. Topical antibiotics should be applied until the epithelium has healed and the danger of infection has passed.

Corneal Lacerations

Any sufficient force can disrupt the ocular coat with a partial or complete tear through the cornea and sclera. Rupture is more likely to occur in areas of thin sclera, such as the insertions of the rectus muscles. It is also more likely to occur in areas of previous surgery or injury; rupture is especially problematic with avascular, clear corneal wounds (eg, cataract, transplantation, refractive incisions), owing to prolonged and incomplete wound healing.

If globe rupture is suspected, a protective metal shield should be placed over the patient's eye pending definitive diagnosis and management. Topical medications are to be avoided if rupture is suspected. It is important to determine if Descemet's membrane has been breached; careful slitlamp examination may reveal this. A Seidel test with 2% fluorescein is performed to detect leakage of the aqueous. Full-thickness lacerations may seal themselves because the corneal stroma swells on contact with aqueous fluid; in this case, the Seidel test may be negative initially. A provocative test with gentle pressure on the upper or lower lid may reveal fluid leakage.[12]

Partial-thickness wounds are treated with antibiotic prophylaxis, such as a broad-spectrum ophthalmic ointment or solution instilled three or four times daily until epithelial healing occurs. A bandage soft–contact lens may also be used to splint the wound. These wounds heal with scar formation, which may impair vision owing to the ensuing opacity or irregularity of the corneal surface. Partial-thickness avulsions or wounds with gaps may require suture closure, as will almost all full-thickness lacerations. Repair of corneal lacerations is addressed in Chapter 9, Sharp Trauma of the Anterior Segment.

Ultraviolet Radiation Keratitis

The cornea transmits most of the visible wavelengths of light between 400 and 800 nm. As the wavelength decreases into the invisible UV portion of the electromagnetic spectrum, more and more of the energy is absorbed by corneal tissue. The wavelengths between 200 and 300 nm are strongly absorbed by corneal cellular elements.[13] UV radiation keratitis occurs with exposure to sunlight, especially in situations with high reflectivity (snow or desert). High-altitude activities and exposure to arc welding or tanning lamps are also common causes of UV radiation keratitis. The corneal epithelium incurs the most damage from UV radiation. The damage typically becomes apparent within 8 to 12 hours after exposure.[13] Symptoms include an FB sensation, pain, and photophobia. Epithelial stippling and epithelial defects seen with fluorescein staining occur with moderate to severe exposure. Resolution occurs in 1 to 2 days.

Protective lenses that absorb UV radiation prevent this injury. Military personnel should be alerted to the increased risk at high altitude and in snow or desert conditions. Treatment of UV injury is similar to that of corneal abrasion: antibiotic ointment, mild cycloplegic agents, and oral analgesics. Pressure patching should be considered on a case-by-case basis.

IRIS

The iris forms a diaphragm that separates the anterior and the posterior chambers of the eye. It consists of an anterior stroma with connective tissue, blood vessels, nerves, and melanocytes; the posterior iris contains a pigment epithelial layer. A sphincter muscle encircles the pupil, controlling light entry into the posterior chamber and maintaining the pupillary contour. A dilator muscle extends from the sphincter muscle to the base of the iris.[14] The iris is diaphanous and easily injured.

Traumatic Iritis

An inflammatory response to blunt trauma begins within hours. Typically, patients present with tearing, photophobia, and pain. Conjunctival injection and reduced vision may be noted. White blood cells are visible in the aqueous, with flare. Medical management of traumatic iritis consists of the application of topical steroid drops until resolution occurs, usually within several days. Prednisolone acetate, 1%, is commonly used three or four times daily. Cyclopentolate, 1%, administered three or four times daily, is sufficient for cycloplegia and offers the advantage of a shorter duration of action than atropine, homatropine, or scopolamine.

Traumatic Mydriasis

Concussion of the anterior segment may damage the iris sphincter muscle, resulting in anisocoria and iris deformity, including a sector defect or an oval pupil. A transient or permanently dilated, nonreactive pupil may be the result. Liberated pigment from the iris pigment epithelium may be deposited on the endothelium, trabecular meshwork, or lens. A circular pigment deposit on the anterior lens capsule due to trauma is known as a Vossius ring.

Iridodialysis

Iridodialysis, separation of the iris root from its scleral attachment (Figure 8-2), may result in bleeding with hyphema. Surgical repair is indicated for a displeasing appearance or polyopia and glare. A small-incision repair is possible with use of a 10-0 polypropylene (Prolene) suture on a double-armed CIF-4 needle (Ethicon, mfg by Johnson & Johnson, Summerville, NJ).[15] The technique is illustrated in Figure 8-3.

HYPHEMA

Characteristics

The presence of precipitated blood cells in the anterior chamber is called *hyphema* (Figures 8-4 and 8-5). Cell suspension in the aqueous is termed microscopic hyphema. Hyphemas may occur for a variety of reasons, including trauma; surgery; bleeding diathesis; neovascularization of the iris or chamber angle; or neoplasia, including juvenile xanthogranuloma.

A direct blow to the anterior globe can indent and shorten the anterior–posterior axis, with an attendant expansion equatorially. The iris–lens diaphragm may be retrodisplaced by the pressure wave. Stretching or shearing of tissues may lead to a tear of the ciliary body or the iris root. A tear in the anterior face of the ciliary body, or traumatic angle recession, is the most common cause of bleeding.[16] In this injury, the circular and oblique muscle fibers of the ciliary body are torn away from the longitudinal fibers, which remain attached to the scleral spur. A tear in this location may disrupt the major arterial circle of the iris or other arteries or veins in the area.[16] Traumatic cyclodialysis with separation of all ciliary body attachments, including the longitudinal fibers, from the scleral spur may also lead to hyphema. Iridodialysis and tears in the iris stroma or sphincter muscle uncommonly produce bleeding.

Small amounts of hemorrhage may circulate as suspended erythrocytes in the aqueous humor or collect as clumps on the iris, lens surface, or corneal endothelium. As the density of red blood cells in the anterior chamber increases, blood settles de-

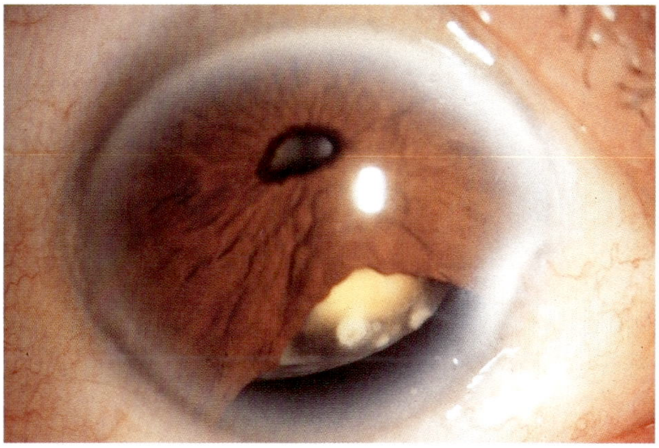

Fig. 8-2. A traumatic iridodialysis is present inferotemporally. A traumatic cataract is evident in the area of iris dehiscence. Photograph: Ms Ellen Foer, Ophthalmic Photographer, Walter Reed Army Medical Center, Washington, DC.

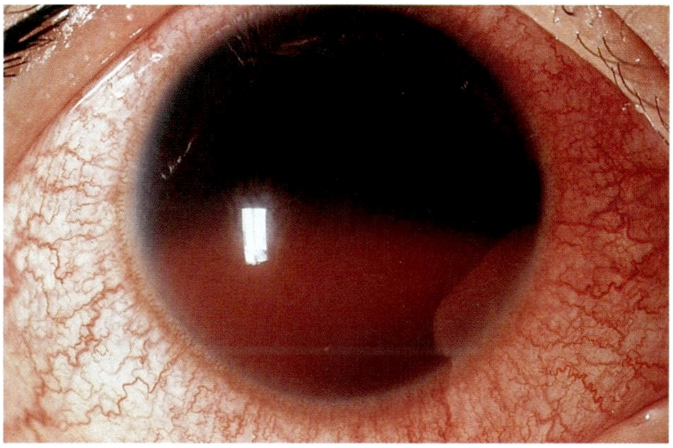

Fig. 8-4. In this hyphema, blood occupies approximately 40% of the anterior chamber following blunt trauma. Photograph: Ms Ellen Foer, Ophthalmic Photographer, Walter Reed Army Medical Center, Washington, DC.

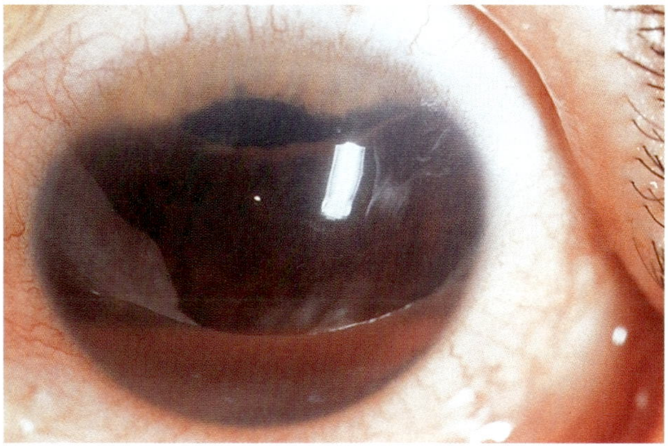

Fig. 8-5. A traumatic hyphema occupies 80% of the anterior chamber. Note the separation of clot and liquid blood (arrow). Photograph: Ms Ellen Foer, Ophthalmic Photographer, Walter Reed Army Medical Center, Washington, DC.

Fig. 8-3. Iridodialysis repair is depicted in the drawings. (**a**) A limbal peritomy and underlying scleral flap are created adjacent to the iridodialysis, and a limbal stab incision is made 180° away. Both needles of double-armed 10-0 polypropylene (CIF-4 needle, Ethicon, mfg by Johnson & Johnson, Summerville, NJ) cross the anterior chamber, engage the edge of the torn iris tissue, and exit through the scleral flap 0.5 mm behind the surgical limbus. (**b**) The suture material is tied with a triple knot and rotated. The scleral flap is closed with 10-0 nylon monofilament suture and the conjunctiva is replaced. Drawings prepared for this textbook by Gary Wind, MD, Uniformed Services University of the Health Sciences, Bethesda, Md.

a

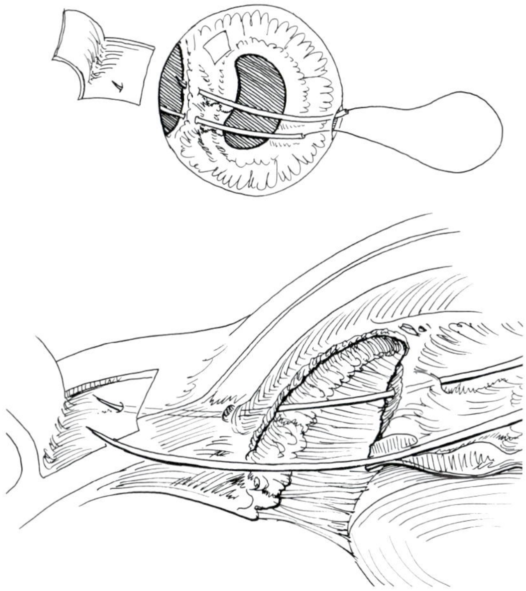

b

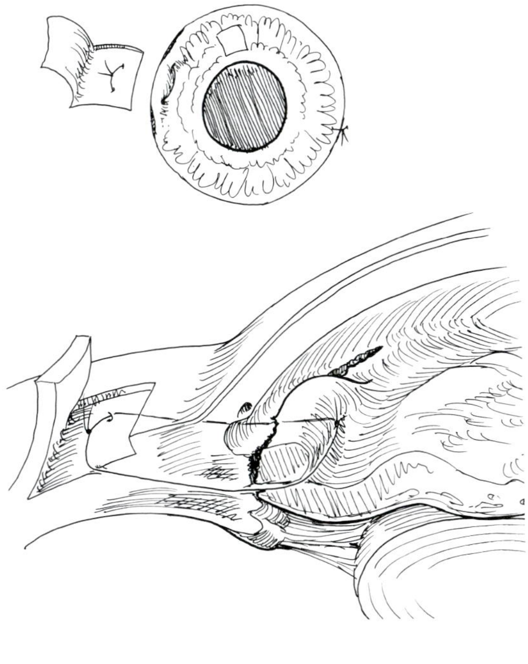

pendently into the inferior chamber angle. Initially, this blood separates into a layered hyphema consisting of solid and plasmoid phases. A fibrin clot eventually forms. Hyphemas are generally graded by the percentage of the anterior chamber volume that they occupy.[17]

Complications

Visual loss may occur secondary to the trauma associated with hyphema. Visually significant complication from hyphema may occur days or weeks after the initial injury and require careful observation.

Rebleeding

Secondary hemorrhage (rebleeding) may complicate hyphema, occurring in 3.5% to 38% of patients, depending on the population studied.[17–21] Rebleeding has been associated with initial hyphema grade II or higher (occupying more than one third of the anterior chamber area),[19,20] although other studies[18,22,23] did not correlate rebleeding with initial hyphema size. Several studies[24–26] suggest that black patients of African descent are at higher risk of secondary hemorrhage. Fresh bleeding, which usually happens 2 to 5 days after the injury, may be caused by clot lysis.[16] Eyes that have rebled have generally been associated with poorer prognoses, although other studies[18,22] suggest that associated ocular injuries, especially retinal abnormalities, may account for this observed tendency.

Elevated Intraocular Pressure

Elevated intraocular pressure (IOP) can occur with hyphema. An acute rise in pressure may follow (1) concussive damage to the trabecular meshwork, with edema or collapse; or (2) obstruction of the outflow channels by formed blood elements and fibrin, or, later, with erythroclasis. Pupillary block by the clot can also occur.[27] A rise in IOP above 25 mm Hg occurs in 25% of patients with hyphema.[26]

Patients with hyphema who are young and whose optic nerves are healthy can withstand moderate rises in IOP without glaucomatous damage. However, patients with sickle cell disease (homozygous SS) or sickle cell trait (heterozygous SC or SA) are at risk of developing high IOP with hyphema. The rigid sickle cells are unable to deform themselves to exit through the trabecular meshwork and therefore clog the pathways, with a consequent pressure spike. Elevated IOP may cause anterior segment ischemia due to hypoperfusion, with acidosis and hypoxia, thereby exacerbating the sickling process.[17] Patients with sickle cell disease or trait are at higher risk for glaucomatous damage, possibly due to vascular occlusion by sickled erythrocytes with hypoperfusion of the optic nerve.[28]

Corneal Bloodstaining

Corneal bloodstaining occurs in 5%[16,26] of hyphema patients. It is associated with larger hyphemas, elevated IOP, prolonged clot duration, corneal endothelium dysfunction, and rebleeding.[16] Hemosiderin and other products of red blood cell degradation are present in the stromal keratocytes. Early signs include a yellowish discoloration in the posterior stroma and reduced definition of the posterior stromal fibrillar structure.[17] Corneal bloodstaining may clear over months to years, beginning peripherally.

Management

Management goals include detection and treatment of other injuries; resolution of the hyphema; and prevention of complications. The risk of deprivation amblyopia must be considered in the pediatric age group. Documentation of vision, IOP, extent of hyphema, and results of anterior and posterior segment examination at presentation is essential. Gonioscopy is not performed as part of the initial examination because manipulation may provoke further bleeding. A metal shield may be used to prevent accidental contact with the injured eye. Because sickling may occur in a patient with either the sickle cell disease or trait, any black patients of African descent with hyphema should undergo a blood test for sickle cell disease or trait and hemoglobin electrophoresis.[17]

Pharmacological Therapy

Inpatient observation has advantages in compliance and follow-up but has not been shown to improve the prognosis of hyphema, compared with outpatients maintained on moderate activity.[29] Discontinuing aspirin and nonsteroidal antiinflammatory oral agents is prudent because of their antiplatelet effects. Acetaminophen is preferred for pain management. Cycloplegic agents, such as a 1% atropine solution, are usually prescribed for twice-daily instillation for patient comfort, prevention of posterior synechiae, and facilitation of posterior pole examination. Cycloplegic agents do not appear to have a beneficial effect on clot resolution or frequency of rebleeding.[18] Topical steroids can reduce associated inflammation and reduce the incidence of rebleeding, possibly through clot stabilization.[18] Prednisolone acetate, 1%, may be administered four times daily to the affected eye. Systemic prednisone has been shown[30] to have an equivalent rate of secondary hemorrhage, compared with oral antifibrinolytic agents, whereas other studies[23] have shown no effect. No study has compared the efficacy of topical versus systemic steroids. The side effects of systemic prednisone must be borne in mind.

Elevated IOP is initially treated medically. Topical timolol maleate, apraclonidine hydrochloride, and oral methazolamide or acetozolamide are used as indicated. Acetozolamide (Diamox, mfg by Lederle Laboratories, Wayne, NJ), which leads to systemic acidosis, hemoconcentration, and elevated ascorbic acid, is contraindicated in patients with sickle cell disease or trait because it causes increased sickling activity. Methazolamide is theoretically preferable in this situation because it produces less acidosis.[17] Miotics are not used because they may increase inflammation.

Systemic antifibrinolytic agents, such as ε-aminocaproic acid and tranexamic acid, have been reported to reduce the incidence of secondary hemorrhage in traumatic hyphema.[23,31–33] Two categories of patients are most likely to benefit: black patients of African descent and those who have been taking aspirin products.[34,35] These agents competitively inhibit the activation of plasminogen (profibrinolysin) to plasmin (fibrinolysin) and prevent early dissolution of clots, presumably allowing healing of injured blood vessels.[33] The usual dosage is 50 to 100 mg/kg orally every 4 hours, up to 30 g/d, for 5 days.[35] Side effects include nausea, vomiting, and postural hypotension.[36] Recently, the use of 30% ε-aminocaproic acid in a topical gel, instilled in the eye four times a day for 5 days, has been reported[37] to be effective without the systemic side effects of oral therapy.

Surgical Intervention

Surgical intervention to remove the clot and the free blood may be indicated in certain patients. Elevated IOP above 50 mm Hg for 5 days or above 35 mm Hg for 7 days, despite use of pressure-lowering agents, has been suggested[17] as an indication for surgery to avoid optic nerve damage. However, a lower threshold is required for patients with sickle cell trait or sickle cell disease or preexisting glaucomatous optic atrophy.[17] Surgery has been recommended[38] if IOP remains higher than 24 mm Hg for 24 hours in a patient with sickle cell disease.

Intervention is warranted if corneal bloodstaining occurs. In patients with total or near-total hyphema and IOP above 25 mm Hg that persists for 5 days, clot evacuation may prevent corneal bloodstaining. Prevention of peripheral anterior synechiae is another consideration: large clots persisting more than several days or total hyphemas lasting more than 5 days may be evacuated.[17] Clot removal in hyphema is not innocuous, however. Risks include damage to the cornea, iris, or lens; inadvertent extraction of the iris; prolapse of intraocular contents; renewed bleeding; formation of synechiae; and postoperative glaucoma.[16]

The simplest and safest technique for hyphema evacuation is an anterior chamber washout through one or two clear corneal limbal paracentesis wounds (Figure 8-6). This procedure allows removal of free blood and fluid and lowers IOP. If bleeding or in-

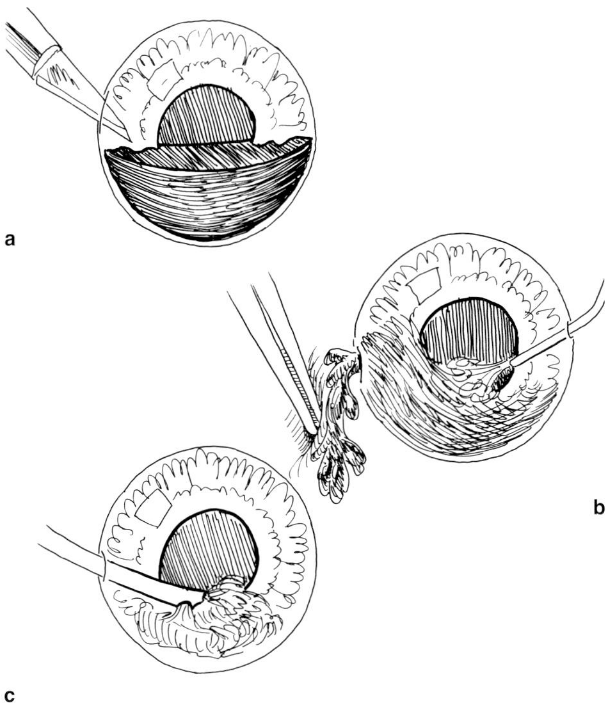

Fig. 8-6. Methods of hyphema evacuation. (**a**) Limbal stab incisions approximately 2 mm wide are made at 10 o'clock and 2 o'clock with a 15° surgical knife. (**b**) Hyphema washout is achieved by irrigation of balanced salt solution into the anterior chamber, while a closed forceps depresses the opposite paracentisis site to allow egress of the fluid and the clot. (**c**) If the washout is insufficient to remove the hyphema, a manual or automated irrigating/aspiration unit is introduced to remove the blood and the clot. Drawings prepared for this textbook by Gary Wind, MD, Uniformed Services University of the Health Sciences, Bethesda, Md.

creased IOP recur, the paracentesis sites may be reopened at the slitlamp with sterile jeweler's or 0.12-mm forceps to "burp" out additional fluid. This procedure leaves the conjunctiva intact in case filtering surgery is required.[17] Large clots may be removed through a limbal incision combined with anterior chamber washout and a peripheral iridectomy, or with trabeculectomy.[27,39]

Disadvantages of surgical intervention include inadvertent delivery of the iris, lens, or vitreous. Automated irrigation/aspiration or automated vitrectomy instruments may be used initially or after conversion from an unsuccessful anterior chamber washout. Tamponade of active bleeding may be obtained by raising the height of the irrigating solution bottle.[17]

SUMMARY

Most blunt trauma and UV radiation injuries are preventable with appropriate protective eyewear, which is available to and should be worn continuously by all military personnel in a theater of action. Blunt trauma to the eye may cause incapacitation through visual loss and pain, adversely affecting the military mission by the loss of a combatant, the use of medical resources, and, in more severe cases, transport of the patient to a rear-echelon facility for surgical management.

In all cases of ocular trauma, a thorough examination is essential to detect occult injury, establish a prognosis, and to formulate a management plan. Most nonperforating injuries to the anterior segment may be treated conservatively, with the goals of therapy to restore vision and ameliorate pain and to prevent secondary complications.

REFERENCES

1. Heier JS, Enzenauer RW, Wintermeyer SF, Delaney M, LaPiana FP. Ocular injuries and diseases at a Combat Support Hospital in support of operations Desert Shield and Desert Storm. *Arch Ophthalmol.* 1993;111:795–798.

2. Holt JE, Holt GR, Blodgett JM. Ocular injuries sustained during blunt facial trauma. *Ophthalmology.* 1983;90:14–18.

3. Maltzman BA, Pruson H, Mund ML. A survey of ocular trauma. *Surv Ophthalmol.* 1976;21:285–290.

4. Schein OD, Hibberd PL, Shingleton BJ, et al. The spectrum and burden of ocular injury. *Ophthalmology.* 1988;95:300–305.

5. Kenyon KR, Wagoner MD. Conjunctival and corneal injuries. In: Shingleton BJ, Hersh PS, Kenyon KR, eds. *Eye Trauma.* St Louis, Mo: Mosby Year–Book; 1991: 63–78.

6. Spencer WH. Cornea. In: Spencer WH, ed. *Ophthalmic Pathology: An Atlas and Textbook.* Vol 3. Philadelphia, Pa: WB Saunders; 1986: 229–388.

7. Clemons CS, Cohen EJ, Arentsen JJ, Donnenfeld ED, Laibson PR. *Pseudomonas* ulcers following patching of corneal abrasions associated with contact lens wear. *CLAO J.* 1987;13:161–164.

8. Kaiser PK. A comparison of pressure patching versus no patching for corneal abrasions due to trauma or foreign body removal. *Ophthalmology.* 1995;102:1936–1942.

9. Kaiser PK, Pineda R. A study of topical nonsteroidal anti-inflammatory drops and no pressure patching in the treatment of corneal abrasions. *Ophthalmology.* 1997;104:1353–1359.

10. Donnenfeld ED, Selkin BA, Perry HD, et al. Controlled evaluation of a bandage contact lens and a topical nonsteroidal antiinflammatory drug in treating traumatic corneal abrasions. *Ophthalmology.* 1995;102:979–984.

11. Slingsby JG, Forstot SL. Effect of blunt trauma on the corneal endothelium. *Arch Ophthalmol.* 1981;99:1041–1043.

12. Hersh PS, Shingleton BJ, Kenyon KR. Management of corneoscleral lacerations. In: Shingleton BJ, Hersh PS, Kenyon KR, eds. *Eye Trauma.* St Louis, Mo: Mosby Year–Book; 1991: 143–158.

13. Hamill WB. Corneal injury. In: Krachmer JH, Mannis MJ, Holland EJ, eds. *Cornea: Cornea and External Disease: Clinical Diagnosis and Management*. St Louis, Mo: Mosby; 1997: 1403–1422.

14. Green WR. The uveal tract. In: Spencer WH, ed. *Ophthalmic Pathology: An Atlas and Textbook*. Vol 3. Philadelphia, Pa: WB Saunders; 1986: 1352–2072.

15. Cockerham GC, Kenyon K, Rapoza PA. Traumatic cataract with other anterior segment injury. In: Albert DM, ed. *Ophthalmic Surgery: Principles and Techniques*. Malden, Mass: Blackwell Science; 1999: 152–162.

16. Wilson FM II. Traumatic hyphema: Pathogenesis and management. *Ophthalmology*. 1980;87:910–919.

17. Shingleton BJ, Hersh PS. Traumatic hyphema. In: Shingleton BJ, Hersh PS, Kenyon KR, eds. *Eye Trauma*. St Louis, Mo: Mosby Year–Book; 1991: 104–116.

18. Ng CS, Strong NP, Sparrow JM, Rosenthal AR. Factors related to the incidence of secondary hemorrhage in 462 patients with traumatic hyphema. *Eye*. 1992;6:309–312.

19. Fong LP. Secondary hemorrhage in traumatic hyphema: Predictive factors for selective prophylaxis. *Ophthalmology*. 1994;101:1583–1588.

20. Kennedy RH, Brubaker RF. Traumatic hyphema in a defined population. *Am J Ophthalmol*. 1988;106:123–130.

21. Volpe NJ, Larrison WI, Hersh PS, Kim T, Shingleton BJ. Secondary hemorrhage in traumatic hyphema. *Am J Ophthalmol*. 1991;112:507–513.

22. Kearns P. Traumatic hyphema: A retrospective study of 314 cases. *Br J Ophthalmol*. 1991;75:137–141.

23. Rahmani B, Jahadi HR, Rajaeefard A. An analysis of risk for secondary hemorrhage in traumatic hyphema. *Ophthalmology*. 1999;106;380–385.

24. Palmer DJ. A comparison of two dose regimens of epsilon aminocaproic acid in the prevention and management of secondary traumatic hyphemas. *Ophthalmology*. 1986;93:102–108.

25. Spoor TC, Hammer M, and Bellosa H. Traumatic hyphema: Failure of steroids to alter its course: A double-blind prospective study. *Arch Ophthalmol*. 1980;98:116–119.

26. Read J, Goldberg MF. Comparison of medical treatment for traumatic hyphema. *Trans Am Acad Ophthalmol Otolaryngol*. 1974;78:799–815.

27. Graul TA, Ruttum MS, Lloyd MA, Radius RL, Hyndiuk RA. Trabeculectomy for traumatic hyphema with increased intraocular pressure. *Am J Ophthalmol*. 1994;117:155–159.

28. Goldberg MF. Sickled erythrocytes, hyphema and secondary glaucoma. *Ophthalmic Surg*. 1979;10:17–31.

29. Shiuey Y, Lucarelli MJ. Traumatic hyphema: Outcomes of outpatient management. *Ophthalmology*. 1998; 105:851–855.

30. Farber MD, Fiscella R, Goldberg MF. Aminocaproic acid versus prednisone for the treatment of traumatic hyphema. *Ophthalmology*. 1991;98:279–286.

31. McGetrick JJ, Jampol LM, Goldberg MF, Frenkel M, Fiscella RG. Aminocaproic acid decreases secondary hemorrhage after traumatic hyphema. *Arch Ophthalmol*. 1983;101:1031–1033.

32. Crouch ER, Frenkel M. Aminocaproic acid in the treatment of traumatic hyphema. *Am J Ophthalmol*. 1976; 81:355–360.

33. Goldberg MF. Antifibrinolytic agents in the management of traumatic hyphema [editorial]. *Arch Ophthalmol*. 1983;101:1029–1030.

34. Teboul BK, Jacob JL, Barsoum-Homsy M, et al. Clinical evaluation of aminocaproic acid for managing traumatic hyphema in children. *Ophthalmology.* 1995;102:1646–1653.

35. Kraft SP, Christianson MD, Crawford JS, Wagman RD, Antoszyk JH. Traumatic hyphema in children: Treatment with epsilon-aminocaproic acid. *Ophthalmology.* 1987;94:1232–1237.

36. Goldberg MF. The treatment of traumatic hyphema with topical ε-aminocaproic acid [editorial]. *Arch Ophthalmol.* 1997;115:1189–1190.

37. Crouch ER, Williams PB, Gray MK, Crouch ER, Chames M. Topical aminocaproic acid in the treatment of traumatic hyphema. *Arch Ophthalmol.* 1997;115:1106–1112.

38. Deutsch TA, Weinreb RN, Goldberg MF. Indications for surgical management of hyphema in patients with sickle cell trait. *Arch Ophthalmol.* 1984;102:566–569.

39. Verma N. Trabeculectomy and manual clot evacuation in traumatic hyphema with corneal blood staining. *Aust N Z J Ophthalmol.* 1996;24:33–38.

Chapter 9

SHARP TRAUMA OF THE ANTERIOR SEGMENT

KRAIG S. BOWER, MD*

*Lieutenant Colonel, Medical Corps, US Army; Cornea and External Disease Section, Ophthalmology Service, Walter Reed Army Medical Center, Washington, DC 20307-5001

INTRODUCTION

Ocular injuries constitute approximately 10% of all injuries that occurred during recent US and foreign conflicts.[1–12] Penetrating eye injuries are commonly seen with blast injuries from terrorist and other bombings,[13,14] and the cornea and anterior segment are commonly involved in ocular trauma. Visual prognosis of eyes with injuries that are limited to the anterior segment is generally better than in those with posterior segment involvement. Isolated anterior segment injuries can often be repaired with excellent results by applying a systematic approach for managing patients with corneal and anterior segment trauma.

This discussion is limited to Zones I and II, as described by the Ocular Trauma Classification Group.[15] Classification of corneal injuries not only gives a framework for discussion but also helps provide a structured approach to surgical repair and an idea of the prognosis postoperatively. The nature and the extent of the injury largely determine the resulting visual potential as well as the set of postoperative complications that may be encountered. Although the degree of overlap varies, certain general categories are defined in the succeeding sections. The surgical approach to each type of injury is discussed later in the chapter.

EXHIBIT 9-1

CLASSIFICATION OF CORNEAL LACERATIONS

- Simple Corneal Lacerations
  - Partial-thickness
  - Full-thickness
  - Stellate
- Complex Corneal Lacerations
  - With tissue loss
  - With uveal prolapse
  - Corneoscleral
  - With intraocular foreign bodies
  - With lens involvement

Corneal rupture is not a common complication of blunt trauma because thinner, weaker areas of the sclera tend to rupture before the cornea. Nevertheless, spontaneous corneal rupture has been reported with thinning disorders such as Terrien's degeneration, Mooren's ulcer, keratoconus, and pellucid marginal degeneration,[16–18] as well as with disorders of collagen metabolism with brittle corneas.[19,20] Postoperative rupture may also occur following penetrating keratoplasty,[21–23] cataract surgery,[24,25] or incisional keratorefractive surgery (radial and astigmatic keratotomy).[26–29]

Sharp trauma of the anterior segment may be classified as *simple* or *complex*. Simple corneal lacerations are those that do not involve significant tissue loss or involvement of other ocular structures. Simple corneal lacerations may be either partial- or full-thickness. In general, simple corneal lacerations, when repaired following the basic principles outlined in this chapter, should result in reasonably good outcomes.

Complex corneal lacerations are not only more difficult to repair but are often associated with a more complicated postoperative course, higher rate of complications, and worse visual prognosis. Complex lacerations include those that have significant tissue loss and those that involve other ocular structures (Exhibit 9-1). Factors that predict poor outcomes include the following[30–34]:

- poor initial visual acuity after the injury,
- type of injury,
- presence of an afferent pupillary defect,
- lacerations longer than 10 mm,
- lacerations extending posterior to the insertions of the rectus muscle,
- lens involvement,
- retinal detachment,
- severe vitreous hemorrhage, and
- the presence of an intraocular foreign body (IOFB).

PATIENT EVALUATION AND PREOPERATIVE MANAGEMENT

Careful evaluation of the trauma patient is essential to correctly identify vision-threatening conditions and to plan the operative intervention. This evaluation includes a thorough history and a complete ocular examination and, in addition, may require laboratory testing and imaging studies. Evaluation of the eye can take place only after life-threatening emergencies have been recognized and treated. Once the patient is medically stable, the goal of the ocular examination should be to identify all eye and ocular adnexal injuries, including the identification and localization of foreign bodies (FBs). Other, less-severe injuries and concurrent medical conditions may influence the ophthalmic care and should be noted. A complete and thorough evaluation provides the treating ophthalmologist with the information necessary to develop a safe and appropriate therapeutic plan.

The evaluation begins with the patient history. If the patient is unable to provide a careful history, any family members or available witnesses to the injury should be interviewed. Detailed documentation of all the information, including the source of the injury, is very important. Military ophthalmologists should always solicit details leading up to and immediately following the trauma, the time interval from the injury to the evaluation, the treatment during that interval, the time of the last meal, past medical and surgical history, past ocular history, and known medication allergies.

A complete eye examination is performed to determine the extent of the injury and rule out an IOFB or infection. The ocular examination should be conducted carefully to avoid further injury to the eye. A Desmarres eyelid retractor may be used to carefully elevate the lid without putting pressure on the globe. If the patient is squeezing the eyelids during the examination or in response to pain, it may be appropriate to administer a facial nerve block. The examination should completely evaluate the visual acuity, pupillary reaction, ocular and adnexal motility, and should include a slitlamp examination of the anterior segment, applanation tonometry, and a dilated funduscopic examination.

If it is immediately evident that a penetrating injury has occurred, as in the case of a flat globe or obvious prolapse of uvea, lens, or vitreous, the examination should then be abbreviated to avoid unnecessary manipulation of the eye. In less-obvious cases, depending on the nature of the injury and with a high index of suspicion, more-subtle signs of a ruptured globe should be sought. Findings predictive of scleral rupture include Light Perception vision or worse, an afferent pupillary defect, hemorrhagic chemosis, intraocular pressure less than 10 mm Hg, asymmetry of anterior chamber depth, or a tented pupil.[35–37]

Ancillary tests are often indicated. Laboratory studies may include cultures, blood alcohol level, blood chemistries, hematocrit, and coagulation indices. Imaging options include ultrasound, plain film radiography, computed tomography, and magnetic resonance, each of which has certain advantages and disadvantages (see Chapter 4, Imaging of Ocular and Adnexal Trauma).

Once the examination is completed and the decision is made to go to the operating room, the goals of management are to minimize further damage to the eye, reduce the risk of infection, minimize risks to the patient's health, and prepare the patient physically and emotionally for surgery. The injured eye must be protected with a rigid shield and the patient started on prophylactic intravenous antibiotics. After the patient provides informed consent, he or she may be given pain medications and sedatives as needed. The ophthalmologist should notify the anesthesia provider and the operating room staff, and if significant posterior segment injury or an FB is present, coordinate surgical repair with a retinal surgeon, if possible.

Prophylactic Antibiotics

Traumatic endophthalmitis makes up approximately 25% of all culture-positive cases of endophthalmitis.[38] Rates of endophthalmitis after penetrating injuries vary from 2% to 17%. Endophthalmitis is more common with posterior segment injuries than with purely corneal wounds.[39] Injuries that occur on the battlefield as well as in rural settings, retained IOFBs, injuries with lens disruption, and delayed primary closure present the greatest risks for an infection.[40–42] The prognosis for eyes that develop endophthalmitis in this setting is quite poor. Prophylactic intravenous antibiotics are, therefore, indicated in all cases of penetrating ocular trauma. The most common organisms isolated from patients with posttraumatic endophthalmitis are *Staphylococcus*, *Bacillus*, and *Streptococcus* species, Gram-negative rods, and various fungal species.[43,44] For further discussion, see Chapter 17, Posttraumatic Endophthalmitis.

Anesthesia

Corneal lacerations should be repaired under general anesthesia. The increased intraorbital volume from a retrobulbar injection may cause pressure on the open globe and increase the risk of extrusion of intraocular contents through the wound. If the patient cannot undergo general anesthesia, a low-volume (5-mL) peribulbar or modified retrobulbar block may be given very slowly while the anesthesia provider and ophthalmologist carefully observe the patient for adverse effects of increased orbital pressure on the injured globe.[45,46] In rare instances, topical anesthesia can be used. When general anesthesia is given, a nondepolarizing muscle relaxant agent is often recommended, because depolarizing agents (eg, succinylcholine) may cause cocontraction of the extraocular muscles and increased intraocular pressure with risk of extrusion of intraocular contents. Patients should be brought out of general anesthesia and extubated with great care to avoid bucking on the endotracheal tube and emesis in the immediate postoperative period.

Patient Preparation

The patient's eye is prepared and draped in sterile fashion, using extreme caution to avoid further trauma. An adherent plastic barrier may be applied to the lashes and cut to expose the globe while it keeps the lashes out of the surgical field. The eyelid speculum should be carefully placed to avoid pressure on the globe. A lid speculum that provides good exposure with little or no pressure on the globe should be used. If a speculum cannot be placed, 4-0 silk retraction sutures may be used. Silk traction sutures placed at the corneoscleral limbus or under the rectus muscles may be necessary to stabilize the globe during repair. Such sutures must be used cautiously, however, because they may exert undue pressure on the open globe, with detrimental results.

GENERAL SURGICAL PRINCIPLES

The primary goal in the initial surgical repair of sharp anterior segment trauma is to reestablish the watertight integrity of the globe.[47,48] Secondary goals are to restore the normal corneal contour and to minimize scarring. When suturing corneal or corneoscleral wounds, familiarity with a few basic surgical concepts will help to obtain the best possible closure with the least corneal astigmatism and scarring, thereby resulting in the best possible visual outcome. The general suggestions in this section pertain to the closure of all corneal or corneoscleral lacerations. Guidelines for repair of specific types of injuries are covered below in this chapter.

Viscoelastic Agents

Before the development of viscoelastic products, ophthalmic surgeons relied on the use of air, gases, and irrigating solutions to try to maintain the anterior chamber spaces in surgery and after a traumatic injury. These older methods often resulted in distortion of visibility, inability to maintain the anterior chamber depth, and inadequate protection of the corneal endothelium.

Modern viscoelastic agents are made from several different materials (eg, sodium hyaluronate, sodium chondroitin sulfate, and hydroxypropylmethyl cellulose) with different molecular weights and viscosities. Agents with higher viscosities tend to maintain the surgical spaces better than those with lower viscosity. By using these materials, we are able to operate on patients while preserving vision with minimal degradation, maintaining tissue planes (ie, keeping the anterior chamber formed), and protecting the corneal endothelium.

TABLE 9-1

SUTURES FOR CORNEAL LACERATION REPAIR

Tissue	Suture Type	Needle	Example
Cornea	10-0 nylon	Spatula-shaped, half-curved	Ethilon CS-175-6
Limbus	8-0 or 9-0 nylon	Spatula-shaped, 160°	Ethilon CS-160-8
Sclera	8-0 nylon	Spatula-shaped	Ethilon CS-160-8

Suture Selection

Corneal lacerations should be sutured using 10-0 monofilament nylon. A spatula-shaped microsurgical needle will allow passage of the suture with minimal tissue damage. A shorter radius of curvature (175°) allows the short, deep bites necessary to achieve the best closure (Table 9-1). The limbus should be reapproximated using 8-0 or 9-0 monofilament nylon on a 160° needle. The longer radius of curvature allows larger bites. 8-0 nylon is used to close sclera.

Suturing Instruments

Suturing corneal or corneoscleral lacerations is not like suturing cataract wounds. The cataract wound is straight or curvilinear and is usually placed in the same location case after case. When suture-closure of the cataract wound is necessary, access and positioning are usually quite easy to accomplish. In contrast, traumatic injuries are frequently located at odd orientations for the surgeon, necessitating awkward hand positions.

EXHIBIT 9-2

EXAMPLE INSTRUMENT SET FOR SURGERY OF ANTERIOR SEGMENT TRAUMA

Jaffe, Park, or similar eyelid speculum	Graefe muscle hook
Straight hemostat	Stevens tenotomy hook
Curved hemostat	Collar button
Towel clamp	Kuglen iris hook and lens manipulator
Dressing forceps	Cyclodialysis spatula
Lester fixation forceps	Lens loop
0.12-mm Castroviejo forceps	Eye scissors
0.3-mm Castroviejo forceps	Vannas scissors
0.5-mm Castroviejo forceps	Long Vannas scissors
0.12-mm Colibri forceps	Blunt Westcott scissors
Straight McPherson tying forceps	Sharp Westcott scissors
Angled or curved McPherson tying forceps	Iris scissors
Straight micro needle holder	Beaver blade handle
Curved micro needle holder	Simcoe irrigating-aspirating (I/A) cannula
Maumenee iris hook	23-gauge anterior chamber cannula

Although surgeon flexibility is helpful, appropriate suturing instruments are essential. Needle holders may be locking or nonlocking, but they should have a fine tip that can be used for tying. Round handles give the surgeon fine control of the instrument and, therefore, the needle tip, by fingertip rotation. Curved tips also give some surgeons greater degrees of mobility than straight tips when working at difficult angles. A 0.12-mm toothed tissue forceps is essential in handling the cornea during the needle pass. Either a Castroviejo or a Colibri style is acceptable, with the Colibri forceps' angled tip offering greater degrees of freedom.

Either forceps style should be equipped with a tying platform. Tying with the needle driver and tissue forceps saves time and allows the case to proceed without the need to pass instruments back and forth between surgeon and surgical scrub technician. This fact is particularly important in situations where the surgeon is operating either alone or with inexperienced assistants. Tying forceps should have fine tips that meet properly. Bent tips make tying more difficult or impossible, and tips that scissor may inadvertently cut the suture, making additional needle passes necessary. Either two straight-tying forceps, or one straight- and one curved-tying forceps should be available. The straight and curved pairs offer more versatility and may facilitate suturing in difficult locations or positions. An example of a standard instrument set for anterior segment trauma repair appears in Exhibit 9-2.

Suture Placement

Tissue should be gently stabilized with 0.12-mm toothed tissue forceps. Take care not to dull the needle tip through contact with the needle driver or tissue forceps, as a dulled needle tip will be difficult to pass, cause tissue distortion, and lead to possible tissue damage. Occasionally, with a formed anterior chamber and well-approximated wound edges, the suture pass may be made in a "no-touch" fashion: follow the curve of the needle. With the appropriate needle selection, this approach generally results in the correct suture placement without distorting the tissue excessively or bending the needle.

Sutures should enter the corneal surface vertically and then exit within the wound horizontally over Descemet's membrane at 90% stromal depth. The needle pass then enters the opposite cut edge horizontally at the same 90% stromal depth and exits the corneal surface vertically (Figure 9-1). Sutures that are too superficial allow gaping of the inner aspect of the wound, but through-and-through sutures can provide (1) a tract for aqueous

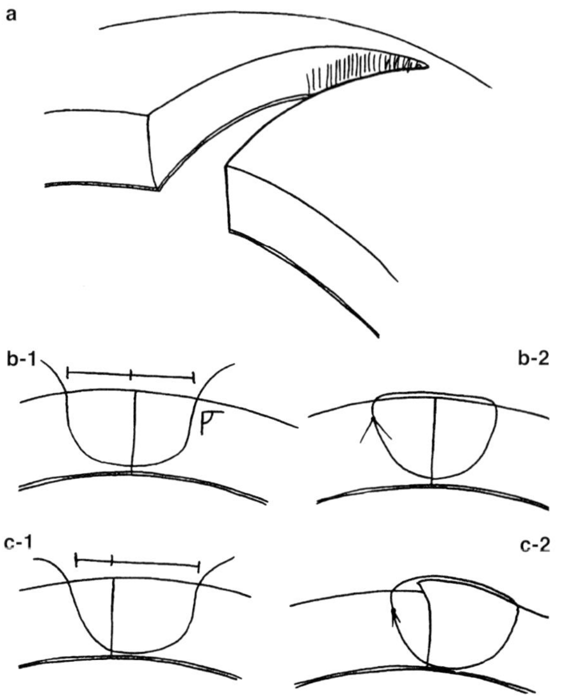

Fig. 9-1. Basic suture principles. (**a**) Full-thickness corneal laceration. (**b**) The ideal suture enters and exits the surface vertically, equidistant from the wound margin, and passes horizontally over Descemet's membrane at 90% stromal depth. (**c**) Uneven bites on either side of the wound lead to overriding of the wound edges. Drawings prepared for this textbook by Gary Wind, MD, Uniformed Services University of the Health Sciences, Bethesda, Md.

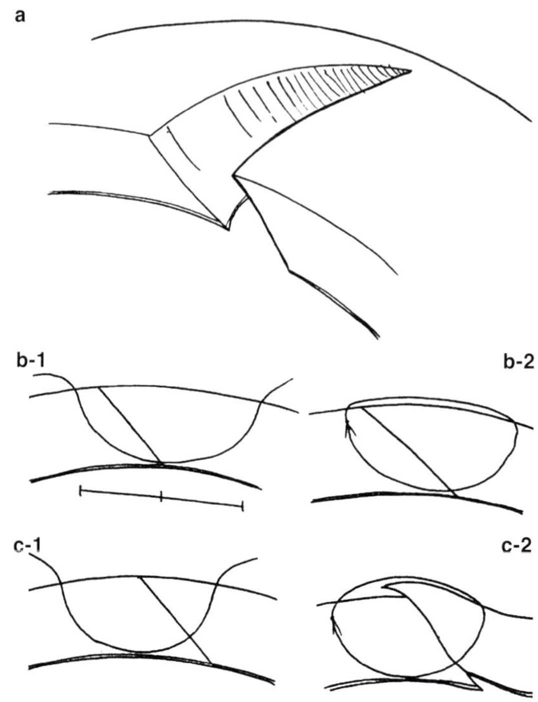

Fig. 9-2. Basic suture principles. (**a**) Shelved corneal laceration. (**b**) The ideal suture distributes the suture bites evenly about the deep portion of the wound to ensure closure without override. (**c**) Spacing the entry and exit points evenly at the surface of a shelved laceration causes overriding of the wound edges. Drawings prepared for this textbook by Gary Wind, MD, Uniformed Services University of the Health Sciences, Bethesda, Md.

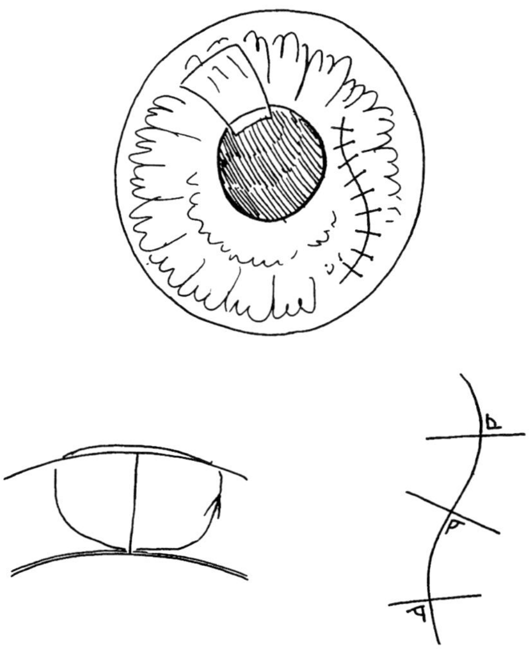

Fig. 9-3. Each suture should be oriented at a right angle to the axis of the wound. Nonradial sutures will cause torque and distortion of the cornea with resulting astigmatism and potential wound leak. Drawings prepared for this textbook by Gary Wind, MD, Uniformed Services University of the Health Sciences, Bethesda, Md.

leakage from the eye and (2) a means for bacterial pathogens to enter, leading to endophthalmitis. Each suture should enter and exit the same distance from the wound edge. Sutures that have uneven bites on either side of the wound lead to overriding of the wound edges. When suturing shelved lacerations, it is important to distribute the suture bites evenly about the deep portion of the wound (Figure 9-2). Inequality of the deep portion of the wound will lead to override, even when the bite appears symmetrical at the surface. Each suture should be at a right angle to the axis of the wound (Figure 9-3). Nonradial sutures will cause distortion and induce astigmatism.

a

b

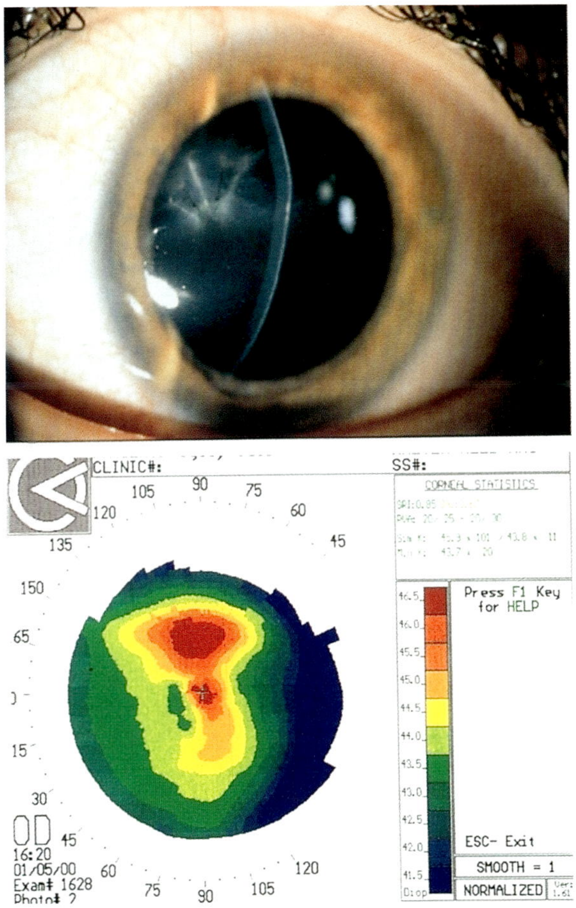

Fig. 9-4. Wound-induced astigmatism. Corneal lacerations disrupt the normal contour of the cornea and induce astigmatism. (**a**) The beam from the slitlamp shows irregularity in the corneal contour after suture closure of a full-thickness corneal laceration. (**b**) Corneal topography depicts irregular astigmatism following corneal trauma sustained in a blast injury. Photograph a: Courtesy of Department of Ophthalmology, University of Pittsburgh Medical Center, Pittsburgh, Pa.

The normal cornea is steeper centrally than at the periphery. Corneal lacerations disrupt this normal contour (Figure 9-4), and suture repair of corneal lacerations should attempt to recreate the normal asphericity. Corneal sutures flatten the area of cornea under the suture, and longer sutures cause a greater degree of flattening. Therefore, to restore the normal corneal contour, peripheral sutures should be longer than those placed centrally.[49,50] In addition to causing less central flattening, shorter suture bites may help minimize scarring in the central visual axis. In general, it is best to avoid passing sutures in or near the visual axis if possible.

Each interrupted suture has an area of tissue compression that is approximately equal to its length. As long as the compression areas of adjacent sutures overlap there will be no wound leak. If sutures are too short or spaced too far apart, wound leaks may occur between sutures (Figure 9-5); therefore, shorter sutures must be spaced closer together.

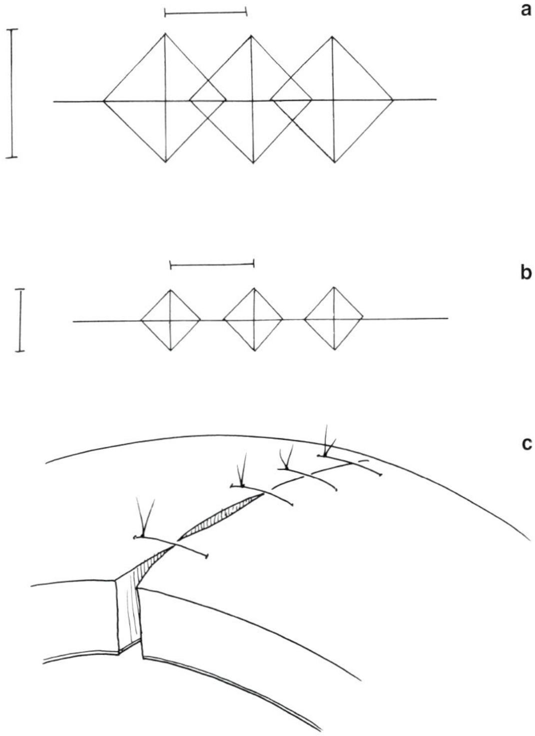

a

b

c

Fig. 9-5. Suture spacing. The area of tissue compression by an interrupted suture is approximately the length of the suture. (**a**) As long as the compression areas of adjacent sutures overlap, there will be no wound leak. If sutures are (**b**) too short or (**c**) spaced too far apart, wound leaks may occur between sutures. Drawings prepared for this textbook by Gary Wind, MD, Uniformed Services University of the Health Sciences, Bethesda, Md.

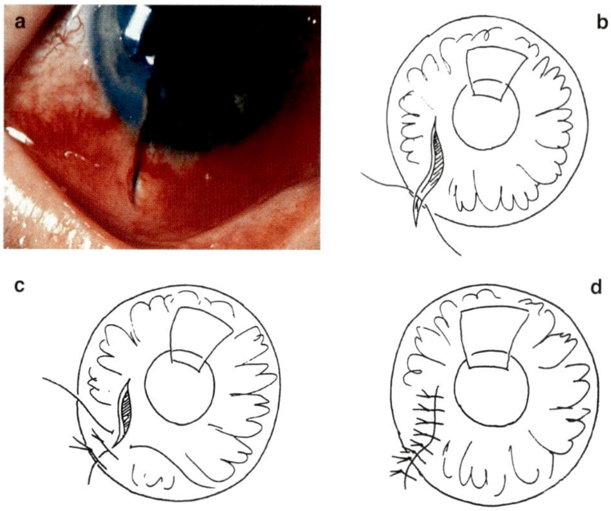

Fig. 9-6. (**a**) Preoperative photograph of a corneoscleral laceration. (**b**) The limbus is aligned first using 8-0 or 9-0 monofilament nylon sutures. (**c**) The corneal component of the laceration is then closed using interrupted 10-0 nylon sutures. (**d**) After exploration to expose the full posterior extent of the wound, the scleral component of the laceration is closed with 8-0 nylon sutures. Drawings prepared for this textbook by Gary Wind, MD, Uniformed Services University of the Health Sciences, Bethesda, Md. Photograph: Courtesy of Department of Ophthalmology, University of Pittsburgh Medical Center, Pittsburgh, Pa.

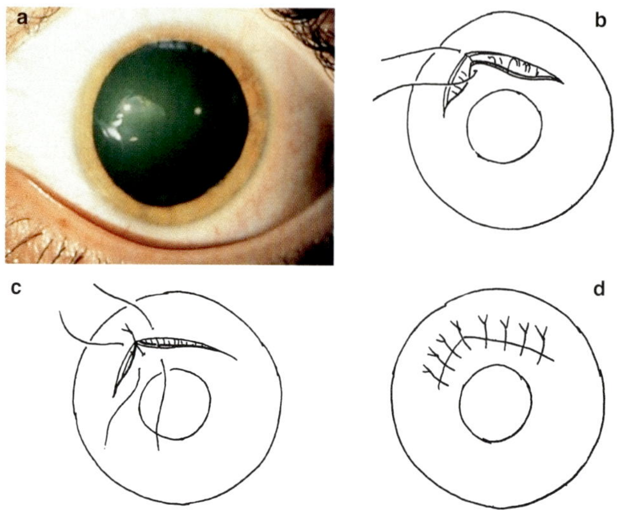

Fig. 9-7. (**a**) Preoperative photograph of an angular corneal laceration. (**b**) Anatomical landmarks, such as the apex of the laceration, can be realigned initially to restore some of the recognizable anatomy of the globe. (**c**, **d**) Once the wound edges have been restored to their basic anatomical position, viscoelastic may be used to reform the anterior chamber, the wound is carefully inspected, and the closure is completed using interrupted sutures. Drawings prepared for this textbook by Gary Wind, MD, Uniformed Services University of the Health Sciences, Bethesda, Md. Photograph: Courtesy of Department of Ophthalmology, University of Pittsburgh Medical Center, Pittsburgh, Pa.

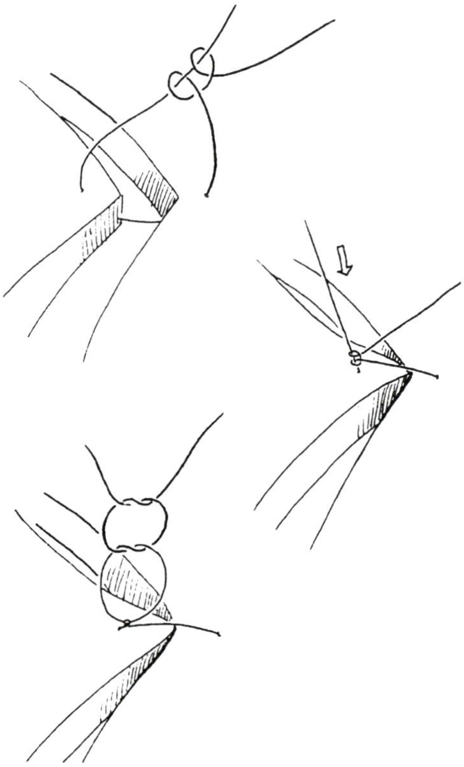

Fig. 9-8. An adjustable slipknot will allow tightening and hold the wound edges under tension. Slipknots are also valuable in corneal laceration closure to adjust wound tension for the control of astigmatism. Drawings prepared for this textbook by Gary Wind, MD, Uniformed Services University of the Health Sciences, Bethesda, Md.

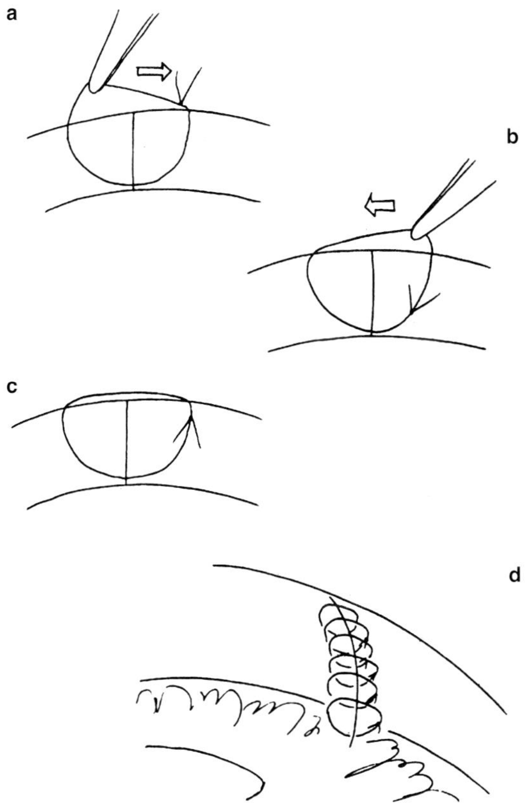

Fig. 9-9. Knots should be buried away from the visual axis by (**a**) grasping the suture with the tips of a nontoothed tying forceps and rotating along the axis of the suture tract. (**b**) Once the knot is buried, rotate the barbs of the cut suture ends away from the corneal surface, (**c**) leaving the knot buried just below the surface (**d**) to facilitate future suture removal. Drawings prepared for this textbook by Gary Wind, MD, Uniformed Services University of the Health Sciences, Bethesda, Md.

It is a good general strategy to reapproximate distinct anatomical landmarks first. Landmarks such as the corneoscleral limbus (Figure 9-6) or angled corners of jagged lacerations (Figure 9-7) can be realigned initially to restore some of the recognizable anatomy of the globe. Then, viscoelastic may be used to reform the anterior chamber and the wound carefully inspected before completing the closure.

Sometimes the initial sutures are difficult to secure when the wound edges are under tension. An adjustable slipknot such as a double half hitch allows tightening and maintains the wound edges under proper tension (Figure 9-8). Once the edges are reunited, the knot can be secured with a square knot. Slipknots are valuable in corneal laceration closure to adjust wound tension for the control of astigmatism. The slipknot secured with a square knot results in a compact knot that is usually easy to bury. If not carefully tied, a 3-1-1-1 surgeon's knot can be bulky and difficult to bury.

Knots should be buried away from the visual axis by using the technique demonstrated in Figure 9-9. Factors that facilitate suture burial include compact knot size, a longer suture tract, a tight suture, a firm globe, and countertraction to stabilize the globe. Lubrication with a small amount of viscoelastic to the suture may also help bury knots. The principles of suture placement for surgical repair of sharp trauma of the anterior segment are summarized in Exhibit 9-3.

Suture Removal

Corneal sutures can safely be removed when the wound has healed and adequate fibrosis has oc-

EXHIBIT 9-3

SUTURE PLACEMENT PRINCIPLES

- Entry and exit points should be equidistant from the wound edge
- Entry and exit should be vertical to the surface
- Sutures should be perpendicular to the wound
- Sutures should be passed through 90% of the corneal thickness but just superficial to Descemet's membrane
- Cornea should be closed from the periphery to the center
- Sutures should be longer near limbus, shorter toward central cornea
- Shorter sutures should be spaced closer together
- Anatomical landmarks (eg, limbus) should be lined up first
- The surgeon should avoid placing sutures in the visual axis
- The surgeon should bury knots superficially, away from the visual axis

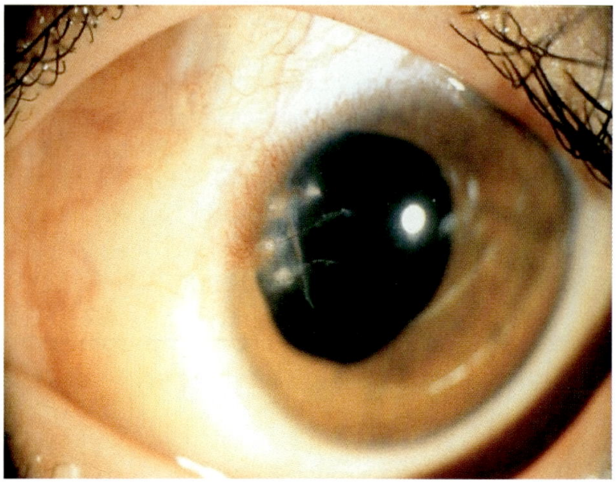

Fig. 9-10. This clinical photograph, taken 2 months after repair of a corneal laceration (the eye of the same patient is seen in Figure 9-21), documents wound fibrosis and corneal vascularization. Two sutures have been removed. Additional signs of healing include spontaneously loosened or broken sutures. Loose or broken sutures should be removed because they prevent epithelialization, cause irritation and discomfort, and pose a risk of infection. Photograph: Courtesy of Department of Ophthalmology, University of Pittsburgh Medical Center, Pittsburgh, Pa.

curred. Wound fibrosis can be seen at the slitlamp using oblique or retroillumination. Although variable, healing generally occurs by 4 to 8 weeks postoperatively. If the iris or vitreous is incorporated in the closure, then healing is often delayed. Additional signs of healing include corneal vascularization and spontaneously loosened or broken sutures (Figure 9-10). Loose or broken sutures should be removed because they prevent epithelialization, cause irritation and discomfort, and pose a risk of infection.

TABLE 9-2

COMMERCIAL SOURCES FOR CYANOACRYLATE TISSUE ADHESIVE

Brand Name	Manufacturer/ Location	Telephone Number
Duodent	Ellman International Hewlett, NY	(800) 835-5355
Nexacryl	Closure Medical Corp. Raleigh, NC	(888) 257-7633
Histoacryl	B. Braun-Dexon GmbH Germany	05663-5030

Tissue Adhesive

Cyanoacrylate tissue adhesive (ie, glue) may be used in certain circumstances instead of, or in addition to, sutures for closing corneal or corneoscleral lacerations.[51,52] Although not yet approved for this

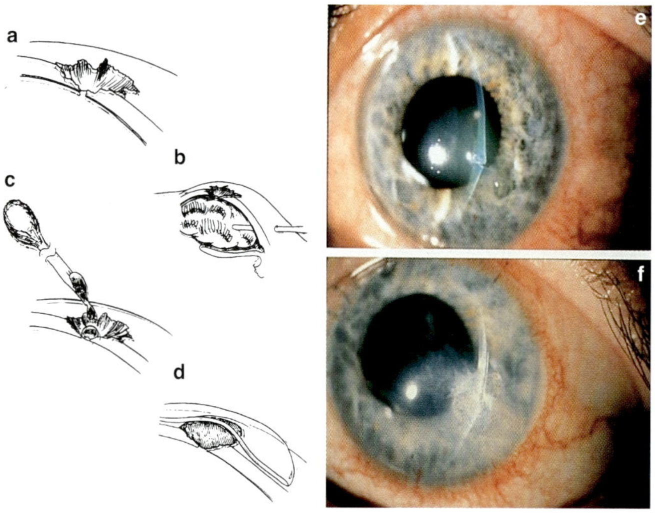

Fig. 9-11. (**a**) Injuries such as this full-thickness laceration with tissue loss often cannot be repaired with sutures alone. Tissue adhesive is also a useful means of closure of small lacerations or wound leaks that may not require sutures. (**b**) A shallow or flat anterior chamber should be reformed with a viscoelastic to avoid gluing intraocular structures. A dry corneal bed and removal of the surrounding epithelium is necessary for the glue to adhere. If there is a continuous aqueous leak from the wound, a cellulose sponge should be used to keep the site dry until immediately before the glue is applied. Remove the sponge just as the glue is brought into position. (**c**) The glue is applied using a micropipette, 30-gauge needle on a 1-cc tuberculin syringe, or by fashioning an applicator from the broken wooden shaft of a cotton swab. (**d**) A bandage contact lens is placed over the glue for comfort and to prevent dislocation of the tissue adhesive. (**e**) Preoperative photograph of a small corneal laceration with a wound leak with slight shallowing of the anterior chamber. (**f**) Postoperative photograph—taken after the wound was sealed—shows the glue plug and a soft contact lens in place. Drawings prepared for this textbook by Gary Wind, MD, Uniformed Services University of the Health Sciences, Bethesda, Md. Photographs e and f: Courtesy of Department of Ophthalmology, University of Pittsburgh Medical Center, Pittsburgh, Pa.

indication by the US Food and Drug Administration, this tissue glue is a valuable tool and is available from domestic and foreign sources (Table 9-2).

Tissue glue may be used for primary closure of small corneal perforations, or to augment closure of stellate lacerations or lacerations with tissue loss that cannot be closed in a watertight fashion using sutures alone (Figure 9-11). It is best to apply the glue in very small amounts, adding as needed to patch the defect. Large glue applications can result in a sizable chunk of glue, which not only causes discomfort to the patient but also is more easily dislodged than is a small piece. Although it is possible to apply the glue at the slitlamp, it is often best to apply the glue with the aid of an operating microscope with the patient lying down. The supine position allows better control of the amount and placement of the tissue glue. Allow adequate time for drying and adhesion of the glue, usually 3 to 5 minutes, and ensure adequate closure by Seidel testing.

The glue should remain in place until the stromal defect is healed. It may spontaneously dislodge when epithelium grows in under the glue, in which case removal is unnecessary. If a peripheral wound has vascularized and shows adequate scarring, the glue may be gently removed with forceps. This can usually be done safely after 6 to 8 weeks; however, central lacerations without vascularization take up to twice as long to heal.

MANAGEMENT OF SIMPLE CORNEAL LACERATIONS

Partial-Thickness Corneal Lacerations

Partial-thickness corneal lacerations should be carefully inspected to verify that Descemet's membrane is intact. Occasionally, a full-thickness corneal laceration self-seals as the stroma hydrates with aqueous and tears. The resulting edema may then tamponade the wound to prevent further leaking. A Seidel test should be performed to check for leaking aqueous (Figure 9-12).

Figure 9-13 depicts both superficial and deeper partial-thickness corneal lacerations. Topical antibiotics (eg, ciprofloxacin or ofloxacin) are indicated, and topical cycloplegics may be used to relieve pain from ciliary spasm. If the laceration is deeper and is associated with mild corneal instability or overriding wound edges, a sturdier bandage contact lens (eg, Bausch & Lomb Plano-T lens) can be used. Frequent topical antibiotics are indicated initially. After 1 to 2 weeks, the frequency may be reduced to one or two drops per day as long as the contact lens is in the eye. Deep partial-thickness lacerations may result in corneal instability with significant wound gape or override or a corneal flap. Such wounds may require sutures and application of a bandage lens until reepithelialization occurs. Topical antibiotics and cycloplegics are also indicated as described above.

Simple Full-Thickness Lacerations

Management of simple full-thickness lacerations depends on the size of the wound, presence of

a

b

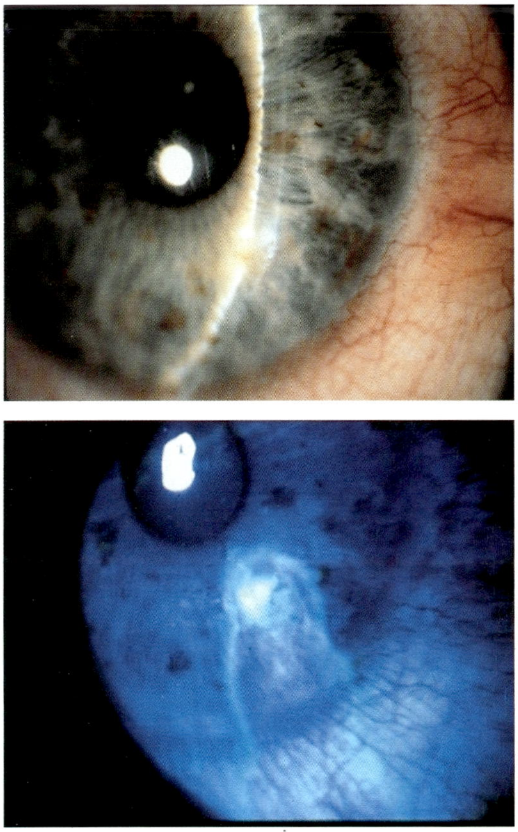

Fig. 9-12. Seidel testing can reveal ocular wound leaks through the use of sterile tetracaine eyedrops and a fluorescein strip. (**a**) Slitlamp photograph of a small corneal laceration with a moderately shallow anterior chamber. Partial-thickness corneal lacerations should be carefully inspected to ensure that Descemet's membrane is intact. (**b**) If the results of the Seidel test are negative, gentle pressure may be applied to the globe to see if the wound leaks from an occult, full-thickness laceration. Photographs: Courtesy of Department of Ophthalmology, University of Pittsburgh Medical Center, Pittsburgh, Pa.

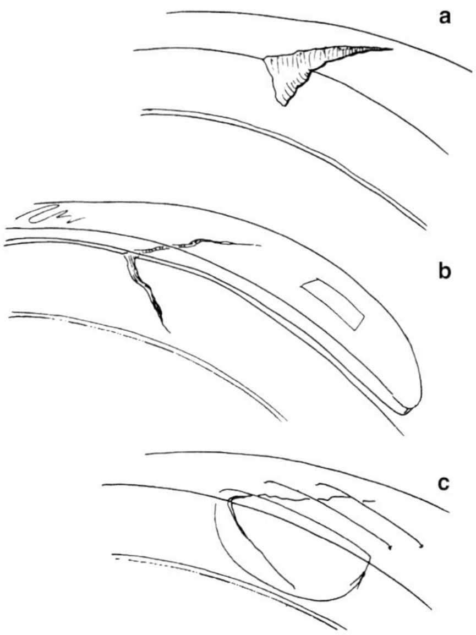

Fig. 9-13. (**a**) Partial-thickness lacerations without significant override or wound gape may be treated with a pressure patch or bandage soft-contact lens until reepithelialization occurs. Topical antibiotics (eg, ciprofloxacin, ofloxacin) are indicated, and topical cycloplegics may be used to relieve pain from ciliary spasm. (**b**) If the laceration is deeper and associated with mild corneal instability or overriding wound edges, a bandage lens will support the cornea until epithelial and stromal healing have occurred, in approximately 4 to 6 weeks. (**c**) Deep partial-thickness lacerations with corneal instability, significant wound gape, override or a corneal flap may require sutures to provide adequate structural support. A bandage lens should be placed over the sutures until reepithelialization occurs. Drawings prepared for this textbook by Gary Wind, MD, Uniformed Services University of the Health Sciences, Bethesda, Md.

wound leak, depth of the anterior chamber, and presence of other ocular injuries. Simple lacerations may be small and self-sealing and require no closure, or they may be larger, requiring multiple sutures. Air, saline, or viscoelastic agent (usually the latter) may be needed to form the chamber while suturing. All full-thickness lacerations, even those that are self-sealing, present an increased risk for endophthalmitis and are an indication for systemic antibiotics.

Small lacerations (< 2–3 mm) that are Seidel-negative may be managed in much the same way as a partial-thickness laceration, with a bandage contact lens, topical antibiotics, and cycloplegics (Figure 9-14). Any laceration that is initially Seidel-negative, however, must be followed closely to ensure that the wound, initially closed by corneal edema, does not develop a leak as the edema resolves. The eye should be protected from reinjury by having the patient wear a protective shield and by limiting physical activity. Admission to a medical treatment facility for close observation should be considered in children and in adult patients for whom compliance is a question.

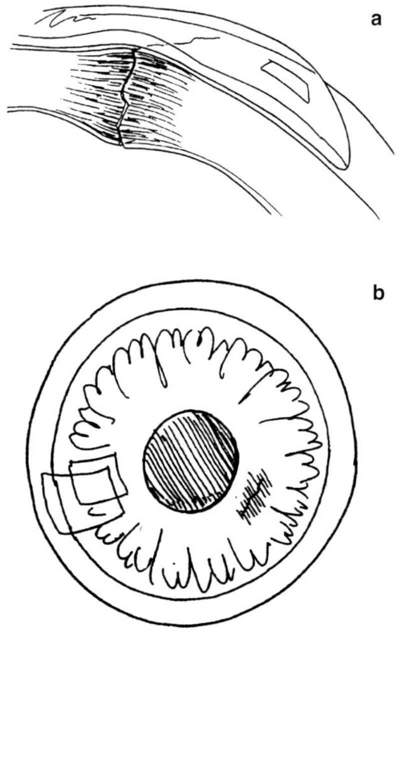

Fig. 9-14. (**a**) Occasionally, a full-thickness corneal laceration will self-seal as the stroma hydrates with aqueous and tears. The resulting edema may then tamponade the wound, preventing further leaking. (**b**) Such injuries may be treated with a bandage soft-contact lens and close follow-up to ensure that the wound does not develop a leak as the edema resolves. Drawings prepared for this textbook by Gary Wind, MD, Uniformed Services University of the Health Sciences, Bethesda, Md.

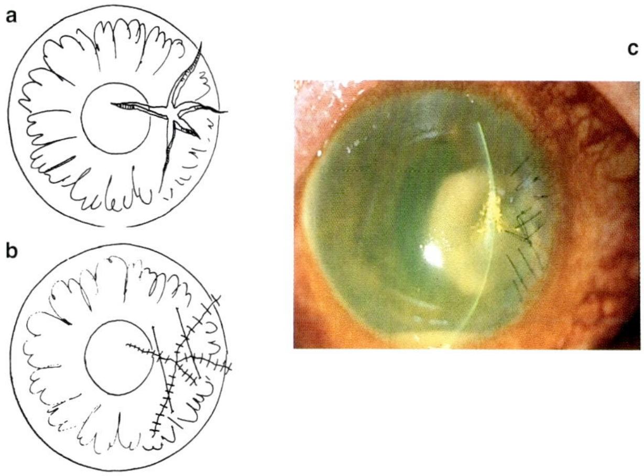

Fig. 9-15. (**a**) Stellate lacerations are often difficult to repair and may result in significant scarring and astigmatism. (**b**) These wounds may require a combination of interrupted, bridging, and mattress sutures to achieve watertight closure. (**c**) Postoperative clinical photograph of a stellate laceration closed with multiple interrupted and bridging sutures. The patient developed fungal keratitis and endophthalmitis postoperatively. Drawings prepared for this textbook by Gary Wind, MD, Uniformed Services University of the Health Sciences, Bethesda, Md. Photograph: Courtesy of Department of Ophthalmology, University of Pittsburgh Medical Center, Pittsburgh, Pa.

Small (< 2–3 mm), Seidel-positive lacerations with a partially or fully formed anterior chamber may be treated with a trial of bandage lens and aqueous suppressant (β-blocker), topical and systemic antibiotics, and very close follow-up. If a partially shallow anterior chamber does not deepen, or if the wound leak does not seal within 48 hours, consider cyanoacrylate glue or closure with sutures (see Figure 9-11). Glue may be particularly useful in a small wound leak from a laceration located in the central cornea, where sutures are likely to induce astigmatism and scarring. Lacerations longer than 2 to 3 mm usually require suture closure and topical and systemic antibiotics.

Stellate Corneal Lacerations

Stellate lacerations are often the most difficult to repair and may result in significant scarring and astigmatism. Combinations of interrupted, bridging, mattress, and purse-string sutures may be necessary to achieve watertight closure (Figure 9-15). Eisner[53] has reported a variation of a mattress suture technique for the repair of stellate lacerations.

PRIMARY REPAIR OF COMPLEX CORNEAL LACERATIONS

Lacerations With Tissue Loss

Corneal tissue may be lost due to avulsion, necrosis, or infection. Small areas of tissue loss may not require replacement as long as the wound can be repaired in a watertight closure with structural integrity. Cyanoacrylate glue may be used to repair small defects. More recently, Ng and colleagues[54] have shown that human fibrinogen (Tisseal, mfg by Baxter HyLand Immuno, Deerfield, Ill) can effectively seal corneal lacerations in an enucleated eye model.

Larger defects may require a lamellar autograft. This procedure may be used for defects smaller than 5 mm and surrounded by nonnecrotic stroma. Larger defects may require a lamellar allograft or rarely, a full-thickness patch graft. Both require donor cornea, but the former has a much lower risk of graft failure and rejection (Figure 9-16). More recently, processed human pericardium (Tutoplast; mfg by Innovative Ophthalmic Products, Inc, Costa Mesa, Calif) has successfully been used to complete the watertight closure on traumatic corneal laceration with tissue loss.[55] After the wound edges have been approximated as much as possible with sutures, the wound with tissue loss may still leak. It is possible to finish the closure by tightly oversewing the wound with pericardium (Figure 9-17).

Corneal Lacerations With Uveal Prolapse

The prolapsed iris should be examined for viability. In general, uveal tissue that has been prolapsed for more than 24 hours should not be reposited because of the increased risk of microbial infection or epithelial seeding into the anterior chamber. Prolonged prolapse or devitalized tissue should be excised and sent for culture. When excising uveal tissue, cut it flush with the corneal surface to preserve as much tissue as possible.

To reposit the prolapsed iris, reform the chamber with viscoelastic through the wound or separate paracentesis. Viscoelastic should be used judiciously, as overinflation of the chamber may cause further prolapse. A temporary suture (superficial) may facilitate chamber formation. Using a fine iris

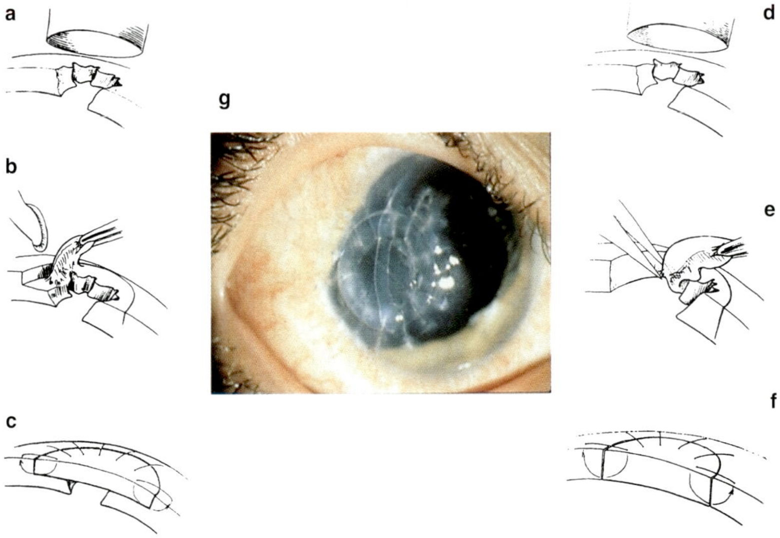

Fig. 9-16. Corneal damage due to avulsion, necrosis, or infection may make watertight closure with sutures alone impossible. Cyanoacrylate glue may be used to repair small defects. Larger defects may require a corneal patch graft. (**a**) Full-thickness laceration with significant tissue loss, prepared for trephination. (**b**) After partial-thickness trephination, a lamellar plane is dissected to excise the anterior cornea. (**c**) Donor cornea is trephined to the same size as the excised cornea and sutured into place with interrupted nylon sutures. For defects smaller than 5 mm and with nonnecrotic stroma, a lamellar autograft may be performed by harvesting donor cornea from the patient's fellow eye. (**d, e, f**) Larger defects may require a lamellar allograft or rarely a full-thickness patch graft. Both require donor cornea, but the former has a much lower risk of graft failure and rejection. (**g**) Postoperative slitlamp photograph of a full-thickness patch graft. Drawings prepared for this textbook by Gary Wind, MD, Uniformed Services University of the Health Sciences, Bethesda, Md. Photograph: Courtesy of Department of Ophthalmology, University of Pittsburgh Medical Center, Pittsburgh, Pa.

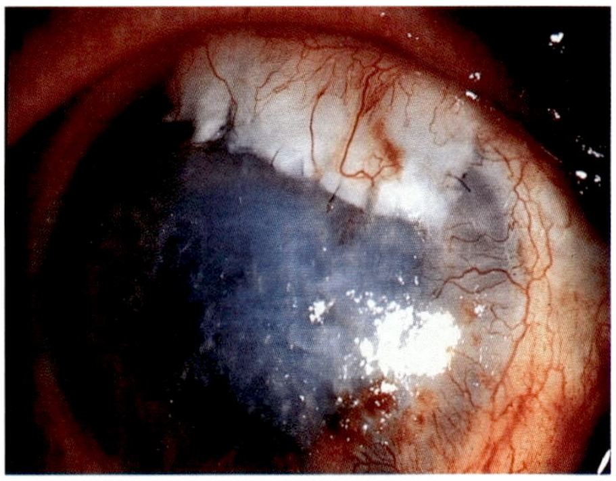

Fig. 9-17. Processed human pericardium (Tutoplast, mfg by Tutogen Medical Inc, Alachua, Fla) has been used to supplement the suture repair of a corneal laceration sustained in a blast injury.

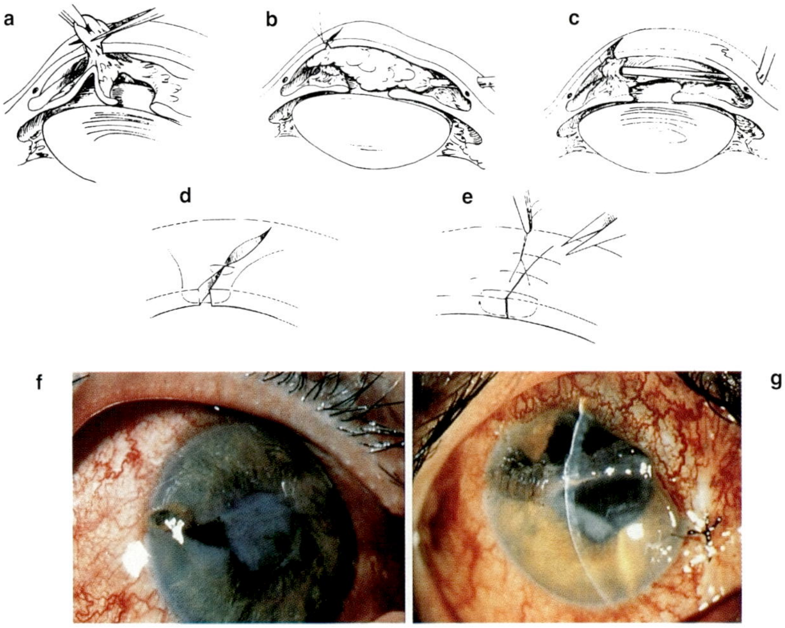

Fig. 9-18. Corneal laceration with uveal prolapse. (**a**) Prolapsed iris should be examined for viability. Devitalized tissue or that which has been prolapsed for 24 hours or longer should be excised and sent for culture. The prolapsed iris is cut flush with the corneal surface to preserve as much tissue as possible. (**b**) The anterior chamber is reformed with viscoelastic through the wound or separate paracentesis, taking care to avoid overinflation and further prolapse of intraocular contents. A temporary suture (superficial) may facilitate chamber formation. (**c**) Prolapsed tissue and that incarcerated in the wound is gently swept from the wound with a cyclodialysis spatula or viscoelastic cannula. After the prolapsed or incarcerated iris has been removed, (**d, e**) the wound is sutured securely, replacing temporary sutures with deeper ones. (**f**) Preoperative photograph of a limbus-to-limbus corneal laceration with collapse of the anterior chamber, iris prolapse temporally, and lens opacification. (**g**) The same eye after surgical repair. Drawings prepared for this textbook by Gary Wind, MD, Uniformed Services University of the Health Sciences, Bethesda, Md. Photographs: Courtesy of Department of Ophthalmology, University of Pittsburgh Medical Center, Pittsburgh, Pa.

spatula through a paracentesis, gently sweep the iris from the wound, and suture the wound securely, replacing temporary sutures with deeper ones (Figure 9-18). A miotic, either Carbastat (carbachol, mfg by Novartis Ophthalmis, Duluth, Ga) or Miochol (acetylcholine chloride, mfg by Novartis Ophthalmis, Duluth, Ga) may be used to facilitate closure of corneal lacerations with iris prolapse near the limbus.

Corneoscleral Lacerations

Lacerations that extend beyond the limbus into the sclera should be carefully explored to determine their full extent. Prolapsed uvea should be managed as previously described. The limbus should be reapproximated first with 8-0 or 9-0 nylon sutures. The corneal component should then be closed. Finally, the sclera should be explored and repaired (Figure 9-19; also see Figure 9-6).

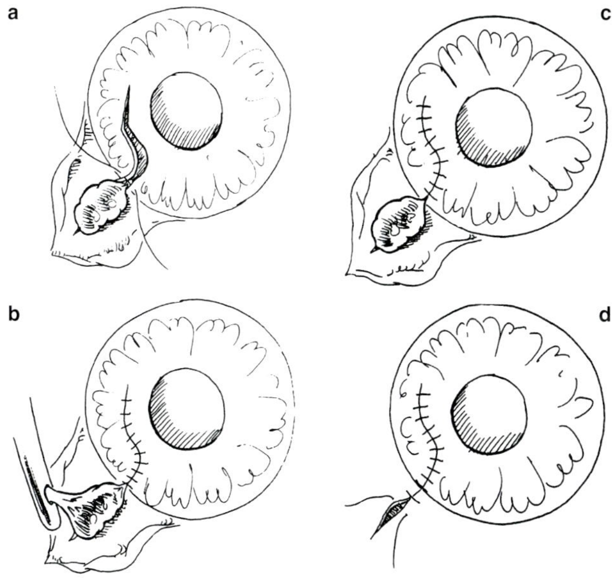

Fig. 9-19. Corneoscleral laceration. (**a**) Repair of a corneoscleral laceration begins by performing a conjunctival peritomy. Then, the sclera is carefully explored to determine the full extent of the laceration. The corneoscleral limbus is an important landmark and is realigned using 9-0 monofilament nylon sutures. (**b**) Any prolapsed uvea or vitreous is carefully reposited or excised. (**c**) The corneal component is then closed using 10-0 nylon sutures. (**d**) Finally, the sclera should be explored and repaired as far posterior as possible using 8-0 nylon sutures. Drawings prepared for this textbook by Gary Wind, MD, Uniformed Services University of the Health Sciences, Bethesda, Md.

Anterior Segment Intraocular Foreign Bodies

The key to diagnosing an IOFB is to maintain a high degree of clinical suspicion. An IOFB should be suspected whenever a patient with anterior segment trauma is examined, particularly if the injury occurred in a high-risk setting (eg, blasts or explosions, broken glass, metal striking on metal, or high-speed machinery) (Figure 9-20).[56,57]

Corneal FBs may occur at any depth and are easily seen at the slitlamp. Vertical abrasions or punctate erosions on the superior cornea suggest one or

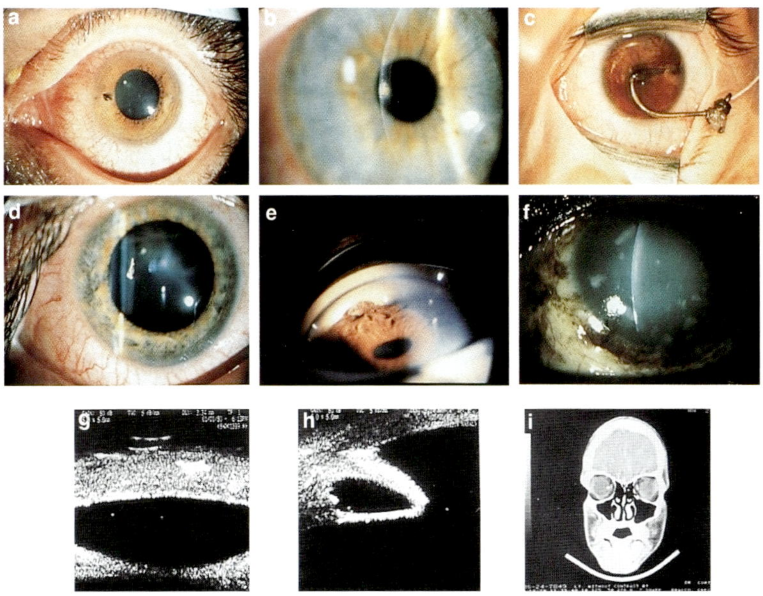

Fig. 9-20. Anterior segment intraocular foreign bodies (IOFBs). (**a**) Superficial corneal metallic foreign body (FB) rests on the corneal epithelium. (**b**) Anterior to midstromal corneal FB. (**c**) Fishhook injury full thickness through the cornea and into the anterior chamber. (**d**) IOFB in the anterior lens as a result of hammering metal on metal. (**e**) Anterior chamber FB viewed in the chamber angle with gonioscopy. Photographs a–e: Courtesy of Department of Ophthalmology, University of Pittsburgh Medical Center, Pittsburgh, Pa.
Blast injury with multiple glass IOFBs. (**f**) Slitlamp photograph of multiple intracorneal FBs and corneal decompensation resulting from a blast injury. (**g**) Ultrasound biomicroscopy of the same eye demonstrates FBs in the cornea and (**h**) the ciliary body. (**i**) Coronal computed tomography (CT) scan demonstrates a metallic FB within the globe.

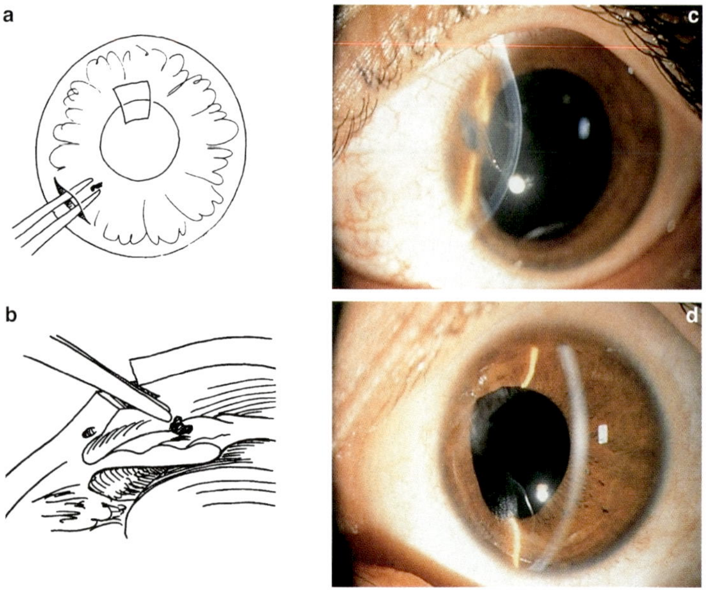

Fig. 9-21. Removal of an anterior chamber intraocular foreign body (IOFB). (**a**) Viscoelastic can be used to reform a shallow anterior chamber and to gently manipulate the foreign body (FB) that is not embedded in iris or angle structures. (**b**) The FB may be carefully removed with forceps directly through the wound. A separate incision may be necessary. (**c**) Preoperative photograph of an anterior chamber FB. (**d**) Postoperative photograph of the same eye (see Figure 9-10). Drawings prepared for this textbook by Gary Wind, MD, Uniformed Services University of the Health Sciences, Bethesda, Md. Photographs: Courtesy of Department of Ophthalmology, University of Pittsburgh Medical Center, Pittsburgh, Pa.

more FBs under the eyelids. Eversion and double eversion should be performed except when an open globe is suspected. Iris or pupil hemorrhage may be seen with an anterior segment IOFB. Careful gonioscopy may reveal an FB in the chamber angle. Dilated examination may reveal an intralenticular or a posterior segment FB, and whenever such is suspected, radiographic and ultrasonic evaluations are performed.

In most cases it is necessary to remove the IOFB. Most FBs are metallic, and most metallic FBs are potentially toxic. Iron-containing FBs result in siderosis. Pure copper usually produces a suppurative response, and alloys of 80% copper or less may lead to chalcosis. Zinc and aluminum are toxic as well. A metallic FB resulting from metal striking on metal, however, is usually sterile because of the heat generated by the striking force.

On the other hand, a tree branch, other vegetable matter, and farm instruments carry a high risk of microbial contamination, and it is usually urgent and mandatory to remove vegetable FBs. A glass, stone, sand, or plastic foreign body may be inert and well-tolerated. They may be left in place if they are nonmobile and nonthreatening to other structures. For further details, please see Chapter 14, Management of Penetrating Injuries With a Retained Intraocular Foreign Body.

An IOFB in the anterior chamber can be removed directly through the wound if the laceration is large enough and in proximity to the final location of the IOFB. Formation of the anterior chamber with viscoelastic will facilitate removal of the IOFB and protect against damage to other ocular structures in the process. Viscoelastic can also be used to gently manipulate the IOFB if it is not embedded in the iris or in angle structures. Forceps are then passed through the wound to grasp the IOFB and remove it from the eye. A separate incision may be necessary (Figure 9-21).

Corneoscleral Laceration With Cataract

Corneal lacerations are frequently accompanied by a traumatic cataract. Cataract extraction is indi-

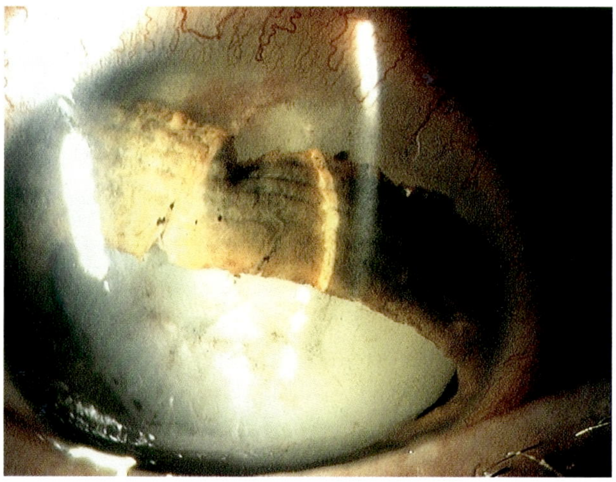

Fig. 9-22. Slitlamp photograph reveals a traumatic cataract with iridodialysis, lens subluxation into the anterior chamber, and collapse of the chamber.

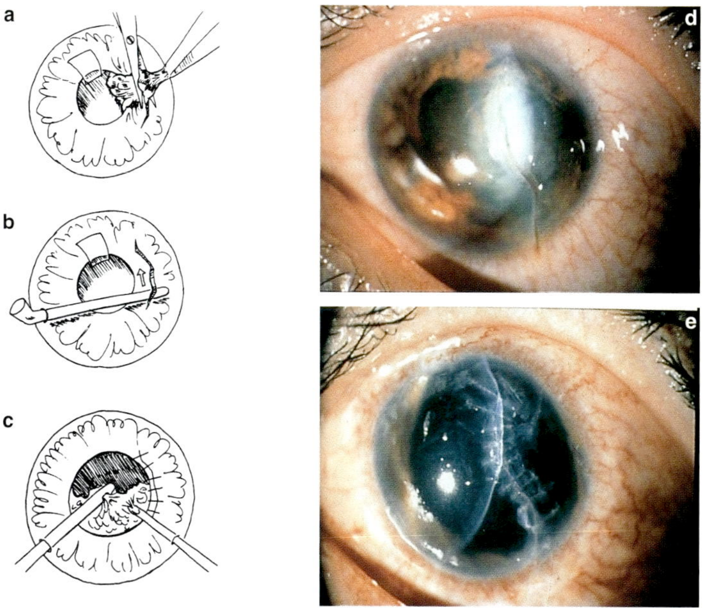

Fig. 9-23. Corneoscleral laceration with cataract. (**a**) The extent of the corneal laceration is explored and prolapsed uvea, lens material, and vitreous are removed from the outer aspect of the wound. (**b**) Incarcerated intraocular contents are gently swept from the inner aspect of the wound and the anterior chamber is reformed with viscoelastic. The corneal laceration is then repaired with a watertight closure. (**c**) The lens may be removed by either an anterior or a posterior approach. (**d**) Preoperative clinical photograph of a corneal laceration with lens disruption and collapse of the anterior chamber. (**e**) This photograph is of the same eye after laceration repair and lens extraction. Drawings prepared for this textbook by Gary Wind, MD, Uniformed Services University of the Health Sciences, Bethesda, Md. Photographs: Courtesy of Department of Ophthalmology, University of Pittsburgh Medical Center, Pittsburgh, Pa.

cated at the time of initial repair when the lens is dislocated into the anterior chamber (Figure 9-22) or is densely clouded, or there is significant capsular disruption.[58–61] The extent of the corneal laceration is explored and repaired, and the anterior chamber is reformed with viscoelastic (Figure 9-23). The lens may be removed by either an anterior or posterior approach. The decision must then be made whether to place an intraocular lens (IOL) or to leave the patient aphakic for possible lens implantation at a later procedure.

Primary IOL insertion may be considered in eyes with clear corneal laceration with good visualization, sufficient zonular/capsular support, no significant vitreous in the anterior chamber, and no evidence of injury or FB in the posterior segment. A staged procedure is indicated when (1) corneal opacity prevents adequate visibility, or (2) vitreous is in the anterior chamber, or (3) an IOFB is present, or (4) the posterior segment is injured. Management of lens injuries is discussed fully in Chapter 10, Trauma of the Crystalline Lens.

POSTOPERATIVE MANAGEMENT

The goal of postoperative management is to prevent, identify, and treat complications that arise as a result of the injury itself or the surgical repair. Potential complications include infection, inflammation, glaucoma, scarring, astigmatism, and pain (Figure 9-24).

Subconjunctival antibiotics (eg, 25 mg vancomycin, 25 mg ceftazidime) should be administered at the conclusion of the surgical case and be followed with postoperative intravenous and topical antibiotics. Cycloplegics as well as systemic analgesics can be used for postoperative pain. Frequent application of topical 1% prednisolone acetate is necessary to reduce postoperative inflammation and scarring. Topical lubricants promote healing of the ocular surface, and a bandage contact lens may be applied over corneal sutures until reepithelialization is complete. β-blockers or carbonic anhydrase inhibitors may be indicated for control of intraocular pressure. Finally, to prevent further injury to the eye, the importance of a rigid eye shield, safety glasses, and appropriate activity limitations are emphasized to the patient.

ANTERIOR SEGMENT RECONSTRUCTION AFTER TRAUMA

It is best to repair the injury primarily and treat the patient medically with antibiotics and steroids. After allowing time to heal, the patient's visual potential should be assessed and rehabilitation of vision pursued. Corneal trauma can reduce vision because of scarring or induced astigmatism. Aphakia may also be present. Often, functional vision may be obtained with the use of a rigid contact lens.[62–65] If a rigid lens alone cannot improve vision because of significant corneal scarring,

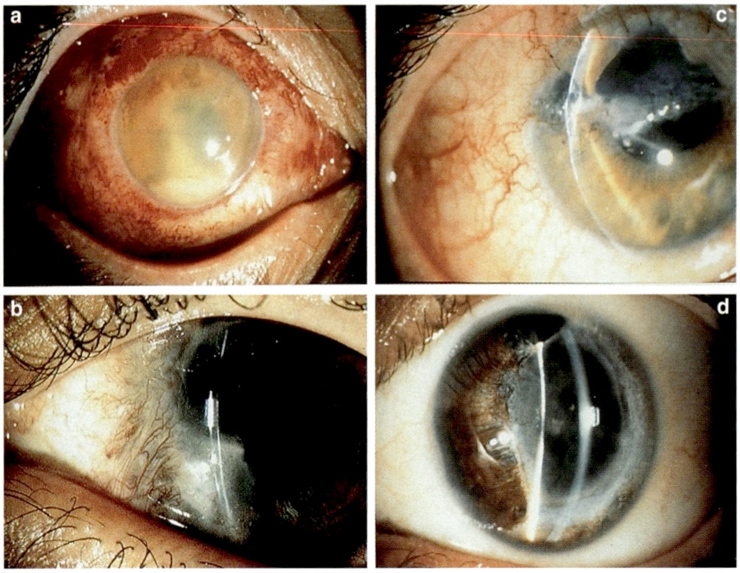

Fig. 9-24. Postoperative complications. (**a**) Streptococcal endophthalmitis after penetrating ocular injury. (**b**) Iris incarceration in repaired corneal laceration. (**c**) Fibrous ingrowth after penetrating injury. (**d**) Iris trauma following open globe injury and repair. Note the significant absence of iris tissue for 180°. Anterior and posterior synechiae and a cyclitic membrane are also present. Photographs: Courtesy of Department of Ophthalmology, University of Pittsburgh Medical Center, Pittsburgh, Pa.

lens opacification, or other anterior segment pathology, or if a successful fit cannot be achieved, then an elective corneal transplant can be performed secondarily on a quiet eye.[66–68] Additional anterior segment reconstruction following trauma may include any combination of the following procedures[69,70]:

- penetrating keratoplasty,
- membrane removal,
- cataract extraction,
- IOL implantation,
- goniosynechialysis,
- iridoplasty, and
- anterior vitrectomy.

SUMMARY

Next to loss of life and alongside loss of limb, the loss of eyesight is one of the most devastating consequences of trauma. The eye is injured in warfare, blast injuries, terrorist attacks, and civilian unrest to an extent disproportionate to its representation in the overall body surface area. Ballistic eye protection is designed to reduce the severity and number of injuries sustained by the soldier in combat situations; however, eye armor is not always available to noncombatants, and even those with access to the protection do not always wear it. For these reasons and many others, eye injuries are likely to continue to be a significant source of morbidity and disability. It is therefore necessary that all military medical personnel at every level and every echelon of care be equipped to handle eye injuries appropriately. Buddy care by the soldier; first aid by the medic; initial evaluation, intervention and evacuation by the battalion surgeon; primary surgical repair by the comprehensive ophthalmologist; and secondary reconstruction and complicated repair by the ophthalmic subspecialist are all important factors that contribute to the ultimate wellbeing of the injured eye.

The vital importance of early and definitive primary closure of the ruptured globe cannot be underestimated. It is therefore imperative that the first ophthalmologist who sees the injured casualty be skilled in the perioperative management and surgical repair of the seriously traumatized but salvageable eye.

REFERENCES

1. Hornblass A. Eye injuries in the military. *Int Ophthalmol Clin*. 1981;21(4):121–138.

2. Wong TY, Seet MB, Ang CL. Eye injuries in twentieth century warfare: A historical perspective. *Surv Ophthalmol*. 1997;41:433–459.

3. Hardy RA. Ocular trauma. *Mil Med*. 1996;161:465–468.

4. Gombos GM. Ocular war injuries in Jerusalem during the 1967 Arab–Israeli conflict. *Am J Ophthalmol.* 1969;68:474–478.

5. Treister G. Ocular casualties in the Six-Day War. *Am J Ophthalmol.* 1969;68:668–675.

6. Hornblass A. Ocular war injuries in South Vietnam. *Surg Forum.* 1973;24:500–502.

7. Belkin M, Treister G, Dotan S. Eye injuries and ocular protection in the Lebanon War, 1982. *Isr J Med Sci.* 1984;20:333–338.

8. Heering SL, Shohat T, Heering AS, Seelenfreund M, Lerman Y. Civil unrest and ocular trauma. *Mil Med.* 1992;157:297–298.

9. Mader TH, Aragones JV, Chandler AC, et al. Ocular and ocular adnexal injuries treated by United States military ophthalmologists during Operations Desert Shield and Desert Storm. *Ophthalmology.* 1993;100:1462–1467.

10. Heier JS, Enzenauer RW, Wintermeyer SF, Delaney M, LaPiana FP. Ocular injuries and diseases at a combat support hospital in support of Operations Desert Shield and Desert Storm. *Arch Ophthalmol.* 1993;111:795–798.

11. Biehl JW, Valdez J, Hemady RK, Steidl SM, Bourke DL. Penetrating eye injury in war. *Mil Med.* 1999;164:780–784.

12. Lashkari K, Lashkari MH, Kim AJ, Carne WG, Jalkh AE. Combat-related eye trauma: A review of 5,320 cases. *Int Ophthalmol Clin.* 1995;35(1):193–203.

13. Mines M, Thach A, Mallonee S, Hildebrand L, Shariat S. Ocular injuries sustained by survivors of the Oklahoma City bombing. *Ophthalmology.* 2000;107:837–843.

14. Thach AB, Ward TP, Hollifield RD, Cockerham K, Birdsong R, Kramer K. Eye injuries in a terrorist bombing: Dhahran, Saudi Arabia, June 25, 1996. *Ophthalmology.* 2000;107:844–847.

15. Pieramici DJ, Sternberg P Jr, Aaberg TM Sr, et al, and the Ocular Trauma Classification Group. A system for classifying mechanical injuries of the eye (globe). *Am J Ophthalmol.* 1997;123:820–831.

16. Orlin SE, Sulewski ME. Spontaneous perforation in pellucid marginal degeneration. *CLAO J.* 1998;24:186–187.

17. Lucarelli MJ, Geldelman DS, Talamo JH. Hydrops and spontaneous perforation in pellucid marginal corneal degeneration. *Cornea.* 1997;16:232–234.

18. Ingraham HJ, Donnenfeld ED, Perry HD. Keratoconus with spontaneous perforation of the cornea. *Arch Ophthalmol.* 1991;109:1651–1652.

19. Izquierdo L Jr, Mannis MJ, Marsh PB, Yang SP, McCarthy JM. Bilateral spontaneous corneal rupture in brittle cornea syndrome: A case report. *Cornea.* 1999;18:621–624.

20. Au YK, Collins WP, Patel JS, Asamoah A. Spontaneous corneal rupture in Noonan syndrome: A case report. *Ophthalmic Genet.* 1997;18:39–41.

21. Topping TM, Stark WJ, Maumanee E, Kenyon KR. Traumatic wound dehiscence following penetrating keratoplasty. *Br J Ophthalmol.* 1982;66:174–178.

22. Agrawal V, Wagh M, Krishnamahary M, Rao GN, Gupta S. Traumatic wound dehiscence after penetrating keratoplasty. *Cornea.* 1995;14:601–603.

23. Tseng SH, Lin SC, Chan FK. Traumatic wound dehiscence after penetrating keratoplasty: Clinical features and outcome in 21 cases. *Cornea.* 1999;18:553–558.

24. Johns KJ, Shiels P, Parrish CM, Elliott JA, O'Day DM. Traumatic wound dehiscence in pseudophakia. *Am J Ophthalmol*. 1989;15:108:535–539.

25. Stevens JD, Claoue CM, Stele AD. Postoperative blunt trauma to 7.5-mm scleral pocket wounds. *J Cataract Refract Surg*. 1994;20:344–345.

26. Binder PS, Waring GO, Arrowsmith PN, Wang C. Histopathology of traumatic corneal rupture after radial keratotomy. *Arch Ophthalmol*. 1988;106:1584–1590.

27. Lee BL, Manche EE, Glasgow BJ. Rupture of radial and arcuate keratotomy scars by blunt trauma 91 months after incisional keratotomy. *Am J Ophthalmol*. 1995;120:108–110.

28. Goldberg MA, Valluri S, Pepose JS. Air bag-related corneal rupture after radial keratotomy. *Am J Ophthalmol*. 1995;120:800–802.

29. Vinger PF, Mieler WF, Oestreicher JH, Easterbrook M. Ruptured globes following radial and hexagonal keratotomy surgery. *Arch Ophthalmol*. 1996;114:129–134.

30. Barr CC. Prognostic factors in corneoscleral lacerations. *Arch Ophthalmol*. 1983;101:919–924.

31. Sternberg P Jr, de Juan E Jr, Michels RG, Auer C. Multivariate analysis of prognostic factors in penetrating ocular injuries. *Am J Ophthalmol*. 1984;98:467–472.

32. Sternberg P Jr, de Juan E Jr, Michels RG. Penetrating ocular injuries in young patients: Initial injuries and visual results. *Retina*. 1984;4:5–8.

33. Esmali B, Elner SG, Schork MA, Elner VM. Visual outcome and ocular survival after penetrating trauma: A clinicopathologic study. *Ophthalmology*. 1995;102:393–400.

34. Pieramici DJ, MacCumber MW, Humayun MU, Marsh MJ, De Juan E Jr. Open-globe injury: Update on types of injuries and visual results. *Ophthalmology*. 1996;103:1798–1803.

35. Russell SR, Olsen KR, Folk JC. Predictors of scleral rupture and the role of vitrectomy in severe blunt ocular trauma. *Am J Ophthalmol*. 1988;105:253–257.

36. Klystra JA, Lamkin JC, Runyan DK. Clinical predictors of scleral rupture after blunt ocular trauma. *Am J Ophthalmol*. 1993;115:530–535.

37. Werner MS, Dana MR, Viana MA, Shapiro M. Predictors of occult scleral rupture. *Ophthalmology*. 1994;101: 1941–1944.

38. O'Brien TP, Choi S. Trauma-related ocular infections. *Ophthalmol Clin North Am*. 1995;8(4):667–679.

39. Duch-Sampler AM, Menezo JL, Hurtado-Sarrio M. Endophthalmitis following penetrating eye injuries. *Acta Ophthalmol Scand*. 1997;75:104–106.

40. Reynolds DS, Flynn HW Jr. Endophthalmitis after penetrating ocular trauma. *Curr Opin Ophthalmol*. 1997;8:32–38.

41. Meiler WF, Ellis MK, Williams DF, Han DP. Retained intraocular foreign bodies and endophthalmitis. *Ophthalmology*. 1990;97:1532–1538.

42. Thompson WS, Rubsamen PE, Flynn HW Jr, Schiffman J, Cousins SW. Endophthalmitis after penetrating trauma: Risk factors and visual acuity outcomes. *Ophthalmology*. 1995;102:1696–1701.

43. Alfaro DV, Roth D, Liggett PE. Posttraumatic endophthalmitis: Causative organisms, treatment, and prevention. *Retina*. 1994;14:206–211.

44. Kunimoto DY, Das T, Sharma S, et al, and the Endophthalmitis Research Group. Microbiologic spectrum and susceptibility of isolates, II: Posttraumatic endophthalmitis. *Am J Ophthalmol*. 1999;128:242–244.

45. Simonson D. Retrobulbar block for open-eye injuries: A report of 19 cases. *CRNA*. 1992;3:35–37.

46. Lo MW, Chalfin S. Retrobulbar anesthesia for repair of ruptured globes. *Am J Ophthalmology*. 1997;123:833–835.

47. Sambursky DS, Azar DT. Corneal and anterior segment trauma and reconstruction. *Ophthalmol Clin North Am*. 1995;8(4):609–631.

48. Hersh PK, Shingleton BJ, Kenyon KR. Management of corneoscleral lacerations. In: Shingleton BJ, Hersh PS, Kenyon KR, eds. *Eye Trauma*. St Louis, Mo: Mosby; 1991: 143–158.

49. Rowsey JJ. Corneal laceration repair: Topographic considerations in suturing techniques. In: Shingleton BJ, Hersh PS, Kenyon KR, eds. *Eye Trauma*. St Louis, Mo: Mosby; 1991: 159–168.

50. Rowsey JJ. Ten caveats of keratorefractive surgery. *Ophthalmology*. 1983;90:148–155.

51. Leahey AB, Gottsch JD, Stark WJ. Clinical experience with N-butyl cyanoacrylate (Nexacryl) tissue adhesive. *Ophthalmology*. 1993;100:173–180.

52. Moschos M, Droutsas D, Boussalis P, Tsioulias G. Clinical experience with cyanoacrylate tissue adhesive. *Doc Ophthalmol*. 1996–1997;93:237–245.

53. Eisner G. *Eye Surgery: An Introduction to Operative Techniques*. New York, NY: Springer-Verlag; 1980.

54. Ng JD. Director, Oculoplastic Surgery, Brooke Army Medical Center, San Antonio, Tex; Personal communication, May 2001.

55. Trudo EW, Bower KS. Processed human pericardium in the treatment of severe eye trauma. Paper presented at: American Academy of Ophthalmology Annual Meeting; October 1999; Orlando, Fla.

56. Smiddy WE, Stark WJ. Anterior segment intraocular foreign bodies. In: Shingleton BJ, Hersh PS, Kenyon KR, eds. *Eye Trauma*. St Louis, Mo: Mosby; 1991: 169–174.

57. Khani SC, Mukai S. Posterior segment intraocular foreign bodies. *Int Ophthalmol Clin*. 1995;35(1): 151–161.

58. Muga R, Maul E. Management of lens damage in perforating corneal lacerations. *Br J Ophthalmol*. 1978;62: 784–787.

59. Lamkin JC, Azar DT, Mead MD, Volpe NJ. Simultaneous corneal laceration repair, cataract removal, and posterior chamber intraocular lens implantation. *Am J Ophthalmol*. 1992;113:626–631.

60. Cohen A, Hersh P, Fleischman J. Management of trauma induced cataracts. *Ophthalmol Clin North Am*. 1995;8(4):633–646.

61. Rubsamen PE, Irvin WD, McCuen BW, Smiddy WE, Bowman CB. Primary intraocular lens implantation in the setting of penetrating ocular trauma. *Ophthalmology*. 1995;102:101–107.

62. Smiddy WE, Hamburg TR, Kracher GP, Gottsch JD, Stark WJ. Contact lenses for visual rehabilitation after corneal laceration repair. *Ophthalmology*. 1989;96:293–298.

63. Boghani S, Cohen EJ, Jones-Marioneaux S. Contact lenses after corneal lacerations. *CLAO J*. 1991;17:155–158.

64. Kanpolat A, Ciftci OU. The use of rigid gas permeable contact lenses in scarred corneas. *CLAO J*. 1995; 21:64–66.

65. McMahon TT, Devulapally J, Rosheim KM, Putz JL, Moore M, White S. Contact lens use after corneal trauma. *J Am Optom Assoc*. 1997;68:215–224.

66. Nobe JR, Moura BT, Robin JB, Smith RE. Results of penetrating keratoplasty for the treatment of corneal perforations. *Arch Ophthalmol*. 1990;108:939–941.

67. Sharkey TG, Brown SI. Transplantation of lacerated corneas. *Am J Ophthalmol*. 1981;91:721–725.

68. Dana MR, Schaumberg DA, Moyes AL, et al. Outcome of penetrating keratoplasty after ocular trauma in children. *Arch Ophthalmol*. 1995;113:1503–1507.

69. Belin MW, Ratliff DC. Anterior segment rehabilitation after trauma. In: Krachmer JH, Mannia MJ, Holland EJ, eds. *Cornea and External Disease: Clinical Diagnosis and Management*. St Louis, Mo: Mosby; 1997: 1947–1955.

70. Hersh PS, Kenyon KR. Anterior segment reconstruction following ocular trauma. In: Shingleton BJ, Hersh PS, Kenyon KR, eds. *Eye Trauma*. St Louis, Mo: Mosby; 1991: 175–184.

Chapter 10

TRAUMA OF THE CRYSTALLINE LENS

JOSEPH PASTERNAK, MD*

*Commander, Medical Corps, US Navy; National Naval Medical Center, 8901 Wisconsin Avenue, Bethesda, Maryland 20889-5600

INTRODUCTION

An estimated 2.4 million ocular injuries occur annually in the United States; of these, 40,000 to 70,000 are serious and vision-threatening. In the setting of ocular injury, injury to the crystalline lens is a frequent and serious consequence of both blunt and penetrating trauma. The National Eye Trauma System (NETS) reports that traumatic cataract occurs in 10% to 40% of reported cases of penetrating ocular trauma.[1] Lens injuries occur in approximately 25% of cases of blunt injury of the globe.[2,3]

In the battlefield setting, the majority of wartime injuries are caused by fragmentation weapons. One third of wartime ocular injuries are corneoscleral lacerations, and associated lens damage is common,[4] occurring in an estimated 27% to 50% of such cases.[5] During the Persian Gulf War, traumatic cataract comprised 9% of reported serious ocular injuries.[6]

Traumatic damage to the crystalline lens has diverse manifestations (Exhibit 10-1). In blunt trauma, the coup–contrecoup theory[7] and the equatorial expansion model[8] account for such diverse injuries as contusion cataracts, capsular disruption, and zonular disruption with resultant subluxation and even dislocation of the lens. Penetrating trauma resulting in anterior and / or posterior capsular disruption can induce a rapid opacification of the lens. Intraocular foreign bodies (IOFBs) can become lodged within the lens itself or cause toxicity through oxidation. Liberation of lens material in both blunt and penetrating trauma can lead to intraocular inflammation and elevation of intraocular pressure (IOP).

EXHIBIT 10-1

MANIFESTATIONS OF TRAUMA TO THE CRYSTALLINE LENS

- Contusion cataract
- Rosette cataract
- Vossius ring
- Complete lens opacification
- Intralenticular foreign body
- Posterior capsular rupture
- Lens involution / Soemmering ring cataract
- Lens subluxation
- Lens dislocation
- Lenticular inflammation / elevated intraocular pressure

Traumatic damage to the lens occurs secondarily to osmotic hydration or dehydration. When the osmolarity of the lens is subject to large variations, a cataract develops. Traumatic laceration of the lens capsule or injury to its adenosine triphosphate–dependent sodium–potassium ion pump results in increased permeability, allowing an influx of sodium and water from the aqueous into the substance of the lens, producing intracellular and extracellular swelling of epithelial cells. Additionally, lens proteins undergo proteolysis, aggregation, and conformational changes, all thought to be factors responsible for lens opacification in acute traumatic cataracts. Capsular integrity is rapidly restored, and—even in the case of observable perforation—opacification may remain localized or even reverse as fibrin seals off the capsular tear.[9] However, the opacity is irreversible once lens fiber swelling and fragmentation occur.

Extremes of heat and cold, electrical shock, and radiation exposure also lead to irreversible protein conformational changes and lens opacification. In cases of significant capsular laceration, the entire lens can rapidly opacify, but the large majority of cataracts in blunt trauma remain localized and morphologically distinct.

BLUNT TRAUMA

Contusion Cataract

A contusion cataract is usually a partial or localized opacification of the lens. It forms days to weeks after the injury and is often transient. The opacification in a contusion cataract is usually stationary and impacts vision in ways that depend on its relationship to the visual axis. Subcapsular opacities may organize into focal, scattered, punctate lesions, or they may coalesce into larger lamellar opacities (Figure 10-1). The morphologic appearance of a concussively induced cataract is often so characteristic as to be diagnostic of previous trauma, even in the absence of a definite history of trauma.

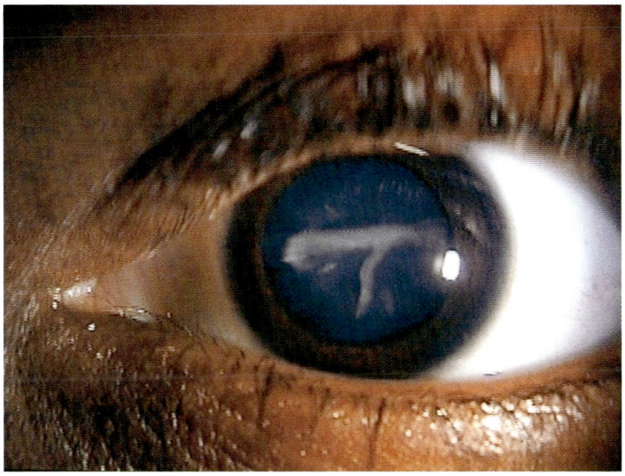

Fig. 10-1. Contusion cataract. Focal traumatic cataract in young man who sustained blunt trauma as a result of being struck by a rock. Although the opacities are focal, their central location caused disabling glare.

An archetypal form of contusion cataract is the rosette (Figure 10-2). A rosette radiates from the central nuclear sutures to the periphery and forms as fluid shifts take place inside an intact capsule. Rosette cataracts are very often visually significant because of their central location. A rosette will occasionally occur years after a traumatic event (Figure 10-3).

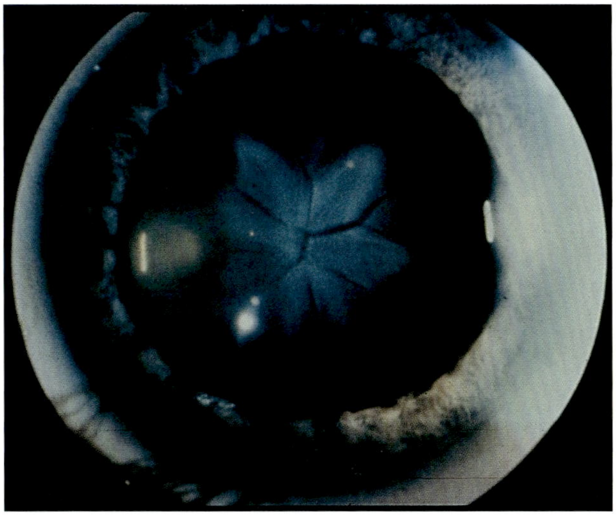

Fig. 10-2. A characteristic rosette cataract seen after blunt trauma, pathognomonic for contusion injury to the lens.

Vossius Ring

A contusion injury may lead to an imprint of pigment from the pupillary border onto the anterior face of the lens. This pigment, termed a Vossius ring, is seen most commonly in young patients and often slowly resolves over time.

Lens Subluxation

The sudden anteroposterior deformation of the globe experienced in severe blunt trauma is associated with rapid circumferential contraction and expansion of the globe. This mechanism accounts for concussive disruption of the iris root, ciliary body, zonules, and even the lens capsule. A subluxation of the lens is a partial zonular dehiscence, with

a

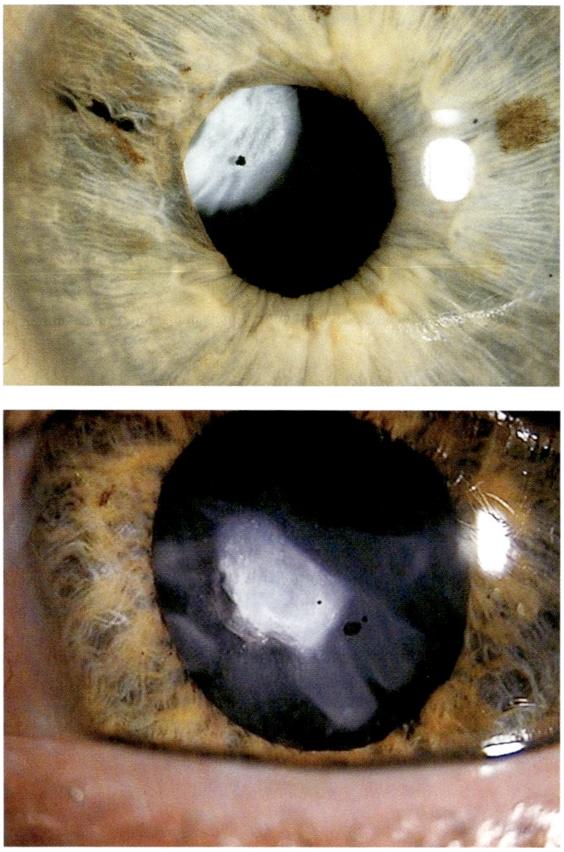

b

Fig. 10-3. Progressive traumatic cataract. (**a**) A focal paraxial contusion cataract, seen here 20 years after blunt injury to the eye (hit with a rock); vision is 20/20. (**b**) Three years later, a rosette cataract developed, dropping vision to 20/200. Rosette formation can occur years after injury, as it did in this case.

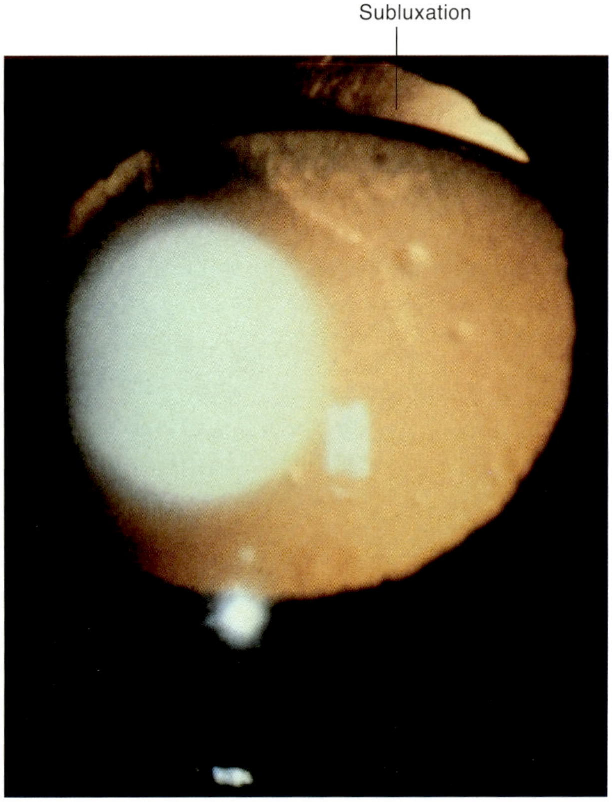

Fig. 10-4. Subluxation of the crystalline lens occurs when a minimum of 25% of the zonules are compromised.

the lens remaining in the pupillary aperture. This phenomenon can cause induced astigmatism, increased myopia, or increased anterior chamber depth. Subluxation occurs when 25% of the zonules are ruptured.

A subluxed lens will often go unnoticed at the time of injury (Figure 10-4), but the presence of iridodonesis or vitreous prolapse into the anterior chamber may indicate its presence. Patients with lens subluxation may complain of fluctuating vision as the lens shifts position, or of monocular diplopia if the lens equator reaches the visual axis.

Lens Dislocation

Lens dislocation occurs only in the setting of a complete zonular dehiscence. Dislocation can allow forward displacement of the lens, causing pupillary block, or even total entrapment in the anterior chamber. The lens can also settle posteriorly and peripherally in the anterior vitreous base. This difficult-to-visualize location may raise the possibility of lens egress from the eye if the globe is open. Rarely, the intact crystalline lens may actually be displaced outside the globe through a limbal rupture, where it becomes deposited subconjunctivally (Figure 10-5).[10,11]

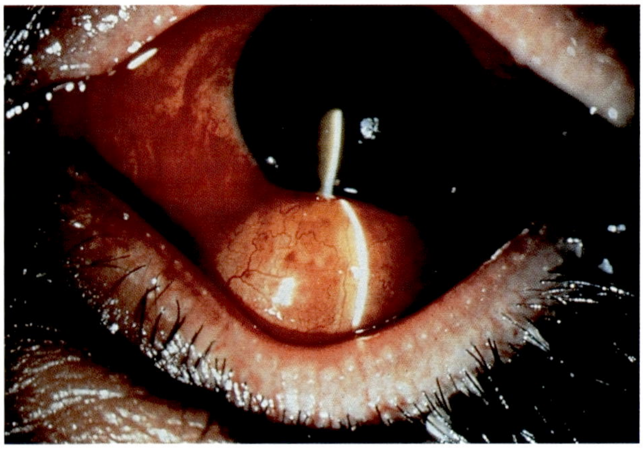

Fig. 10-5. This photograph demonstrates a crystalline lens deposited in the subconjunctival space following globe rupture. When the lens has been totally dislocated from its normal anatomical position, a careful, dilated peripheral posterior segment examination should be performed to determine whether the lens remains intraocular. Its presence will often be revealed in the far-equatorial anterior vitreous.

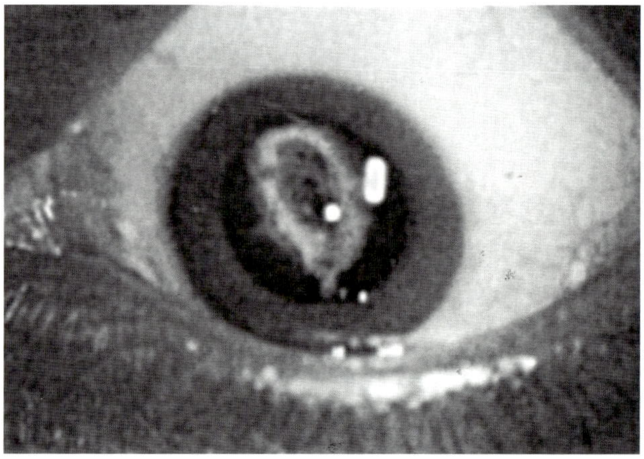

Fig. 10-6. Fibrosed edges of posterior capsular break seen after blunt trauma. Contusion injury may result in isolated posterior capsular breaks because the posterior capsule is thinner, anatomically, than the anterior. Reproduced with permission from Thomas R. Posterior capsular rupture after blunt trauma. *J Cataract Refractive Surg.* 1998;24:284.

Posterior Disruption

Rapid equatorial expansion of the globe sometimes causes a tear or break in the lens capsule. The posterior capsule, which is the thinnest, is often the site of rupture. Capsular tears may occur in conjunction with zonular disruption or as an alternative to it. Two distinct presentations of posterior capsular rupture have been described (Figure 10-6).[12,13] A Type 1 tear is a break in the capsule with thick, fibrous opaque margins and associated posterior capsular opacification. A Type 2 tear, on the other hand, has thin, transparent margins without associated lens opacification.

Differences in the two types of capsular breaks appear to be time dependent. When surgical intervention was delayed (1 mo–2 y postinjury), lenses show Type 1 tears, with clinical evidence of attempted healing of the defect. This type of capsular break does not tend to enlarge intraoperatively. When early surgical intervention is required (3–7 d postinjury), lenses exhibit Type 2 tears, which behave similarly to fresh intraoperative breaks. Type 2 tears tend to enlarge during irrigation or aspiration and need to be managed by viscoelastic plugging, dry aspiration, and adequate vitrectomy.

PENETRATING TRAUMA

Anterior Capsule Injury

In perforating wounds in which the lens capsule is directly injured, a large proportion of cases show localized and morphologically distinctive opacities rather than rapid, generalized opacification. Histologically, a cap of fibrin forms over the rent and the local epithelial cells rapidly degenerate, but neighboring subcapsular epithelium soon grows over the defect. These cells eventually decrease in size and become replaced by a homogeneous matrix, which then becomes covered by normal epithelium, which secretes a hyaline membrane.

If the tear occurs in the region of the iris, the reconstitution of the injured area is reinforced by fibroblasts from the iris tissue, and sometimes pigment from the iris is incorporated in the scar. In this way the tear can be completely and rapidly closed. Even with an observable tear, the preliminary local clouding of the lens may disappear if the tear itself is rapidly sealed off by fibrin while the imbibition of fluid is still reversible.[14] If a tear is larger and compromise of the lens capsule exceeds its mechanisms for repair, a rapid and complete opacification of the lens will occur (Figure 10-7).

Lens Absorption (Involution)

In younger patients, usually in the first decade of life, a laceration of the anterior lens capsule can result in an intense inflammatory response with

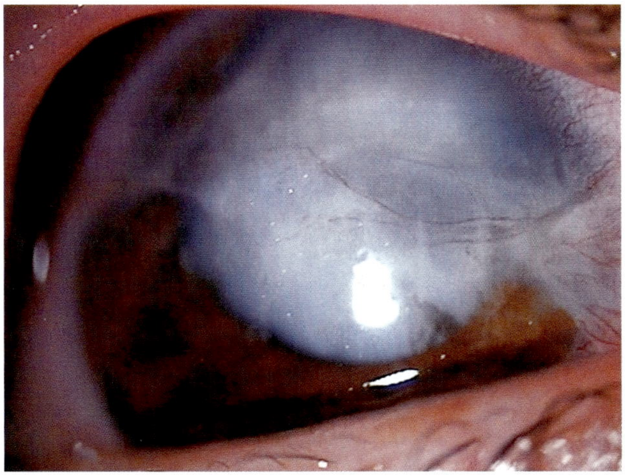

Fig. 10-7. Penetrating trauma often results in combined injury of the anterior segment. Corneal lacerations are commonly seen with concomitant anterior capsular disruption. Rapidly progressive or delayed lens opacification may result, as it did in this case of penetrating trauma from needle-nosed pliers.

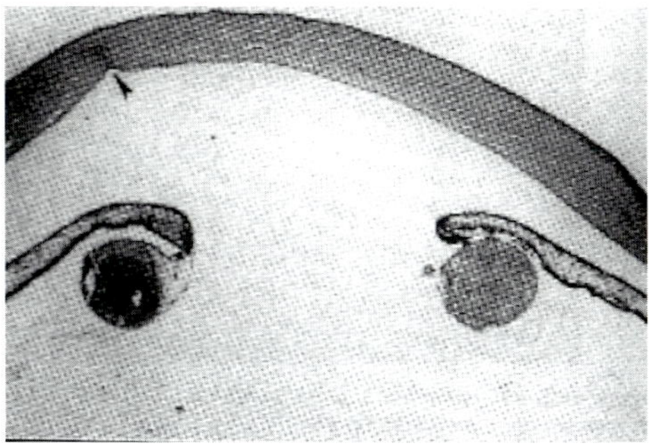

Fig. 10-8. Soemmering's ring cataract developed in this patient following penetrating corneal laceration (arrow). Reproduced with permission from Streeter BW. Pathology of the lens. In: Albert DM, ed. *Principles and Practice of Ophthalmology*. Vol 4. Philadelphia, Pa: WB Saunders; 1994: 2208.

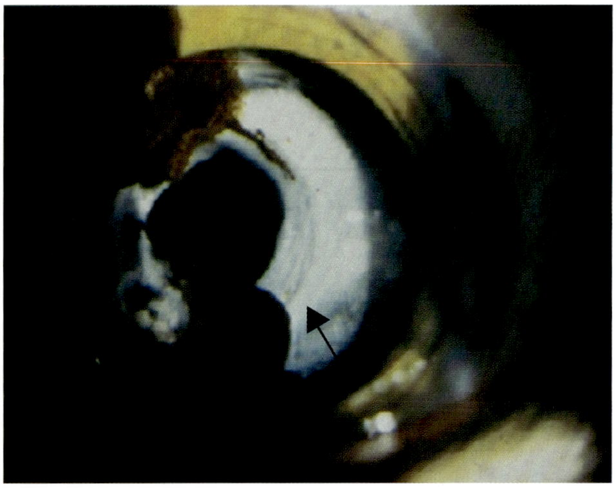

Fig. 10-9. This patient, a 24-year-old man, sustained blunt trauma to his eye with anterior capsular rupture. Despite minimal inflammation, his lens material spontaneously involuted, leaving behind a Soemmering's ring cataract (arrow) and an "aphakically" corrected eye with 20/20 vision.

spontaneous absorption of the entire lens nucleus, rendering the eye aphakic. Typically, a remnant of lens capsule and cortex will remain, forming a yellow-white ring called a Soemmering ring cataract (Figure 10-8).[15] Laser capsulotomy can aid in clearing of the visual axis, and treatment of aphakia can render excellent visual correction (Figure 10-9).

Intraocular Foreign Body

When a traumatic foreign body enters the eye, a cataract can be induced by either direct injury to the lens or through the toxic action of oxidized metal. Products of oxidation slowly invade the lens and produce characteristic lens discoloration or opacification. Sunflower cataracts arise from copper-containing foreign bodies (chalcosis; see Figure 15-11 in this textbook) and brown discoloration from iron deposits of the capsular epithelium (siderosis lentis; also see Figures 15-3 and 15-4). Cilia, glass, and nonoxidizing metals can occasionally enter the lens and may be well-tolerated for long periods with only localized opacification (Figure 10-10).[16]

Lenticular Glaucoma

Lens-induced inflammation results from the release of lens proteins into the anterior chamber. In the setting of a hypermature cataract, this release can occur through microscopic leaks in the lens capsule (ie, phacolytic glaucoma). After traumatic laceration of the capsule, macroscopic lens particles are liberated into the aqueous and may elicit a macrophage response, with subsequent deposition of high-density lens material and bloated macrophages in the trabecular meshwork. Medical therapy is required to control inflammation and check acute rises in IOP. The severity of the glaucoma is proportional to the amount of free cortical material in the aqueous humor.[17] Eyes with preexisting decreased outflow facility are more likely to develop increased IOP with lens protein in the aqueous.[18] Lens-particle-induced inflammation and IOP management often require urgent extraction of the lens to restore the eye to its normal state.[19]

In the setting of lens subluxation or dislocation, a mobilized lens can move forward, producing pupillary block with angle closure. With a complete dislocation of the lens posteriorly, the pupil may become blocked with vitreous, which can also produce a pupillary-block, angle-closure glaucoma.[19] Treatment of this form of glaucoma is directed at relieving the pupillary block, often with laser

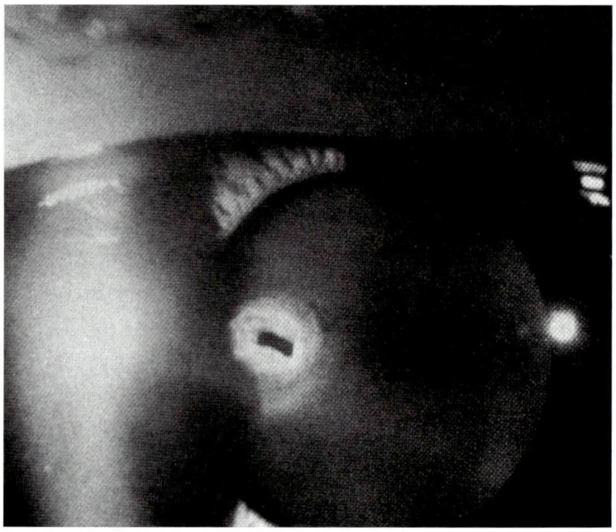

Fig. 10-10. The glass particle, seen here in the anterior lens capsule, remained stable and inert for 10 years since injury; the patient's vision remained 20/20. Reproduced with permission from Cowden JW. Anterior segment trauma. In: Spoor TC, Nesi FA, eds. *Management of Ocular, Orbital and Adnexal Trauma.* New York, NY: Raven Press; 1988: 48.

iridotomy or surgical iridectomy. Lensectomy should be undertaken only when other methods of visual rehabilitation prove unsuccessful or if pupillary block recurs. Occasionally a trauma-induced cataractous lens becomes intumescent. Such swollen lenses can subsequently cause angle-closure glaucoma as a result of pupillary block or result in direct-angle compromise by mass effect.[15]

EVALUATION

History

In the setting of ocular trauma, the mechanism of injury is a critical determinant of the type of the ocular damage sustained and is, therefore, the cornerstone of the medical history. In the battlefield setting, explosions account for the majority of ocular injuries, many of which are sustained concurrently with other major trauma. Fragmentation injury can cause both blunt and perforating ocular trauma, depending on the size of the fragment and the velocity at which it reaches the eye. Timing of the injury is also important.

Although a perforating injury most often brings about immediate evaluation, many patients who have sustained blunt trauma to the globe and develop contusion cataract or lens subluxation do not seek immediate medical care. They may later develop inflammation or experience a delayed onset of fluctuating or decreased vision from subluxation of the lens or progressive cataract. A past medical history should be obtained to establish any preexisting ocular or systemic conditions, such as glaucoma, previous ocular surgery, or diabetes, that may affect outcome.

Examination

Examination of the patient with eye trauma should always begin with the determination that the patient has stable respiratory and cardiovascular systems. Only then should attention be turned to the eye. The eye examination begins with assessment of the vision. In many cases of ocular trauma, the visual acuity on presentation is a predictor of visual outcome.[20]

Establishing whether media opacities or retinal or optic nerve pathology is responsible for visual loss is of immediate importance. Opacification of the lens can progress rapidly after the traumatic insult, and the initial evaluation may provide the only opportunity to evaluate the posterior pole. Retinoscopy can help detect an unsuspected shift in astigmatism or myopia in the case of a subluxed lens. A subtle subluxation may only be identifiable using a retroillumination biomicroscopic view after wide dilation. A deep anterior chamber and iridodonesis may be suggestive of subluxation, and a narrowing of the angle may indicate forward displacement of the lens. Prolapse of vitreous into the anterior chamber confirms the presence of lens subluxation. If corneal edema or blood in the anterior chamber preclude visualization of the lens, ultrasound can be useful in determining its position (Figure 10-11). If lenticular opacification prevents visualization of the retina, B-scan ultrasonography can be used to evaluate vitreous hemorrhage or retinal detachment. Ultrasound is also helpful in determining the presence of a foreign body.

A low IOP is potentially helpful in determining the presence of a ruptured globe, whereas an elevated pressure can indicate subluxation of the lens with pupillary blockade, disruption of the angle, the inflammatory effects of lens particles, or angle closure secondary to an intumescent lens.

When severe ocular injuries are seen with associated head and facial trauma, radiographic studies may be indicated. Plain film radiography can be useful in localizing foreign bodies, and a computed tomography (CT) scan is ideal for defining bony anatomy of the orbit and offers a greater deal of precision in foreign body localization. A CT scan

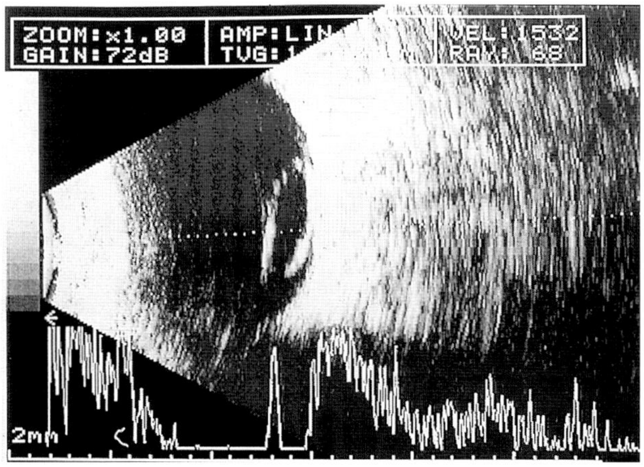

Fig. 10-11. After blunt trauma, the dislocated crystalline lens was visualized using B-scan ultrasound. Corneal edema precluded viewing with indirect ophthalmoscopy.

can also provide information about the state of lens opacification. Signal attenuation may be seen in a lens that is cataractous, even before clinical lens opacification.[21]

SURGICAL MANAGEMENT

After the casualty has been stabilized, the ophthalmologist's attention is directed to the management of ocular trauma. There are a few indications for immediate surgical intervention for isolated lenticular injury:

- dislocation of the lens into the anterior chamber with corneal touch,
- pupillary block due to anterior lens displacement,
- angle closure secondary to an intumescent lens,
- uncontrollable inflammation, and
- elevation of IOP secondary to lens-particle release.

Initial surgical intervention for lens injury can generally be delayed; further evaluation and monitoring are usually indicated. With a localized, eccentric contusion cataract, pharmacological therapy can be tried first to decrease pupil size and clear the visual axis. If the lens is markedly subluxed, miosis can render a patient effectively aphakic, and the vision can then be improved with a contact lens.

Surgical management is indicated for the emergent indications previously described, or it can be offered electively for visual rehabilitation. Elevated IOP and any inflammation should be fully treated before any elective cataract removal. The primary consideration when planning surgical removal of a traumatic cataract or a subluxed lens is the possibility of vitreous loss.[19]

To optimize the surgical outcome and minimize complications, a decision must be made between an anterior (limbal) and a posterior (pars plana) surgical approach. An anterior approach is preferred to remove a traumatic cataract in the presence of an intact posterior capsule or if the lens has been dislocated completely into the anterior chamber. A posterior approach is preferable if the posterior capsule has been ruptured, if the lens is dislocated posteriorly, or if there is a traumatic rupture of the zonules with vitreous presenting anteriorly. Removal of a minimally subluxed lens can be made through a limbal incision; however, anterior vitrectomy and a possible conversion to a pars plana incision may be required. If a lens has been completely dislocated out of the visual axis and is causing no inflammation or elevation of IOP, surgical removal can be delayed indefinitely.

Anterior Approach (Limbal Incision)

An anterior approach to traumatic cataract or traumatic subluxation is indicated in the following situations:

- lens opacification with no apparent zonular compromise and an intact posterior capsule,
- lens opacification with minimal zonular compromise, no displacement of the lens, and no vitreous present in the anterior chamber, and
- dislocation of the lens into the anterior chamber.

Many ocular injuries occur in younger people, and their opacified lens material is relatively soft and easy to remove. If the capsule and zonules are intact, performing a capsulorrhexis is identical to standard cataract surgery. Small compromises in the anterior capsule can potentially be converted directly into a capsulorrhexis. If compromise of the posterior capsule or zonules is occult and a conversion to extracapsular surgery is needed, relaxing incisions can be made at 3 o'clock and 9 o'clock in the capsulorrhexis.[20] It is common in trauma-related cataract surgery that previously unrecognized compromises in the zonules or capsule become manifest during surgery, and the surgeon should anticipate the need to modify the procedure as a case progresses. It is very important to make an adequately sized capsulotomy so that if extracapsular delivery is necessary, expression of the nucleus does not lead to further disruption of the zonules and prolapse of the vitreous.

A standard limbal approach is as follows. Create limbal entry sites at the limbus at the 10 o'clock and 2 o'clock positions. Opposing incisions allow manipulation of the globe, and bimanual technique allows both for finer control of aspiration and for the lowest possible amount of irrigant, which minimizes hydration of the vitreous cavity through any potential zonular interruption. In a lens with intact zonules, a capsulotomy is fashioned with bent-needle cystotome and continued with capsular for-

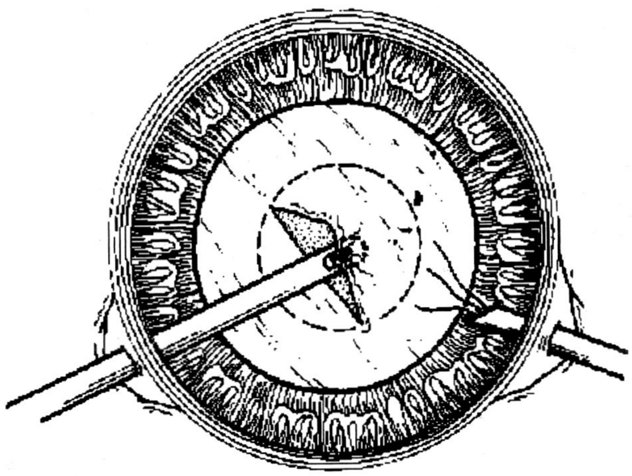

Fig. 10-12. If visualization is poor because of opacification of the lens cortex or if zonular compromise limits the ability to perform capsulorrhexis, an anterior vitrector can be introduced through a capsular opening and used to easily create a well-defined anterior capsulotomy. Reproduced with permission from Irvine JA, Smith RE. Lens injuries. In: Shingleton BJ, ed. *Eye Trauma.* St Louis, Mo: Mosby–Year Book; 1991: 131.

ceps. If visualization is poor, the capsulotomy is fashioned using a can-opener technique with the cystotome, or it can be augmented with Vannas scissors.

When an adequate red reflex is lacking, visualization of the capsule can be enhanced with an off-axis light with a retinal light pipe. Alternatively, a capsulotomy can be started with a Ziegler knife or MVR (micro-vitreo-retinal) blade, and an anterior vitrectomy handpiece that is introduced through the nasal incision is used to cut away the central anterior capsule (Figure 10-12). During mechanical capsulorrhexis, generous use of viscoelastic is advisable to stabilize the anterior capsular plane of the lens and to aid in visualizing the full extent of any capsular tears. Iris retracting hooks can be used to further visualize the lens to the equator, or they can be placed in the advancing tear of a capsulorrhexis to provide countertraction of the capsular bag in areas of zonular weakness.

In a young patient, whose lens is soft, lens removal is performed with the aspiration port of the anterior vitrectomy unit. A separate infusion port is placed through the 2 o'clock incision, using a 23-gauge butterfly needle for chamber maintenance. Maximum aspiration of 150 mm Hg is usually sufficient. In an older patient with more-advanced nuclear sclerosis, routine phacoemulsification may be performed. Careful attention should be given to performing a hydrodissection of the lens with balanced salt solution through a small-gauge cannula. This procedure enables manipulation and removal of the nucleus to be completed with a minimum of traction on the zonules. After removal of the lens nucleus, cortical removal is performed. Manual aspiration through a fine cannula allows carefully controlled cortical removal and can even be performed in areas of zonular dehiscence.

An intracapsular fixation ring (mfg by Morcher, Munich, Germany) is now available that can be placed into the equator of the capsular bag before lens removal. By distributing tension over 360°, countertraction is provided in areas where weak or missing zonules do not provide sufficient tension for adequate stripping of the cortex. Using a curved cannula, bending the cannula, or switching limbal entry sites can all aid in cortical removal in areas of the lens nucleus that are difficult to access, such as under the iris at the 12 o'clock position.

Efforts should be made to ensure that no vitreous is present in the anterior chamber. Viscoelastic tamponade may be helpful in preventing vitreous

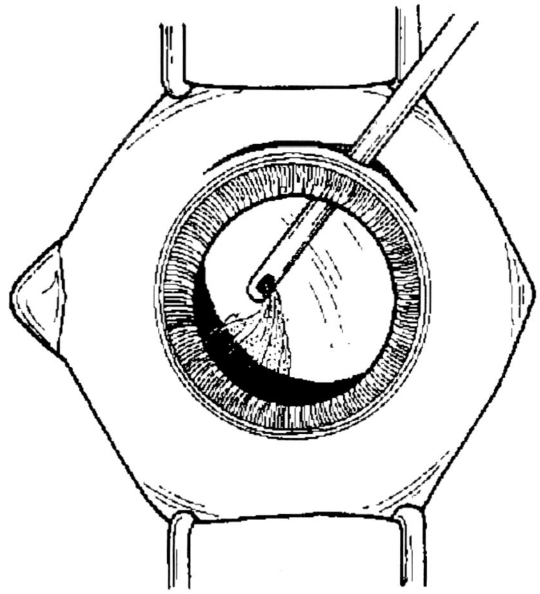

Fig. 10-13. Vitreous presenting into the anterior chamber through an area of zonular compromise should be removed before surgically approaching the lens. Limiting irrigation as much as possible minimizes hydration of the vitreous. A separate site for irrigation may facilitate anterior chamber stability. After vitreous cleanup, viscoelastic is used to tamponade further anterior migration of vitreous. Reproduced with permission from Cohen A, Hersh PS, Fleischman JA. Management of trauma-induced cataracts. *Ophthalmic Clinics of North America.* 1995;8:641.

prolapse in areas of known zonular dehiscence. If partial subluxation of the lens is present and vitreous has presented into the anterior chamber, a vitrectomy should be performed before the lens is removed (Figure 10-13). A separate infusion port is used, keeping the anterior chamber formed with the least amount of fluid possible. If lens removal has been completed, then an intracameral miotic should be instilled, and peaking of the pupil may indicate that vitreous is presenting to the incision. Air can be infused to replace fluid in the anterior chamber to aid in visualization of vitreous strands. A cyclodialysis spatula is introduced through the limbal incision and is used to sweep from the angle toward the pupil in order to free the vitreous strands from the incision site (Figure 10-14). Further vitrectomy and repeated sweeping might be needed to completely free the trapped vitreous strands. If lens material has fallen posteriorly, it is inappropriate and even dangerous to attempt anterior removal of the lens pieces.[22]

Rarely, when a lens is dislocated anteriorly into the anterior chamber and is abutting the endothelium, a topical miotic should be instilled preoperatively and then intracamerally through a limbal paracentesis to prevent posterior migration of the lens. Viscoelastic is injected to protect the corneal endothelium. In a younger patient, the lens can be removed entirely by cutting and aspirating with a vitrectomy handpiece. If the lens is more sclerotic, the limbal incision is extended and the lens delivered intracapsularly through the extended incision. An irrigating vectus can be used to aid expression of the lens. The incision is then closed using interrupted nylon sutures (Figure 10-15).

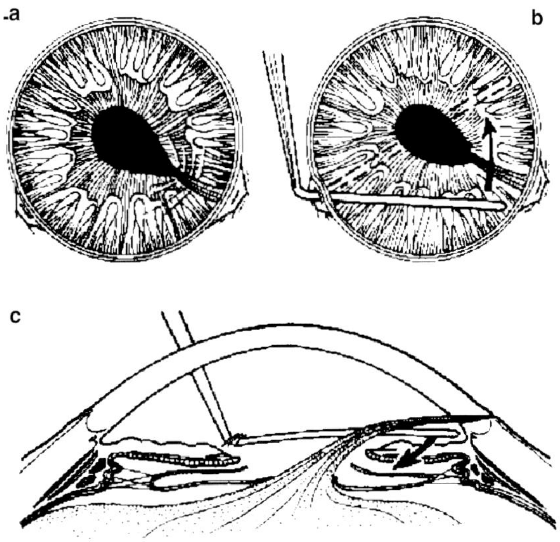

Fig. 10-14. Sweeping of vitreous with cyclodialysis spatula. (**a**) After introduction of an intracameral miotic, constriction of the pupil reveals peaking secondary to vitreous presenting to the wound. (**b, c**) The vitreous may be removed from the angle by passing a sweep or spatula from the opposite port. This procedure may be done under fluid, air, or viscoelastic material. Reproduced with permission from Irvine JA, Smith RE. Lens injuries. In: Shingleton BJ, ed. *Eye Trauma.* St Louis, Mo: Mosby–Year Book; 1991: 132.

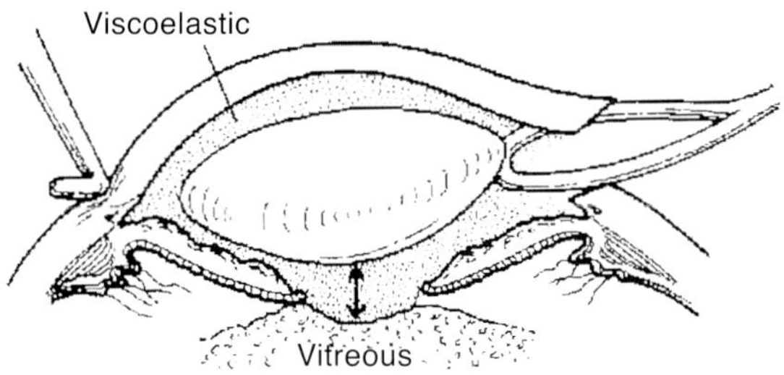

Fig. 10-15. Pharmacological miosis aids in trapping the anteriorly dislocated lens in the anterior chamber, thereby preventing posterior migration. Lens removal then may be achieved via aspiration or limbal delivery. Reproduced with permission from Cohen A, Hersh PS, Fleischman JA. Management of trauma-induced cataracts. *Ophthalmic Clinics of North America.* 1995;8:642.

Posterior Approach (Pars Plana Incision)

A pars plana technique and a posterior approach can be used if there is posterior subluxation or dislocation of the lens or disruption of the posterior capsule with lens fragments in the anterior vitreous.

The following is a standard pars plana approach. A limbal peritomy is performed, allowing for sclerotomies at 10 o'clock, 2 o'clock, and the inferotemporal positions. With an MVR blade, sclerotomies are made 3 mm posterior to the limbus, allowing for a passive infusion port at the inferotemporal position. Care must be taken in placing the infusion cannula, as lens opacification may interfere with adequate visualization of the port, and subchoroidal infusion of irrigating fluid may occur. The bottle height of the balanced salt solution irrigant is adjusted to maintain appropriate chamber depth and IOP.

Twenty-gauge instrumentation is used to perform a core anterior vitrectomy and lensectomy of posteriorly displaced lens materials (Figure 10-16). A bimanual crushing of harder nuclear material (Figure 10-17) may be necessary in older patients,

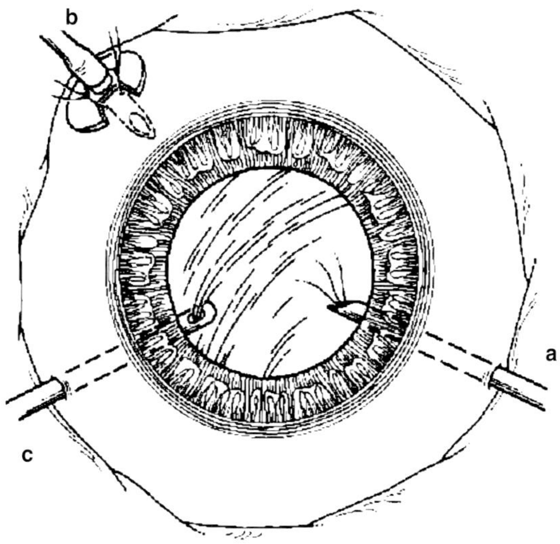

Fig. 10-16. Placement of instrumentation for pars plana lens removal. Sclerotomies are made 3 mm posterior to the limbus. (**a**) The supranasal incision may be used temporarily for a handheld infusion until (**b**) the infusion cannula is sewn into place infratemporally. (**c**) The cutting tip is introduced via the supratemporal sclerotomy. Site "a" can then be used for a second instrument to permit bimanual manipulation of the posterior segment. Reproduced with permission from Irvine JA, Smith RE. Lens injuries. In: Shingleton BJ, ed. *Eye Trauma.* St Louis, Mo: Mosby–Year Book; 1991: 133.

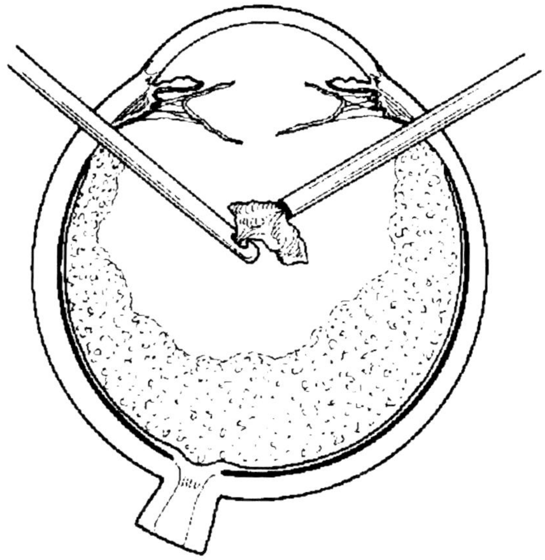

Fig. 10-17. Gentle suction brings posteriorly dislocated lens fragments to a midvitreous location where they can then be removed by a bimanual crush technique or with an ultrasound fragmatome. Reproduced with permission from Cohen A, Hersh PS, Fleischman JA. Management of trauma-induced cataracts. *Ophthalmic Clinics of North America.* 1995;8:643.

or an ultrasonic fragmatome may be required. Contact between lens material and the retina should be assiduously avoided. A limited core vitrectomy is usually adequate, and any lens pieces that are close to the retina should be aspirated off the cushion of remaining vitreous and removed in the midvitreous.[19] Cautious cortical and capsular removal should be performed with the vitrector, with careful attention to leaving behind a ring of capsular remnant to provide for intraocular lens (IOL) support in the sulcus.

Primary Intraocular Lens Placement

The timing of lens removal in the setting of coexisting ocular trauma is controversial. Primary surgical management is often dictated by the extent of corneal and scleral injury in addition to the injury to the lens. When the lens alone is injured, delayed removal has been favored historically.[8] Arguments against acute lens removal include the following:

- the extent of visual compromise can be difficult to assess accurately,
- acute trauma is often repaired by relatively inexperienced surgeons, and
- emergency trauma can take place in a less-controlled setting (eg, after hours, with fatigued operating teams).

Nevertheless, experience is increasing with early lens removal and primary or secondary IOL placement, and numerous reports suggest good results.[23–27] Once the decision to remove the lens has been made, the judgment as to whether to leave the patient aphakic must be weighed carefully against the placement of a primary IOL. Reluctance about placing an implant at the time of primary repair and lens removal is based on the concern that the IOL will be a nidus for infection and a potential aggravant of intraocular inflammation.[28] Some surgeons[29] believe that an implant potentiates the risk of posttraumatic glaucoma, but others[30] refute this claim. A pseudophakic eye can also be more difficult to operate on if further posterior segment repair becomes necessary after the original anterior segment restoration.[31] Advocates[23–35] argue that there is minimal risk of increased posttraumatic endophthalmitis from a sterile implant, that increased inflammation and glaucoma have not been observed, and that posterior segment surgeons are becoming more experienced with procedures on pseudophakic eyes.

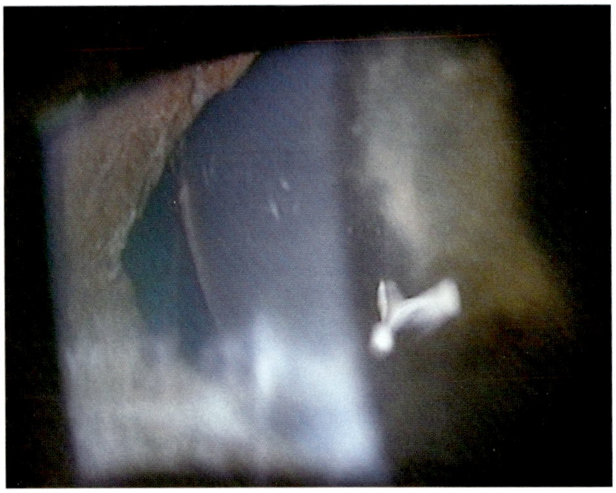

Fig. 10-18. Traumatic cataract and lens subluxation with primarily repaired corneal laceration. At primary closure of this corneal laceration (due to knife injury), the lens was noted to be clear. By 6 months later, a posterior subcapsular cataract (PSC) had developed, and inferonasal subluxation was apparent. Cataract surgery planning was complicated by elevated intraocular pressure secondary to angle disruption; irregular corneal curvature, which made keratometry measurement problematic; and lens opacification, which disrupted measurement of axial length with A-scan biometry.

When planning cataract removal and lens implantation in an eye with concurrent corneal injury, the status of the cornea must be taken into account. It is sometimes impossible to obtain keratometry and axial length measurements because of corneal scarring and irregularity and the poor quality of biometry through an opacified lens (Figure 10-18). Measurements of the nontraumatized eye can guide selection of the lens implant.

Choices for lens fixation include (*a*) in-the-bag, (*b*) sulcus-fixated, and (*c*) anterior chamber lenses. In patients whose eyes have small posterior breaks, direct in-the-bag fixation can be considered without scleral fixation; alternatively, single haptic fixation may be adequate. In patients with incomplete posterior capsule support, posterior chamber IOLs can be implanted with both haptics transsclerally fixated. However, this technique causes more damage to the eye and may lead to more complications.[32] An anterior chamber lens may be considered as a preferable option, depending on the status of the iris and the cornea. Ultrasound examination before surgery can reveal the status of the posterior capsule and aid in optimal decision making with regard to IOL implantation, anterior vitrectomy, or prevention of retinal detachment.[36]

POSTOPERATIVE COMPLICATIONS

Surgery to repair a traumatic cataract has a higher rate of postoperative complications than standard cataract surgery does. The loss of lens material into the posterior segment is the most commonly encountered intraoperative complication.[20] Loss of zonular support or enlargement of posterior capsule breaks can contribute to this risk. Lens material should be left in place for spontaneous absorption or for secondary removal through a pars plana approach.

Bleeding from a ciliary body is a risk when sulcus-fixated lenses are placed. Postoperative complications include hyphema, transient IOP elevation or transient hypotension, posterior iris synechiae, iris capture, subluxation of lens implant, endothelial cell loss, and cystoid macular edema.

SUMMARY

Lens injury is a frequent consequence of trauma to the eye. Blunt injury can result in contusion cataracts, either acutely or as late sequelae of the trauma. Disruption of the zonules can result in subluxation and dislocation of the lens. Penetrating trauma often results in combined anterior segment laceration and traumatic cataract. Management of lens injury and timing of surgery are based on location and morphology of the lens opacity, stability of vision, presence of intraocular inflammation, IOP control, and ability to examine the posterior segment. Modern advances in microsurgical techniques have enhanced the results of lens removal. Primary IOL implantation has achieved excellent visual results in an increasingly large number of patients. Careful examination and accurate diagnosis are critical in surgical decision-making, both in the choice of the most appropriate timing for surgery and the selection of the best surgical technique.

REFERENCES

1. Parver LM, Dannenberg AL, Blaklow B, Fowler CJ, Brechner RJ, Tielsch JM. Characteristics and causes of penetrating injuries reported to the national eye trauma system registry, 1985–91. *Public Health Rep.* 1993;108(5):625–633.

2. Shaffer RV. Comparison of cataract incidence in normal and glaucomatous population. *Am J Ophthalmol.* 1970;69:386–370.

3. Eagling EM. Ocular damage after blunt trauma to the eye: Its relationship to the nature of the injury. *Br J Ophthalmol.* 1974;58:126–140.

4. Mader TH. *Lessons Learned From Operations Desert Shield and Desert Storm.* Bethesda, Md: Tri-Service Ocular Trauma Course, Uniformed Services University of the Health Sciences; May 1997.

5. Muga R, Maul E. The management of lens damage in perforating corneal lacerations. *Br J Ophthalmol.* 1978; 62:784–787.

6. Mader TH, Aragones JV, Chandler AC, et al. Ocular and ocular adnexal injuries treated by United States military ophthalmologists during Operations Desert Shield and Desert Storm. *Ophthalmology.* 1993;100:1462–1467.

7. Wolter JR. Coup-contrecoup mechanism of ocular injuries. *Am J Ophthalmol.* 1963;56:785–796.

8. Weidenthal DT, Schepens CL. Peripheral fundus changes associated with ocular contusion. *Am J Ophthalmol.* 1966;62:465–477.

9. Duke-Elder S, ed. *System of Ophthalmology.* Vol 14. St Louis: Mosby–Year Book; 1972: 121–142.

10. Albal MV, Kalyani RS. Subconjunctival dislocation of lens: A case report. *Indian J Ophthalmol.* 1977;24:31–32.

11. Napora C. Commander, Medical Corps, US Navy (Ret). Personal communication; 1994.

12. Vajpayee RB, Angra SK, Honavar SG, Titiya JS, Sharma YR, Sakhuja N. Pre-existing posterior capsule breaks from perforating ocular injuries. *J Cataract Refract Surg.* 1994;20:291–294.

13. Thomas R. Posterior capsular rupture after blunt trauma. *J Cataract Refract Surg.* 1998;24:283–284.

14. Tasman W, ed. *Duane's Clinical Ophthalmology.* Vol 1. Philadelphia, Pa: Lippincott; 1994: Chap 73.

15. Albert DM, ed. *Principles and Practice of Ophthalmology.* Vol 4. Philadelphia, Pa: Saunders; 1994: 2208.

16. Spoor TC, Nesi FA, eds. *Management of Ocular, Orbital and Adnexal Trauma.* New York, NY: Raven Press; 1988: 48.

17. Shields MB, ed. *The Glaucomas.* St Louis, Mo: Mosby–Year Book; 1989: 334.

18. Savage JA, Thomas JV, Belcher CD, Simmons RJ. Extracapsular cataract extraction and posterior chamber intraocular lens implantation in glaucomatous eyes. *Ophthalmology.* 1985;92:1506–1516.

19. Shingleton BJ, ed. *Eye Trauma.* St Louis, Mo: Mosby–Year Book; 1991: 126–135.

20. Cohen A, Hersh PS, Fleischman JA. Management of trauma-induced cataracts. *Ophthalmol Clin North Am.* 1995;8:633–645.

21. Boorstein JM, Titelbaum DS, Patel Y, Grossman RI. CT diagnosis of unsuspected traumatic cataracts in patients with complicated eye injuries: Significance of attenuation value of the lens. *Am J Roentgenol.* 1995;164:181–184.

22. Lambrou FH, Stuart MW. Management of dislocated lens fragments: Pars plana vitrectomy and trans-scleral fixation of posterior chamber lens implants. *Vit Surg Technol*. 1992;4:5–6.

23. Anwar M, Bleik JH, von Noorden GK, el-Maghraby AA, Attin F. Posterior chamber lens implantation for primary repair of corneal lacerations and traumatic cataracts in children. *J Pediatr Ophthalmol Strabismus*. 1994;31:157–161.

24. Sinskey RM, Stoppel JO, Amin P. Long-term results of intraocular lens implantation in pediatric patients. *J Cataract Refract Surg*. 1993;19(3):405–408.

25. Prochazkova L, Rozsiva P. Cataract operations and implantation of intraocular lenses in children and adolescents. *Cesk Slov Oftalmol*. 1992;8:331–337.

26. Bienfait MF, Pameijer JH, Wildervanck-de-Blecourt-Devilee M. Intraocular lens implantation in children with unilateral traumatic cataract. *Ophthalmology*. 1990;14:271–276.

27. Insler MS, Helm CJ. Traumatic cataract management in penetrating ocular injury. *CLAO J*. 1989;15:78–81.

28. Lamkin JC, Azar DT, Mead MD, Volpe NJ. Simultaneous corneal laceration repair, cataract removal, and posterior chamber intraocular lens implantation. *Am J Ophthalmol*. 1992;113:626–631.

29. Schein OD, Hibbard PI, Shingleton BJ, et al. The spectrum and burden of ocular injury. *Ophthalmology*. 1988;95:300–305.

30. Blum M, Tetz MR, Greiner C, Voekker HE. Treatment of traumatic cataracts. *J Cataract Refract Surg*. 1996;22:342–346.

31. Blankenship GW, Flynn HW Jr, Kokame GT. Posterior chamber intraocular lens implantation during diabetic pars plana vitrectomy. *Ophthalmology*. 1989;96:603–610.

32. Zou Y, Yang W, Li S, You L. Primary posterior chamber intraocular lens implantation in traumatic cataract with posterior capsule breaks. *Yen Ko Hsueh Pao*. 1995;11(3):140–142.

33. Rozsival P, Hakenova J. Results of 52 operations for traumatic cataracts. *Cesk Slov Oftalmol*. 1992;48:325–330.

34. Kora Y, Inatomi M, Fukado Y, Marumori M, Yaguchi S. Long-term study of children with implanted intraocular lenses. *J Cataract Refract Surg*. 1992;18:485–488.

35. Gupta AK, Grove AK, Gurha N. Traumatic cataract surgery with intraocular lens implantation in children. *J Pediatr Ophthalmol Strabismus*. 1992;29(2):73–78.

36. Clemens S, Kroll P, Buss H. Echography of the posterior lens capsule before implantation of an artificial lens. *Klin Monatsbl Augenheilkd*. 1987;191(2):110–112.

Chapter 11

GLAUCOMA ASSOCIATED WITH OCULAR TRAUMA

NEIL T. CHOPLIN, MD*

*Captain, US Navy (Ret); Eye Care of San Diego, 3939 Third Avenue, San Diego, California 92103; Adjunct Clinical Professor of Surgery, Uniformed Services University of Health Sciences, 4301 Jones Bridge Road, Bethesda, Maryland 20814-4799; formerly, Chairman, Department of Ophthalmology, Naval Medical Center, San Diego, California

INTRODUCTION

The definition of glaucoma has undergone considerable change in the last 20 years. As commonly used today, *glaucoma* refers to a diverse group of eye disorders characterized by progressive loss of axons from the optic nerve, resulting in loss of visual function as manifested in the visual field.[1] The structural changes in the optic nerve head are recognizable, and the patterns of visual field damage are characteristic but not specific. Glaucoma may thus be considered to be an optic neuropathy. For purposes of this discussion, the term *glaucoma* is used to describe conditions resulting in high intraocular pressure (IOP); eventual optic neuropathy is presumed to be the long-term result if the elevated IOP is not adequately lowered.

In the population without glaucoma, approximately 95% of people have IOPs between 11 and 21 mm Hg. An IOP above 24 mm Hg is considered elevated. Although the exact etiology of glaucomatous optic neuropathy is not known, many risk factors have been identified, with elevated IOP considered to be one of the most important. The risk of glaucoma increases with the level of IOP, and the risk of disease progression decreases as the pressure is lowered. Nevertheless, not all patients with elevated IOP develop glaucoma, and not all patients with glaucoma have elevated IOP. In the context of ocular trauma, patients with glaucoma *may* present with optic neuropathy but *almost assuredly will* present with elevated IOP. Because changes in the eye following trauma can result in significant elevations of IOP, it is presumed that optic nerve damage will occur if the pressure remains high enough long enough, even if the optic nerve is normal at the time of presentation.

Although glaucomatous optic neuropathy may take some time to develop, elevated IOP after ocular trauma can occur immediately after the injury or at any time in the future, even years later. Conditions associated with elevated IOP at the time of injury include the following:

- alterations in outflow from inflammation and inflammatory byproducts,
- hyphema with or without pupillary block,
- subluxation of the lens, and
- increased episcleral venous pressure.

Elevated IOP may also be a consequence of changes in ocular tissues due to chemical injuries or from damage to nonocular structures. Weeks, months, or years following injury, IOP may become elevated due to chronic use of corticosteroids for control of inflammation, secondary angle closure, ghost cells, scar tissue formation, effects of retained foreign bodies, or damage to the drainage structures (angle recession). For purposes of this discussion, *early* refers to the period from the time of injury through the first 2 weeks following injury, whereas *late* refers to any time after the first 2 weeks.

GLAUCOMA OCCURRING EARLY FOLLOWING OCULAR TRAUMA

Inflammation

Inflammation of varying degrees invariably follows any injury to the eye. Although iritis and iridocyclitis usually cause lower IOP because of decreased aqueous formation, elevated IOP may occur through a variety of mechanisms.[2] Leakage of proteins into the anterior chamber from the increased vascular permeability that accompanies inflammation may result in elevated IOP through the osmotic influx of water. Inflammatory cells and other particulate debris (eg, blood, fibrin, iris pigment, lens material, vitreous) can mechanically block the outflow pathways. Figure 11-1 shows a typical inflammatory reaction in the anterior chamber with fibrin formation, which may lead to pupillary block and secondary angle closure, or an open-angle glaucoma due to outflow pathway obstruction. Blunt trauma can also cause direct damage to trabecular endothelial cells or to meshwork extracellular components, resulting in elevated IOP.[3]

Alterations in Lens Position

Blunt trauma may cause zonular disruption, resulting in dislocation of the lens. Partial subluxation may allow prolapse of vitreous into the anterior chamber. This process may, in itself, result in elevated IOP, probably by an osmotic mechanism. Anterior movement of vitreous may also cause a pupillary block with secondary angle closure. Partial subluxation of the lens is illustrated in Figure 11-2. Complete dislocation of the lens into the anterior chamber may result in pupillary block and angle closure as shown in Figure 11-3.

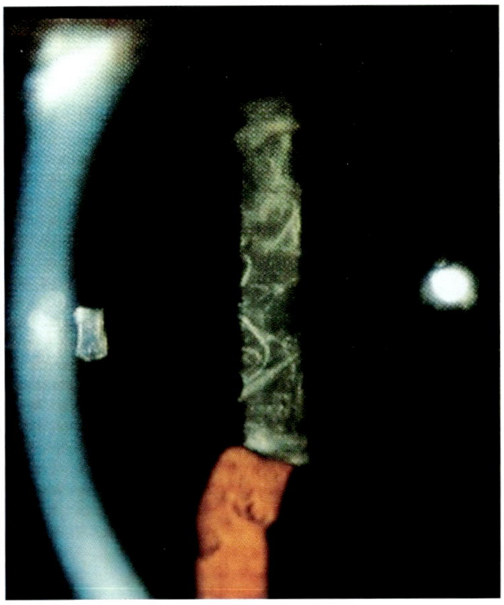

Fig. 11-1. Intraocular inflammation. Severe intraocular inflammation, as can occur following trauma, may result in the formation of a fibrinous exudate, seen here. Fibrin, inflammatory debris, and cells may obstruct the outflow pathways and cause elevated intraocular pressure. Reproduced with permission from Meyer J, Katz L. Secondary open-angle glaucomas. In: Choplin NT, Lundy DC, eds. *Atlas of Glaucoma.* London, England: Martin Dunitz, Ltd; 1998: Figure 9.14(a).

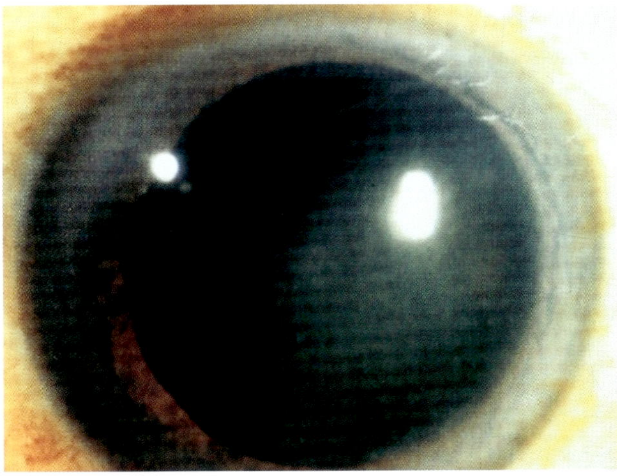

Fig. 11-2. Blunt trauma may rupture zonules and cause total or partial dislocation of the crystalline lens. This lens is partially dislocated inferiorly and temporally. Vitreous may come around the edge of the lens and cause a pupillary block or direct elevation of intraocular pressure. Reproduced with permission from Meyer J, Katz L. Secondary open-angle glaucomas. In: Choplin NT, Lundy DC, eds. *Atlas of Glaucoma.* London, England: Martin Dunitz, Ltd; 1998: Figure 9.13.

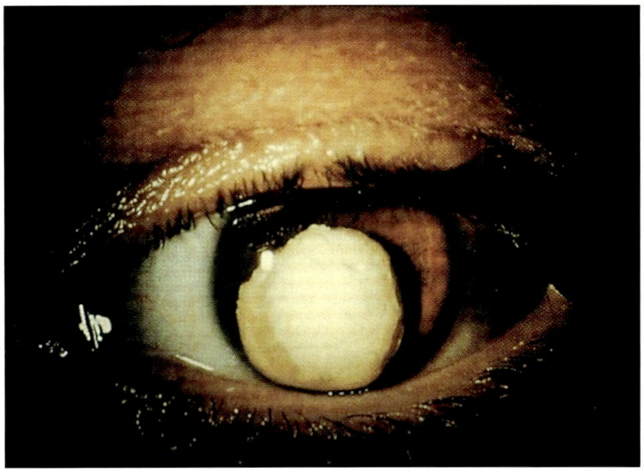

Fig. 11-3. This photograph shows subluxation of the lens into the anterior chamber, causing pupillary block and secondary angle closure glaucoma. Reproduced with permission from Liebmann JM, Ritch R, Greenfield DS. The angle-closure glaucomas. In: Choplin NT, Lundy DC, eds. *Atlas of Glaucoma.* London, England: Martin Dunitz, Ltd; 1998: Figure 10.6.

Hyphema

Bleeding into the anterior chamber, or hyphema (Figure 11-4), is discussed in detail in Chapter 8, Blunt Trauma and Nonpenetrating Injuries of the Anterior Segment. Blood in the anterior chamber may cause elevated IOP by mechanically blocking outflow channels. A total, or "eight-ball," hyphema

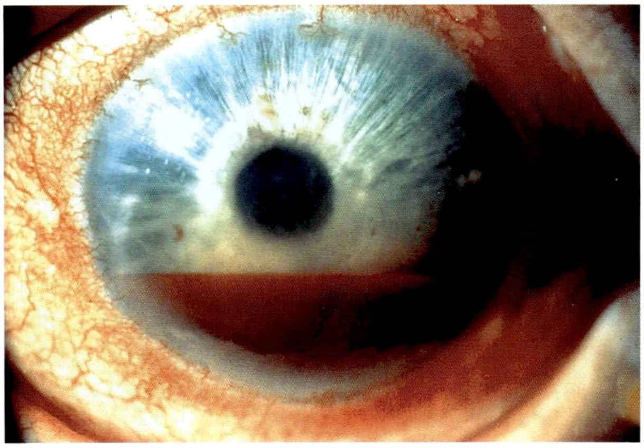

Fig. 11-4. Hyphema. Blood in the anterior chamber from trauma may elevate intraocular pressure by blocking outflow pathways or by causing pupillary block and secondary angle closure. Reproduced with permission from American Academy of Ophthalmology. *Ophthalmology Study Guide.* San Francisco, Calif: American Academy of Ophthalmology; 1987: Figure 42.

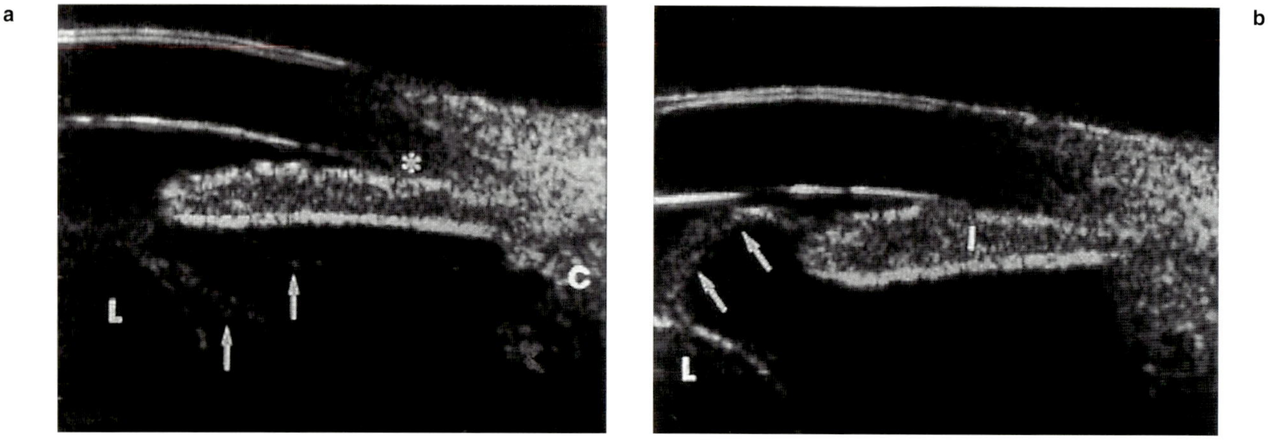

Fig. 11-5. Ultrasound biomicroscope image of an eye following blunt trauma. (**a**) This image shows a subluxed lens (L) and broken zonules (arrows), disinserted from the ciliary body (C). The angle is closed (indicated with an asterisk) due to pupillary block caused by the clotted blood and (**b**) anteriorly displaced vitreous (arrows). The iris (I) is pushed up against the cornea. Reproduced with permission from Berinstein DM, Gentile RC, Sidoti PA, et al. Ultrasound biomicroscopy in anterior ocular trauma. *Ophthalmic Surg Lasers.* 1997;28:201–207.

or an organized clot of sufficient size can cause pupillary block. Figure 11-5[4] is an ultrasound biomicroscope image from an eye with a subluxed lens with clotted blood and anterior movement of vitreous, resulting in pupillary block. The iris is apposed to the trabecular meshwork, resulting in secondary angle closure.

Phacoanaphylactic Glaucoma

Lens protein is normally sequestered within the capsular bag from the time of embryonic development. If the lens is ruptured by trauma (usually penetrating trauma), the immune system reacts to the released lens protein with a granulomatous inflammatory response, often associated with elevated IOP. This phenomenon is illustrated in Figure 11-6.

Increased Episcleral Venous Pressure

Orbital hemorrhage from trauma may result in proptosis and marked congestion within the orbit, compressing the orbital veins and preventing drainage from the outflow channels. The resulting increase in episcleral venous pressure may cause a significant rise in IOP.

Glaucoma Following Chemical Injuries

Alkali burns can cause extensive damage to the anterior segment; glaucoma may result acutely from the inflammatory response accompanying the injury. Alkali can also cause direct damage to the outflow pathways, leading to elevated IOP.[5] However, elevation of IOP may occur almost immediately following the injury, due to scleral shrinkage and pros-

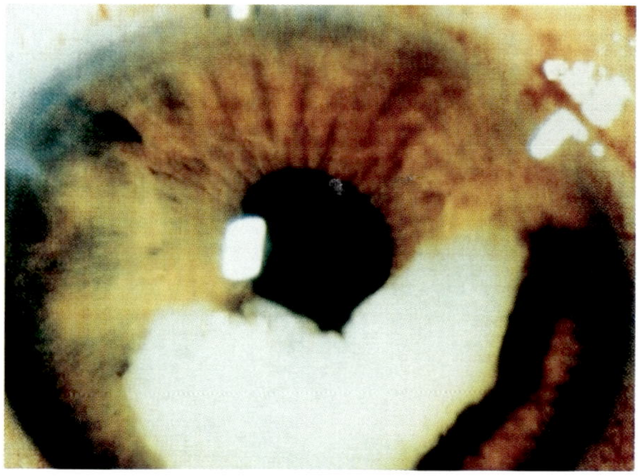

Fig. 11-6. Phacoanaphylactic uveitis and glaucoma. The lens in this eye has been ruptured; cortical material has been released into the anterior chamber, resulting in a massive inflammatory response. The inflammation, along with the osmotic effect of the lens protein's pulling water into the anterior chamber, may cause marked increases in intraocular pressure. Reproduced with permission from Meyer J, Katz L. Secondary open-angle glaucomas. In: Choplin NT, Lundy DC, eds. *Atlas of Glaucoma.* London, England: Martin Dunitz, Ltd; 1998: Figure 9.26(d).

taglandin-mediated alterations in ocular blood flow.[6] See Chapter 7, Chemical Injuries of the Eye, for a more extensive discussion of chemical injuries of the eye.

Glaucoma Due to Trauma to Nonocular Structures

Anything that impedes venous drainage from the head can cause increased episcleral venous pressure and elevated IOP. Theoretically, a chest injury causing a superior vena caval syndrome or a neck injury with jugular vein obstruction may increase IOP. A more common occurrence is secondary glaucoma due to development of a carotid-cavernous sinus fistula following head trauma. Figure 11-7 demonstrates the vascular congestion that may be seen with the high-flow type of arteriovenous shunt that occurs with a carotid-cavernous sinus fistula.[7] The arterialization of the venous drainage increases resistance to drainage of blood from the eye, and, as the "sewer" backs up, the drainage of aqueous humor is also impeded. This can result in very high IOP.

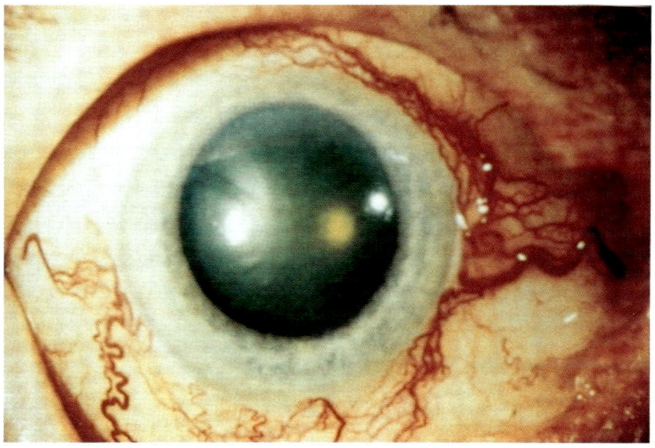

Fig. 11-7. Carotid–cavernous sinus fistula. Intense vascular congestion with engorgement of episcleral veins is seen in this external view. The resulting increase in episcleral venous pressure may cause marked increases in intraocular pressure. Patients with this condition are also at risk for ocular ischemia, possibly leading to neovascular glaucoma. Reproduced with permission from Meyer J, Katz L. Secondary open-angle glaucomas. In: Choplin NT, Lundy DC, eds. *Atlas of Glaucoma.* London, England: Martin Dunitz, Ltd; 1998: Figure 9.38.

GLAUCOMA OCCURRING LATE FOLLOWING OCULAR TRAUMA

Steroid-Induced Glaucoma

Glaucoma following trauma may occur as a result of the treatment as well as from the injuries to the eye. Prolonged use of corticosteroids may elevate IOP and lead to glaucomatous optic neuropathy in susceptible individuals, even in the absence of trauma.[8] Figure 11-8 shows the appearance of the visual field in one eye from a patient with steroid-induced glaucoma. The patient was a physician who self-medicated with steroid drops for ocular allergy. Elevated IOP from chronic steroid use may occur from the accumulation of fibrillar material within the intertrabecular and intratrabecular spaces. Enzymes that would normally clear this material are thought to be inhibited by the corticosteroids.

Secondary Angle Closure

Organization of anterior chamber blood, inflammatory products, or both, may result in the formation of both anterior (between the iris and angle structures) and posterior (between the pupillary border and the lens) synechiae. Three hundred sixty degrees of posterior synechiae, resulting in seclusion of the pupil, will cause pupillary block. These conditions may lead to secondary permanent clo-

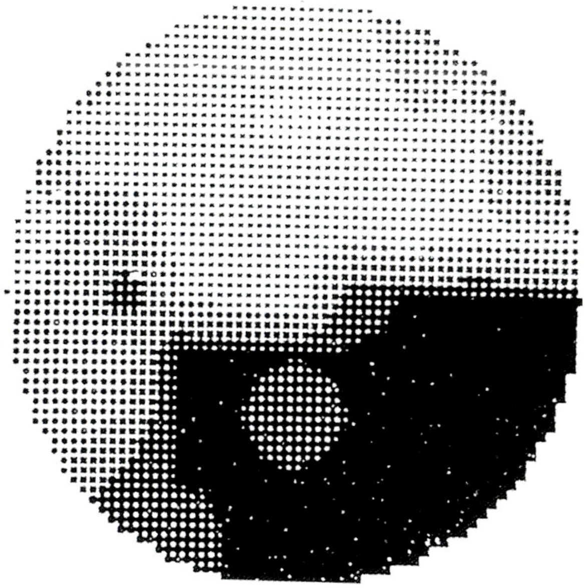

Fig. 11-8. Visual field from the left eye of a physician who self-prescribed topical steroids for allergic eye disease for many years, resulting in steroid glaucoma. Reproduced with permission from Meyer J, Katz L. Secondary open-angle glaucomas. In: Choplin NT, Lundy DC, eds. *Atlas of Glaucoma.* London, England: Martin Dunitz, Ltd; 1998: Figure 9.17.

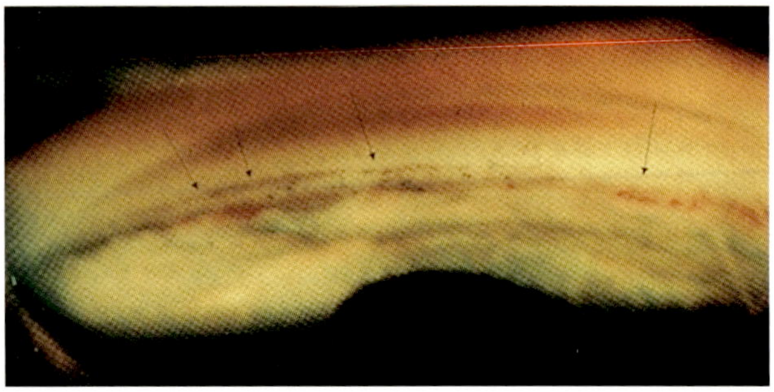

Fig. 11-9. Peripheral anterior synechiae, showing the types of adhesions (arrows) that can occur between the peripheral iris and the anterior chamber angle structures following chronic inflammation in the eye. When synechiae extend around the angle for 360°, outflow is extremely compromised and secondary angle closure glaucoma develops. Reproduced with permission from Fellman RL. Gonioscopy. In: Choplin NT, Lundy DC, eds. *Atlas of Glaucoma*. London, England: Martin Dunitz, Ltd; 1998: Figure 5.12(c).

sure of the anterior chamber angle, resulting in late glaucoma following trauma. Untreated pupillary block from subluxation or dislocation of the lens can also result in permanent angle closure. Peripheral anterior synechiae with partial secondary angle closure is demonstrated in Figure 11-9.

Ghost Cell (Hemolytic) Glaucoma

Following long-standing vitreous hemorrhage or hyphema, red blood cells, having undergone normal senescence, lose their hemoglobin and their normal cell membrane malleability. The resulting "ghost" cells lose the ability to flex and move through the intertrabecular spaces of the trabecular meshwork, becoming trapped within the meshwork and reducing aqueous outflow. This phenomenon increases IOP and leads to a secondary type of open-angle glaucoma known as ghost cell glaucoma.[9] The trapped ghost cells and the inflammatory response to them may be seen in Figure 11-10.

Posttraumatic Angle Deformity (Angle Recession)

The transient rise in IOP that occurs at the time of a blunt injury may abruptly force aqueous into the anterior chamber angle and cause tears in the face of the ciliary body at its insertion into the scleral spur. The amount of tearing and the percentage of the angle involved is highly variable and not necessarily correlated to the specific type of injury. The gonioscopic appearance of this type of angle damage is that of an apparent widening of the ciliary body band in the involved area, usually with a noticeable drop-off between the normal and recessed areas. Variable

a

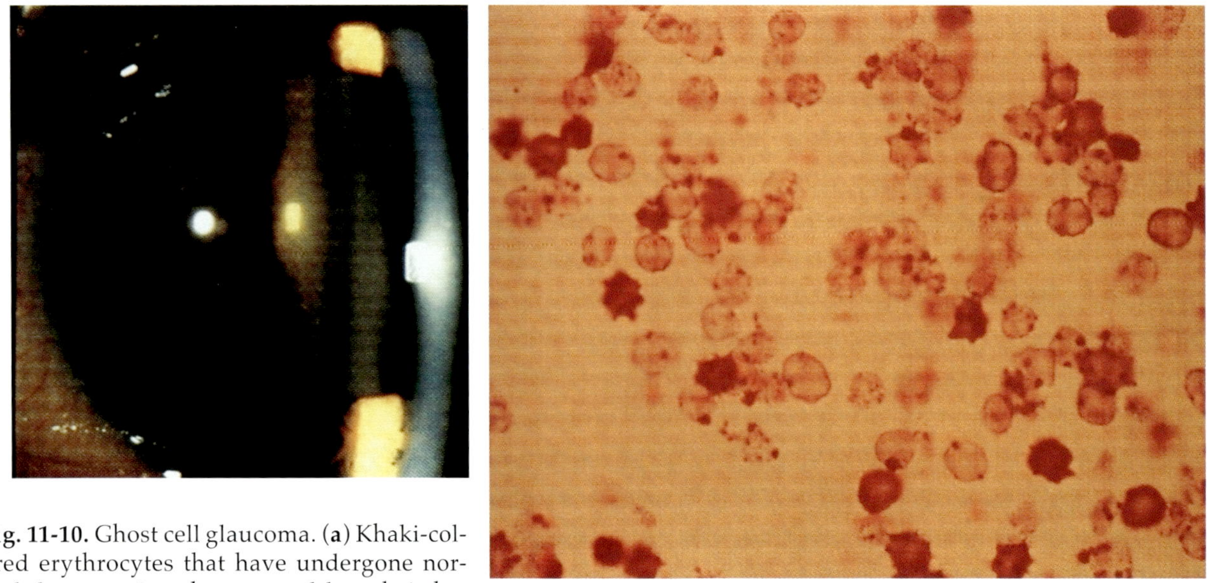

Fig. 11-10. Ghost cell glaucoma. (**a**) Khaki-colored erythrocytes that have undergone normal degenerative changes and lost their hemoglobin may be seen in the anterior chamber and anterior vitreous on slitlamp examination. (**b**) Ghost cells, along with the macrophage response, are seen in this vitrectomy specimen. Reproduced with permission from Meyer J, Katz L. Secondary open-angle glaucomas. In: Choplin NT, Lundy DC, eds. *Atlas of Glaucoma*. London, England: Martin Dunitz, Ltd; 1998: Figure 9.22.

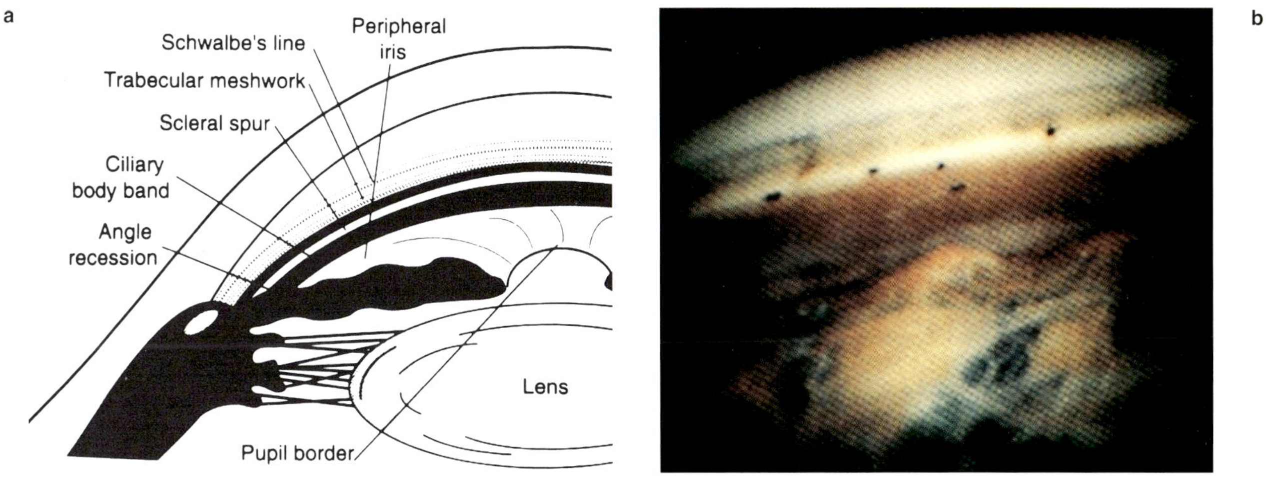

Fig. 11-11. (**a**) Posttraumatic angle deformity (angle recession). (**b**) In this photomicrograph, the widened appearance of the recessed angle is evident by the visible sclera anterior to the iris root. Scattered pigmentation is also seen in the angle. Reproduced with permission from Fellman RL. Gonioscopy. In: Choplin NT, Lundy DC, eds. *Atlas of Glaucoma.* London, England: Martin Dunitz, Ltd; 1998: Figure 5.17.

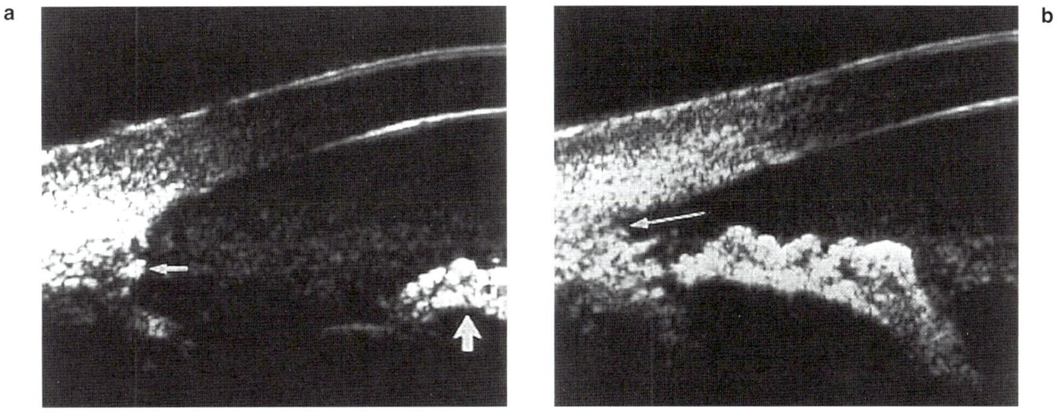

Fig. 11-12. Ultrasound biomicroscope image of angle recession. (**a**) The large arrow (right) points to an area of iridodialysis following blunt trauma, with a small remnant of iris attached to the ciliary body indicated by the small arrow (left). (**b**) The arrow (left) points to an area of angle recession in the same eye. Reproduced with permission from Berinstein DM, Gentile RC, Sidoti PA, et al. Ultrasound biomicroscopy in anterior ocular trauma. *Ophthalmic Surg Lasers.* 1997;28:201–207.

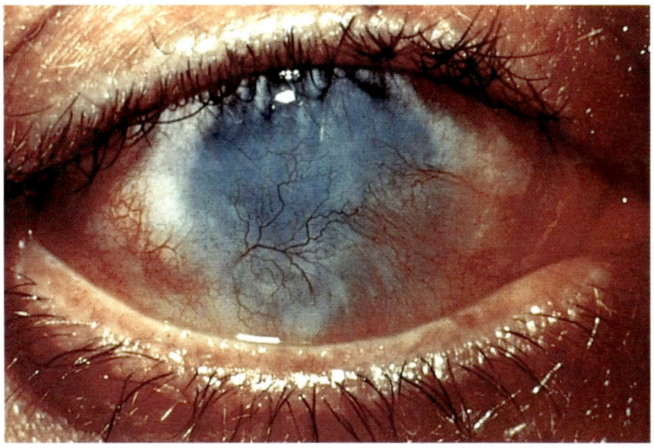

Fig. 11-13. Scarring following an alkali injury. This photograph shows the typical appearance of an eye following an alkali burn after the healing process is completed, with vascularization of the cornea and marked disruption of the anterior segment. Glaucoma may result from scleral shrinkage. Reproduced with permission from American Academy of Ophthalmology. *Ophthalmology Study Guide.* San Francisco, Calif: American Academy of Ophthalmology; 1987: Figure 45.

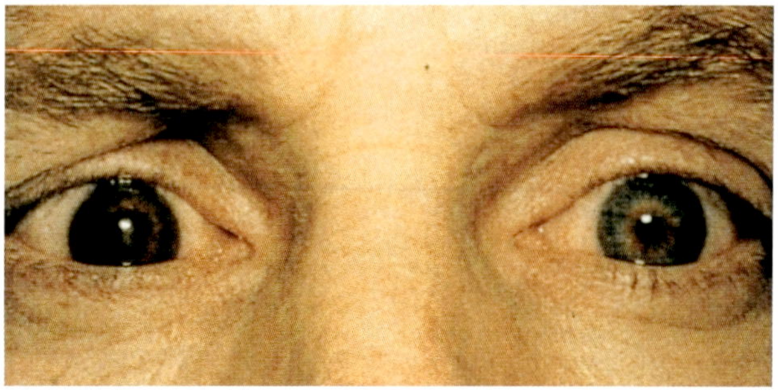

Fig. 11-14. Heterochromia from siderosis bulbi. The iris of this patient's affected right eye shows darkening compared with the normal (left) eye because of the deposition of iron from a retained intraocular foreign body. Reproduced with permission from Kanski JJ, Nischal KK. *Ophthalmology: Clinical Signs and Differential Diagnosis.* London, England: Harcourt Publishers Ltd; 2000: 189.

changes in pigmentation in the angle are also seen.

The mechanism by which IOP becomes elevated in eyes with angle recession is not clear, and which eyes with angle recession will later develop increased IOP with glaucoma cannot be predicted. It is possible that the increase in IOP is due in part to sclerosis within the trabecular meshwork, or it may be due to the change in forces exerted on the meshwork by the ciliary muscle that has been damaged. One study[10] detected glaucoma in only 8% of eyes with 360° of recession. In addition, patients who develop angle recession glaucoma may have an underlying predisposition to glaucoma; one study[11] showed that 50% of patients with angle recession glaucoma had evidence of glaucoma in the fellow (nontraumatized) eye.

Glaucoma has been reported[12] to occur up to 20 years after injury, and it is therefore necessary for patients who have had blunt eye trauma to have periodic eye examinations for the remainder of their lives.

Population-based studies[13] suggest that the risk of developing glaucoma in an eye with some degree of angle recession is up to 6%, which may be lower than that observed following perforating injuries. Figure 11-11 shows an area of posttraumatic angle deformity in a traumatized eye and a schematic drawing of the angle illustrating the concept of angle recession. Figure 11-12 demonstrates the findings of an ultrasound biomicroscopy study in an eye with angle recession.

Chemical Injuries

Elevated IOP and glaucoma may occur because of inflammatory changes and scarring that follow a chemical injury. Alkali burns can cause scleral shrinkage. Figure 11-13 shows the extensive type of anterior segment disruption that may occur after such an injury.

Glaucoma Following Penetrating and Perforating Injuries

All mechanisms that can elevate IOP after blunt trauma can also lead to increased IOP in eyes that have had penetrating or perforating injuries. In addition, eyes that have been ruptured may have fibrous ingrowth, epithelial downgrowth, or retained foreign bodies that may cause elevated IOP by different mechanisms.[14]

Siderosis Bulbi

Iron from retained metallic foreign bodies may deposit in the anterior segment, causing siderosis bulbi and retinal dysfunction, as well. The iris may become darker in color (Figure 11-14), and the IOP may become elevated from deposition of iron in the outflow pathways, resulting in inflammation and sclerosis.

TREATMENT

The general principles for the treatment of secondary glaucomas also apply to glaucomas associated with ocular trauma. Therapy should be directed first at the underlying cause of the glaucoma and second at lowering IOP. Thus, if inflammation is the primary problem, topical (and systemic, if necessary) corticosteroids should be used judiciously and then tapered to discontinuance as the conditions allow. Strong consideration should be given to cycloplegia as well, which not only may alleviate discomfort by relieving ciliary spasm but may also increase uveoscleral outflow and lower IOP. The guidelines for the treatment of hyphema (see Chapter 8, Blunt Trauma and Nonpenetrating Injuries of the Anterior Segment) should be followed as to the timing of evacuation of the blood. Pupillary block should be treated with iridotomy, and dislocated lenses should be removed.

The mainstay of medical therapy for secondary glaucoma is the use of aqueous suppressants such as β-adrenergic antagonists, carbonic anhydrase inhibitors (topical or systemic, as appropriate), and α_2 agonists. Adrenergic agonists (eg, dipivefrin and epinephrine) may also prove useful in the management of glaucoma associated with inflammation owing to their vasoconstrictive properties. Miotics should be avoided, as they tend to further disrupt the blood–aqueous barrier, may shallow the anterior chamber, and can hasten the formation of synechiae. Prostaglandin analogues should probably be avoided as well, at least in the early glaucomas, because the effect of these agents on conditions associated with inflammation are not yet well established.

Should medical therapy fail, consideration should be given to surgery, depending on the level of IOP and the condition of the optic nerve. In general, argon laser trabeculoplasty does *not* work in secondary glaucoma and may even make the IOP worse. Increased failure rates from standard filtering procedures should be anticipated, and filtering surgery should be undertaken with the concomitant use of an antimetabolite, such as mitomycin-C or 5-fluorouracil. Consideration should also be given to the use of an aqueous shunt, especially if the eye is pseudophakic.

SUMMARY

Glaucoma must be considered as a possibility with every ocular injury, and it can occur by a variety of mechanisms at the time of the injury or anytime thereafter. Treatment must be directed at the underlying injuries, with the suppression of inflammation, removal of foreign material, and restoration of normal anatomy being the mainstays. Treatment of elevated IOP should rely on aqueous suppressants (β-adrenoreceptor antagonists, α_2 agonists, and carbonic anhydrase inhibitors); miotics and prostaglandin analogues, which have the potential for exacerbating inflammation in the early postinjury period, should be avoided. Surgery may be necessary for control of IOP if medical therapy fails, depending on the level of IOP and the assessed risk for glaucomatous optic neuropathy.

Decisions regarding return to duty must be individualized and based on the degree of injury, visual function, and the need (and availability) for continued medical treatment. Most likely it is the nature of the injury and not the IOP that determines if the service member is removed from the theater of operations or if he or she may be treated in theater. Each military service has its own guidelines regarding medical evacuation.

REFERENCES

1. Choplin NT, Lundy DC, eds. *Atlas of Glaucoma.* London, England: Martin Dunitz, Ltd; 1998.
2. Folberg R, Parrish RK. Glaucoma following ocular trauma. In: Tasman W, Jaeger E. *Duane's Ophthalmology.* Philadelphia, Pa: Lippincott-Raven; 1996: Chap 54C, 1–7.
3. Herschler J, Cobo M. Trauma and elevated pressure. In: Ritch R, Shields MB, eds. *The Secondary Glaucomas.* St Louis, Mo: CV Mosby; 1982: 307–319.
4. Berinstein DM, Gentile RC, Sidoti PA, et al. Ultrasound biomicroscopy in anterior ocular trauma. *Ophthalmic Surg Lasers.* 1997;28:201–207.
5. Paterson CA, Pfister RR. Intraocular pressure changes after alkali burns. *Arch Ophthalmol.* 1974;91:211–218.
6. Paterson CA, Pfister RR. Prostaglandin-like activity in aqueous humor following alkali burns. *Invest Ophthalmol.* 1975;14:177–183.
7. Hitchings RA. Secondary glaucoma. In: Spalton DJ, Hitchings RA, Hunter PA, eds. *Slide Atlas of Ophthalmology.* London, England: Gower Medical Publishing Ltd; 1984: Section 8: 8.1–8.22.
8. Hodapp EA, Kass MA. Corticosteroid-induced glaucoma. In: Ritch R, Shields MB, eds. *The Secondary Glaucomas.* St Louis, Mo: CV Mosby; 1982: 258–268.
9. Campbell DG, Simmons RJ, Grant WM. Ghost cells as a cause of glaucoma. *Am J Ophthalmol.* 1976;81:441–450.
10. Herschler J. Trabecular damage due to blunt anterior segment injury and its relationship to traumatic glaucoma. *Trans Am Acad Ophthalmol Otolaryngol.* 1977;83:239–248.

11. Kaufman JH, Tolpin DW. Glaucoma after traumatic angle recession: A ten-year prospective study. *Am J Ophthalmol*. 1974;78:648–654.

12. Salmon JF, Mermoud A, Ivey A, Swanevelder SA, Hoffman M. The detection of post-traumatic angle recession by gonioscopy in a population-based glaucoma survey. *Ophthalmology*. 1994;101:1844–1850.

13. Wolff SM, Zimmerman LE. Chronic secondary glaucoma associated with retrodisplacement of iris root and deepening of the anterior chamber angle secondary to contusion. *Am J Ophthalmol*. 1962;54:547–562.

14. Allen JC. Epithelial and stroma ingrowths. *Am J Ophthalmol*. 1968;65:179–182.

Chapter 12

BLUNT INJURY OF THE POSTERIOR SEGMENT

DAVID O. MAZUR, MD*

*Captain, Medical Corps, US Navy; Chairman, Department of Ophthalmology, National Naval Medical Center, 8901 Wisconsin Avenue, Bethesda, Maryland 20889-5600

INTRODUCTION

Instruction in the management of ocular trauma usually emphasizes dramatic injuries such as penetration of the eye wall, retention of foreign bodies, and associated adnexal consequences. Nonpenetrating injuries, however, are far more common and can be disastrous to visual function. They have been consistently documented as a wartime injury, both from direct actions of combat and from the associated industrial hazards of the support environment.[1,2]

These blunt injuries may challenge the diagnostic acumen of the clinician and pose vexing therapeutic questions. In addition, the eye may display significant consequences in the fundus of injuries that are completely remote from the globe. The ophthalmologist treating combat casualties will benefit from a review of posterior segment manifestations of such injuries, including injury mechanisms, damage to the various tissue layers, and the sequelae of remote injury.

MECHANISM OF POSTERIOR SEGMENT INJURY

Direct blows to the eye transmit energy to the adjacent tissues as they produce compression, shearing, and tensile strains. The globe and orbital anatomy predispose the temporal fundus to such direct contact, although the variety of methods and locations of ocular injury seem unlimited. The terms *coup* and *contrecoup*[3] have been used to distinguish the effects of trauma on immediately adjacent tissues (coup) from the effects of forces transmitted to more distant portions of the eye (contrecoup). Clinical and experimental observations on such transmitted forces in the eye and in the brain confirm a consistent pattern of injury location at interfaces with significant differences in density (impedance mismatch). Common ocular sites are the lens–vitreous interface and the posterior vitreo–retinal–scleral interface.

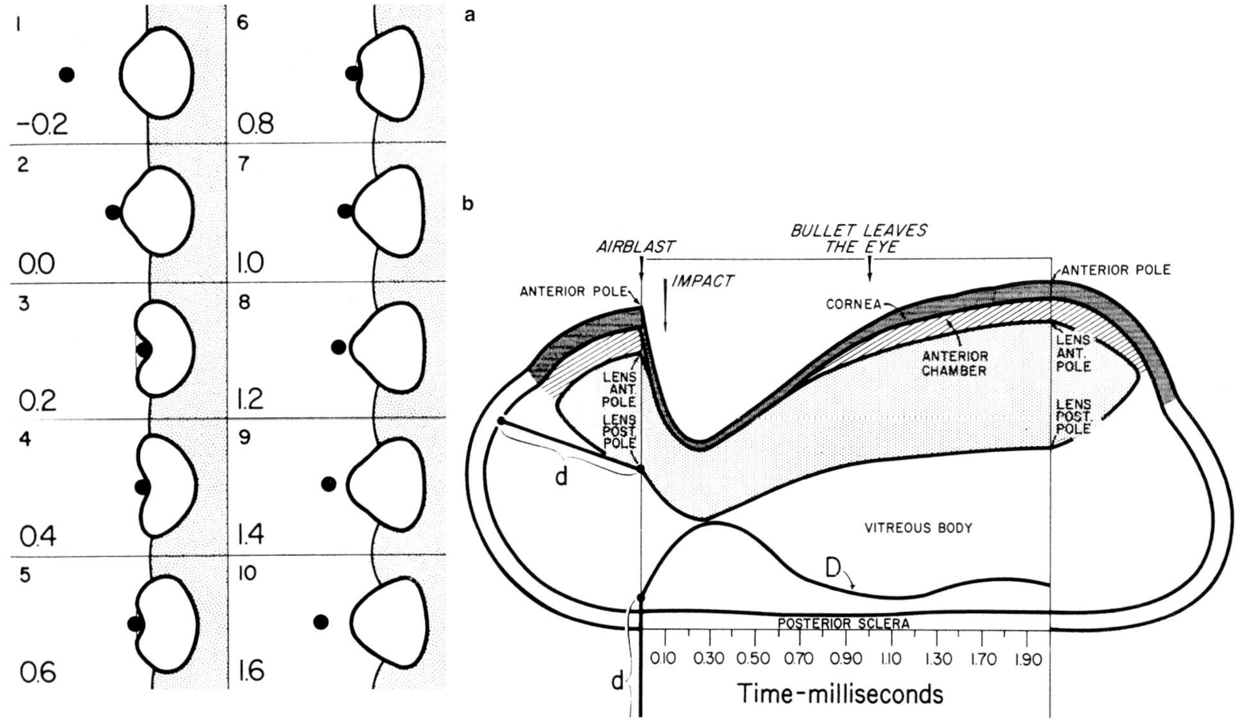

Fig. 12-1. (**a**) Schematic illustration of globe deformation sequence during high-speed impact and recoil (in milliseconds) demonstrates the occurrence of dramatic axial compression and transverse elongation, placing tension on the vitreous base. (**b**) The posterior indentation of anterior segment structures is accompanied by a simultaneous equatorial expansion. The vitreous base dimension *D* is maximally elongated at approximately 0.30 milliseconds, exerting forces on the peripheral retina that may produce retinal dialysis. Reproduced with permission from Delori F, Pomerantzeff O, Cox M. *Invest Ophthalmol.* 1969;8:294, 300.

Delori, Pomerantzeff, and Cox[4] studied globe deformation and injury under high-speed impact and were able to document the dramatic difference the speed of injury makes in ocular trauma. Ocular tissues are viscoelastic materials that exhibit the phenomenon of rate dependence. This means that "increased deformation rates result in increased levels of stress in the deformed tissues."[5(pp197–198)] For example, high-velocity projectiles caused retinal dialyses and other injuries, while low-velocity deformations—even with greater amounts of energy—caused no equivalent peripheral fundus injury.

High-speed impact creates impressive ocular indentation and other deformation (Figure 12-1). The impact site is displaced posteriorly while the globe's equatorial diameter dramatically expands. A 28% expansion of the vitreous base radius was documented 0.4 milliseconds after deformation begins.[4] The indentation process is followed, in nonpenetrating injury, by a recovery (recoil) that includes dampening oscillations of these structures. In addition, the anterior structures are displaced posteriorly during the first 0.3 milliseconds, followed by a more-gradual recovery phase with some overshoot displacement anteriorly. Measurements of the vitreous base (from the posterior pole of the lens to the insertion of the vitreous base) are maximal during the peak corneal indentation. The results include impressive inward tension exerted on the vitreous base, which is opposed by the high intraocular pressure that compresses the retina against the choroid. The resultant great shearing forces are usually strongest at the posterior border of the vitreous base, and a linear tear of the retina may result. If traction is strongest at the anterior border of the vitreous base, the nonpigmented ciliary epithelium is torn. Strong traction at both the anterior and posterior borders may produce vitreous base avulsion, which is pathognomic of ocular contusion.

Weidenthal and Schepens[6] used an experimental model that controlled these globe distortions by encasing the globe in rigid shells of variable geometry. When the equatorial expansion of the globe following impact was prevented, the damaging effects on the peripheral retina were dramatically reduced. Because these direct and indirect forces affect each tissue differently, the resulting injuries are discussed in this chapter based on the specific tissue layers involved.

RETINAL INJURY WITHOUT BREAKS

In 1873, Berlin[7] described retinal opacity (commotio retinae) following blunt ocular trauma that was assumed to represent extracellular retinal edema. However, Sipperley[8] documented in an owl monkey injury model that the outer retinal opacification, or whitening, corresponded with photoreceptor outer segment disruption (Figure 12-2). Histological evidence indicated that neither intracellular nor extracellular edema was present. This photoreceptor disruption was followed by phagocytosis of the fragmented outer segments by cells of the retinal pigment epithelium (RPE) and subsequent migration of these cells into the retina. Fluorescein angiography and vitreous fluorophotometry

a b

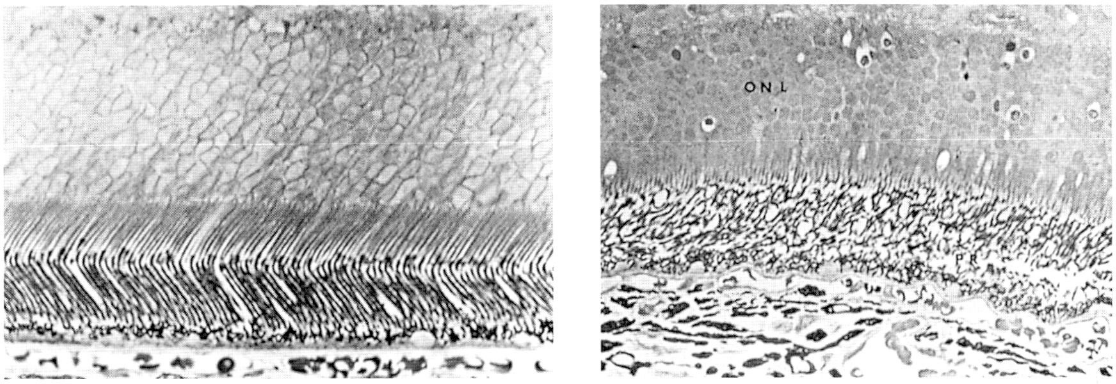

Fig. 12-2. Photomicrographs of (**a**) a normal owl monkey retina, contrasting with (**b**) the damage observed to the experimental animal 4 hours after blunt trauma. The photoreceptor outer segments are disrupted and disorganized, and the outer nuclear layer (ONL) demonstrates pyknotic nuclei. The pathological appearance corresponds with clinically observed retinal opacification. Reproduced with permission from Sipperley JO, Quigley HA, Gass JDM. *Arch Ophthalmol.* 1978;96:9226.

Fig. 12-3. Commotio retinae observed in the peripheral fundus of a patient seen 1 day following blunt injury. The zone of whitened retina is characteristically sharply demarcated, and associated retinal hemorrhage is seen. The outer retinal whitening obscures choroidal detail, but the view of the more superficial retinal vessels is unaffected.

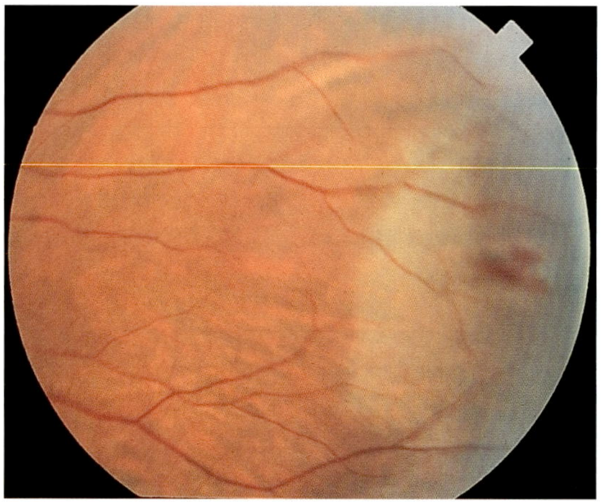

a

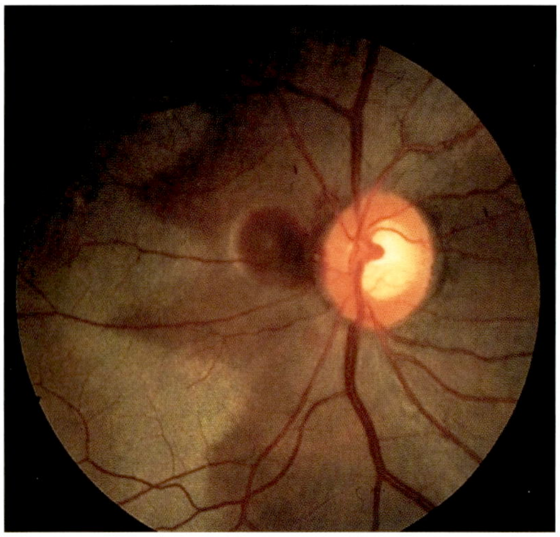

b

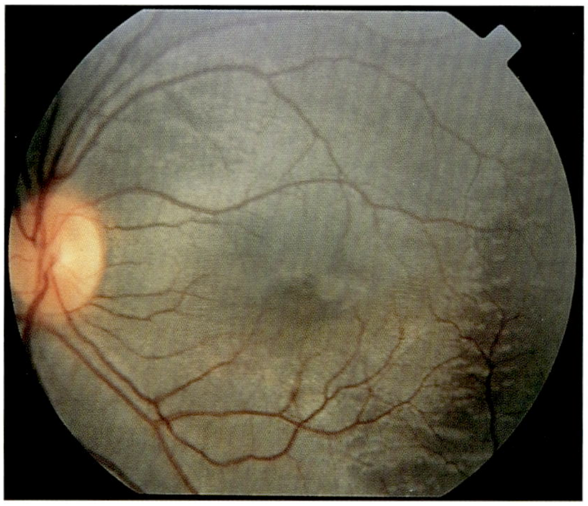

Fig. 12-4. (**a**) Retinal opacification in the posterior pole reveals a typical gray-white hue and sharply demarcated margins, which here have assumed a peculiar geometric pattern of scalloping. Peripapillary hemorrhage is also seen. (**b**) Fundus appearance 3 days after blunt injury reveals a large zone of outer retinal whitening affecting the macula, with sharp, geometric borders. The patient's vision was reduced to 20/400.

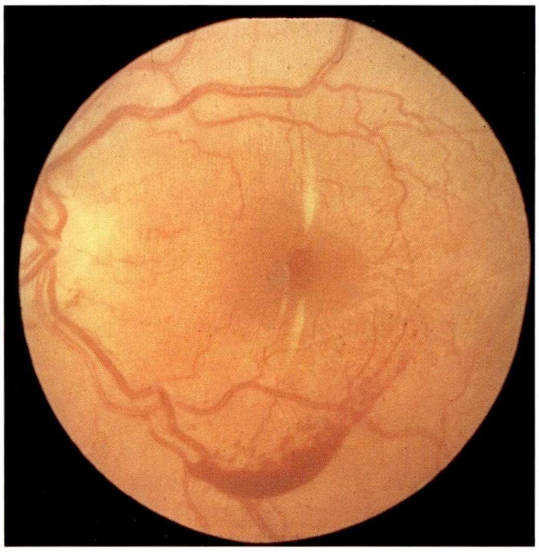

Fig. 12-5. This macular hole was noted 1 week after blunt injury. A macular hole may be seen as an immediate consequence of trauma or observed after a latent interval. Patients with an interval of better vision prior to macular hole development are more likely to benefit from macular hole surgery.

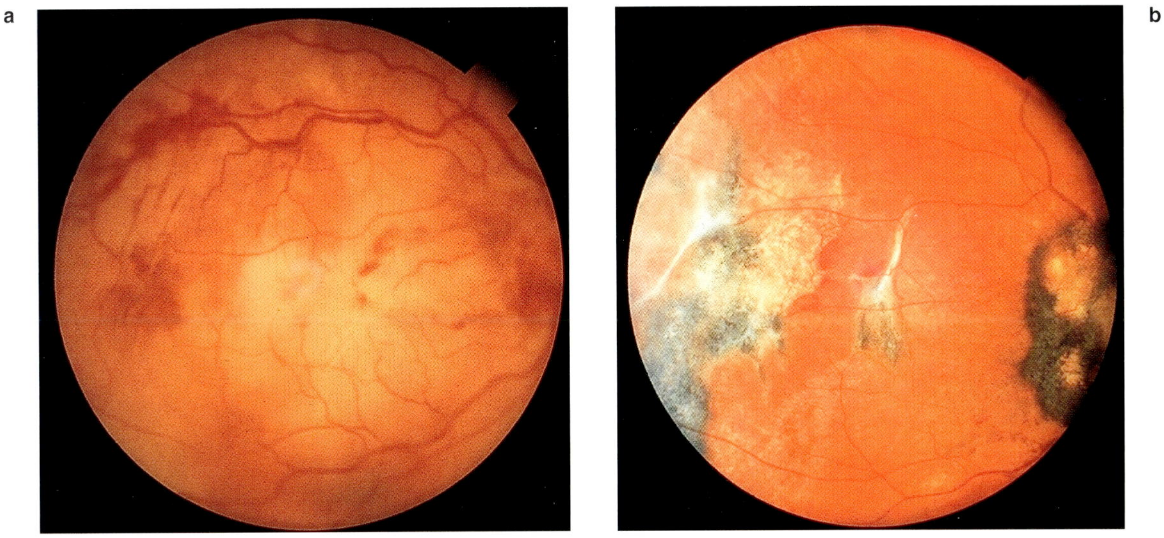

Fig. 12-6. (**a**) Retinal pigment epithelial contusion injury shows a cream-colored change at the level of the retinal pigment epithelium (RPE), associated with shallow overlying neurosensory retinal detachment and areas of retinal and vitreous hemorrhage. (**b**) By 4 months after the injury, the same patient had widespread retinal pigment epithelial hyperplasia and migration. Vision remained stable at 20/400.

confirmed the intact blood–retinal barrier.

Clinically, opacification may develop peripherally,[9] often at the site of impact (Figure 12-3) or in the posterior pole (Figure 12-4). The patient's visual loss, which depends on the location and the degree of the photoreceptor disruption, occurs promptly, and delayed visual loss should lead to investigation for other origins. The peripheral opacification may resemble either white without pressure or retinal detachment. Because foveal anatomy essentially includes only photoreceptors and their axons, extensive foveal photoreceptor loss results in significant risk of macular hole formation (Figure 12-5). Contusion of the RPE may present a confusing differential diagnosis. This cream-colored change in the RPE develops within 48 hours of injury (Figure 12-6), shows leakage and staining on fluorescein angiography, and may have serous elevation of the RPE or neurosensory retina. Resolution of edema and elevation is commonly accompanied by development of pigmentary migration and hyperplasia.

RETINAL BREAKS

Retinal breaks may be subdivided into two categories: (1) those caused by *vitreous traction,* which have such manifestations as dialyses, horseshoe tears, or operculated tears, and (2) those *without apparent vitreous traction,* with typical appearances including inferotemporal retinal defects of varied size.

Breaks Due to Vitreous Traction

The most common break produced by traumatic vitreous traction is the retinal dialysis. Tension on the vitreous base may result in tears at any location, but the inferotemporal and supranasal quadrants strongly predominate, representing approximately 60% of all traumatic retinal tears. Several clinical series[10,11] have demonstrated that the inferotemporal quadrant is most commonly affected; however, the presence of a clear history of antecedent trauma was less consistent than that noted in patients with supranasal dialyses. This distinction has suggested an anatomical predisposition of the inferotemporal quadrant to develop dialysis in milder injuries. Such a tendency—or even the possible spontaneous occurrence of such defects—may contribute to the bilaterality of inferotemporal dialyses, emphasizing the critical need for the examiner to study the peripheral fundus of both eyes in every patient with an eye injury.

Vitreous base avulsion is present in about 15% of dialysis patients but is pathognomic of trauma when present; multiple small dialyses or giant retinal tears may also be seen (Figure 12-7).

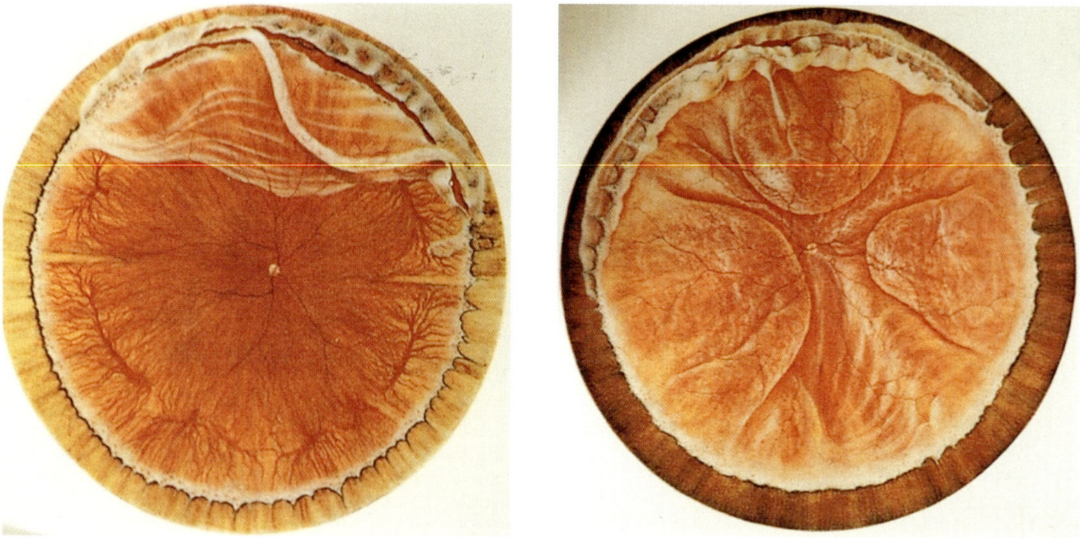

Fig. 12-7. Retinal breaks following contusion injury. (**a**) Supranasal retinal dialysis. The "bucket handle" avulsion of the vitreous base is pathognomic of trauma. Retinal tearing is seen both at the ora serrata and in the nonpigmented ciliary epithelium of the pars plana. (**b**) Retinal detachment. Careful peripheral fundus scrutiny with scleral depression is required to demonstrate the responsible linear tears located anterior to the ora serrata. Reproduced with permission from Weidenthal DT, Schepens CL. *Am J Ophthalmol.* 1966;62:465–477.

Detachment caused by dialysis occurs immediately following ocular contusion only in 12% of cases and typically presents after a latent interval: within 1 month (30% of cases), within 8 months (50% of cases), or within 2 years (80% of cases).[12] This delay in presentation affords an opportunity for effective prophylactic therapy using cryopexy or photocoagulation. When detachment does develop from dialysis, it has characteristics that differentiate it from nontraumatic rhegmatogenous detachments. These detachments are seldom bullous; they are usually smooth, thin, and transparent. Star folds or other stigmata of proliferative vitreoretinopathy (PVR) are rare. Features of chronicity are common (Figure 12-8), such as intraretinal cysts (20%) and demarcation lines (50%, often multiple). Detachment from dialysis is not related to refractive error. It seldom flattens with bed rest, so activity or position restrictions during transport of such patients are normally not valuable. The surgical prognosis is generally very good.

Tension on the vitreous base may also produce more-typical flap (horseshoe) or operculated breaks, usually at the posterior margin of the vitreous base or at the site of abnormal vitreoretinal attachments.

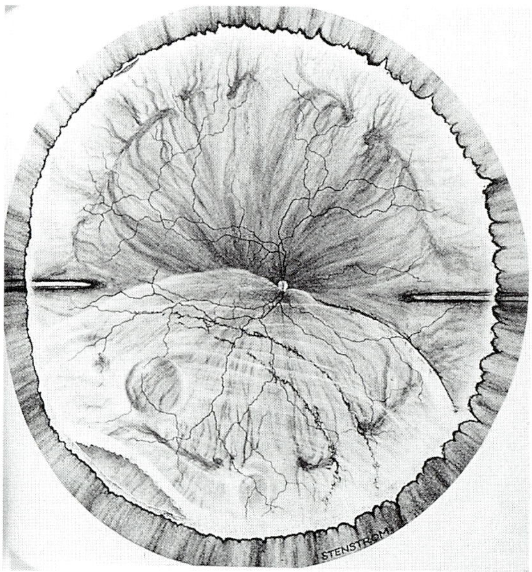

Fig. 12-8. Artist's depiction of typical findings of retinal detachment due to inferotemporal retinal dialysis. Parallel rows of demarcation lines ("high-water marks") are seen, along with retinal macrocyst formation. The absence of features of proliferative vitreoretinopathy is characteristic. Reproduced with permission from Hagler WS, North AW. *Arch Ophthalmol.* 1968;79:381.

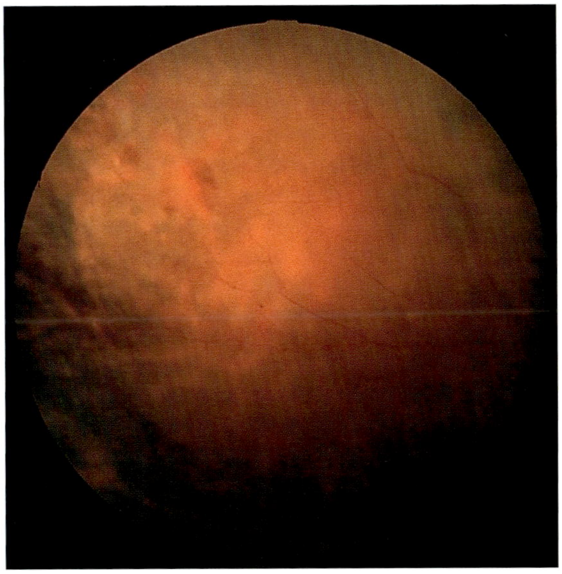

Fig. 12-9. A cluster of small, round retinal holes with localized retinal detachment is noted in the temporal periphery of an 11-year-old patient seen 1 week after injury from a soccer ball. Although the retinal holes are produced at the time of impact, the development of retinal detachment from traumatic holes may be delayed by a lengthy latent interval, or detachment may not occur at all.

Breaks Without Apparent Vitreous Traction

Traumatic retinal breaks may also occur in a sectoral or ovoid configuration, usually inferotemporal.[13] These defects are associated with extensive hemorrhage, ragged edges, and fragments of retina suspended in the overlying vitreous. Configurations vary from clustered, small, round holes (Figure 12-9) to a single, enormous defect (Figure 12-10). Choroidal ruptures may accompany the lesions, and the retina itself may be opaque. (Although the kinds of injuries seen in Figures 12-13 and 12-14 were initially [historically] suspected of being due to necrosis or a delayed effect of hemorrhage, they seem on reflection to be an immediate consequence of severe rapid deformation.) The retina and often the choroid are ruptured and both may retract leaving a zone of exposed bare sclera. (The choroid is not well anchored to the sclera in the anterior fundus.) The overlying hyaloid is usually not ruptured, explaining the usual absence of retinal detachment at presentation. Late detachment may occasionally develop, especially in association with PVR, but recent evidence[5] suggests that prophylactic treatment of these often very large breaks is ill-advised.

A macular hole may occur following contusion necrosis[14] or as a consequence of hemorrhage or vitreous traction.[15] Unlike spontaneous macular holes, the presence of associated photoreceptor disruption (suggested by severe vision loss immediately following the injury) may limit the value of any surgical intervention. In contrast, patients exhibiting visual decline due to delayed macular hole development may benefit from surgical efforts to close the macular hole.[16]

Traumatic retinal breaks generally occur at the time of injury. The production of these varied types of breaks seems to depend largely on the point of impact and the speed of deformation. The locations

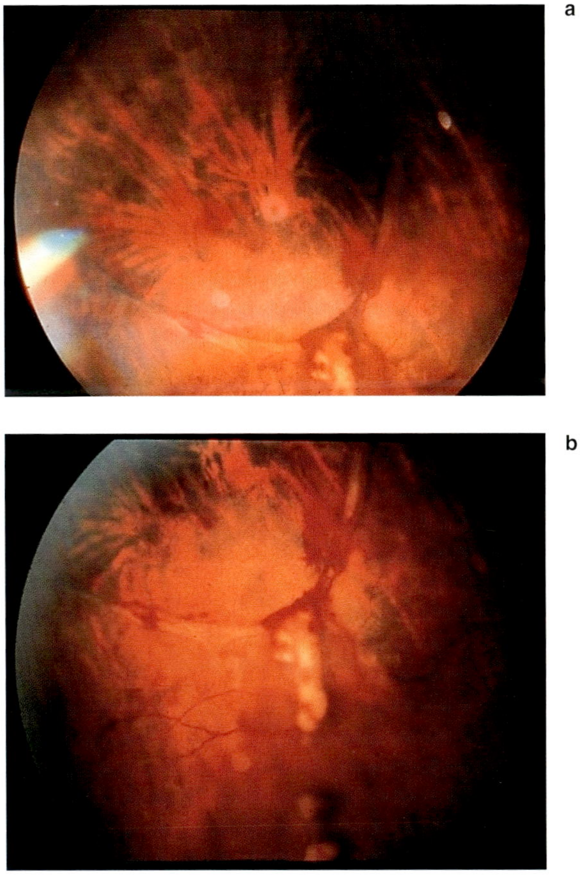

Fig. 12-10. Enormous retinal defect seen in the supratemporal periphery of a 22-year-old patient examined 1 day after being struck in the eye during a basketball game. (**a**) Note that the underlying choroid is intact in contrast to the defects seen in sclopetaria injuries. The retina remains attached. (**b**) Posterior extent of the same injury. Note the clumped material within the vitreous, which seems to descend from the retinal injury. This material may include blood, fibrin, and remnants of disrupted retina. The retina remained attached without treatment.

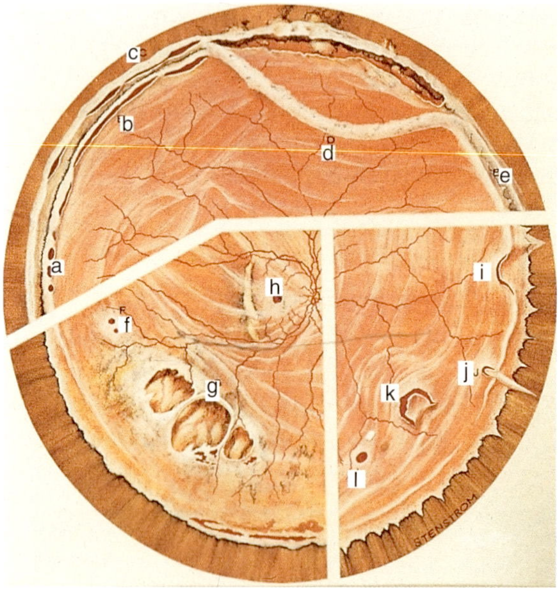

Fig. 12-11. This composite illustration depicts the variety of retinal breaks seen following contusion injury. The top portion depicts tears of the (**a**) anterior and/or (**b**) posterior margins of the vitreous base, including (**c**) complete dialysis, (**d**) small consecutive breaks, and (**e**) avulsion of the vitreous base. The lower left portion depicts breaks without apparent relationship to vitreous traction, including (**f**) small clustered round holes, (**g**) large ovoid breaks, and (**h**) a macular hole. The lower right portion (**i-l**) shows traumatic breaks associated with abnormal vitreoretinal traction, resulting in defects indistinguishable from most nontraumatic breaks. Reproduced with permission from Cox M, Schepens C, Freeman H. *Arch Ophthalmol.* 1966;76:678–685.

of retinal breaks in contusion injuries are elegantly summarized in Figure 12-11.

Head trauma without associated ocular trauma has been alleged to induce retinal breaks. Although such injury may be the precipitating event in some predisposed individuals, a clinical study of 247 cases of severe head trauma found that no retinal breaks were induced.[17]

CHOROIDAL RUPTURE

Choroidal rupture is a common manifestation of blunt injury, reflecting the mechanical vulnerability of Bruch's membrane. The retina is relatively elastic and the sclera mechanically strong, but Bruch's membrane does not share these characteristics. When ruptured, the choriocapillaris and the RPE also tear, and injury may extend through the full thickness of the retina.[18] Choroidal ruptures may be seen in the peripheral fundus (Figure 12-12), where they are caused by adjacent injury forces, or in the posterior pole (Figure 12-13), where indirect forces are transmitted to produce injury that is usually concentric to the optic nerve and temporally located.[19] The visual prognosis is variable and depends on the location, extent of rupture, associated hemorrhage, and subsequent fibrosis or vascularization. Ruptures may initially be obscured by extensive hemorrhage, which can also detach the choroid or retina or dissect into the vitreous (Figures 12-14 and 12-15). The proper therapy for these extensive hemorrhages remains controversial. Most such hemorrhages clear spontaneously, but poor vision following extensive hemorrhage under the fovea may be the result of the initial injury itself or due to photoreceptor loss or fibrosis caused by the hemorrhage.

Vitreous surgery to remove these extensive hemorrhages has significant associated risks and often is unsuccessful in fully evacuating the hemorrhage. The use of pneumatic displacement techniques, with or without intravitreous tissue plasminogen activator (tPA) injection to promote clot lysis, may successfully diminish foveal hemorrhage with less surgical risk.[20] A recently suggested approach[21] utilizes gas injection and positioning alone, followed in 24 to 48 hours by intravitreal tPA injection if hemorrhage is not displaced from the fovea. This approach is particularly appealing for the military ophthalmologist with limited equipment, although the impact of intraocular gas on subsequent aeromedical transport must be considered.

Neurosensory retinal detachments may be noted shortly after injury in some patients with extensive choroidal ruptures (Figure 12-16), but these normally resolve after several days. Late development of neurosensory detachment may herald subretinal neovascular membrane formation (Figure 12-17). Focal photocoagulation is usually appropriate for neovascular membranes not located under the foveal center.

Chorioretinitis sclopetaria is a term introduced into the German literature to describe a concussion injury to the globe that occurs adjacent to the path of an orbital missile (Figure 12-18). The term probably relates to

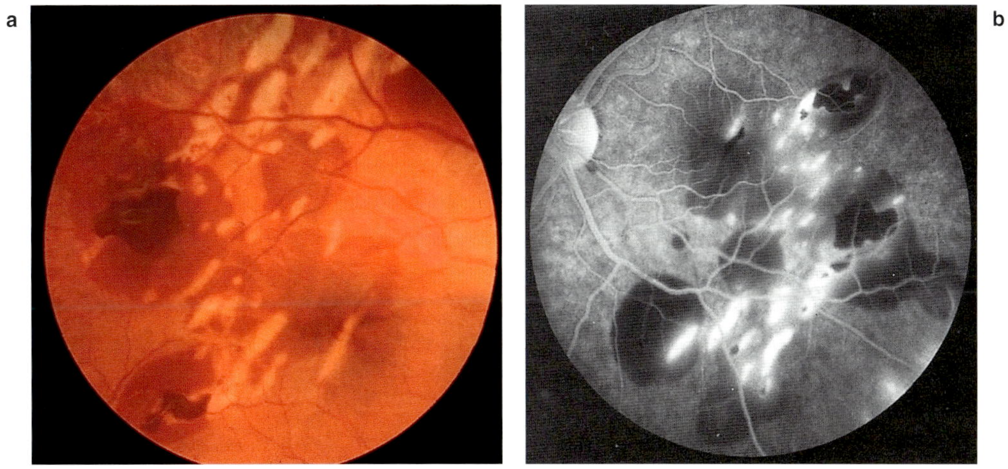

Fig. 12-12. Following contusion injury to the temporal globe, (**a**) multiple choroi dal ruptures are seen and extend from the temporal macula to the equator. The linear ruptures are accompanied by subretinal and preretinal hemorrhage. (**b**) The fluorescein angiography of the fundus demonstrates intense fluorescence at sites of choroidal rupture that leaks into adjacent pools of hemorrhage and a shallow neurosensory retinal detachment. This fluorescein leakage typically ceases within several weeks, but transmission defects and blocking defects may remain indefinitely.

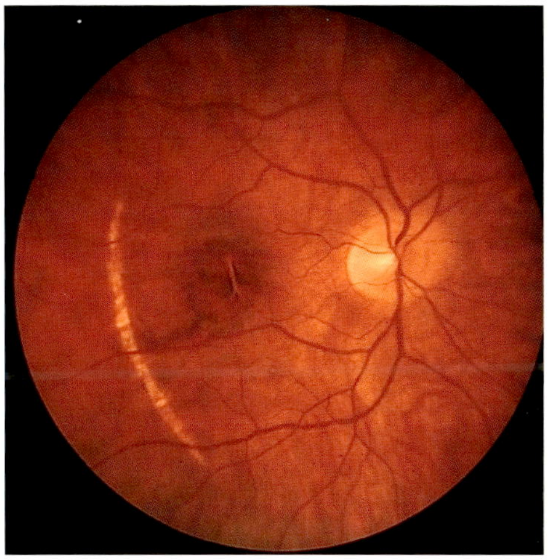

Fig. 12-13. Late appearance of two choroidal ruptures in the posterior pole. The curvilinear geometry is characteristic. Final visual outcome may depend primarily on the location of injury, such as the small foveal rupture seen here.

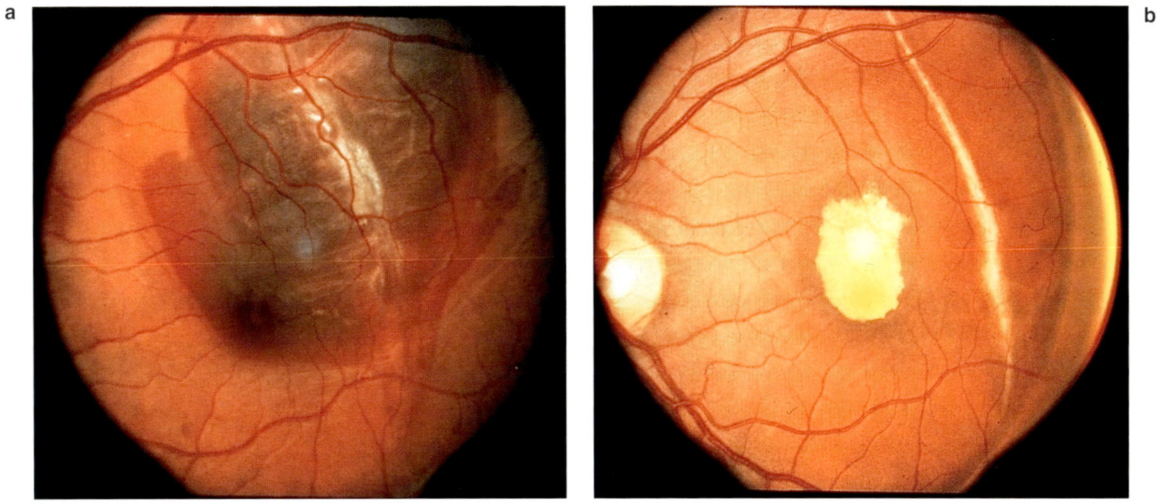

Fig. 12-14. (**a**) Large subretinal hemorrhage in the posterior pole following contusion injury extends to the foveal area. The underlying choroidal rupture responsible for the hemorrhage is largely obscured by the blood. (**b**) One month after the injury, the hemorrhage has cleared, exposing a large temporal choroidal rupture. A central macular scar and collection of absorbing hemorrhage elements is associated with persistently reduced vision of 20/400.

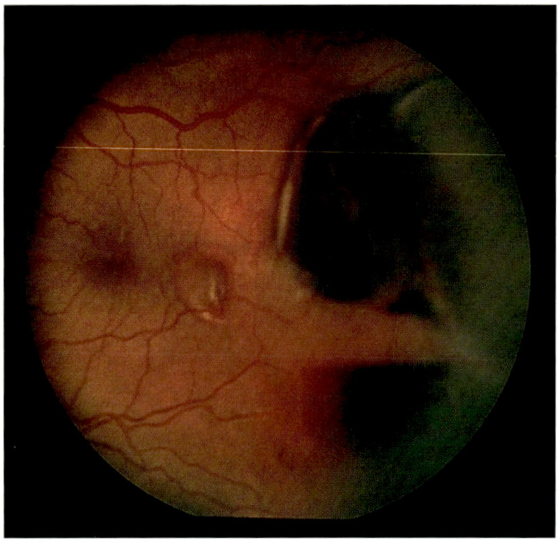

Fig. 12-15. A large, bullous subretinal hemorrhage is present in the temporal fundus obscuring the underlying choroidal ruptures. A meniscus separating blood and clear subretinal fluid is visible in the inferior balloon of hemorrhage. The fovea is spared from the hemorrhage, and visual acuity was 20/20.

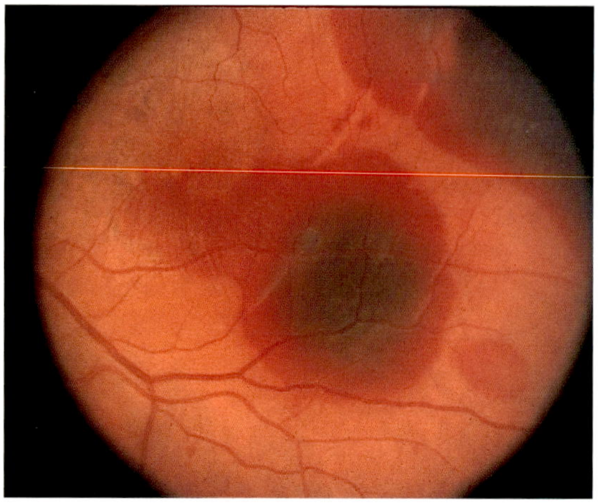

Fig. 12-16. Multiple, widespread bilateral choroidal ruptures are seen in a patient injured by a bomb blast. The partially obscured ruptures are accompanied by shallow neurosensory retinal detachments. Retinal striae have produced a fingerprint pattern to the shallow macular hemorrhage. The hemorrhage and detachments resolved over 1 month.

a

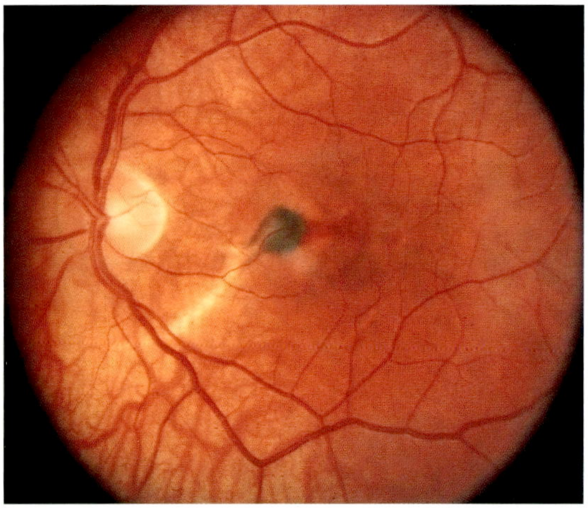

b

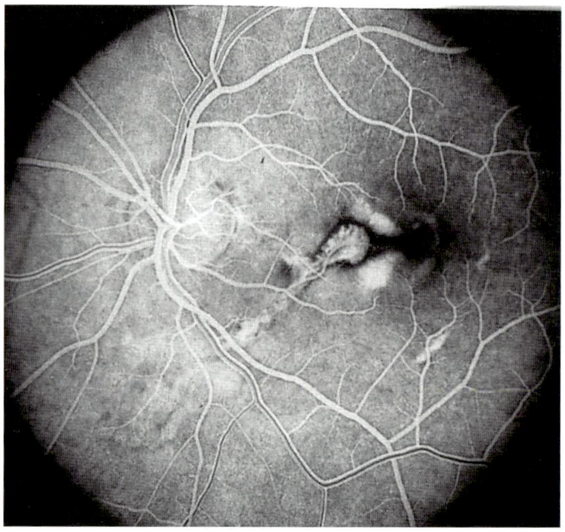

Fig. 12-17. A 23-year-old Marine noted reduced vision 11 months after being struck in the eye. (**a**) Neurosensory retinal detachment and subretinal hemorrhage were present. A previously unrecognized choroidal rupture is visible inferotemporal to the disc, with a choroidal neovascular membrane extending from the rupture to the edge of the fovea. (**b**) Fluorescein angiography of the fundus reveals a well-defined, classic, juxtafoveal neovascular membrane arising from the choroidal rupture site. The neovascularization was successfully treated with argon laser photocoagulation.

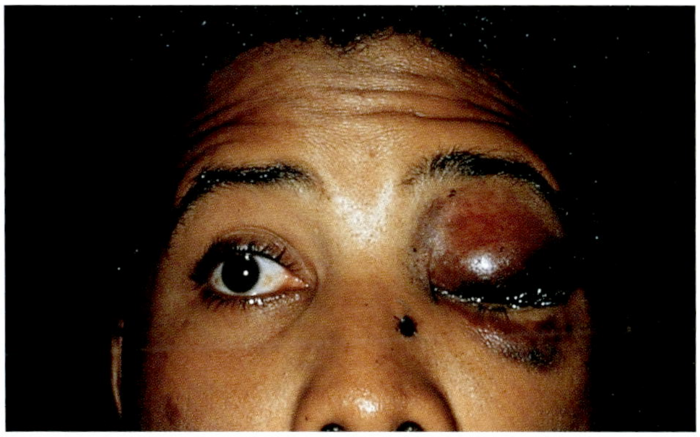

Fig. 12-18. A gunshot wound of the nasal orbit produced marked orbital edema and ecchymosis. The missile path avoided direct contact with the globe but resulted in retinitis sclopetaria injury to the peripheral fundus.

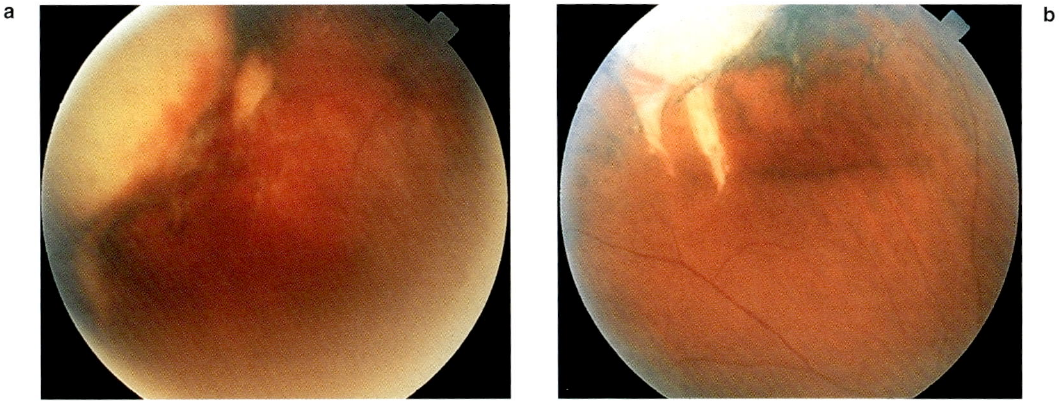

Fig. 12-19. A 20-year-old patient sustained an orbital missile wound that resulted in retinitis sclopetaria. (**a**) The large defect in the retina and choroid has a characteristic rolled and thickened posterior margin, representing retracted tissue. Despite the size of the defect, no treatment was applied. (**b**) The fundus is seen 6 weeks later, with maturation of the scarring process. The retina remained attached. Characteristic radial, claw-like scars are noted extending posteriorly from the large retinal and choroidal defect.

an old description of the claw-like breaks in Bruch's membrane and the RPE noted in many patients. Associated rupture and retraction of both choroid and retina may accompany severe injuries, but the posterior hyaloid commonly remains intact, substantially reducing the likelihood of retinal detachment.[5] Despite the impressive appearance of the retinal defects (Figure 12-19), treatment usually is not required.

SCLERAL RUPTURE

Scleral rupture must be strongly suspected in every significant contusion injury, and surgical exploration must be strongly considered even in the absence of hypotony.[22] Characteristic presenting features include very poor vision (hand motions [HM], light perception [LP]), marked hemorrhagic chemosis, severe hyphema, lacrimation, and loss of ocular motility (Figure 12-20).[23,24]

Optic nerve avulsion from the sclera (Figure 12-21) is an uncommon but disastrous event that has been well documented as a wartime injury.[1] The avulsion can be partial or complete with varying degrees of intraocular hemorrhage. The nerve head may be absent and the retinal circulation arrested. Imaging of the orbit reveals that the optic nerve sheath is usually intact.[25] No therapy is beneficial.

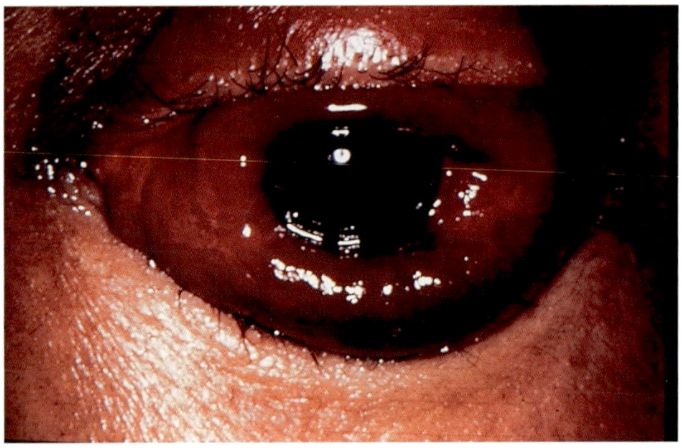

Fig. 12-20. A patient who sustained a blunt injury to the globe has massive hemorrhagic chemosis and a total "eight-ball" hyphema. Reduced ocular motility was noted. Surgical exploration disclosed a large posterior scleral rupture.

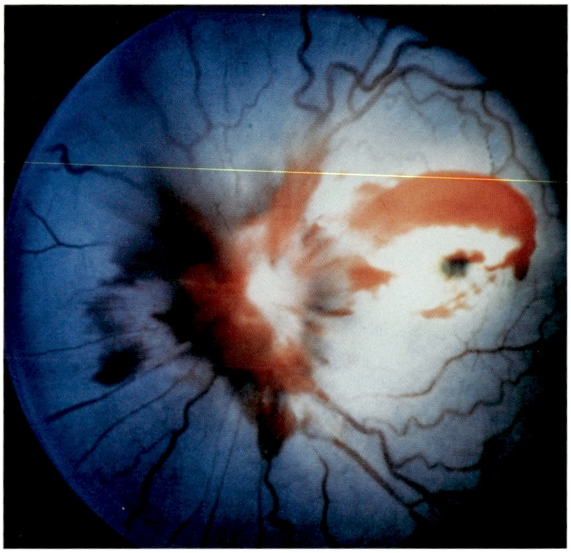

Fig. 12-21. Peripapillary and retinal hemorrhage, retinal edema, and arterial circulatory obstruction are seen in a patient with avulsion of the optic nerve. The dramatic variation in the inferotemporal diameter of the retinal arterioles confirms the interruption of the arterial circulation.

POSTERIOR SEGMENT EFFECTS OF REMOTE TRAUMA

Circulatory Influences

Remote effects may reflect venous, arterial, and mixed circulatory influences on the posterior segment. Valsalva retinopathy[26] follows a sudden rise in intraabdominal or intrathoracic pressure, including performance of Valsalva's maneuver. The rapid rise of venous pressure in the eye reflects the absence of competent venous valvular protection. Patients may have a history of coughing or straining, or they may not be able to relate the visual symptoms to any activity.

Rupture of retinal capillaries produces typical posterior pole preretinal hemorrhage (Figure 12-22), which may detach the internal limiting membrane. Intraretinal hemorrhage or vitreous hemorrhage may be seen. A fluid level (Figures 12-23 and 12-24) often develops over days before gradual, spontaneous clearing of the blood. Vision usually returns to normal. Investigation for predisposing circulatory defects may be appropriate, especially in the absence of a supportive history, but is commonly unrewarding. An extreme instance of venous pressure increase occurs in the compression cyanosis syndrome[27] (Figure 12-25), originally described as a consequence of bail-out from high-speed aircraft but now recognized in many traumatic settings where chest compression occurs, such as in trampling injuries.

Fat Embolism

Fat embolism occurs in approximately 5% of patients with fractures of the long bones and may be fatal in severe cases. About half of affected patients have retinal manifestations, including nerve fiber layer infarcts and blot hemorrhages (Figure 12-26). Recognition of the ophthalmic features can help establish the diagnosis and guide therapy of this condition.

Purtscher's Retinopathy

Purtscher (as cited in Marr and Marr[28]) described a retinopathy occurring after severe head trauma that appears to actually be more common after severe thoracic or abdominal injury. Within hours or days, the patient develops multiple patches of superficial whitening of the retina, which usually surround the nerve and may reflect the distribution of the radial peripapillary capillary plexus (Figure 12-27). These white patches are significantly larger than those seen in fat embolism. Retinal hemorrhages and disc edema may be seen. Intravenous fluorescein angiography shows capillary nonperfusion and leakage. The lesions slowly clear, often leaving optic atrophy, vessel attenuation, and variable visual defects.

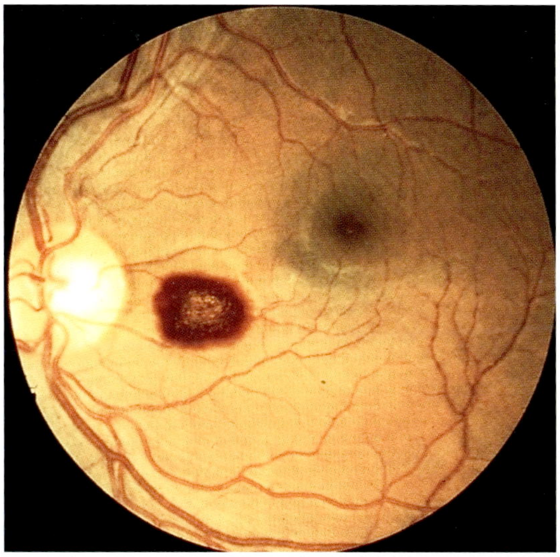

Fig. 12-22. Localized preretinal hemorrhage is seen in a 23-year-old Marine who noted a scotoma after completing a forced march with a 70-pound backpack. The hemorrhage cleared uneventfully, with vision remaining 20/20.

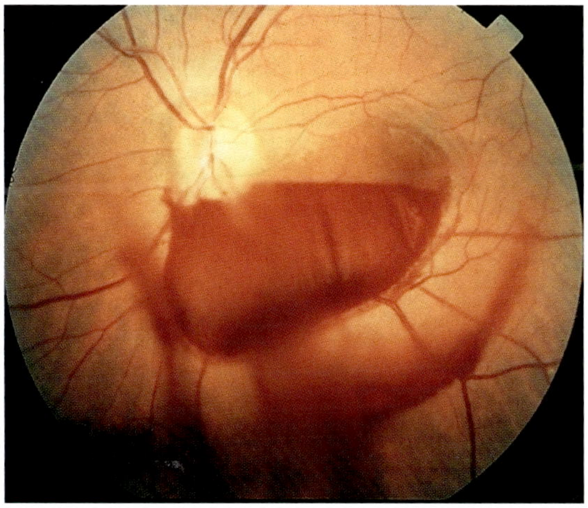

Fig. 12-23. Preretinal and vitreous hemorrhage due to Valsalva retinopathy. The hemorrhage cleared without treatment.

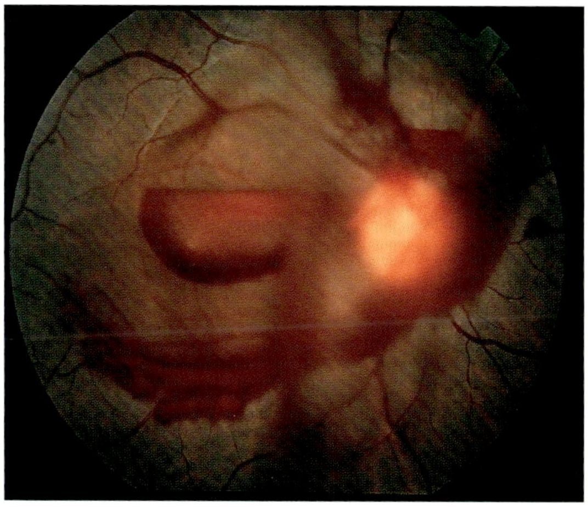

Fig. 12-24. Extensive retinal, subretinal, and vitreous hemorrhage is present in a 21-year-old patient with Valsalva retinopathy. Vision acutely was reduced to 20/400 but recovered to 20/20 over a 4-month period.

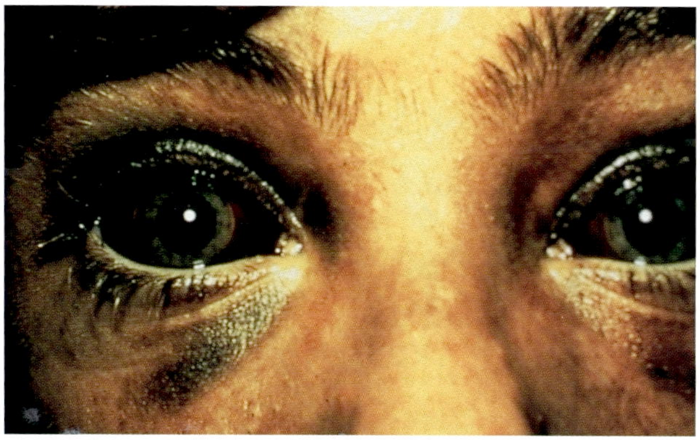

Fig. 12-25. Generalized ecchymosis of the head, neck, and thorax was seen in this patient with compression cyanosis syndrome following chest compression injury. Subconjunctival hemorrhage is present bilaterally.

Purtscher's retinopathy may be related to C5a complement activation and granulocyte aggregation resulting in embolic occlusion. This mechanism has reproduced the Purtscher's retinopathy clinical picture in animal models.[29] Similar lesions are also seen in patients with pancreatitis[30] and other illnesses with a presumably similar mechanism. Interestingly, a number of patients with unilateral Purtcher's retinopathy[31] have been observed. High-dose steroid therapy has been suggested for patients in whom the disorder is recognized early, although the efficacy of this approach has not been demonstrated.

Other Causes

Ocular effects of remote injury may also be seen in Terson's syndrome, in which subretinal, intraretinal, or vitreous hemorrhage develops in patients who have either spontaneous or posttraumatic sub-

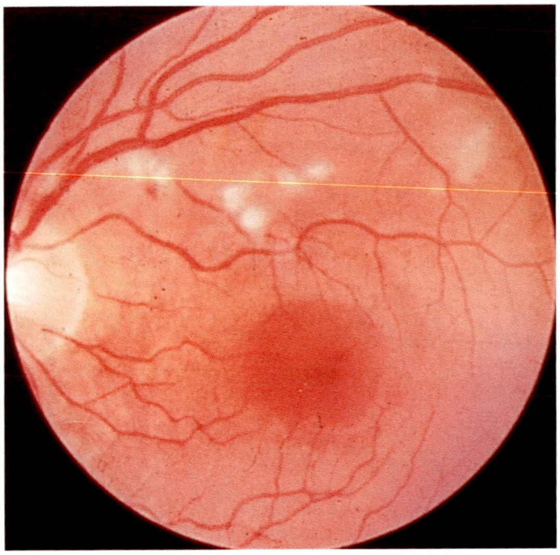

Fig. 12-26. Multiple white retinal lesions that are indistinguishable from nerve fiber layer infarcts are noted in this 22-year-old patient with long-bone fractures and fat embolism.

a

b

c

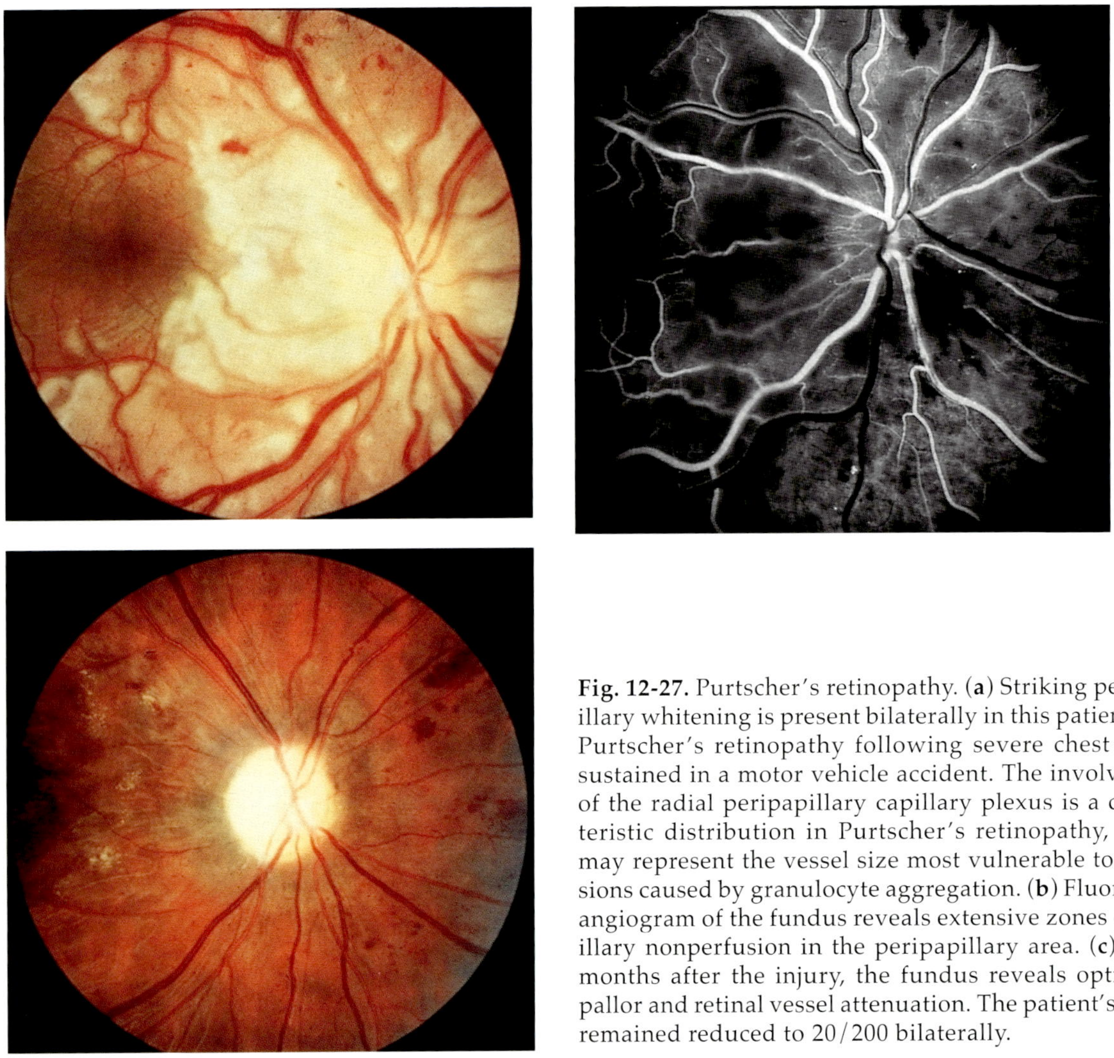

Fig. 12-27. Purtscher's retinopathy. (**a**) Striking peripapillary whitening is present bilaterally in this patient with Purtscher's retinopathy following severe chest injury sustained in a motor vehicle accident. The involvement of the radial peripapillary capillary plexus is a characteristic distribution in Purtscher's retinopathy, which may represent the vessel size most vulnerable to occlusions caused by granulocyte aggregation. (**b**) Fluorescein angiogram of the fundus reveals extensive zones of capillary nonperfusion in the peripapillary area. (**c**) Three months after the injury, the fundus reveals optic disk pallor and retinal vessel attenuation. The patient's vision remained reduced to 20/200 bilaterally.

arachnoid hemorrhage. Spontaneous clearing of the hemorrhage is common, and surgical intervention to evacuate the hemorrhage is only rarely indicated.[32]

Severe flexion–extension of the head and neck may generate macular changes in the form of whiplash maculopathy. This entity produces mild reduction in visual acuity (20/30) promptly after injury, with development of a subtle gray foveal change and a foveolar pit. The pathophysiology is not known, although speculation includes forceful avulsion of superficial foveal tissue from forces exerted on the hyaloid. No treatment is required.

MILITARY IMPLICATIONS

The variety and, sometimes, the subtlety of posterior segment manifestations of ocular trauma challenge the acumen of any clinician. For military ophthalmologists managing combat casualties, these difficulties may be aggravated by the challenges of simultaneously managing many patients with multisystem injuries, addressing complex disorders with a modest equipment inventory, and being isolated from consultation assistance. The following principles may be particularly helpful in managing casualties with posterior segment trauma:

- Consider posterior segment injury early in the patient management. Fundus examination opportunities at presentation may be lost to subsequent hemorrhage, lens opacification, and so forth.
- Careful peripheral depressed examination is imperative either primarily or, when appropriate, as a deferred follow-up examination.
- Do not overlook examination of the fellow eye.
- Clinical examination provides the overwhelming amount of useful information. Simple findings such as the presence of an afferent pupillary defect may be more valuable than imaging studies.
- Ultrasonography is a helpful and readily available mode with which to assess injured eyes with opaque media. Electrophysiology, in contrast, is unlikely to contribute useful findings.
- Despite their dramatic clinical appearance, many lesions of the posterior segment are best managed conservatively.

REFERENCES

1. Lister W. Some concussive changes met with in military practice. *Br J Ophthalmol.* 1924;8:305.
2. Caiger H. Ocular injuries resulting from the war. *Trans Ophthalmol Soc U K.* 1941;61:54–73.
3. Wolter J. Coup–contrecoup mechanism of ocular injuries. *Am J Ophthalmol.* 1963;56:785–796.
4. Delori F, Pomerantzeff O, Cox, M. Deformation of the globe under high-speed impact: Its relation to contusion injuries. *Invest Ophthalmol.* 1969;8:290–301.
5. Martin DF, Awh CC, McCuen BW, Jaffe GJ, Slott JH, Machemer R. Treatment and pathogenesis of traumatic chorioretinal rupture (sclopeteria). *Am J Ophthalmol.* 1994;117:190–200.
6. Weidenthal DT, Schepens CL. Peripheral fundus changes associated with ocular contusion. *Am J Ophthalmol.* 1966;62:465–477.
7. Berlin R. Zur sogenannten commotio retinae. *Klin Monatsbl Augenheilkd.* 1873;1:42–78.
8. Sipperley JO, Quigley HA, Gass JDM. Traumatic retinopathy in primates: The explanation of commotio retinae. *Arch Ophthalmol.* 1978;96:2267–2273.
9. Blight R, Hart JC. Structural changes in the outer retinal layers following blunt mechanical non-perforating trauma to the globe: An experimental study. *Br J Ophthalmol.* 1977;61:573–587.
10. Hagler WS, North AW. Retinal dialyses and retinal detachment. *Arch Ophthalmol.* 1968;79:376–388.
11. Ross W. Traumatic retinal dialyses. *Arch Ophthalmol.* 1981;99:1371–1374.

12. Cox M, Schepens C, Freeman H. Retinal detachment due to ocular contusion. *Arch Ophthalmol.* 1966;76:678–685.

13. Cox M. Retinal breaks caused by blunt nonperforating trauma at the point of impact. *Trans Am Ophthalmol Soc.* 1980;78:414–466.

14. Yanagiya N, Akiba J, Takahashi M, et al. Clinical characteristics of traumatic macular holes. *Jpn J Ophthalmol.* 1996;40(4):544–547.

15. Gass JDM. *Stereoscopic Atlas of Macular Diseases: Diagnosis and Treatment.* 4th ed. St Louis, Mo: Mosby–Year Book; 1997:740.

16. Garcia-Arumi J, Corcostegui B, Cavero L, Sararols L. The role of vitreoretinal surgery in the treatment of post-traumatic macular hole. *Retina.* 1997;17:372–377.

17. Doden W, Stark N. Retina and vitreous findings after serious indirect trauma. *Klin Monatsbl Augenheilkd.* 1974;164:32.

18. Aguilar JP, Green WR. Choroidal rupture: A histopathologic study of 47 cases. *Retina.* 1984;4:269–275.

19. Wood CM, Richardson J. Indirect choroidal ruptures: Aetiological factors, patterns of ocular damage, and final visual outcome. *Br J Ophthalmol.* 1990;74:208–211.

20. Hassan AS, Johnson MW, Schneiderman TE, et al. Management of submacular hemorrhage with intravitreous tissue plasminogen activator injection and pneumatic displacement. *Ophthalmology.* 1999;106:1900–1906. Discussion 1906–1907.

21. Ohji M, Saito Y, Hayashi A, Lewis JM, Tano Y. Pneumatic displacement of subretinal hemorrhage without tissue plasminogen activator. *Arch Ophthalmol.* 1998;116:1326–1332.

22. Cherry P. Indirect traumatic rupture of the globe. *Arch Ophthalmol.* 1978;96:252–256.

23. Russell SR, Olsen KR, Folk JC. Predictors of scleral rupture and the role of vitrectomy in severe blunt ocular trauma. *Am J Ophthalmol.* 1988;105:253–257.

24. Klystra JA, Lamkin JC, Runyan DK. Clinical predictors of scleral rupture after blunt ocular trauma. *Am J Ophthalmol.* 1993;115:530–535.

25. Williams DF, Williams GA, Abrams GW, Jesmanowicz A, Hyder JS. Evulsion of the retina associated with optic nerve evulsion. *Am J Ophthalmol.* 1987;104:5–9.

26. Duane T. Valsalva hemorrhagic retinopathy. *Trans Am Ophthalmol Soc.* 1972;70:298–313.

27. Ravin JG, Meyer RF. Fluorescein angiographic findings in a case of traumatic asphyxia. *Am J Ophthalmol.* 1973;75:643–647.

28. Marr W, Marr E. Some observations on Purtscher's disease: Traumatic retinal angiopathy. *Am J Ophthalmol.* 1962;54:693–705.

29. Lai JC, Johnson MW, Martonyi CL, Till GO. Complement-induced retinal arteriolar occlusions in the cat. *Retina.* 1997;17:239–246.

30. Shapiro I, Jacob HS. Leukoembolization in ocular vascular occlusion. *Ann Ophthalmol.* 1982;14:60–62.

31. Burton TC. Unilateral Purtscher's retinopathy. *Ophthalmology.* 1980;87:1096–1105.

32. Schultz PN, Sobol WM, Weingeist TA. Long-term visual outcome in Terson syndrome. *Ophthalmology.* 1991;98:1814–1819.

Chapter 13

PRIMARY REPAIR OF THE POSTERIOR SEGMENT: PENETRATING, PERFORATING, AND BLUNT RUPTURE INJURIES

GORDON A. BYRNES, MD*

*Captain, Medical Corps, US Navy; Department of Ophthalmology, National Naval Medical Center, 8901 Wisconsin Avenue, Bethesda, Maryland 20889-5600

INTRODUCTION

Successful repair of a scleral laceration resulting from operational casualties requires an understanding of the mechanisms of combat eye injury and a hierarchy of surgical repair goals. Once globe penetration is suspected, timely surgical exploration and repair are required to prevent infection, tissue necrosis, sympathetic ophthalmia, and tissue downgrowth. Proper wound exposure greatly facilitates globe closure. The initial repair should succeed in creating a watertight closure, free of entrapped tissues and foreign bodies (FBs). Reconstructive efforts should be minimized during the initial repair. Following primary repair, the patient should be evacuated for further evaluation, removal of FBs from the eye, and reconstructive surgery.

OPERATIONAL EYE INJURY

Ocular injuries sustained in the battlefield have become increasingly common throughout the 1900s as weaponry has favored blast fragmentation munitions. Most of these injuries occur in the setting of multiple trauma, reflecting the effectiveness of modern weapons,[1] and in recent conflicts, 13% of all those wounded have had injuries to the eyes.[2] Small, high-velocity fragments easily penetrate exposed soft tissues, including the eyes and adnexal structures. The depth of particle penetration depends on the shape, mass, and velocity of the FB. Most FBs that penetrate and remain within the eye are 5 mm or less in size[3,4]; larger particles tend to perforate the eye and travel deeper into the orbit or adjacent tissues (Figure 13-1).

Penetrating and perforating injuries account for 20% to 50% of all wartime ocular injuries,[5] and approximately 15% to 25% of injuries are bilateral.[1,6–8] The most common weapons responsible for fragmentation ocular injuries are shells, rockets, grenades, and mines. Roughly 55% of combat FBs are nonmagnetic, reflecting the nonferrous composition of mines and secondary missiles.[5] The mortality of close-proximity shell injuries is very high; most ocular injuries occur at a distance of 150 feet or more from highly explosive blasts.[9] Rifle bullets and large projectiles are less often responsible for isolated ocular injuries because of such injuries' high mortality when they occur in the head region. Antipersonnel mines commonly produce severe extremity and ocular injuries,[10] and from the perspective of maintaining the fighting strength, the data are even grimmer: 75% of soldiers who suffered ocular injuries during the Vietnam War were unable to return to duty.[11]

Regardless of the setting, ocular trauma that results in globe rupture tends to derive from mechanisms that include projectile penetration, sharp laceration, and blunt contusion.[12] Combat blast injuries threaten the eye through release of high-velocity missiles, direct concussion effects, or architectural collapse leading to sharp laceration or blunt injury of the globe.

Ocular injuries that occur during peacetime operational settings more closely reflect those commonly encountered in the industrial workplace. The National Eye Trauma System Registry reports that 65% of these injuries result from projectiles, 24% from sharp injury, 9% from blunt objects, and 3% from blasts.[13] The majority of both civilian and peacetime military ocular injuries are preventable and occur in individuals who fail to wear adequate eye protection.[14]

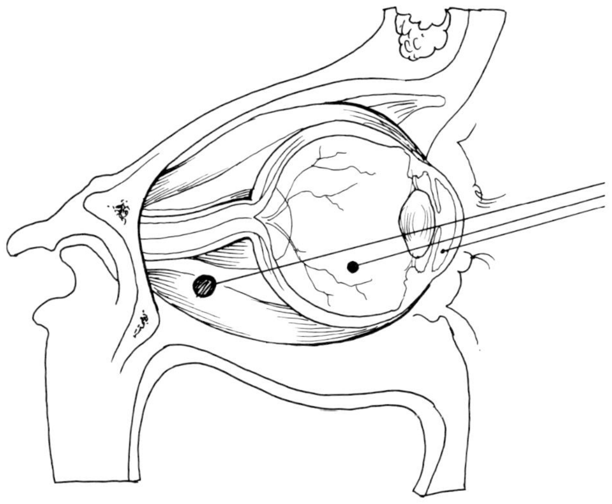

Fig. 13-1. *Penetrating* globe injuries result from a foreign body's (FB's) entering and remaining within the globe, commonly within the posterior segment. In general, the larger the FB, the more likely it will travel deep into the eye. Most FBs that penetrate and lodge within the eye are 5 mm or less in size. A *perforating* eye injury results from an FB's passing entirely through the eye and lodging within the orbital tissues. Drawing prepared for this textbook by Gary Wind, MD, Uniformed Services University of the Health Sciences, Bethesda, Md.

MECHANISMS OF OCULAR INJURY

High-velocity projectiles are responsible for most battlefield globe ruptures. Aside from the fragmentation produced directly by munitions, particles of glass, metal, stone, or vegetable matter may become secondary missiles in a blast (Figure 13-2). In the Iran–Iraq War (1982–1988), roughly 22% of intraocular foreign bodies (IOFBs) were composed of organic materials.[15] Metal striking metal also commonly leads to high-velocity metallic fragments with enough energy to penetrate the eye. Small projectiles may become lodged within the globe or perforate the globe and travel into the orbit. Between 80% and 90% of wartime IOFBs are located in the posterior segment.[8,15–17] By location and frequency, 15% of IOFBs are found in the anterior chamber (look in the inferior angle), 8% in the lens, 70% in the posterior chamber, and 7% in the orbit.[18]

Large, high-velocity projectiles (eg, bullets) can generate an associated shock wave within the surrounding tissue at impact and may rupture the globe despite an adjacent but noncontiguous penetration site. Bullet injuries directly impacting an eye produce devastating and often irreparable damage.

Although high-velocity, metallic FBs are usually sterile, secondary missiles produced by a blast injury are likely to increase the risk of endophthalmitis. The wartime incidence of endophthalmitis (6.9%–7.9%) is slightly higher than that documented in civilian industrial reports.[1,3,4] Vegetable matter carries the largest risk for introducing infectious contamination into the wound. Debris associated

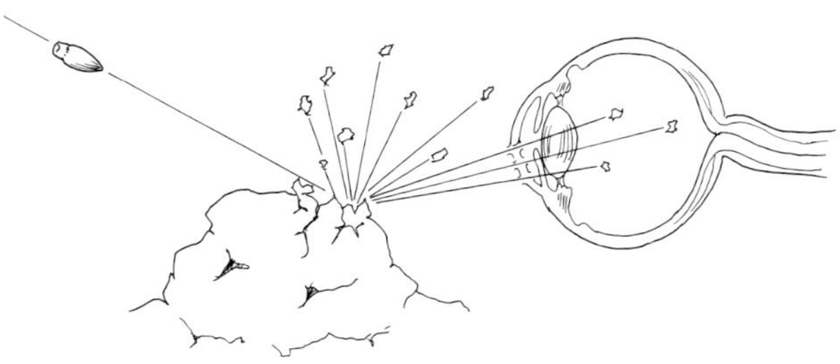

Fig. 13-2. Secondary missiles are produced when a high-velocity projectile strikes a stationary object, causing it to shatter into many high-velocity particles. In combat, secondary missiles are often responsible for tissue injury and typically are composed of such materials as rock, soil, glass, vegetable matter, clothing, or metal. Drawing prepared for this textbook by Gary Wind, MD, Uniformed Services University of the Health Sciences, Bethesda, Md.

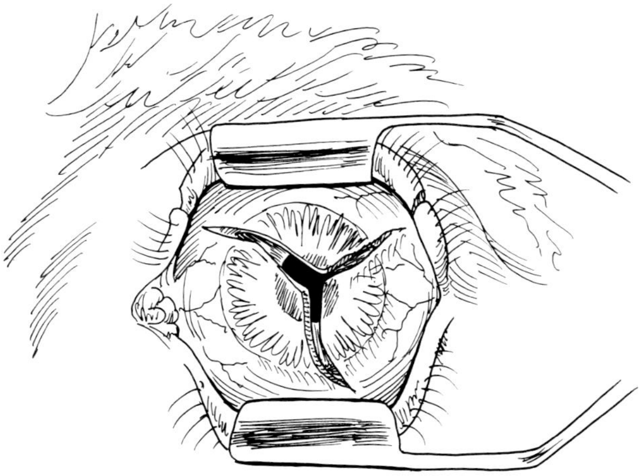

Fig. 13-3. Ocular injuries resulting from a sharp laceration commonly involve multiple tissue layers, including the eyelids and anterior segment. In evaluating an eyelid laceration, a careful inspection of the globe must be completed to exclude an associated ocular injury. Drawing prepared for this textbook by Gary Wind, MD, Uniformed Services University of the Health Sciences, Bethesda, Md.

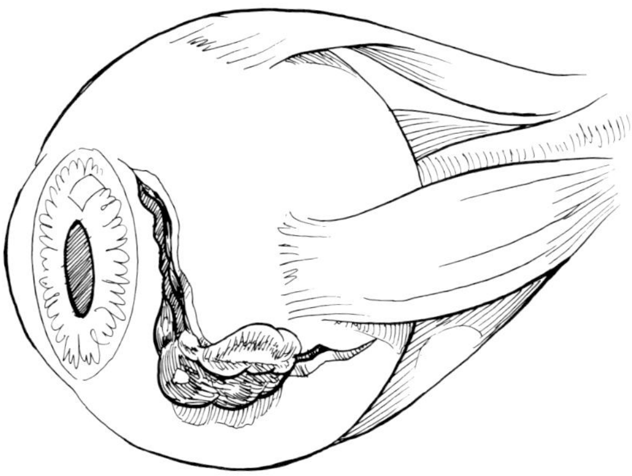

Fig. 13-4. Marked deformation of the eye occurs during blunt compression of the globe, generating tremendous intraocular pressure. A rupture occurs when the weakest portion of the globe gives way as the strength of the eye wall is exceeded by rising intraocular pressure. Common sites for globe rupture include the limbus, the area beneath the rectus muscles, and at the site of prior surgical scars. Drawing prepared for this textbook by Gary Wind, MD, Uniformed Services University of the Health Sciences, Bethesda, Md.

with mine blasts accounted for 40% of endophthalmitis cases in the Vietnam War.[19] Approximately 20% of these infections were attributed to *Bacillus* species, which causes severe infection with devastating visual effects.

Laceration to the globe from knives, glass, or sharp structural elements usually involves multiple tissue layers and frequently disrupts the eyelids and cornea (Figure 13-3). Despite severe tissue derangement, sharp lacerations often approximate precisely and carry a more favorable prognosis than some other forms of injury. Residue (eg, rust, glass fragments, paint) from the instrument of injury should be considered during wound debridement before globe repair.

With blunt compression, the globe undergoes marked deformation before rupture.[20,21] The weakest portions of the globe give way as the compressed intraocular structures generate tremendous intraocular pressure. Common sites for blunt rupture include the limbus, beneath the rectus muscles, or within the site of a prior surgical scar[12] (Figure 13-4). Many blunt ruptures extend parallel to the limbus and then turn sharply beneath a rectus muscle. The blunt mechanism of injury rarely induces more than one continuous rupture site.

INJURY HISTORY AND EVALUATION

If it is possible to obtain a history, the examining physician should seek to understand the mechanism and time course of the ocular injury. Details about the chronology of events will influence decisions on surgical management, and knowledge about the mechanism of injury will guide the preoperative investigation.

Intraocular tissues that prolapse through a rupture site often have limited viability. The decision whether to reposit or to amputate a prolapsed tissue is influenced by the duration of the extraocular exposure. When an FB is suspected, it is important to consider the possible materials involved (eg, glass, steel, copper, lead). Small, inert FBs may be carefully observed over time for infection and staining, whereas reactive materials such as copper require early removal from the eye.

Before assessing an ocular injury, the patient must be stabilized with regard to associated injuries. The physician should approach the patient with as complete an examination as is practical. The assessment will determine whether the globe should be explored and whether further studies should be performed to search for IOFBs. The physician should always maintain a high index of suspicion for a more serious injury than is readily apparent. Clinical signs of globe rupture by various mechanisms are listed in Table 13-1.

TABLE 13-1

CLINICAL SIGNS OF GLOBE RUPTURE

Mechanism and/or Location of Rupture	Clinical Signs
Corneal Laceration and Perforation	Shallow anterior chamber Seidel-positive wound Uveal incarceration Self-sealing tract
Posterior Scleral Rupture	Decreased motility Deep anterior chamber Hemorrhagic chemosis Vitreous hemorrhage Hypotony
Intraocular Foreign Body	Direct visualization (early in the examination, offers the best chance for locating and characterizing the foreign body) External penetration site Lens injury Tract within the vitreous Other sign of foreign body

Large projectiles often produce marked derangement of the globe with obvious perforation and extrusion of intraocular contents. The impact of a high-velocity missile can cause massive loss of ocular and adnexal tissue. The large mass of these missiles results in deeper penetration and greater damage to underlying and adjacent tissues.

Penetration of the globe by minute projectiles may cause minimal signs of overt injury at presentation (Figure 13-5). A high index of suspicion is often necessary to identify the FB and repair the injury. The examiner must search carefully for wound tracts, conjunctival lacerations, vitreous blood, and lens damage. If the view permits, indirect ophthalmoscopy affords the best opportunity to identify the composition, size, and shape of the projectile (Figure 13-6). Ancillary testing with computed tomography (CT) is helpful in detecting small, metallic FBs when visualization is not possible. Nonmetallic FBs are best visualized with magnetic resonance imaging (MRI) scanning. B-scan ultrasonography can help detect an FB but should not be used if an obvious rupture exists. Interpretation of the B-scan is often difficult owing to numerous tissue interfaces and artifacts in the blood-filled eye. Plain film radiographs are useful in determining the shape of radiodense FBs but lack the accuracy to precisely locate the object in three dimensions.

Sharp lacerations leading to globe rupture frequently involve deep puncture or lacerations through the eyelids and adnexal structures. Hemorrhage and blood clots from the eyelid laceration often obscure the globe injury. Full assessment of ocular integrity may require surgical exploration at the time of lid repair.

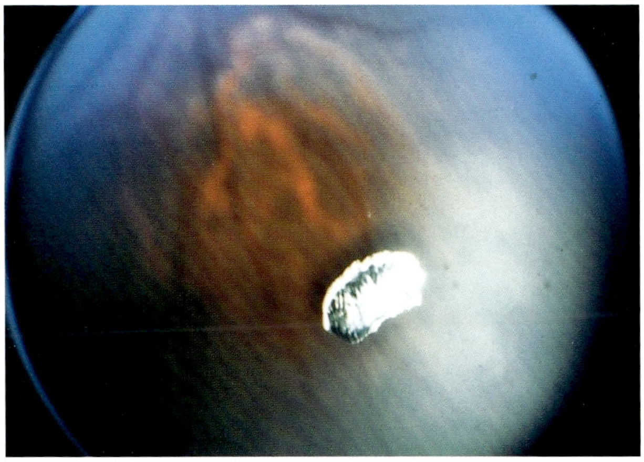

Fig. 13-6. An intraocular foreign body such as this metal fragment located in the vitreous (arrow) is often visible by ophthalmoscopy in the early postinjury period. Direct visualization of the foreign object offers the best opportunity to determine the size, shape, and composition of the projectile.

Blunt posterior globe rupture often produces hemorrhagic chemosis, deep anterior chamber, reduced ocular motility, vitreous hemorrhage, and increased tearing (Figure 13-7). Although intraocular pressure is usually low, ocular tension may be normal or elevated. Visualization of a clear vitreous cavity with an intact retina and choroid excludes the diagnosis of blunt posterior rupture. Any eye suspected to have a possible posterior globe rupture should be surgically explored to determine whether the integrity of the eye has been compromised.

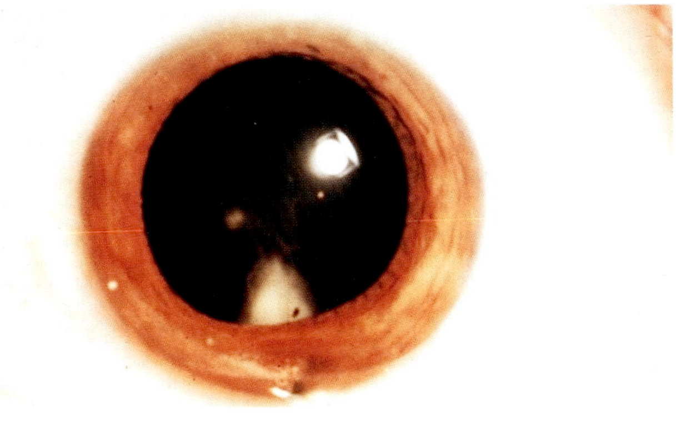

Fig. 13-5. Occult globe penetration by a foreign body may be revealed when the pupil is dilated. In this example, the small foreign body (FB) passed through the limbus and lens before lodging in the posterior segment. The white triangle at the 6 o'clock position is the lens opacity induced by the FB's passing through the eye.

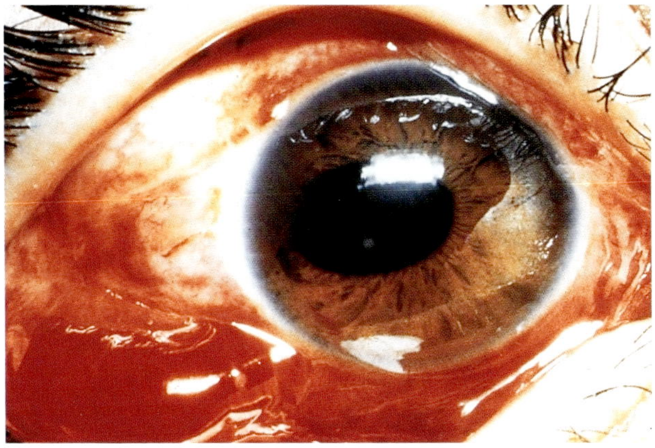

Fig. 13-7. This eye with a blunt posterior globe rupture demonstrates hemorrhagic chemosis and a deep anterior chamber. A low intraocular tension and reduced ocular motility were associated with the injury.

SURGICAL MANAGEMENT

Surgical Goals

Delayed closure of a ruptured globe is *not* a viable option in ocular surgery; prompt repair reduces the risk of endophthalmitis, tissue downgrowth, and tissue necrosis. Because all subsequent ocular reconstructive surgeries depend on a strong, watertight closure, the goals of the 3rd-echelon ophthalmologist are to

- identify the extent of injury,
- rule out an IOFB if possible,
- close the open globe primarily,
- limit reconstruction as much as is practical, and
- guard against infection, sympathetic ophthalmia, and tissue downgrowth.

Although FB identification is important, removal is usually not practical in this arena. Steps to identify FBs (eg, CT scan, ultrasonography) may also be deferred to the 4th echelon if they are impractical to perform at the 3rd echelon of care.

The ophthalmologist should surgically explore any eye suspected to be ruptured, identify the extent of injury, and complete a precise closure of the wound. FBs presenting at the injury site during closure should be removed (Figure 13-8). Ensuring that the injury site is clean of debris and well approximated helps prevent infection, sympathetic ophthalmia, and tissue downgrowth. Reconstructive efforts are rarely necessary during the initial repair and should be avoided. Both corneal edema and a greater tendency for ocular bleeding make reconstruction surgery ill-advised in the acutely injured eye. Marked inflammation and vascular engorgement increase the risk of hemorrhage in the first several days following trauma. Delaying reconstruction for several days significantly reduces the risks of surgery. Eyes known or suspected to have a retained FB should be repaired primarily and promptly evacuated to the next level of care for removal of the FB.

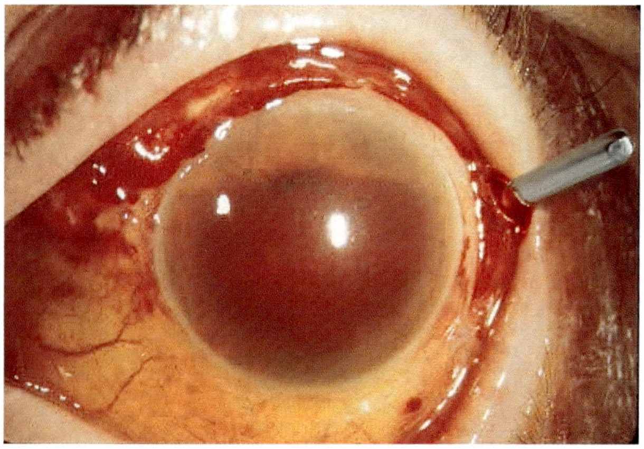

Fig. 13-8. Foreign objects, such as this aluminum shard lodged within the sclera, should be removed at the time of initial surgical repair. Intraocular foreign bodies that cannot be visualized directly by the surgeon should not be removed during the initial repair but should be addressed at the 4th-echelon level of care.

When an open globe is suspected, prophylactic intravenous antibiotics should be started as soon as is practical. Most authors recommend antibiotic coverage with a first-generation cephalosporin in combination with an aminoglycoside for wounds that are not heavily contaminated.[22–25] Vancomycin also offers a broad range of coverage and is often substituted for cephalosporin. Intravenous clindamycin should be added to the antibiotic regimen to cover *Bacillus* species if the injury has been contaminated with soil or vegetable matter.

Preoperatively, the ophthalmologist should avoid the use of topical and subconjunctival antibiotics that might enter the ruptured eye and cause retinal toxicity. The concentration of standard topical and subconjunctival antibiotics is roughly 10-fold higher than the toxic threshold level tolerated by the retina. A protective shield should be applied over the injured eye until definitive repair is possible.

The surgeon should never enucleate an eye primarily unless restoration of the globe is impossible. No light perception (NLP) vision should *not* be used as an early enucleation criterion, because several reports of patients with initial NLP indicate that they later recovered some level of vision.[26] Methodical repair can reconstruct many eyes that initially appear unsalvageable.

Step-by-Step Repair

1. Under general anesthesia, gently retract the eyelids of the injured eye with either a lid speculum or eyelid-retraction suture. Pressure on the globe should be avoided.
2. Perform a 360° limbal conjunctival peritomy beginning in a quadrant away from the suspected rupture site and working toward the rupture (Figure 13-9). Care must be taken to avoid engaging the prolapsed tissues or wound edge.

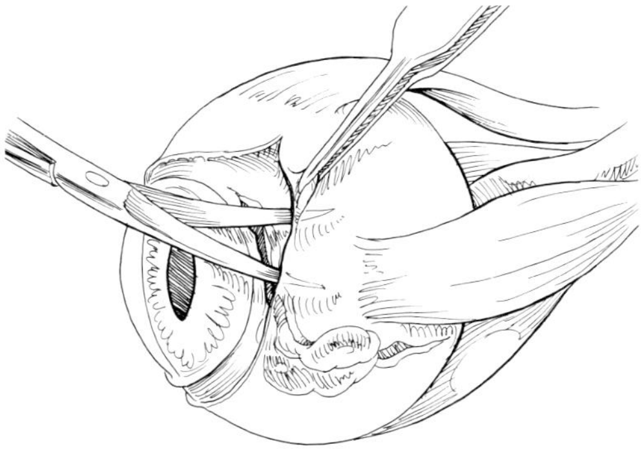

Fig. 13-9. A 360° limbal conjunctival peritomy is performed to explore for globe rupture. Care must be taken in completing the dissection to avoid engaging prolapsed intraocular tissue or wound edges. Drawing prepared for this textbook by Gary Wind, MD, Uniformed Services University of the Health Sciences, Bethesda, Md.

3. Irrigate and identify tissue, cleaning the wound of debris. Handle tissues carefully, as prolapsed uveal tissue may resemble foreign matter or clotted blood and will bleed freely if injured.
4. Gain control of the eye using a 4-0 silk traction suture placed through the limbus distal from the wound or by looping individual rectus muscles with 2-0 silk bridle suture. Before passing the bridle suture beneath the rectus muscle, the sclera must be carefully inspected to avoid manipulation of the rupture site. Extreme care must be exercised in using a muscle hook near the injury to guard against inadvertent wound penetration (Figure 13-10).

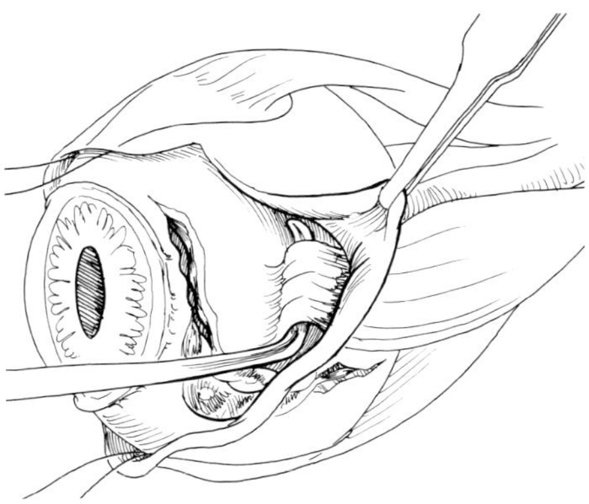

Fig. 13-10. Globe rotation is greatly facilitated by placement of 2-0 silk traction sutures beneath the rectus muscles or 4-0 silk suture through the limbus. To avoid inadvertent wound penetration, extreme care must be exercised in using a muscle hook under the rectus muscle. Drawing prepared for this textbook by Gary Wind, MD, Uniformed Services University of the Health Sciences, Bethesda, Md.

5. Identify the path and course of the rupture. Carefully remove any foreign material lodged within the wound. Inspect tissue before considering removal of any clotted blood or debris from the scleral wound, because the tissue actually may be choroid or retina. Send any excised tissue to pathology for identification. Attempt to reposit all viable exposed tissues.
6. Proper wound exposure greatly aids in both the identification and the repair of the injury. If the injury cannot be adequately exposed using traction sutures, the surgeon should consider tagging and temporarily reflecting a rectus muscle to enhance globe rotation (Figure 13-11). A 5-0 double-armed Vicryl suture woven through the muscle tendon, incorporating "locking bites" on either end, secures the muscle before the tendon is cut from the sclera.

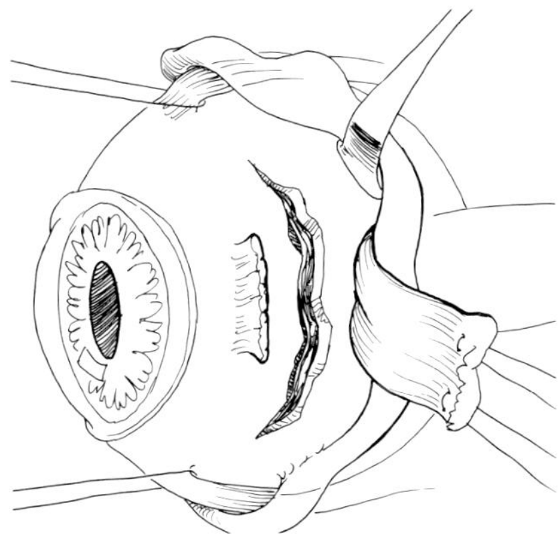

Fig. 13-11. In certain circumstances, reflecting a rectus muscle provides superior wound exposure and can greatly improve globe rotation. Before transecting the muscle from its scleral insertion, a double-armed 5-0 Vicryl suture should be woven through the muscle tendon with "locking bites" taken on either end. Drawing prepared for this textbook by Gary Wind, MD, Uniformed Services University of the Health Sciences, Bethesda, Md.

7. Injuries through the limbus should be approximated with a 9-0 nylon interrupted suture to maintain tissue orientation.
8. Close the corneal wound with 10-0 nylon (see Chapter 9, Sharp Trauma of the Anterior Segment).
9. Inspect the scleral wound edges for corresponding defects and begin the posterior repair by approximating these landmarks. Repair sclera with 8-0 nylon in an interrupted or baseball suture pattern by passing the needle through each side of sclera separately to a depth of 75% of the scleral thickness (Figure 13-12). Try to avoid passing the

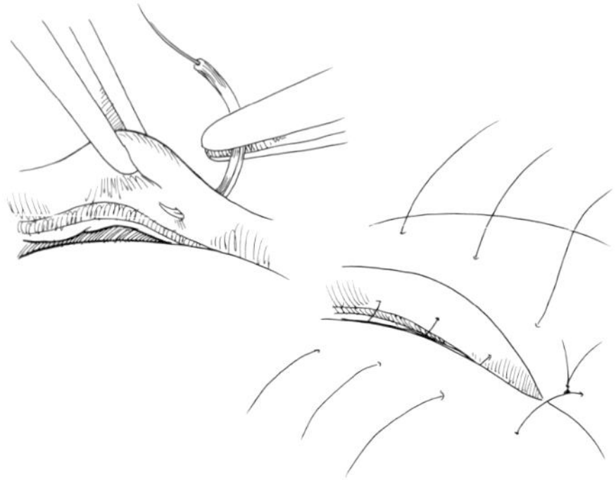

Fig. 13-12. The sclera is repaired with an interrupted or baseball suture pattern passed through each side of the sclera to a 75% depth. Closure is facilitated when an assistant can depress choroid and vitreous while the wound is approximated and tied. Drawings prepared for this textbook by Gary Wind, MD, Uniformed Services University of the Health Sciences, Bethesda, Md.

needle through the full thickness of sclera, as this maneuver often results in uveal incorporation within the closure. The assistant uses a spatula to depress choroid and vitreous while the surgeon approximates the wound edges and the sutures are tied.

10. Vitreous should be cut flush with the choroidal tissue using either an automated vitrectomy instrument or a cellulose sponge and fine scissors (Figure 13-13). Vitrectomy cut rates of 400 to 600 cuts per minute are optimal to remove vitreous and reduce the tendency to incorporate uvea or retinal tissue within the vitrectomy port. The vitrectomy instrument should not be placed directly into the eye, thus avoiding retinal injury, but may be used along the wound to remove residual vitreous as the wound is approximated. Vitreous and clotted blood will likewise adhere to a cellulose sponge, allowing the surgeon to exert gentle traction on the tissues and trim them close to the wound with fine scissors.

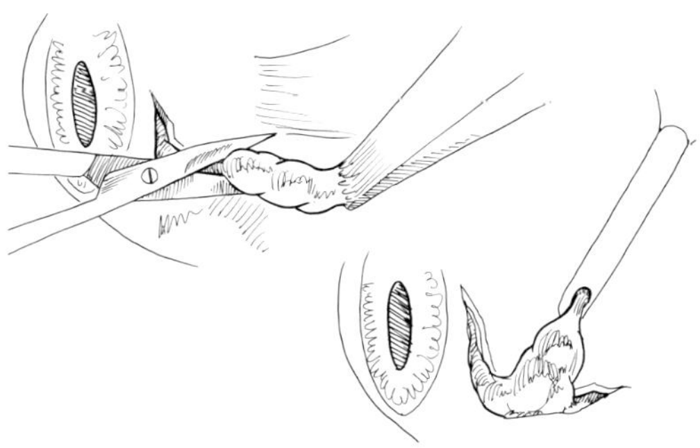

Fig. 13-13. Vitreous should be cut flush with the choroidal tissue using either a cellulose sponge and fine scissors or an automated vitrectomy instrument. Care must be taken to avoid cutting the choroid or retina during this procedure. Drawing prepared for this textbook by Gary Wind, MD, Uniformed Services University of the Health Sciences, Bethesda, Md.

11. When wounds extend beneath the rectus muscle, the muscle should be tagged with a double-armed 5-0 Vicryl suture and reflected from its scleral insertion. Following the scleral repair, the rectus muscle should be reattached by making partial-thickness scleral passes with the Vicryl sutures that attach the muscle to its original position.

12. Wounds should be repaired posteriorly as far as is practical without putting excessive pressure on the globe. Exposure may be greatly enhanced by reflecting one of the rectus muscles (as mentioned above). Posterior wounds should be left unrepaired, as manipulation to expose the area may result in expulsion of the intraocular contents. The nonsutured posterior wound generally becomes watertight by 10 days following the globe repair.

13. When scleral tissue is missing from the wound, the eye cannot be closed without creating significant deformation of the globe. To avoid globe irregularity and still seal the wound, a tissue patch may be fashioned and sewn over the defect using multiple interrupted sutures to span the gap. Banked sclera, fascia lata, preserved pericardial tissue, or scleral buckle material may each be used in this fashion to close the wound. With an interrupted horizontal mattress suture pattern, the wound is compressed and will likely achieve watertight closure (Figure 13-14). Smaller leaks may be sealed with cyanoacrylate tissue adhesive (tissue glue),

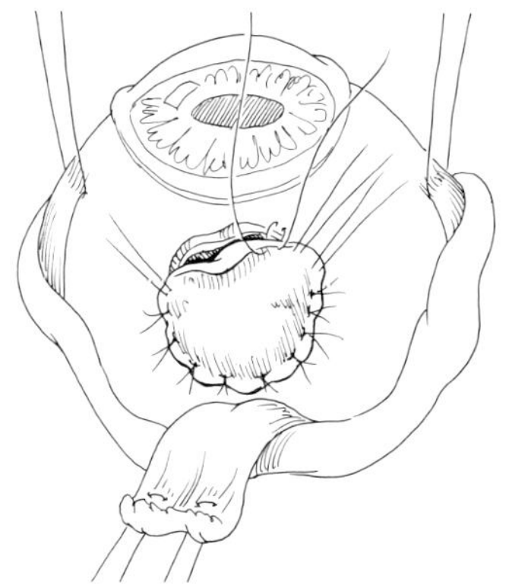

Fig. 13-14. When, owing to missing tissue, a scleral wound cannot be sealed, a patch graft can be fashioned from banked sclera, fascia lata, preserved pericardium, or scleral buckle material, and used to oversew the wound. By using interrupted horizontal mattress sutures through the graft and globe, the wound is compressed and a watertight seal can be obtained. Drawing prepared for this textbook by Gary Wind, MD, Uniformed Services University of the Health Sciences, Bethesda, Md.

applied with cotton-tipped applicators after the wound has been temporarily dried. Tissue adhesive should never be applied to wounds that are actively leaking or bleeding, because adhesion will not occur.

14. Once the identified laceration is repaired, thoroughly examine the remainder of the globe for any additional injuries.

15. Reform the globe using a balanced salt solution injected through the anterior chamber or pars plana (away from the rupture site). Check for wound leaks along the sutured wound and ensure that the eye maintains inflation. The surgical goal of wound closure is to achieve a strong, watertight wound repair that can withstand additional reconstructive surgery within days of the initial repair.

16. Close the conjunctiva using interrupted 7-0 Vicryl or 6-0 plain gut suture and bury knots to avoid ocular irritation.

17. Administer prophylactic subconjunctival antibiotic away from the wound repair. If a posterior rupture site remains open, subconjunctival antibiotics should be avoided.

Because of the difficulty in distinguishing pain and inflammation of trauma from early endophthalmitis, the initial diagnosis of endophthalmitis is often overlooked or delayed. Posttraumatic endophthalmitis has been reported in up to 7.9% of ocular injuries with retained FBs.[19] Patients should therefore routinely receive intravenous, topical, and subconjunctival antibiotics. The use of prophylactic intravitreal antibiotics is controversial and is generally reserved for cases of suspected early endophthalmitis or eyes with markedly contaminated FBs.

Factors associated with poor visual outcomes in scleral laceration include poor initial visual acuity, afferent pupillary defect, vitreous hemorrhage, and wounds extending posterior to the rectus muscles or greater than 10 to 12 mm in length.[27,28] The initial sensory status of the eye is more important in foretelling outcome than are anatomical factors. Eyes injured by limited sharp laceration or small FBs tend to have a more favorable prognosis than eyes ruptured by blunt compression or large foreign objects.[27]

POSTSURGICAL CONSIDERATIONS

Postoperative Care

Following wound repair and stabilization, the patient should be evacuated to the 4th echelon for observation and reconstructive care. Particular attention should be directed toward observing signs of endophthalmitis, sympathetic ophthalmia, and retinal detachment. Intravenous and topical antibiotics are continued for the first 3 to 5 days, then tapered if no signs of infection are evident. Aggressive use of topical steroids reduces anterior segment inflammation, corneal edema, and fibrin formation. The use of tissue plasminogen activator (tPA) in the treatment of total hyphema or anterior segment fibrin should be avoided when possible because of the increased risk of inducing secondary vitreous hemorrhage.[29] When the posterior chamber view is limited by corneal edema or blood, the retinal status may be assessed postoperatively through periodic B-scan ultrasonography.

Pathophysiology of Posttraumatic Retinal Detachment

Severely traumatized eyes with posterior penetration or rupture commonly develop retinal detachment. Traumatic retinal breaks may lead to detachment at the time of injury or weeks after the trauma, once liquefied vitreous has gained access to the subretinal space. A more onerous form of retinal detachment may develop days to weeks following the injury in response to fibrocellular proliferation and membrane contraction.

Following severe, penetrating trauma, a prominent inflammatory reaction occurs in the posterior segment. The presence of both intravitreal hemorrhage and inflammation stimulates the proliferation of myofibroblasts within the vitreous gel, resulting in the formation of fibrocellular membranes.[30] Serum components including fibronectin and platelet-derived growth factor enhance cell migration and proliferation of these membranes.[31,32] As the fibrocellular membranes mature and contract, traction develops across the vitreous, pulling the retina centrally and anterior. Severe traction results in the retina's being pulled into a funnel configuration with dense membranes located centrally.

In most ophthalmology textbooks written before 1985, cryotherapy was reported to reduce the risk of subsequent retinal detachment in penetrating trauma by surrounding the wound with a form of retinopexy. Although the benefit of this procedure has never been established, experimental models indicate that the application of cryotherapy to a lacerated eye promotes the formation of a fibrocellular response and induces complex retinal detachment.[33] Although cryotherapy may create a strong posttraumatic chorioretinal adhesion in some cases, the risk for fibrocellular membrane proliferation and vitreous hemorrhage make the use of this tool inadvisable in the setting of globe rupture.

Timing of Secondary Surgical Intervention

In considering the surgical repair of posttraumatic retinal detachment, scleral buckling alone is generally insufficient to overcome the traction generated by the fibrocellular response. Vitrectomy and membrane peeling are, therefore, essential elements of retinal repair and serve to restore retinal architecture by reducing retinal traction. The addition of an encircling band at the time of surgery redirects tractional forces that may develop during the postoperative period and reduces the risk for subsequent macular detachment (Figure 13-15).[34] In most reported case series, placement of an encircling band at the time of vitrectomy repair reduced the risk for subsequent retinal detachment by more than 50%.[35–37]

The decision of when to surgically intervene in the posterior segment of a traumatized eye remains controversial. Indications for vitrectomy in the posttrauma setting include

- removal of an FB,
- repair of retinal detachment,
- removal of lens fragments,
- removal of hemorrhage,
- surgical exploration, and
- treatment of endophthalmitis.

The urgency of such procedures varies from patient to patient and must be carefully weighed against the increased surgical risks of early intervention.

In the first several days following significant ocular trauma, the eye is inflamed and tends to bleed easily and profusely if surgically damaged. The vitreous gel is firmly attached to the retina in most cases and difficult to remove, enhancing the risk of bleeding. Corneal edema is commonly present and may necessitate the use of a temporary keratoprosthesis for surgical visualization. Hyphema, if present, requires surgical evacuation for visualization posteriorly. Additionally, an eye with one or more penetrating injuries may have posterior exit wounds that interfere with maintaining fluid control during the procedure.

After 7 to 14 days of observation, the eye is less inflamed and the tendency to bleed is significantly reduced.[34] A spontaneous vitreous detachment occurs by this time in most patients and greatly enhances the ease of vitrectomy surgery. The cornea and anterior chamber often clear spontaneously, avoiding the need for a keratoprosthesis. Posterior penetration wounds usually self-seal by this time, allowing for proper intraocular pressure control during vitrectomy.

Most surgeons agree with early intervention for retained IOFBs to limit their potential toxicity and prevent encapsulation. Additionally, endophthalmitis in the trauma setting warrants early vitrectomy and intravitreal antibiotics. The timing of surgical intervention for other conditions, including retinal detachment, remains controversial. Some authors[38,39] have advocated early vitrectomy to reduce the risk of intraocular membrane formation by removing the scaffold for cellular proliferation. Although these authors have reported improved surgical outcomes with early vitrectomy, comparison groups were either not reported or not comparable to the delayed surgical group. Other investigators have reported either serious choroidal bleeding with early surgery,[40,41] or no statistically significant visual difference between early or late vitrectomy for cases of retinal detachment, or IOFB following penetrating trauma.[42]

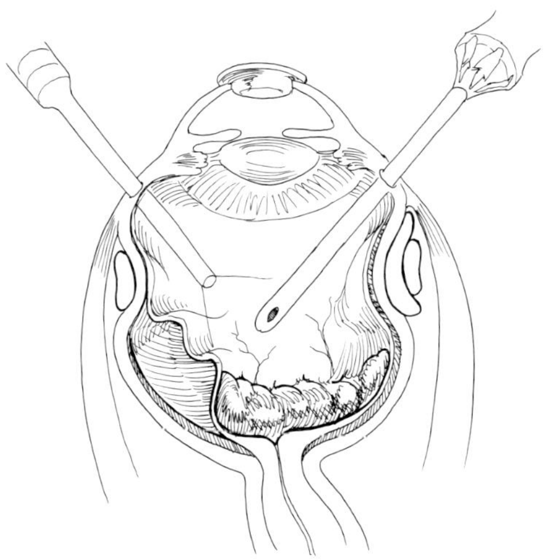

Fig. 13-15. The repair of a complex retinal detachment following penetrating trauma generally requires the removal of intravitreal fibrocellular membranes using vitrectomy and membrane peeling techniques. The addition of an encircling band reduces the risk for subsequent retinal detachment by redirecting tractional forces within the eye. A temporary keratoprosthesis aids intraocular visualization for eyes with persistent corneal edema or severe corneal scarring. Drawing prepared for this textbook by Gary Wind, MD, Uniformed Services University of the Health Sciences, Bethesda, Md.

SUMMARY

The fragmentation munitions used by combatants in modern warfare have generated a high incidence of multiple traumas, with ocular casualties comprising 13% of all injuries during recent conflicts. Aside from projectile injury, combat is associated with globe rupture from sharp laceration, blunt contusion, and secondary shock wave injury. The implementation of fragmentation weaponry has resulted in a substantial number of bilateral ocular penetration injuries, many of which could have been avoided through the proper use of protective eyewear. The social and economic consequences of wartime ocular injuries have been enormous, as reflected by the fact that 75% of soldiers suffering ocular injury during the Vietnam War were unable to return to active duty.

Restoring sight to injured patients begins with timely recognition of the ocular injury and completion of a precise, well-approximated closure of the ocular wound at the 3rd echelon of care. The first repair of the globe is the most important, setting the stage for further reconstruction efforts once inflammation, corneal edema, and visualization have improved. Following the primary globe repair, patients are typically evacuated to the 4th echelon, where additional evaluation and IOFB removal takes place. Although early surgical intervention is warranted for IOFBs and endophthalmitis, other reconstruction efforts are usually delayed for 1 to 2 weeks.

The visual prognosis for patients managed in this manner depends primarily on their initial visual acuity, the mechanism of injury, and the extent of damage. Complications that can further jeopardize visual outcome include endophthalmitis, hemorrhage, retinal detachment, tissue downgrowth, and sympathetic ophthalmia. Proper wound closure, appropriate use of antibiotics, and timely reconstruction efforts help limit additional damage to the eye during the healing process and optimize the soldier's chance for visual recovery.

REFERENCES

1. Treister G. Ocular casualties in the 6 Day War. *Am J Ophthalmol.* 1969;68:669–675.

2. Heier JS, Enzenauer RW, Wintermeyer SF, Delaney M, LaPiana FP. Ocular injuries and diseases at a combat support hospital in support of Operations Desert Shield and Desert Storm. *Arch Ophthalmol.* 1993;111:795–798.

3. Bellows JG. Observations on 300 consecutive cases of ocular war injuries. *Am J Ophthalmol.* 1947;30:309–323.

4. Moisseiev J, Belkin M, Bartov E, Treister G. Severe combat eye injuries in the Lebanon war, 1982. *Isr J Med Sci.* 1984;20:339–344.

5. Wong TY, Seet B, Chong–Lye A. Eye injuries in twentieth century warfare: A historical perspective. *Surv Ophthalmol.* 1997;41(6):433–459.

6. Belkin M. Ocular injuries in the Yom Kippur War. *J Ocul Therapy Surg.* 1983;2:40–49.

7. Dansey-Browning GC. The value of ophthalmic treatment in the field. *Br J Ophthalmol.* 1944;28:87–97.

8. Scott GI, Michaelson IC. An analysis and follow-up of 301 cases of battle casualty injury to the eyes. *Br J Ophthalmol.* 1946;30:42–55.

9. Blake PM. Injuries to the eyes or to the intracranial visual paths in air raid casualties admitted to hospital. *Br J Ophthalmol.* 1945;29:1–5.

10. Hornblass A. Eye injuries in South Vietnam. *Surg Forum.* 1973;24:500–502.

11. Tredici TJ. Management of ophthalmic casualties in south-east Asia. *Mil Med.* 1968;133:355–362.

12. Shingleton BJ, Hersh PS, Kenyon KR, eds. *Eye Trauma.* St Louis, Mo: Mosby–Year Book; 1991:204–211.

13. Dannenberg AL, Parver LM, Brechner RJ, Khoo L. Penetration eye injuries in the workplace. The National Eye Trauma System Registry. *Arch Ophthalmol.* 1992;110(6):843–848. Review.

14. Stewart GM. Eye protection against small high speed missiles. *Am J Ophthalmol.* 1961;51:80–87.

15. Lashkari K, Lashkari MH, Kim AJ, Crane WG, Jalkh AE. Combat-related eye trauma: A review of 5,320 cases. *Int Ophthalmol Clin.* 1995:35:193–203.

16. Belkin M, Ivry M. Explosive intraocular foreign bodies. *Am J Ophthalmol.* 1978;85:676–678.

17. Haik GM. The management of intraocular foreign bodies in military practice. *Am J Ophthalmol.* 1946;29:815–827.

18. Duke-Elder S, MacFaul PA. *Injuries.* Vol 14. In: Duke-Elder S, ed. *System of Ophthalmology.* St. Louis, Mo: Mosby–Year Book; 1972: 482–483.

19. Anderson WD. Prophylactic antibiotics and endophthalmitis in Vietnam. *Am J Ophthalmol.* 1973;75:481–485.

20. Weidenthal DT, Schepens CL. Peripheral fundus changes associated with ocular contusion. *Am J Ophthalmol.* 1966;62:465–477.

21. Delori F, Pomerantzeff O, Cox MS. Deformation of the globe under high speed impact: Its relation to contusion injuries. *Invest Ophthalmol.* 1969;8:290–301.

22. Affeldt JC, Flynn HW, Forster RK, Mandelbaum S, Clarkson JG, Jarus GD. Microbial endophthalmitis resulting from ocular trauma. *Ophthalmology.* 1987;94:407–413.

23. Brinton GS, Topping TM, Hyndiuk RA, Aaberg TM, Reeser FH, Abrams GW. Post-traumatic endophthalmitis. *Arch Ophthalmol.* 1984;102:547–550.

24. Parrish CM, O'Day DM. Traumatic endophthalmitis. *Int Ophthalmol Clin.* 1987;27:112–119.

25. Kunimoto DY, Das T, Sharma S, et al. Microbiologic spectrum and susceptibility of isolates, II: Posttraumatic endophthalmitis. Endophthalmitis Research Group. *Am J Ophthalmol.* 1999;128(2):242–244.

26. Morris RE, Witherspoon CD, Helms HA Jr, Feist RM, Byrne JB Jr. Eye Injury Registry of Alabama (preliminary report): Demographics and prognosis of severe eye injury. *South Med J.* 1987;80(7):810–816.

27. de Juan E, Sternberg P, Michels RG. Penetrating ocular injuries: Types of injuries involving the posterior segment. *Trans Ophthalmol Soc UK.* 1975;95:335–339.

28. Hutton WL, Fuller DG. Factors influencing final visual results in severely injured eyes. *Am J Ophthalmol.* 1984;97:715–722.

29. Kim MH, Koo TH, Sah WJ, Chung SM. Treatment of total hyphema with relatively low-dose tissue plasminogen activator. *Ophthalmic Surg Lasers.* 1998;29:762–766.

30. Cleary PE, Minckler DS, Ryan SJ. Ultrastructure of traction retinal detachment in rhesus monkey eyes after a posterior penetrating ocular injury. *Am J. Ophthalmol.* 1980;90:829–845.

31. Campochiaro PA, Jerdan JA, Glaser BM. Serum contains chemoattractants for human retinal pigment epithelial cells. *Arch Ophthalmol.* 1985;103:1830–1833.

32. Campochiaro PA, Glaser BM. Platelet-derived growth factor is chemotactic for human retinal pigment epithelial cells. *Arch Ophthalmol.* 1984;102:576–579.

33. Campochiaro PA, Gaskin HC, Vinores SA. Retinal cryopexy stimulates traction retinal detachment formation in the presence of an ocular wound. *Arch Ophthalmol.* 1987;105:1567–1570.

34. Spalding SC, Sternberg P. Controversies in the management of posterior ocular trauma. *Retina.* 1990;10:S76–S82.

35. Brinton GS, Aaberg TM, Reeser FH, Topping TM, Abrams GW. Surgical results in ocular trauma involving the posterior segment. *Am J Ophthalmol.* 1982;93:271–278.

36. Hutton WL, Fuller DG. Factors influencing final visual results in severely injured eyes. *Am J Ophthalmol.* 1984;97:715–722.

37. Miyake Y, Ando F. Surgical results of vitrectomy in ocular trauma. *Retina.* 1983;3:265–268.

38. Coles WH, Haaik GM. Vitrectomy in intraocular trauma: Its rationale and its indications and limitations. *Arch Ophthalmol.* 1972;87:621–628.

39. Coleman DJ. Early vitrectomy in the management of the severely traumatized eye. *Am J Ophthalmol.* 1982; 93:543–551.

40. Deutsch TA, Feller DB. *Paton and Goldberg's Management of Ocular Injuries.* Philadelphia, Pa: WB Saunders; 1985: 161–162.

41. Ryan SJ, Allen AW. Pars plana vitrectomy in ocular trauma. *Am J Ophthalmol.* 1979;88:483–491.

42. Dalma-Weiszhausz J, Quiroz-Mercado H, Morales-Canton V, Oliver-Fernandez K, De Anda-Turati M. Vitrectomy for ocular trauma: A question of timing? *Eur J Ophthalmol.* 1996;6:460–463.

Chapter 14

MANAGEMENT OF PENETRATING INJURIES WITH A RETAINED INTRAOCULAR FOREIGN BODY

WENDALL C. BAUMAN, JR, MD*

*Colonel, US Air Force, Medical Corps; Assistant Chief, Department of Surgery; Chief, Retina Service, Brooke Army Medical Center, Fort Sam Houston, Texas 78234-6200; Staff, Retina Service, 59th MDW/MCST, Lackland Air Force Base, Texas 78256-5300

INTRODUCTION

Penetrating ocular injuries with an associated retained intraocular foreign body (IOFB) constitute a significant portion of ocular trauma in the military. A steady increase in eye-related injuries, from 2% during World War I and World War II to 13% in the Persian Gulf War, could be attributed to the evolution of modern warfare this century.[1,2] The lethality to the eye has increased, owing to the use of new technology in weapon systems such as improved fragmentation munitions, which produce large numbers of tiny fragments. With this increase in ocular trauma, penetrating injuries with associated IOFBs account for 31% to 85% of significant injuries to the eye (Table 14-1).

In the past 2 decades, advances in understanding the pathophysiology of traumatic injuries to the retina and vitreous as well as new vitreoretinal surgical techniques have made management of traumatized eyes with IOFBs more predictable. With the evolution of these advancements, a new expediency in diagnosis and management of retained IOFBs challenges today's military ophthalmologists. Whether timely and prompt management will save or improve vision in those who sustain eye injuries in future armed conflicts remains to be determined.

The setting and occurrence of penetrating injuries with retained IOFBs have evolved as society and industrialization evolved in the 20th century. With the emergence of an industrial base, occupational eye injuries were far more common in the city, compared with rural agrarian settings. From a military perspective, non-warfare-related injuries mirrored those of occupational and accidental injuries. The setting of warfare-related eye injuries, however, was directly related to the type and use of armaments generating high-velocity metal fragments.

TABLE 14-1

INTRAOCULAR FOREIGN BODIES IN WAR

War	Penetrated Eyes With Retained IOFBs (%)	Nonmagnetic IOFBs (%)	Enucleation Resulting From IOFBs (%)
WW2 (US Army)[1]	63.7	55.4	30.8
WW2 (British Army: Libyan campaign 1941–1943)[2]	75.3	—	25.4
Vietnam[3]	32.7	22.2	—
Arab–Israeli Six-Day War (in Jerusalem)[4]	65.3	17.6	11.8
Arab–Israeli Six-Day War (compiled record, all cases)[5]	42.9	23.8	—
Lebanon[6]	84.6	66.7	27.3
Iran–Iraq[7]	31.1	90	—
Persian Gulf[8]	32.7	—	—

—: data not reported
IOFB: intraocular foreign body
Data sources: (1) Bellows JG. Observations on 300 consecutive cases of ocular war injuries. *Am J Ophthalmol.* 1947;30:309–323. (2) Dansey-Browning GC. The value of ophthalmic treatment in the field. *Br J Ophthalmol.* 1944;28:87–97. (3) Hoefle FB. Initial treatment of eye injuries. *Arch Ophthalmol.* 1968;79:33–35. (4) Gombos GM. Ocular war injuries in Jerusalem. *Am J Ophthalmol.* 1969;68:474–478. (5) Treister G. Ocular casualties in the Six-Day War. *Am J Ophthalmol.* 1969;68:669–675. (6) Moisseiev J, Belkin M, Bartov E, Treister G. Severe combat eye injuries in the Lebanon War. *Isr J Med Sci.* 1984;20:339–344. (7) Lashkari K, Lashkari M, Kim A, Crane WG, Jalkh AE. Combat-related eye trauma: A review of 5,320 cases. *Int Ophthalmol Clin.* 1995;35:193–203. (8) Mader TH, Aragones JV, Chandler AC, et al. Ocular and ocular adnexal injuries treated by United States military ophthalmologists during Operations Desert Shield and Desert Storm. *Ophthalmology.* 1993;100:1462–1467.

Occupational and Domestic Perspectives

Since antiquity, open globe injuries with a retained IOFB have intrigued and dismayed those caring for the eye. In industrialized European cities at the turn of the 20th century, the incidence of retained IOFBs was one per 1,000, but in rural cities the incidence was markedly lower. Worldwide, the percentage of ocular injuries with a retained IOFB has remained remarkably consistent over the years. In an industrial series out of the Munich Clinic[3] in 1933, penetrating injuries with a retained IOFB accounted for 39.2% of cases, with two thirds of IOFBs located in the posterior segment. More recently, the National Eye Trauma System Registry[4] reported a retained IOFB present in 35% of the injured workers between 1985 and 1991, with a trend toward stable or improved vision following treatment.

From an occupational or accidental viewpoint, the etiology of most retained IOFBs was an isolated metal projectile generated by hammering metal on metal. Less-frequent causes were handling wire, welding, drilling, grinding, and working with machinery; wood was an even less frequent source of IOFBs. In the occupational setting, an injury involving both eyes with IOFBs or one eye with multiple IOFBs is rare.[5]

In the military, the nature of IOFBs unrelated to combat mirror those in the occupational series. An unpublished series from Brooke Army Medical Center,[6] for example, showed that 50% of IOFBs resulted from metal striking metal. Explosions producing fragments accounted for another 29% of IOFBs (Figure 14-1).

Military Perspective

Warfare-related wounds, on the other hand, tend to be different from occupational and accidental trauma. War-induced, penetrating ocular injuries typically result from shell fragments, grenades, bullets, mines, booby traps, and armored warfare. Clearly, the risk of ocular injury during modern warfare depends on the strategy through which commanders utilize their forces and weapons. Not surprisingly, the incidence of IOFBs is higher in situations involving armor, artillery, and mine warfare. Exploding fragmentation munitions cause multiple, high-velocity, fragment injuries not only adjacent to but also up to several hundred feet away from the blast. These injuries typically involve multiple IOFBs, affect the posterior segment, and often result in bilateral ocular injuries. The incidence of

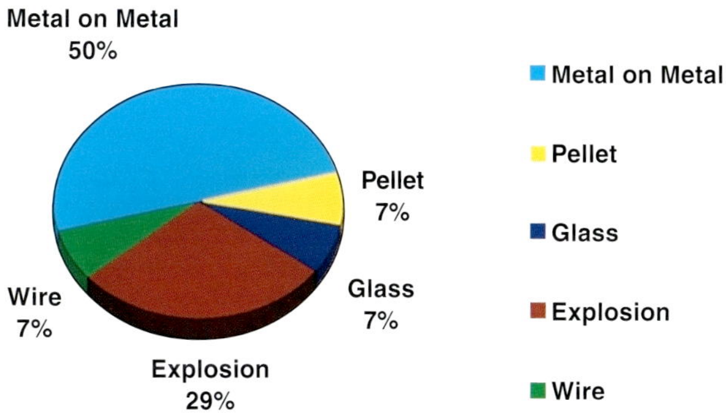

Fig. 14-1. Etiology of penetrating intraocular foreign bodies managed at Brooke Army Medical Center from 1982 to 1993.

these injuries with IOFBs can be modified by the aggressive use of eye protection (eye armor) introduced in the 1980s to protect the warrior's vision.

The composition of the IOFB in warfare has major treatment implications. Whereas only 10% of retained IOFBs in the industrial and accidental setting are nonmagnetic, up to 90% are nonmagnetic in war (see Table 14-1).[7,8] These nonmagnetic IOFBs cannot be removed with external magnets. For example, landmines are increasingly composed of plastic and synthetic materials, making detection of IOFBs more difficult.[9]

As in occupational settings, the size and shape of the IOFB has a direct effect on visual outcome. The concussion of a large IOFB severely disrupts all layers of the eye. Larger, blunt IOFBs frequently result in a poorer visual prognosis, whereas small, sharp projectiles may penetrate cleanly with minimal disruption of ocular architecture.[10,11]

Penetrating ocular injuries with retained IOFBs are usually associated with multisystem trauma and generally occur on battlefields remote from specialists. Frequently, definitive treatment tends to be delayed. These wounds require initial stabilization by a multispecialty team performing surgery to save life and limb. The ophthalmologist contributes with repairs to the open globe and ocular adnexa within the theater. Current medical doctrine advocates prompt aeromedical evacuation to permit a vitreoretinal specialist located in the communication zone to remove the IOFB and manage any other vitreoretinal complications associated with the initial trauma. The delay in final repair and the means of transport must be considered when managing penetrating eye injuries with an IOFB.

The introduction of pars plana vitrectomy in the 1970s resulted in new techniques to permit controlled access to IOFBs and related intraocular complications. Only recently have modern vitreoretinal techniques been used to treat penetrating war injuries with IOFBs.[8,12] With changing strategies in managing war injuries, miniaturization of instrumentation, and changing medical doctrine, specialists are now available closer to the battlefield to manage serious ocular injuries. Time will tell whether the new technologies will improve the outcome from potentially blinding battlefield wounds.

POTENTIAL COMPLICATIONS

The severity of complications related to an IOFB in conjunction with a penetrating injury is generally related to the site of the initial impact, size of the entry wound, composition of the IOFB, and presence of an exit wound. A smaller IOFB usually results in fewer complications and better visual results.[13] These complications and their management have an impact on salvaging vision and the globe.

Anterior segment complications include corneal and corneoscleral lacerations, iris penetration or perforation, lenticular perforation, cataract, retained IOFB within the anterior chamber, hyphema, and angle recession. Most projectiles associated with combat-related ocular injuries have relatively high mass and velocity, causing them to perforate the anterior segment or sclera or both and come to rest in the posterior segment.[8,14,15]

With posterior segment involvement, the ocular complications are frequent and the resultant vision often worse.[7,16] Posterior segment complications typically involve vitreous or preretinal hemorrhage, retinal tear, retinal detachment, incarcerated retina, endophthalmitis, epiretinal membrane formation, the physiological effects of a retained IOFB, and sympathetic ophthalmia. Typically, vitreous or preretinal hemorrhage accompanies the retained IOFB, often obscuring retinal details. This vitreous hemorrhage may be extensive, preventing identification of the foreign body (FB) and associated retinal damage such as retinal holes, tears, or detachments. Ancillary testing is vital for determining the presence of an IOFB or associated complications when confronted with opaque vitreous. The findings of additional complications on ancillary testing determine the course and timing of surgical intervention.

Vitreous Hemorrhage

Vitreous hemorrhage initially does not cause damage. However, the organization of the hemorrhage, its fibrocellular contents, and inflammatory elements from the initial injury within the vitreous scaffold promote the development of fibrous contractile tissue. This tissue contracts over time, causing either traction on the retina and ciliary body and subsequent tractional retinal detachment or hypotony. This retinal traction, which can be anterior–posterior, circumferential, or subretinal, is directly attributable to the initial penetrating injury.[17]

Retinal Tears and Detachments

A retinal tear or break occurs either when the IOFB strikes or embeds in the retina or from the mechanical blunt trauma of the IOFB striking the globe. This complication may be obscured by a dense vitreous hemorrhage and so may not be detected initially. Unrecognized retinal tears or breaks can be the source for rhegmatogenous (rhegma, Greek for *rent*) retinal detachments. Early recognition of these tears or breaks and appropriate management may prevent retinal detachments (Figure 14-2).

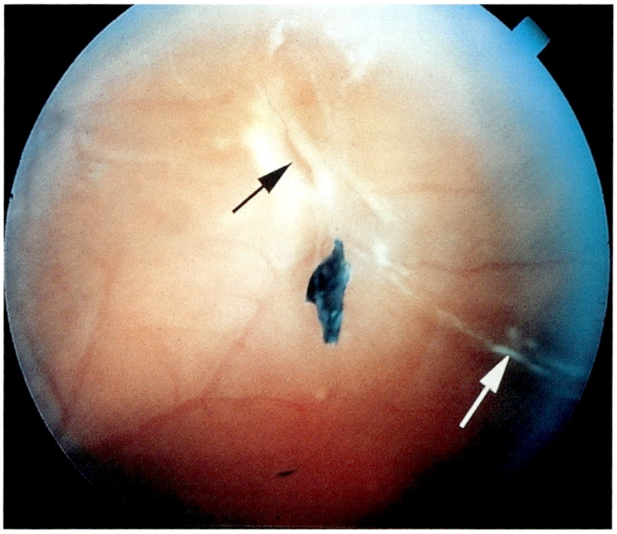

Fig. 14-2. This posterior segment photograph reveals a black retained metallic intraocular foreign body (IOFB, center) within the vitreous and the associated retinal detachment. The IOFB struck the retina, creating a retinal hole (dark arrow) causing this retinal detachment. A track of old vitreous blood is seen streaking from the entry wound to the retinal hole (white arrow). Photograph: Courtesy of Ophthalmology Service, Brooke Army Medical Center, Fort Sam Houston, Tex.

Retinal detachments, either rhegmatogenous or tractional, can complicate these penetrating injuries. Tractional detachments typically occur days to weeks after the injury. A rhegmatogenous retinal detachment is frequently a result of the initial trauma. This complication results from retinal lacerations or retinal breaks as a result of the mechanical disruption of the retina, the vitreous, or both.

Although an acute retinal detachment may be obscured by dense vitreous hemorrhage, it can easily be detected with echography. Echography should be performed as soon as safety permits, because the detection of an early retinal detachment would prompt pars plana vitrectomy. These detachments frequently do well with vitreoretinal surgery. Reactivation of intraocular bleeding during early repair of traumatic retinal detachment usually portends a poorer prognosis and can frequently be avoided if vitrectomy is delayed from 7 to 14 days.[18]

Incarceration of the retina, specifically posteriorly, through the sclera generally has a poorer prognosis. Either posterior extraction of the subretinal or intraretinal IOFB or impaction of the FB into the sclera causes retinal incarceration. This incarceration results in retinal traction, which frequently leads to retinal tears and detachment. This complication is repaired using scleral buckling, vitreoretinal techniques, or both.

Endophthalmitis

Infectious endophthalmitis is an uncommon but urgent concern when associated with a retained IOFB. The incidence of endophthalmitis with a retained IOFB is approximately 7% to 13%.[13,19] Compounding this complication is the difficulty in diagnosing endophthalmitis in the setting of acute trauma.[7,19–23] Several factors determine whether the severely injured eye develops clinical endophthalmitis. One series[22] reported 26% of eyes with positive surveillance intraocular cultures, although only 13% developed culture-proven endophthalmitis. Of particular note, a high incidence of *Bacillus cereus* endophthalmitis associated with retained IOFB has been reported[7,24] with rapid clinical onset and abysmal loss of vision and the eye. *Bacillus cereus* endophthalmitis is associated with organic contamination of the IOFB from the soil, which may be of particular military significance because of the increased use of landmines.[20] (For additional information, interested readers should consult Chapter 17, Posttraumatic Endophthalmitis, in this textbook.)

Inflammatory Changes and Physiological Effects

Epiretinal membranes are fibrocellular sheets on the surface of the retina that are composed of a variety of cells such as fibrous astrocytes, fibrocytes, retinal pigment epithelial (RPE) cells, macrophages, and fibrous tissue. The formation of an epiretinal membrane is frequently caused by penetrating injuries and is due to the presence of blood in the vitreous, choroidal hemorrhage under the retina, or a hole or tear in the retina. The contraction of these cellular elements contorts the retinal surface and distorts central vision. Cystoid macular edema and retinal traction can also result from these membranes. Epiretinal membranes may account for poor central vision despite successful IOFB removal.[25]

The physiological effects of a retained IOFB depend on its composition and whether it generates an inflammatory response (Exhibit 14-1). An acute inflammatory reaction surrounding the IOFB can obscure its location or cause adhesion between the vitreous and the retina. This fibrous tissue can cause traction or rhegmatogenous retinal detachments. An IOFB composed of iron or copper retained for a prolonged period of time can result in siderosis (iron) or chalcosis (copper), as discussed in Chapter 15, Metallosis Bulbi.

Although initial management of metallic IOFBs frequently involves their removal, recent evidence suggests that in certain cases, patients with retained IOFBs may do well with careful observation and monitoring.[26] The indication for removal depends more on the associated trauma created by the IOFB than the FB itself. The presence of mitigating factors, such as a small, peripheral entry site, minimal vitreous hemorrhaging, absence of traumatic cataract, lack of retinal holes or tears, or minimal peripheral vitreoretinal traction would allow close observation rather than immediate removal of the IOFB. However, a large entry site, significant vitreous hemorrhage, possible retinal holes or tears, retinal traction, or retinal detachment would suggest intervention with pars plana vitrectomy and IOFB removal.

Sympathetic Ophthalmia

Sympathetic ophthalmia is a rare complication of penetrating injuries with an IOFB; there have been no reported cases in military conflicts since World War II.[27–30] Five enucleated eyes from World War II were examined at the Armed Forces Institute of Pathology. Four eyes contained nonmagnetic

EXHIBIT 14-1

COMPOSITION OF INTRAOCULAR FOREIGN BODIES

Inert or Precious Metals
- Glass
- Porcelain
- Plastic
- Gunpowder
- Sand
- Coal
- Concrete
- Rubber (organic)
- Silver
- Quartz
- Stone
- Rock
- Cordite
- Clay
- Carbon
- Solder (two parts lead to one part tin)
- Gold
- Platinum

Somewhat Inert
- Lead (shot)
- Zinc
- Aluminum
- Cotton fiber

Inflammatory
- Copper
- Nickel
- Steel
- Iron
- Mercury
- Vegetable matter (contaminated)

Source: Duke-Elder S, MacFaul P. Inert materials. In: Duke-Elder S, ed. *System of Ophthalmology*. Vol 14. St Louis, Mo: CV Mosby; 1972: 501–551.

IOFBs, whereas the fifth contained a metallic IOFB. Most of the patients involved had retained the IOFBs for 2 months to 36 years with vague clinical histories.[31] Clearly, advances in managing penetrating trauma have nearly eliminated this devastating complication. (For further information, interested readers should see Chapter 16, Sympathetic Ophthalmia, in this textbook.

CLINICAL HISTORY AND EXAMINATION

Military ophthalmologists should understand and utilize the latest classification for mechanical injuries of the eye, such as the Ocular Trauma Classification Group[32] or the proposed Madigan Eye and Orbit Trauma Scale (MEOTS),[33] which are used to standardize how ocular trauma is classified and how outcomes are reported. (For further information, see Chapter 6, Ocular Trauma Scales.) For example, the Ocular Trauma Classification Group system uses the type of injury, the grade of visual acuity, pupil reactivity, and the location of injury for purposes of standardization and prognostic significance. Using this classification, an eye with a retained IOFB would be classified as an open globe injury with laceration and IOFB. The grade is based on the visual acuity, the presence or absence of an afferent pupillary defect, and the location of the penetration by zone. Consistent use of one or the other classification groups can improve communication between specialists.

History

Although basic techniques in the ocular history and examination were covered previously (see Chapter 3, Ocular Trauma: History and Examination), specific salient features related to IOFBs are important for proper management. A complete accounting of the nature and circumstances of the initial and associated injuries is vital. This information should be obtained directly from the patient, indirectly from accompanying individuals, or from the triage card accompanying the soldier. The circumstances surrounding the initial injury are helpful when discerning the risk of an IOFB (eg, was the patient using a tool while repairing a vehicle, working with explosives, or surrounded by exploding shells and gunfire?). It is also helpful to know if protective eyewear or glasses were worn.

While documenting the ocular history, the past ocular history is important for determining the visual prognosis. A history of poor vision from preexisting disease or trauma is common and may be related to a history of amblyopia (crossed eyes or lazy eye), previous ocular trauma, or surgery. For disability and medicolegal considerations, determining a preinjury visual acuity is beneficial.

Previous ocular surgical interventions related to the initial injury must be clearly documented as the patient proceeds through the military health care system. From the time of injury until final disposition, a careful detailed accounting of procedures, including tetanus history and diagnostic tests, should be documented and transferred with the patient. The details and timing of primary globe repair, observations at the time of surgery to include the extent of the wound, management of prolapsing intraocular contents, and associated complications during the repair need to be documented clearly. Should intraocular tissue be removed during the initial repair of the globe, the histopathological findings should be forwarded with the patient's record. This information is essential when determining further management. The use of prophylactic antibiotics, route of administration, duration, and type should be documented for assisting subsequent management. Notation of the best visual acuity following initial repair is also beneficial when determining subsequent management.

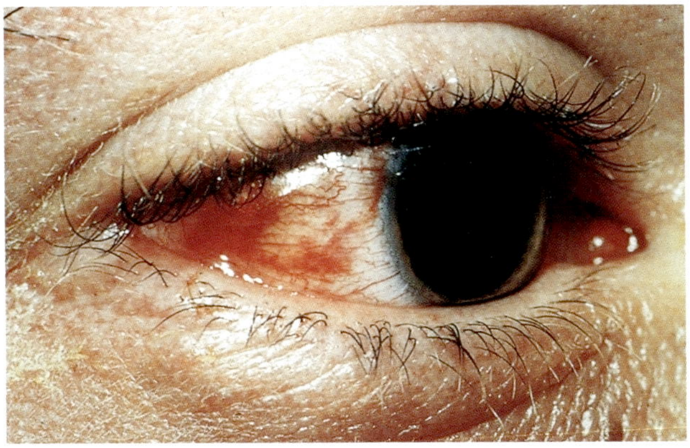

Fig. 14-3. External photograph showing a subconjunctival hemorrhage covering the penetration site of a retained intraocular foreign body (IOFB). A penetration site from a small foreign body frequently appears harmless; a high index of suspicion based on clinical history leads to a dilated posterior segment examination with discovery of the IOFB or other signs suggestive of the presence of a foreign body. Photograph: Courtesy of Ophthalmology Service, Brooke Army Medical Center, Fort Sam Houston, Tex.

Examination

A complete ocular examination is critical to determine the extent and degree of the injury. Direct visualization is the best diagnostic method for determining type, quantity, and potential composition of the IOFB. General anesthesia may be required to perform a thorough eye examination safely without further extruding intraocular contents.

All traumatic ocular injuries need to have an initial visual acuity documented. The presenting visual acuity is the most important prognostic indicator for final visual outcome. Since an initial vi-

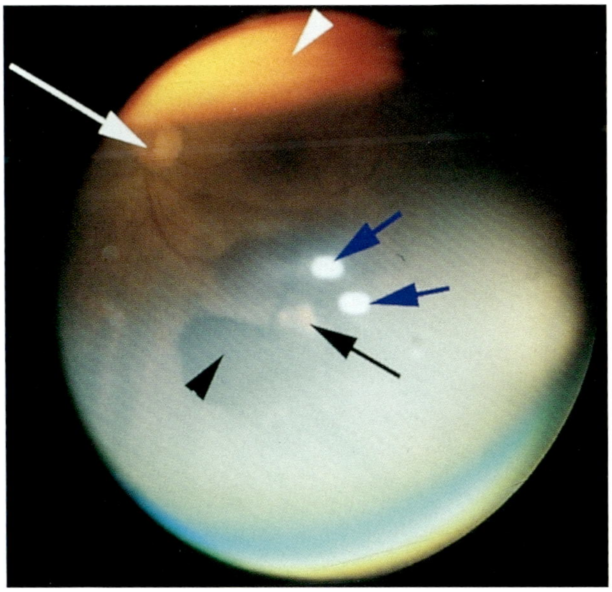

Fig. 14-4. This fundus photograph through a 20-diopter lens shows a fresh preretinal hemorrhage (black arrowhead) nearly covering a retained intraocular foreign body (IOFB; black arrow). Prompt retinal examination through a dilated pupil is critical to visualize the IOFB before hemorrhage, inflammation, or cataract obscures the view. The optic nerve (white arrow) and retinal arteries and veins are noted. The two elliptical white spots (blue arrows) and the orange ellipse (white arrowhead) are light reflections. Photograph: Courtesy of Ophthalmology Service, Brooke Army Medical Center, Fort Sam Houston, Tex.

sual acuity of no light perception (NLP) carries a grave prognosis, assessment using the light source from the indirect ophthalmoscope set on high intensity is essential. Careful attention in patching the uninjured eye or covering it well when eliciting light perception is important in verifying NLP of the injured eye.

The presence or absence of an afferent pupillary defect (APD) also has prognostic implications. Some series suggest a worse prognosis for patients presenting with an initial APD.[12]

Clues from the motility and slitlamp examinations can support the presence of an open globe. The motility of the eye may be restricted because of a lack of scleral integrity from the perforation or penetration. Slitlamp biomicroscopy aids in detecting subtle conjunctival chemosis, subconjunctival hemorrhage (Figure 14-3), penetration or laceration of the cornea or limbus, deepened anterior chamber, microscopic or frank hyphema, as well as FBs of the cornea, anterior chamber, iris, and crystalline lens. Careful inspection of the anterior vitreous may reveal hemorrhage or stranding of the vitreous mixed with blood extending from the site of ocular penetration into the eye.

Prompt fundus examination of ocular trauma is imperative. Delay in examining a penetrating injury with a retained IOFB may result in an obscured view of the IOFB or retina from hyphema, cataract formation, or vitreous hemorrhage (Figure 14-4). Other complications such as a retinal tear, detachment, or dialysis may be missed or unsuspected. The examiner should note all IOFBs and their locations. A drawing of the retina to document the location and size of the IOFBs and associated complications is beneficial. This drawing should accompany the patient. A clue to the location of the IOFB is stranding of the vitreous and blood tracking to the resting location of the IOFB within the vitreous, retina, choroid, or exit site from the globe (see Figure 14-2).

DIAGNOSTIC IMAGING

In addition to the complete ocular examination, imaging of an ocular penetrating injury to rule out the presence of an IOFB is critical to the visual outcome of the eye. If corneal edema, hyphema, traumatic cataract, or vitreous hemorrhage preclude a thorough posterior segment evaluation for a retained IOFB, ancillary studies such as echography, radiographic imaging, or computed tomography (CT) should be performed to exclude a retained FB. Magnetic resonance imaging (MRI) should be discouraged because the strong magnetic fields generated can shift iron-containing FBs and create further intraocular damage. However, should a CT confirm a nonmetallic IOFB, an MRI would be superior to CT for detecting a piece of wood or plastic ranging in size from 3 to 5 mm.[34]

Plain Film Radiography

When used in conjunction with a clinical examination suggesting a possible IOFB, plain film radiographs are useful for identifying and localizing the object. Bray and Griffiths[35] reported that in no case was an IOFB detected on plain film radiograph without evidence of ocular penetration. The presence of any media opacification to the posterior segment should alert the examiner to the potential for an IOFB.

In battlefield settings, the use of dental film with dental X-ray capability can determine the presence or absence of a metallic IOFB. Wood and plastic are not visualized as easily.

Computed Tomography

As was discussed in Chapter 4, Imaging of Ocular and Adnexal Trauma, localization of an IOFB by CT is considered the standard. Thin, 1.5-mm axial sections at 1-mm intervals provide overlapping images (called stacks) and can frequently detect even the smallest IOFBs. CT imaging can detect an IOFB as small as 0.048 mm^3 for metallic objects and 1.82 mm^3 for automobile glass.[36,37] Advantages of CT scanning include the need for only minimal patient cooperation, no need for contact with the globe, the ability to localize anterior FBs, and the ability to image nonopaque materials such as wood, plastic, and glass.[38]

Nevertheless, CT scanning can miss multiple, small IOFBs that are masked by scanning artifacts cast by larger adjacent IOFBs (Figure 14-5). Wood and plastic are poorly imaged, and IOFBs that either are embedded in the retina or located posterior to the globe are frequently missed.[39,40] One report[40] suggests that metallic IOFBs smaller than 1 mm in size are difficult to image.

Echography

Echography (or ultrasonography) is excellent for detecting and localizing an IOFB and for assessing intraocular complications. However, *direct-contact echography of a suspected open globe is contraindicated for fear of expelling intraocular contents.* With the ad-

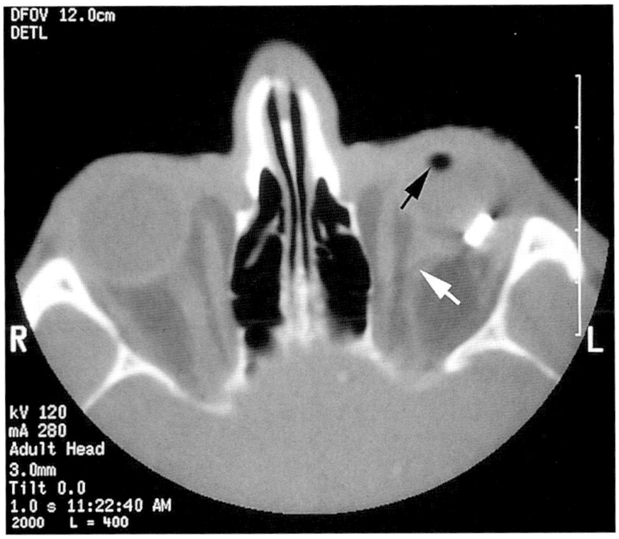

Fig. 14-5. A computed tomography (CT) scan of a large retained intraocular foreign body (IOFB, white rectangle) with intraocular air (black arrow) and radiating scanning artifact from the metallic IOFB (white arrow). Computed tomography scan: Courtesy of Ophthalmology Service, Brooke Army Medical Center, Fort Sam Houston, Tex.

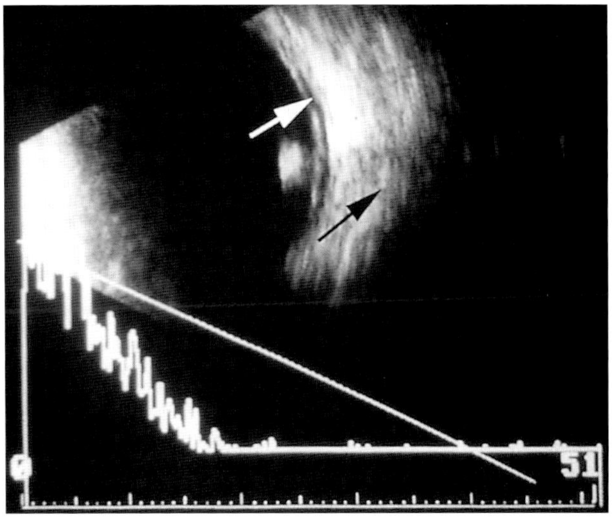

Fig. 14-7. A combined A- and B-scan ultrasound of a penetrating injury with retained metallic intraocular foreign body (IOFB). The vector line for the A-scan has been moved to show the shadowing behind the IOFB and the anechoic zone extending into the sclera (black arrow). Note the low-lying retinal detachment caused by a hole from the IOFB (white arrow). Echography scan: Courtesy of Ophthalmology Service, Brooke Army Medical Center, Fort Sam Houston, Tex.

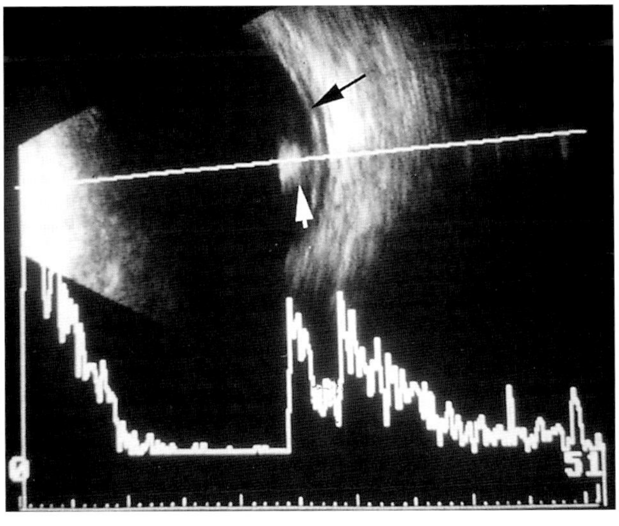

Fig. 14-6. A combined A- and B-scan ultrasound of a penetrating injury with retained metallic intraocular foreign body (IOFB). The vector line for the A-scan passes through the metallic foreign body and indicates an initial high reflectivity spike and high internal echoes, indicated by the A-scan scale at the bottom of the scan. On the B-scan, the white arrow demonstrates "tailing" of echoes posterior to the metallic foreign body. The black arrow shows a low-lying retinal detachment. Echography scan: Courtesy of Ophthalmology Service, Brooke Army Medical Center, Fort Sam Houston, Tex.

vances in electronic miniaturization, portable echography is readily available at forward locations on the battlefield to evaluate ocular injuries with an IOFB. Ultrasonic characteristics of an IOFB include

- high initial reflectivity,
- high internal echoes,
- tailing of echoes behind the IOFB, and
- shadowing behind the FB from absorbed sound waves, which result in an anechoic zone behind the IOFB (Figures 14-6 and 14-7).

The IOFB can be located by using as landmarks other ocular structures or tissue changes such as vitreous hemorrhage, choroidal detachment, and retinal detachment.

Studies also show that echography can determine the extent of such injuries as retinal detachment, subretinal hemorrhage, massive choroidal effusions, and hemorrhage that affect the visual prognosis. This information affects decisions about the surgical removal of the IOFB.[41,42] Echography after globe repair is also helpful for establishing other complications such as retinal detachment.

MANAGEMENT

The meticulous, prompt closure of any breach of the globe is a prerequisite for successful management of a retained IOFB. Whether IOFB removal is immediate or delayed, the importance of reestablishing ocular anatomical integrity is vital to ensure return of most physiological functions of the eye while awaiting further surgical management. Furthermore, the longer the globe remains open or decompressed, the greater the risk of complications (eg, expulsion of intraocular contents, serous or hemorrhagic exudation, corneal decompensation, expulsive hemorrhage, fibrous/endothelial downgrowth, endophthalmitis, progressing cataract formation, ciliary body detachment or hemorrhage, retinal detachment, proliferative vitreo-retinopathy). All these complications related to delayed globe repair often result in poorer visual prognoses.

Prompt closure also promotes healing and fibrosis at the entry site. These wounds must be made watertight to permit further reparative procedures such as scleral buckling and pars plana vitrectomy. Finally, reestablishment of ocular integrity permits safe evacuation to tertiary care facilities for management of complications secondary to the penetrating injury and the IOFB.

Primary Management

Immediate Globe Closure Without Primary Removal of IOFB

The decision whether to remove an IOFB in conjunction with the primary repair of the penetrating injury hinges on several factors. The primary ophthalmologist may lack the experience, proper microsurgical equipment, or ancillary support for managing the ocular complications of the initial injury or from the IOFB. Vitreoretinal surgeons, on the other hand, are trained to manage IOFBs and associated intraocular complications but are rarely located at forward medical care areas. Therefore, patients with this type of injury require prompt evacuation to support areas.

The primary ophthalmologist should close the globe primarily and evacuate the patient—as soon as he or she is stable for transport—for further reparative and rehabilitative care. The patient should not be given anticoagulants or antiplatelet agents because these could cause further intraocular hemorrhage and complications. Following the initial globe repair, complications (eg, hyphema, endophthalmitis, lens-induced glaucoma) should be monitored closely and treated promptly prior to evacuation. The primary ophthalmologist should consider prophylactic treatment of these complications, because patients are not accompanied by ophthalmologists en route to tertiary care facilities. *There is no monitoring of vision-threatening complications during patient transport in the aeromedical evacuation system.*

Some benefits may be realized by delaying removal of retained IOFBs. The literature suggests that delayed vitrectomy surgery (defined as more than 3 d but within 14 d of the initial repair) may be beneficial. By delaying surgery, the vitreous hemorrhage may promote a posterior vitreous detachment that can simplify the vitrectomy and other microsurgical techniques in removing an IOFB or repositioning a detached retina.

If the IOFB is not removed primarily following primary globe repair, the use of broad-spectrum prophylactic intravenous, subconjunctival, and topical antibiotics is indicated. Penetrating ocular injuries with an IOFB have a 7%[19] to 26%[20] risk of endophthalmitis. Unlike normal eyes, in which intravenous antibiotics have poor intravitreal penetration, in eyes with a penetrated globe, bactericidal levels are achieved when treating posttraumatic endophthalmitis caused by Gram-positive microorganisms.[43] Furthermore, adequate prophylaxis should be considered because the patient will spend many hours or days in the aeromedical evacuation system without observation by an ophthalmologist for endophthalmitis.

The disadvantages of delayed removal of IOFBs include development of media opacification from the cornea, hyphema, lens opacification, vitreous hemorrhage, and reactive inflammation. In addition, encapsulation of the IOFB may complicate later removal. These disadvantageous are, in general, manageable with modern vitreoretinal techniques.

Immediate Globe Closure With Primary Removal of IOFB

Factors to consider in primary removal of an IOFB in conjunction with wound repair include the complexity of the injury, the location of the IOFB, the experience of the surgeon, the availability of micro-vitreoretinal instruments, the ability to ensure proper repositioning of intraocular contents, and the ability to handle complications of such removal. Some authors[44] suggest removing an IOFB immediately during primary repair of an open globe, reasoning that the IOFB can incite intraocular inflammation, which can result in encapsulation of the IOFB and cause a difficult future removal. An additional indication for primary removal is to reduce local toxic effects of the IOFB.

A more compelling reason for immediate removal is that there is an increased incidence of endophthalmitis associated with IOFBs. In the setting of penetrating trauma, diagnosing endophthalmitis is difficult. Associated findings from the penetrating injury itself include severe eyelid edema, conjunctival chemosis, corneal haze, hypopyon, vitreous inflammation, and/or retinal necrosis, all of which mask the key features of endophthalmitis. Should the appropriate personnel and equipment be present for IOFB removal, and if the IOFB is easily accessible at the time of primary closure, then early IOFB removal at that time is acceptable.

Observation

The removal of an IOFB is based on balancing the risk of ocular complications against the benefits of potential vision. Clearly, a reactive IOFB (usually copper or iron) should be removed promptly to avoid metal toxicity and intense inflammation. Also, an IOFB contaminated with organic material poses an increased risk of bacterial endophthalmitis. Inert materials (see Exhibit 14-1) pose a difficult management decision. In the absence of complications or symptoms, observation of an IOFB is indicated for small, inert, or chronically encapsulated IOFBs. Reports from the Iran–Iraq War (1980–1988)[8] and Israel[26] suggest that careful observation of retained IOFBs may be safe without secondary complications and with preservation of visual acuity of 20/80 or better, despite the presence of an IOFB over several years.

External Magnet Extraction of Retained IOFB

Improved intraocular vitreoretinal techniques permit a controlled and direct means of removing an IOFB and dealing with intraocular complications. Intraocular removal of an IOFB has generally replaced external magnetic techniques for removing an IOFB. However, before modern vitreoretinal techniques came into use, immediate removal of the IOFB was facilitated with external magnets. These magnets are either electromagnetic or of rare earth metals. Considerable literature exists supporting the use of external magnets for the prompt removal of a magnetic IOFB, although most vitreoretinal surgeons consider that the use of magnets has been superseded by modern intraocular techniques. The Bronson magnet is a cumbersome, handheld device still in use in many locations (Figure 14-8). Its advantages include powerful graduated force with interchangeable tips. It is particularly good for anterior segment IOFBs. The disadvantages include bulkiness, possibility of incorrect use, and the fact that

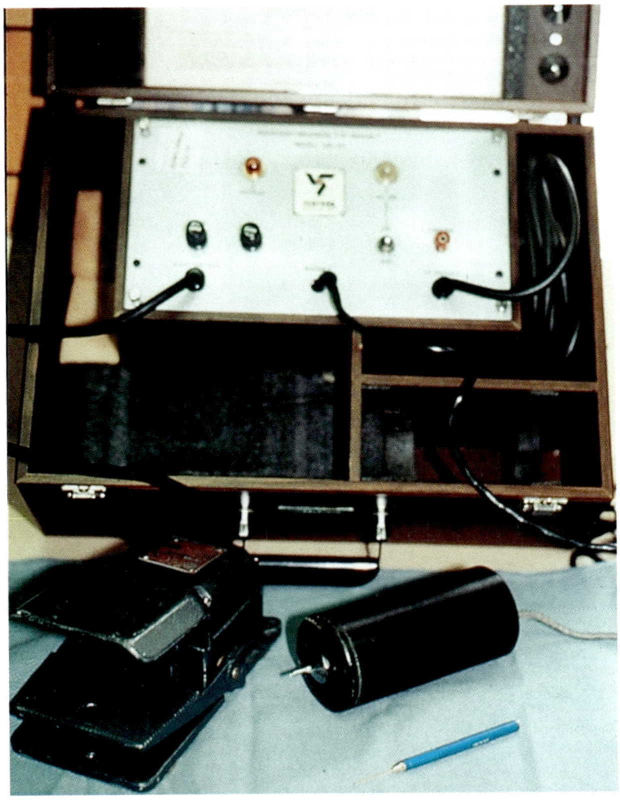

Fig. 14-8. The Bronson electromagnet, consisting of the amplifier box, foot pedal, and a large, handheld magnet.

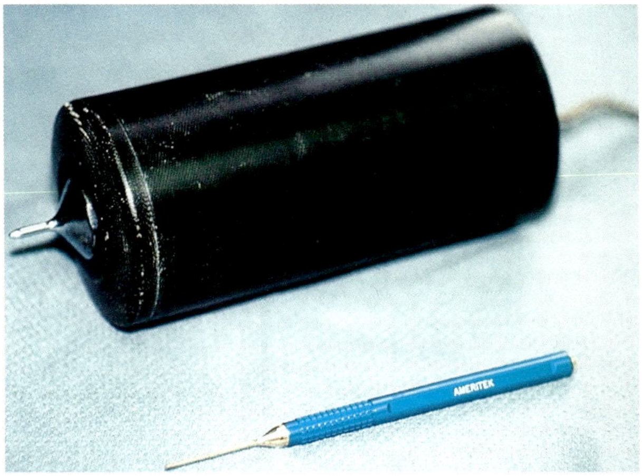

Fig. 14-9. The large Bronson electromagnet with the fine point attachment (top) is compared with the rare earth intraocular magnet (bottom).

no metallic items can be near the eye during use. A smaller electromagnetic magnet is the JEDMED, which sacrifices power for size. Intraocular rare earth magnets lose up to 15% of their force per year and require remagnetizing yearly (Figure 14-9).

An IOFB in the posterior segment is more challenging to properly remove using the external magnet. Careful case selection is important. Small, posterior-segment IOFBs that are positioned within the midvitreous, located anteriorly, and associated with minimal vitreous hemorrhage are ideal candidates for extraction through a sclerotomy at the pars plana. IOFB removal in eyes with intraretinal hemorrhage, fibrous encapsulation, or copious amounts of vitreous hemorrhage should be avoided. When the IOFB is encased in fibrous tissue or lying directly on the retina, manipulation with an external magnet can result in retinal tears and detachments.[45]

Enucleation

Following a penetrating injury with IOFB, an eye may appear to be severely and irreparably damaged. Careful inspection, however, often reveals no loss of scleral or corneal tissue. Generally, eyes with retained pellets or BBs have a poor visual prognosis, although the globe may be salvaged. As a general principle, *do not enucleate an injured eye primarily unless restoration of the globe is impossible.*

Careful documentation of NLP vision as outlined previously is important. Although the prognosis of an eye with an initial vision of NLP is poor, the globe may be salvageable. Useful vision has been regained in eyes with dense vitreous hemorrhages and small IOFBs after pars plana vitrectomy. The use of the intense indirect ophthalmoscope light is very important in evaluating for NLP.

Summary of Primary Management

Although there may be subtle variations in the primary management of a penetrating globe injury with retained IOFB, the principles of prompt globe repair and referral to an experienced posterior-segment surgeon are key for salvaging any useful vision. A summary and decision tree on the management of these injuries is seen in Figure 14-10.

Secondary Management

Anterior Segment Management

Numerous factors play important roles in the decision about when to remove an IOFB. Generally, the eye is surgically closed and the decision to extract the IOFB is left to the vitreoretinal specialist, who is qualified in the instrumentation and manipulation of the retina. Should the eye recover somewhat normal anatomical and physiological function following initial repair of the penetrating or perforating site, the patient is transported within 72 hours or when deemed stable to a vitreoretinal specialist for definitive care.

The postoperative visual acuity following the initial repair of the penetrated or perforated globe weighs heavily in the decision to pursue additional reparative processes. If the preoperative and postoperative vision assessments are NLP, and if there is no anatomical reconstitution of the globe, then the military vitreoretinal surgeon should consider performing an enucleation to decrease the risk of sympathetic ophthalmia. Improved vitreoretinal techniques now offer the possibility of ocular preservation and visual restoration in cases previously considered hopeless. In most situations, however, a patient with prolonged NLP vision does not recover any vision and is usually managed with an enucleation.

Using vitreoretinal techniques, the vitreoretinal surgeon secures and stabilizes structures beginning from the anterior segment proceeding to the posterior segment. Thus, the integrity of the cornea, anterior chamber, iris, and lens is ensured before the posterior segment is addressed. Failure to stabilize structures in the anterior segment frequently limits the visualization of the posterior segment. Without good visualization, vitreoretinal techniques are of limited value.

Should the cornea be cloudy from endothelial folds or decompensation from the initial trauma or repair, a period of watchful waiting to permit recovery of corneal endothelium function can facilitate the view of the posterior segment. On average, in a healthy person and in the absence of any preexisting corneal disease, the cornea may regain its clear translucent appearance within 3 to 7 days to permit adequate viewing of the posterior segment. During this watchful waiting, sutured penetrated sites can continue to heal and scar. These fibrosed sites can then tolerate the higher internal pressure required by pars plana vitrectomy. In addition, this waiting can allow clearing of blood in the anterior chamber and reestablishment of the blood-aqueous barrier. On the other hand, factors against waiting for this clearing process include violation of the lens capsule, which can leak a high concentration of lens protein. The lens protein attracts inflammatory cells, resulting in intense anterior chamber inflammation

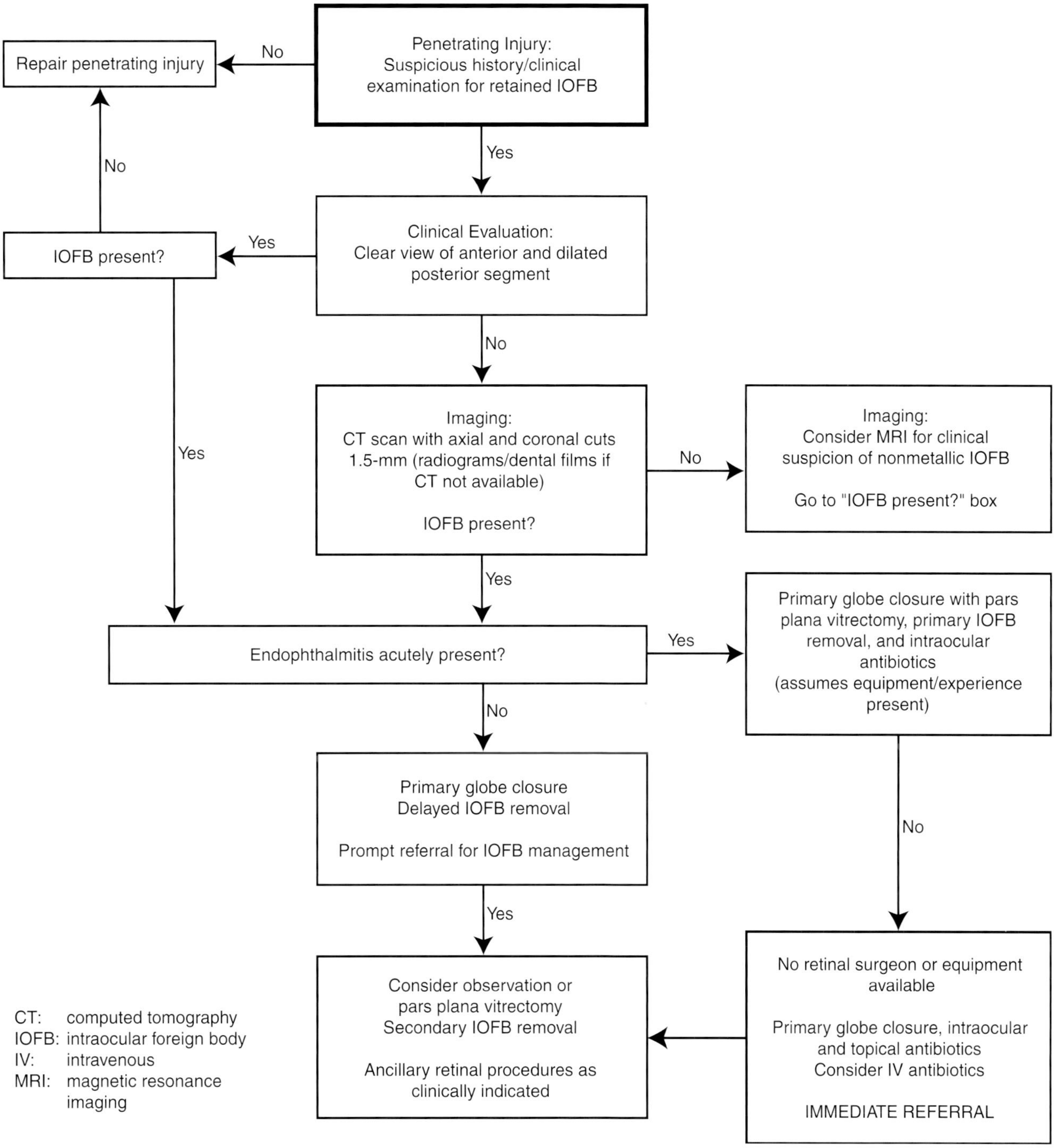

Fig. 14-10. Decision tree: Primary management of penetrating injuries with retained intraocular foreign bodies.

and a rise in the intraocular pressure. This inflammatory glaucoma compromises the corneal endothelium. To maintain a clear cornea, in this scenario, surgery must occur sooner.

When circumstances require intervention sooner or when the view of the posterior segment is compromised, the native cornea may be centrally excised and replaced with a temporary keratoprosthesis (KP). This highly refractive glass or silicon lens is secured with sutures and allows a clear view to the posterior segment for delicate vitreoretinal work (Figure 14-11). After the removal of the native cornea and before the placement of the KP lens, any blood, lens particles, or inflammatory debris is

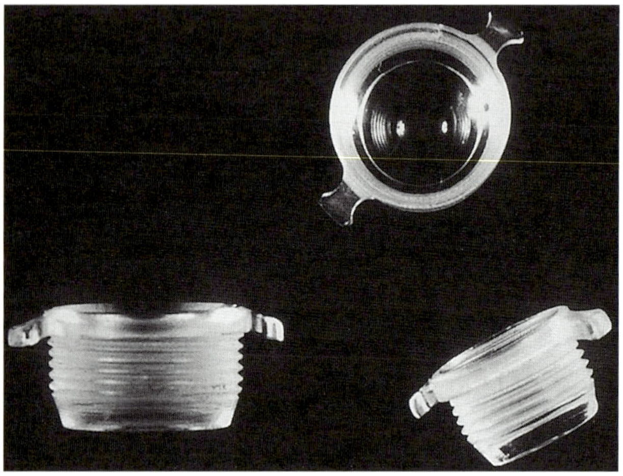

Fig. 14-11. Examples of the high-index, glass Landers-Foulks temporary keratoprosthesis (KP). Note the two flanges on the surface for suturing the KP to the globe.

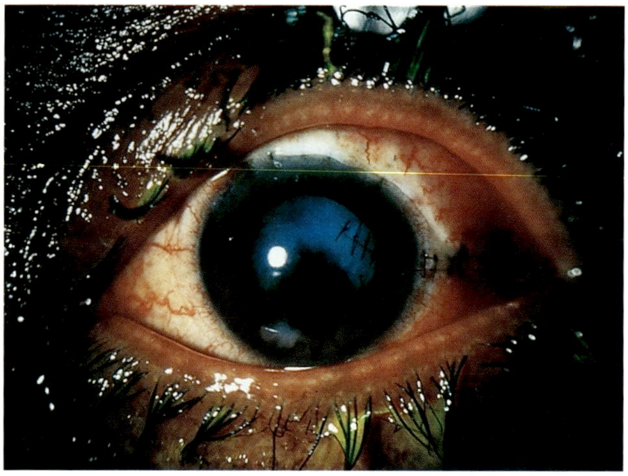

Fig. 14-12. An external photograph shows a sutured corneoscleral laceration with a white traumatic cataract. Note the fluffy cortex in the inferior anterior chamber. A black aperture is noted along the inferior margin of the cataract where the intraocular foreign body (IOFB) perforated the lens. Photograph: Courtesy of Ophthalmology Service, Brooke Army Medical Center, Fort Sam Houston, Tex.

removed from the anterior chamber. The surgeon avoids incising the iris to prevent uncontrolled bleeding and further visual compromise. Once in place, the KP permits a clear, unobstructed view of the posterior segment. In addition, the KP facilitates a closed pressurized system for intraocular surgery and allows multiple vitreoretinal techniques to be performed during one surgery.

The KP offers a chance to salvage otherwise doomed eyes. For large IOFBs, one flange of the KP is released to permit retrieval anteriorly through the open cornea. Smaller IOFBs are removed at the pars plana. Once the intraocular surgery is completed, the KP is replaced with a donor cornea secured in place with 10-0 nylon sutures (ie, penetrating keratoplasty). Results in the use of the KP are mixed, due primarily to the severity of the initial trauma. Using the Landers-Foulks KP, 60% of noncombat eyes retained some vision, whereas 60% of the combat injuries had no vision,[46] although these results most likely reflect the severity of the initial injury rather then the use of the KP.

The next anatomical barrier to successful removal of IOFBs is the crystalline lens. In those cases where the IOFB entry site spares the lens, preserving lens integrity improves the chances of visual recovery. Therefore, surgical removal of the IOFB through the pars plana frequently preserves lens clarity. Successful removal of the IOFB, maintenance of lens clarity, and restoration of normal retina anatomy with no complications can preserve good visual acuity. However, should the anatomical integrity of the lens be compromised by the initial trauma, the primary surgical repair, or the secondary repair, then the lens can be removed in its entirety to permit visualization of the posterior segment and prevent the complications of lens-induced glaucoma (Figure 14-12). The surgical approach for the lentectomy (lensectomy) can be either anterior (through the anterior chamber) or posterior via the pars plana. Generally, the pars plana approach is preferred by vitreoretinal surgeons because (1) additional manipulation of the anterior segment can be avoided and (2) it allows universal access to both the posterior and the anterior segments (Figure 14-13). In certain cases, preservation of the anterior lens capsule during the pars plana lensectomy facilitates placement of an intraocular lens concurrently or at a later date.

An additional barrier to visualization of the posterior segment is at the iris plane. Frequently, a traumatized eye dilates poorly. Management of a miotic pupil is facilitated by flexible iris retractors or sutured retraction of the iris. Both methods are used in aphakic or traumatic cataract eyes. The placement of iris retractors in a phakic eye is avoided to prevent an iatrogenic anterior capsule tear or cataract formation. In addition, a transpupillary fibrin membrane can easily form from a hyphema or inflammation. The membrane can be dissolved with an intraocular injection of tissue plasminogen activator (tPA), surgically sectioned and aspirated, or it

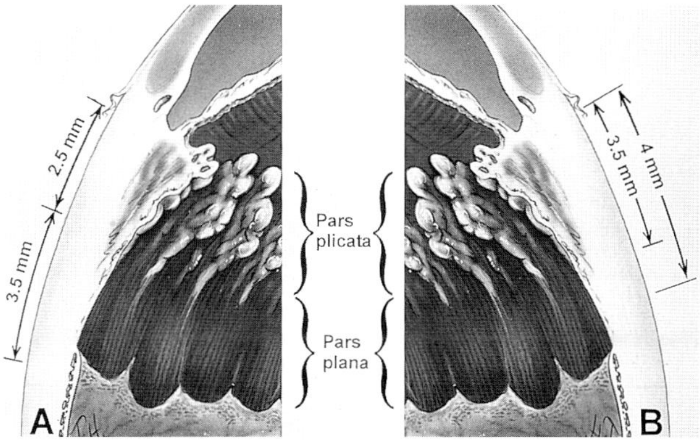

Fig. 14-13. Pars plana anatomy and locations of sclerotomies for vitreoretinal surgery. (**a**) The ciliary body is 7.0 mm in length and is composed of the anterior pars plicata ciliaris and the posterior pars plana ciliaris. The pars plicata measures 2.5 mm in length, whereas the pars plana measures 3.5 mm. The ora serrata, anterior edge of the retina, begins at the posterior margin of the pars plana. (**b**) Safe placement of sclerotomies for access to the vitreous is important to prevent iatrogenic injury to the pars plicata, anterior retina, or the crystalline lens. Sclerotomies are placed 3.5 mm posterior to the surgical limbus (noted by the anterior arrow) for aphakic (without a crystalline lens) and 4.0 mm for phakic (with crystalline lens) eyes. Avoid touching the crystalline lens to prevent an iatrogenic cataract and clouding of the lens during vitreoretinal surgery. Adapted with permission from Wilkinson CP, Rice TA. Anatomy and physiology. In: *Michels Retinal Detachment.* St Louis, Mo: CV Mosby; 1997: 8.

can be sectioned and removed with a vitreoretinal hook or pick to clear the pupillary space. Caution is necessary with the use of tPA because it can cause recurrent bleeding if used soon after the initial trauma.

Posterior Segment Management

Vitreoretinal surgery was modernized in the early 1970s with the introduction of closed intraocular surgery at the pars plana. The pars plana permits a safe posterior approach to the vitreous and retina. It is located between the ciliary body and the ora serrata (the leading edge of the retina). Incision of the sclera at this location is atraumatic and bloodless to the retina and ciliary body. Placement of an infusion cannula, fiberoptic light device, and microsurgical instrumentation (three-port divided instrumentation concept) through scleral incisions permits a closed, pressurized, well-controlled environment for manipulating the intraocular contents and removing the IOFB. Anterior vitrectomy for managing IOFBs is reserved for those cases where removal of the crystalline or damaged lens is anticipated or where the IOFB is so large that removal from an enlarged pars plana sclerotomy would jeopardize the anterior retina, vitreous base, or ciliary body. Anterior vitrectomy enters the eye at or near the corneal limbus. Vitreoretinal surgeons prefer the pars plana approach.

A principal concept of vitrectomy is the extensive removal of the vitreous gel, hemorrhage, and fibrous proliferation in trauma surgery. As mentioned previously in regard to managing penetrating injuries, removal of the vitreous scaffolding reduces the risk of fibrous proliferation and later contraction, which can cause tractional retinal detachment. Timely pars plana vitrectomy decreases the risk of retinal detachment associated with vitreous hemorrhage.[17] The significance of an extensive vitreous hemorrhage in the visual prognosis has been well described[7,10,47] and is discussed in the Prognosis section of this chapter. Furthermore, to remove the IOFB, vitreous attached to the IOFB must be excised, as well as any hemorrhage and inflammatory debris, to avoid direct traction on and potential tearing of the retina.

After all the attached vitreous and debris have been cautiously amputated (with the vitreous cutter), the IOFB, now freely mobile, is transported by intraocular forceps either to a pars plana incision or anteriorly through a corneal limbal incision. Frequently, the pars plana sclerotomy or the corneal limbal incision must be enlarged to ensure adequate space for removing the IOFB. Failure to have an adequate opening can cause the IOFB to be displaced from the forceps; a falling IOFB can strike and possibly damage the retina.

Several intraocular instruments have been used to secure IOFBs. Weak, rare earth intraocular magnets are used through a pars plana sclerotomy to attract a metallic IOFB and transport it to the midvitreous, away from the retina. Then, using intraocular microforceps, the IOFB is firmly grasped in the midvitreous and removed from the eye. The choice of microforceps depends on the size of the IOFB. Microforceps can also be used to retrieve nonmetallic IOFBs from the surface of the retina. The Wilson foreign body forceps has a retractable wire configuration permitting entry through the 1.2-mm pars plana sclerotomy and subsequent deployment of its three prongs for engaging the IOFB (Figures 14-14 and 14-15). A diamond-dusted IOFB forceps is used for larger IOFBs. Careful removal of the forceps and IOFB through the sclerotomy prevents damage to the retina, vitreous base, and ciliary body.

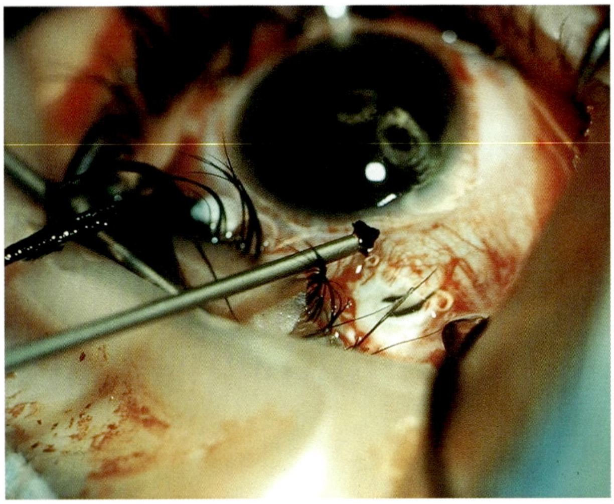

Fig. 14-14. This intraoperative photograph shows the extraction of an intraocular foreign body (IOFB) through the pars plana. The IOFB is shown captured at the end of the Wilson foreign body forceps after its extraction from the globe. Photograph: Courtesy of Ophthalmology Service, Brooke Army Medical Center, Fort Sam Houston, Tex.

Site selection, whether anterior or posterior, for removing the IOFB is important to prevent complications. If the IOFB is smaller than 1.5 mm, removal through the sclerotomy is preferred; to aid removal, the surgeon can enlarge the sclerotomy in a circumferential or in a T-shaped fashion. If the IOFB is larger than 3.0 mm, removal through the limbus or clear cornea can avoid damage to peripheral retina, vitreous base, or ciliary body. In those cases, removal through the anterior segment prevents excessive enlargement of the sclerotomy. Anterior removal is facilitated by the absence of the lens (Figure 14-16).

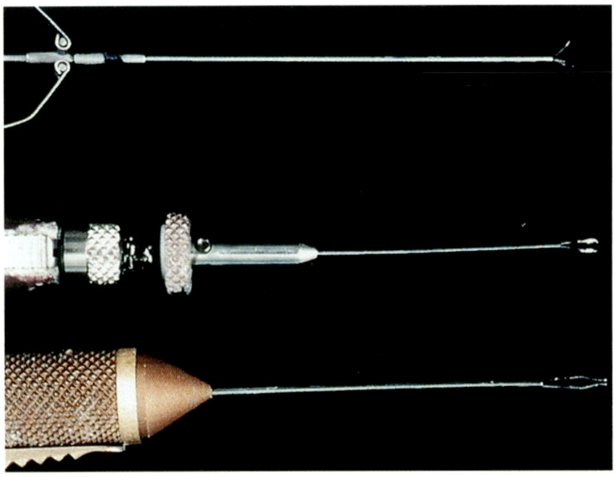

Fig. 14-15. Microforceps commonly used for removing an intraocular foreign body (IOFB). (**a**) The Wilson foreign body forceps with the delicate three-pronged wires deployed. (**b**) An L-shaped microforceps. (**c**) A diamond-dusted forceps for larger IOFBs.

After its removal, appropriate handling of the IOFB is important. An accurate measurement of the size and shape should be made and recorded (this information is helpful for accessing outcomes). The IOFB is then cultured for aerobic organisms (helpful when selecting prophylactic antibiotics or treating endophthalmitis).

Management of Intraocular Complications

The treatment of retinal breaks associated with IOFBs is controversial. Some authors[25,48] suggest some form of retinopexy—either cryopexy or laserpexy—in addition to retinal tamponade with air or gas. The use of cryoretinopexy can disperse intravitreal RPE cells, resulting in epiretinal membranes, proliferative vitreoretinopathy, or tractional retinal detachment. Laser retinopexy may also stimulate fibrous proliferation with epiretinal mem-

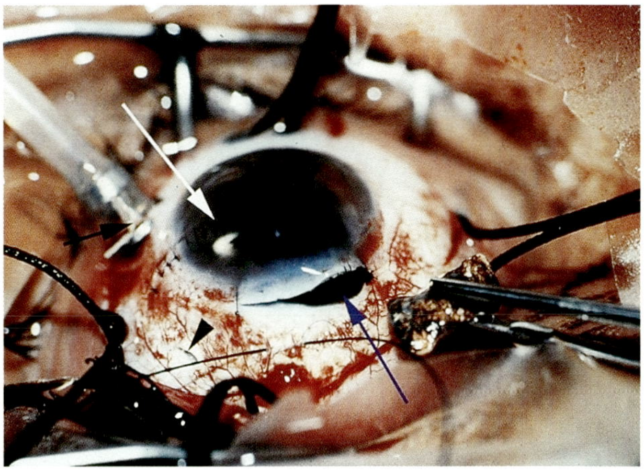

Fig. 14-16. This intraoperative photograph shows the removal of a large intraocular foreign body (IOFB) through a corneal-limbal incision. Note the infusion port (black, left-most arrow), which maintains intraocular pressure during surgery. Vitreoretinal tools are introduced into the eye through the pars plana sclerotomy (dark arrowhead). The iris is prolapsed through the corneal-limbal incision, where this large IOFB was extracted (blue arrow). After successful vitreoretinal surgery, the patient's vision returned to 20/25. The white arrow shows a light reflex. Photograph: Courtesy of Ophthalmology Service, Brooke Army Medical Center, Fort Sam Houston, Tex.

brane formation, but this is more likely with cryoretinopexy. Other authors,[49] however, suggest that posterior segment breaks with associated subretinal hemorrhage can spontaneously develop a chorioretinal adhesion without the need for any mechanical tamponade or cryo/laser retinopexy. A handheld laser probe inserted through the pars plana sclerotomy is used in laser retinopexy within the eye (endolaser). Endolaser is used to create a chorioretinal adhesion between the retina and RPE.

The use of a prophylactic scleral buckle is controversial when managing a penetrating injury with a retained IOFB. A scleral buckle is used mainly to support the retina at the vitreous base to prevent a tractional retinal detachment as fibrous tissue pulls and detaches the peripheral retina. No controlled clinical trials have investigated this issue. One series, which included war injuries, found that the use of a prophylactic scleral buckle resulted in a higher rate of retinal reattachment.[12] Should extensive hemorrhage exist or if the vitreous cannot be removed close to the vitreous base, then a scleral buckle encircling the globe can relieve fibrous traction and potentially prevent a tractional retinal detachment.

The use of prophylactic antibiotics is controversial, as well. To use prophylactic antibiotics appropriately, the surgeon must understand the main causative agents of posttraumatic endophthalmitis: *Staphylococcus epidermidis*, *Bacillus* species, and *Streptococcus* species. Topical, subconjunctival, and intravenous antibiotics are recommended for posttraumatic endophthalmitis prophylaxis.[43] Intracameral or intravitreal antibiotics are not recommended for routine prophylaxis. However, aeromedical personnel must be trained (1) to evaluate the signs and symptoms of endophthalmitis while evacuating the patient to a tertiary care facility and (2) to promptly refer suspected cases for immediate treatment.

Adjuvants for use in vitreoretinal surgery include intraocular agents for temporary tamponade and flattening of the retina. Perfluorocarbon liquids are heavier than water and can be used to reposition the retina. The perfluorocarbon liquid is subsequently removed and replaced with either air, expansile gases (eg, C_3F_8 or SF_6), or silicon oil at the conclusion of the surgery. In some cases, the perfluorocarbon liquid can float the IOFB off the surface of the retina, permitting the vitreoretinal surgeon to grasp it with microforceps and remove it. Caution should be used, however, because the IOFB can slide off the meniscus of the perfluorocarbon liquid and impale the retina, creating a hole or a hemorrhage.

Intraocular expansile gases are reserved for longer tamponade of retinal detachment. After the retina is repositioned against the RPE and lasered, air replaces the aqueous in the posterior segment. To help the retina adhere to the RPE, the air is exchanged for the longer-acting expansile gases. This gas stays within the eye for 2 to 8 weeks, depending on the type and concentration of the gas. *Unfortunately, patients treated with expansile gas should not travel by air because the gas can expand and increase intraocular pressure to dangerous levels, thereby compromising blood supply to the central retinal artery.*[50]

If the retina is firmly adhered to the RPE, the retina remains attached as the gas is resorbed and the poster segment filled with the patient's own aqueous. On the other hand, if fibrous tractional forces are stronger than the chorioretinal adhesion, or if new retinal breaks form or old breaks fail to close, the retina can detach. On occasion, silicon oil is used for long-acting tamponade. This tamponade lasts months but at some point—usually 6 months after the original surgery—the silicon oil is removed to prevent intraocular complications. One of the advantages of using silicon oil is that the patient is able to travel by air.

Postoperative management of vitreoretinal procedures for removing an IOFB includes monitoring for vitreous hemorrhage, endophthalmitis, elevated intraocular pressure, and retinal detachment. Should the lens be salvaged, careful observation for cataract formation and lens-induced glaucoma is important. Prophylactic topical antibiotics, corticosteroids, and cycloplegic agents are used to control postoperative inflammation and pain.

PROGNOSIS

Evaluating the prognosis of penetrating injuries with a retained IOFB is difficult. Frequently, the inciting injury itself causes ocular damage in addition to that resulting from the presence of an IOFB. This damage, too, affects the final visual acuity. The nature, location, extent, and complications from the initial injury frequently have a greater impact on visual outcome or even necessitate enucleation. Although an IOFB itself can cause chemical toxicity or an inflammatory reaction, most series on the management of penetration with an IOFB cite the characteristics of the initial injuries as determinants of prognosis.

With the advent of vitreoretinal surgery, controlled IOFB removal generally has replaced external magnet removal. In a small, uncontrolled study comparing primary external magnetic extraction with pars plana vitrectomy, visual outcomes seemed to favor external magnetic extraction.[51] However, Williams and colleagues[13] found no statistical difference in the postoperative visual acuity when comparing the two methods of removing the IOFB. Case selection, based on the location of the IOFB; its size, composition, and type; the extent of the associated ocular injury; and the experience of the surgeon, are all important for both techniques.

Several factors can determine visual prognosis, including

- the location of the perforation,
- the type of injury,
- initial visual acuity,
- the presence of afferent pupillary defect,
- prolapse of intraocular contents,
- the presence of an IOFB, and
- the presence of vitreous hemorrhage.

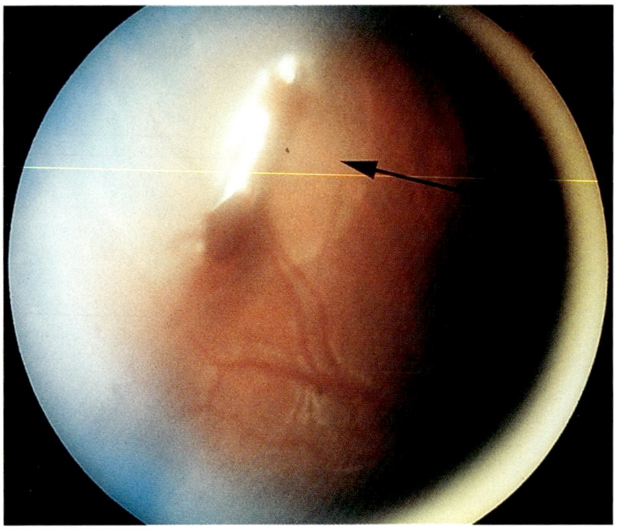

Fig. 14-17. A sharp, pointed metallic intraocular foreign body (IOFB) rests on the retina, covered by a small amount of vitreous hemorrhage in this photograph of the fundus. Note the ring of commotio retinae (arrow) under the IOFB, a result of the initial impact when the IOFB struck the retina. Photograph: Courtesy of Ophthalmology Service, Brooke Army Medical Center, Fort Sam Houston, Tex.

A perforation of the posterior segment frequently portends a poorer visual prognosis, compared with the anterior segment.[10,12,52] Factors that portend a better prognosis include good initial visual acuity; the absence of an afferent pupillary defect; and a small, sharp IOFB (Figure 14-17). A presenting visual acuity of 20/40 to 5/200 is a good prognostic indicator for final visual acuity. Interestingly, if the postoperative visual acuity was better then 5/200, then the chances of obtaining 20/50 vision or better are 40% to 90%.[10,13]

The factors associated with an adverse prognosis include blunt injury, prolapsing intraocular tissue, larger IOFB (> 3 mm in size), larger laceration size, and the presence of extensive vitreous hemorrhage. Penetrating injuries from spherical objects, such as BBs, are known to portend a poorer visual prognosis.[10,12,52]

Few reports directly compare visual outcomes following penetrating injuries with an IOFB sustained in an occupational or domestic setting with those sustained in combat. The effectiveness of modern vitreoretinal techniques, when compared with historical norms in managing these complex cases, suggests that final visual acuity may differ between these groups. Two recent series[8,12] suggest that even with modern vitreoretinal techniques, the visual prognosis of war injuries with an IOFB is worse than for occupational and domestic cases. Frequently, the nature of the injuries and the severe concussive effect of large and multiple missiles is cited in the poorer outcomes.[8,12]

What have improved are enucleation rates for severely traumatized eyes with an IOFB. In the previtrectomy era, occupational and industrial enucleation rates were as high as 20% to 23%, but these have been reduced recently to 3% to 6%.[12,13,53] In combat-related IOFB injuries, there appears to be a trend toward fewer IOFB-related enucleations (see Table 14-1). Reduced enucleation rates may be attributed to vitreoretinal techniques that address secondary complications of the initial injury, the use of intraocular antibiotics, and the combination of vitrectomy and antibiotics in managing posttraumatic endophthalmitis.

SUMMARY

Ocular injuries, although infrequent, are increasing in number as the sophistication of warfare evolves. The management of penetrating ocular injuries with a retained IOFB has also evolved since the 1980s. Maintaining a high index of suspicion, making an early diagnosis, promptly closing open globes, and referring patients without delay to vitreoretinal specialists have all improved the management and outcomes of these serious injuries. Although the nature and extent of the initial injury usually portends the prognosis of vision, newly developed vitreoretinal surgical techniques may save or improve vision from these potentially devastating injuries in future armed conflicts. The actions taken by the general ophthalmologist during the initial management of these ocular injuries are important for salvaging eyesight.

REFERENCES

1. Shimkin NI. Ophthalmic injuries in war. *Br J Ophthalmol.* 1940;24:265–285.

2. Heier JS, Enzenauer RW, Wintermeyer SF, Delaney M, La Piana F. Ocular injuries and diseases at a combat support hospital in support of Operations Desert Shield and Desert Storm. *Arch Ophthalmol.* 1993;111:795–798.

3. Duke-Elder S, MacFaul PA. Retained foreign bodies. In: *Injuries*. Vol 14. In: Duke-Elder, S, ed. *System of Ophthalmology.* St Louis, Mo: CV Mosby; 1972: Chap 4: 477.

4. Dannenberg AL, Parver LM, Brechner RJ, Khoo L. Penetrating eye injuries in the workplace. *Arch Ophthalmol.* 1992;110:843–848.

5. Patel BCK, Morgan LH. Work-related penetrating eye injuries. *Acta Ophthalmol.* 1991;69:377–381.

6. Bauman WC. Intraocular foreign bodies treated at Brooke Army Medical Center, 1982–1993. Unpublished.

7. Brinton GS, Aaberg TM, Reeser FH, Topping TM, Abrahms GW. Surgical results in ocular trauma involving the posterior segment. *Am J Ophthalmol.* 1982;93:271–278.

8. Lashkari K, Lashkari M, Kim A, Crane WG, Jalkh AE. Combat-related eye trauma: A review of 5,320 cases. *Int Ophthalmol Clin.* 1995;35:193–203.

9. Doucet I. The coward's war: Landmines and civilians. *Medicine and War.* 1993;9:304–16.

10. DeJuan E Jr, Sternberg P Jr, Michels RG. Penetrating ocular injuries. *Ophthalmology.* 1983;90:1318–22.

11. Potts AM, Distler JA. Shape factor in the penetration of intraocular foreign bodies. *Am J Ophthalmol.* 1985;100:183–7.

12. Ahmadieh H, Soheilian M, Sajjadi H, Azarmina M, Abrishami M. Vitrectomy in ocular trauma. *Retina.* 1993;13:107–113.

13. Williams DF, Mieler WF, Abrahms GW, Lewis H. Results and prognostic factors in penetrating ocular injuries with retained intraocular foreign bodies. *Ophthalmology.* 1988;95:911–916.

14. Belkin M, Ivry M. Explosive intraocular foreign bodies. *Am J Ophthalmol.* 1978;85:676–678.

15. Haik GM. The management of intraocular foreign bodies in military practice. *Am J Ophthalmol.* 1946;29:815–827.

16. Martin DF, Meredith TA, Topping TM, Sternberg P Jr, Kaplan HJ. Perforating (through-and-through) injuries of the globe. *Arch Ophthalmol.* 1991;109:951–956.

17. Cleary PE, Ryan SJ. Vitrectomy in penetrating eye injury: results of a controlled trial of vitrectomy in an experimental posterior penetrating eye injury in the rhesus monkey. *Arch Ophthalmol.* 1981;99:287–292.

18. Hutton WL. Retinal detachments associated with intraocular foreign bodies. *Mod Probl Ophthalmol.* 1979;20:260–263.

19. Thompson JT, Parver LM, Enger CL, Mieler WF, Liggett PE. Infectious endophthalmitis after penetrating injuries with retained intraocular foreign bodies. *Ophthalmology.* 1993;100:1468–1474.

20. Boldt HC, Pulido JS, Blodi CF, Folk J, Weingeist T. Rural endophthalmitis. *Ophthalmology.* 1989;96:1722–1726.

21. Duch-Samper AM, Menezo JL, Hurtado-Sarrio M. Endophthalmitis following penetrating eye injuries. *Acta Ophthalmol Scand.* 1997;75:104–106.

22. Mieler WF, Ellis MK, Williams DF, Han DP. Retained intraocular foreign bodies and endophthalmitis. *Ophthalmology.* 1990;97:1532–1538.

23. Verbraeken H, Rysselaere M. Post-traumatic endophthalmitis. *Eur J Ophthalmol.* 1994;4:1–5.

24. Schemmer GB, Driebe WT Jr. Post-traumatic *Bacillus cereus* endophthalmitis. *Arch Ophthalmol.* 1987;105:342–344.

25. Slusher MM, Sarin LK, Federman JL. Management of intraretinal foreign bodies. *Ophthalmology.* 1982;89:369–373.

26. Neumann R, Belkin M, Loewenthal E, Gorodetsky R. A long-term follow-up of metallic intraocular foreign bodies, employing diagnostic x-ray spectrometry. *Arch Ophthalmol.* 1992;110:1269–1272.

27. Bell RW. Diagnosis and treatment of intraocular foreign bodies incurred in Vietnam. *Surg Forum.* 1973;24:498–499.

28. Gombos GM. Ocular war injuries in Jerusalem. *Am J Ophthalmol.* 1969;68:474–478.

29. Moisseiev J, Belkin M, Bartov E, Treister G. Severe combat eye injuries in the Lebanon War. *Isr J Med Sci.* 1984;20:339–344.

30. Treister G. Ocular casualties in the Six-Day War. *Am J Ophthalmol.* 1969;68:669–675.

31. Wilder HC. Intraocular foreign bodies in soldiers. *Am J Ophthalmol.* 1948;31:57–64.

32. Pieramici DJ, Sternberg P Jr, Aaberg TM Sr, et al, and The Ocular Trauma Classification Group. Perspective: A system for classifying mechanical injuries of the eye (globe). *Am J Ophthalmol.* 1997;123:820–831.

33. Ainbinder DA, Sanford EG, Raymond WR IV, et al. Madigan Eye and Orbit Trauma Scale. Presented at the Annual Meeting of the American Academy of Ophthalmology; October 1999; Orlando, Fla.

34. Lobue TD, Deutsch TA, Lobick J, Turner DA. Detection and localization of nonmetallic intraocular foreign bodies by magnetic resonance imaging. *Arch Ophthalmol.* 1988;106:260–261.

35. Bray LC, Griffiths PG. The value of plain radiograph in suspected intraocular foreign body. *Eye.* 1991;5:751–754.

36. Chacko JG, Figueroa RE, Johnson MH, Marcus DM, Brooks SE. Detection and localization of steel intraocular foreign bodies using computed tomography. *Ophthalmology.* 1997;104:319–323.

37. Tate E, Cupples H. Detection of orbital foreign bodies with computed tomography. *Am J Roentgenol.* 1981;137:493–495.

38. Lobes LA Jr, Grand MG, Reece J, Penkrot RJ. Computerized axial tomography in the detection of intraocular foreign bodies. *Ophthalmology.* 1981;88:26–29.

39. Topilow HW, Ackerman AL, Zimmerman RD. Limitations of computerized tomography in the localization of intraocular foreign bodies. *Ophthalmology.* 1984;91:1086–1091.

40. Gaster RN, Duda EE. Localization of intraocular foreign bodies by computed tomography. *Ophthalmic Surg.* 1980;11:25–29.

41. Rubsamen PE, Cousins SW, Winward KE, Byrne SF. Diagnostic ultrasound and pars plana vitrectomy in penetrating ocular trauma. *Ophthalmology.* 1994;101:809–814.

42. Bronson NR. Intraocular foreign bodies: Ultrasonic localization. *Int Ophthalmol Clin.* 1968;8(1):199–203.

43. Alfaro DV, Roth D, Liggett PE. Posttraumatic endophthalmitis. *Retina.* 1994;14:206–211.

44. Sternberg P Jr. Trauma: Principles and techniques of treatment. In: Ryan SJ, ed. *Retina.* 2nd ed. St Louis, Mo: Mosby–Year Book; 1994:2361.

45. Amalong RJ. Retinal detachment after manipulation of magnetic foreign body. *Am J Ophthalmol.* 1970;70:10–13.

46. Soheilian M, Ahmadieh H, Sajjadi H, Azarmina M, Miratashi AM, Peyman GA. Temporary keratoprosthesis for surgical management of complicated combined anterior and posterior segment injuries to the eye: Combat versus noncombat injury cases. *Ophthalmic Surg.* 1994;25:452–457.

47. Percival SPB. Late complications from posterior segment intraocular foreign bodies. *Br J Ophthalmol.* 1972; 56:462–468.

48. Vine AK. Endolaser photocoagulation in penetrating and perforating intraocular foreign bodies. *Eur J Ophthalmol.* 1991;1:119–122.

49. Ambler JS, Meyers SM. Management of intraretinal metallic foreign bodies without retinopexy in the absence of retinal detachment. *Ophthalmology.* 1991;98:391–394.

50. Dieckert JP, O'Connor PS, Schacklett DE, et al. Air travel and intraocular gas. *Ophthalmology.* 1986;93:642–645.

51. Shock JP, Adams D. Long-term visual acuity results after penetrating and perforating ocular injuries. *Am J Ophthalmol.* 1985;100:714–718.

52. Punnonen E, Laatikainen L. Prognosis of perforating eye injuries with intraocular foreign bodies. *Acta Ophthalmol (Copenh).* 1989;66:483–491.

53. Roper-Hall MJ. Review of 555 cases of intra-ocular foreign body with special reference to prognosis. *Brit J Ophthalmol.* 1954;38:65–99.

Chapter 15

METALLOSIS BULBI

PETER H. CUSTIS, MD*; AND TIM B. HOPKINS, MD†

*Captain, US Navy; Director, Retina Service, Department of Ophthalmology, Naval Medical Center San Diego, San Diego, California 92134-2202; and Clinical Assistant Professor, Department of Surgery, Uniformed Services University of Health Sciences, 4301 Jones Bridge Road, Bethesda, Maryland 20814-4799

†Lieutenant Commander, Medical Corps, US Navy; Department of Ophthalmology, US Naval Hospital Great Lakes, Great Lakes, Illinois 60088

INTRODUCTION

Modern weaponry, favoring blast fragmentation munitions, has resulted in an increase in ocular injuries in the battlefield. These often small, high-velocity fragments can easily penetrate the surface of the eye, remaining as a retained intraocular foreign body (IOFB). Damage that occurs to the eye as a direct result of retained metallic IOFBs is called *metallosis bulbi*, and changes that result from this damage are distinct from the changes caused by injuries concomitant with the ocular trauma. Over a period of months to years, toxic effects of metal ions that are taken up by various structures in the eye result in characteristic clinical findings with variable effects on visual function. Although most metallic foreign bodies (FBs) are alloys, or mixtures of metals, the two most common components are iron and copper.

Diagnosis of a retained metallic IOFB can be established in some cases by direct ophthalmoscopic examination. Alternatively, ancillary tests, such as plain film radiography, computed tomography (CT) scanning, ultrasonography, and electroretinograms, can be useful. Decisions regarding management of these cases are usually made in conjunction with other indications for vitreoretinal surgery. In most cases, surgical extraction of the FB is appropriate, although timing is rarely a critical issue.

METALLOSIS BULBI

Metallosis bulbi is defined as tissue damage to ocular structures as a direct result of retained metal particles following penetrating globe injury by an IOFB. In contrast to other sequelae of ocular trauma, most of the damage that ensues in metallosis is not inflammatory or immune-mediated. Instead, the mechanism of damage is thought to be electrolytic dissociation of the metal followed by oxidation and other chemical reactions with surrounding tissues and fluids.[1,2] These effects cause enzyme liberation from lysosomes and increased cellular permeability, resulting in the characteristic damage associated with metallosis.

Metallosis can occur as a consequence of numerous types of metals, but iron and copper alloys are the two most common. When an IOFB contains iron, the form of metallosis that develops is referred to as *siderosis*. Copper-containing IOFBs with less than 85% copper content cause *chalcosis*. Table 15-1 summarizes the most significant differences between siderosis and chalcosis. When copper content exceeds 85%, a sterile endophthalmitis ensues, which is not considered to be part of the spectrum of chalcosis.

Metallosis is a process that develops slowly over a period of months to years after injury—except when an IOFB contains very pure concentrations of copper (> 85%). Therefore, prevention of metallosis is generally not a significant issue that influences decision making in the primary surgical management of ocular trauma. Ferromagnetic objects are the most common cause of posterior segment IOFBs (Figure 15-1), accounting for approximately 80% of such injuries.[3] Copper and aluminum, respectively, are next on the list of common causes of posterior segment IOFBs.[4]

Factors Influencing Damage From IOFBs

The extent of ocular damage is determined by (*a*) mechanical factors and (*b*) the metal composition of the IOFB. Mechanical factors, including the IOFB's size, shape, velocity, final resting location, and concomitant injuries, are discussed extensively in other chapters. Larger objects and those with irregular shapes are associated with more-extensive initial damage. Velocity influences the depth of penetration after impact. To reach the posterior segment, an FB must have sufficient momentum and energy. Therefore, most posterior segment IOFBs are metallic.[1,5,6] In addition to velocity, the site of entry contributes to both the initial extent of injury and the final resting location of the IOFB. IOFBs that penetrate the sclera retain the highest momentum upon reaching the posterior segment, whereas IOFBs that traverse the cornea and anterior segment structures lose some of their momentum before reaching the posterior segment.[7]

Although the initial concomitant injuries to the anterior and posterior segment affect ultimate vision potential, the IOFB's final resting location also has a significant effect on the time course and severity of metallosis bulbi because the tolerance of different ocular tissues for IOFB fragments is variable. In general, the more vascular the tissue and the higher its metabolic activity, the lower its tolerance.[2] This observation is supported by animal studies[8] that demonstrated that iron-containing IOFBs con-

TABLE 15-1

FINDINGS IN SIDEROSIS AND CHALCOSIS

Findings	Siderosis	Chalcosis
Ocular Anatomical Features		
Cornea	Usually normal, but the stroma may develop a diffuse brown haze late in the clinical course	Kayser-Fleischer ring
Iris	Heterochromia with the affected side having a brown discoloration	Heterochromia with the affected side having a greenish color
Lens	Diffuse, brownish discoloration of the anterior capsule and generalized yellowing of cortex	Classic sunflower cataract of the anterior capsule
Retina	RPE degeneration affecting peripheral fundus first and posterior segment later	Refractile deposits in the macular region, with sparing of the periphery
Vitreous	Brownish opacification	Copperlike opacification
Magnetic Properties of IOFB	Yes	No
ERG	Supernormal b-wave, followed by eventual 100% loss of amplitudes	No supernormal b-wave; extent of ERG amplitude reduction usually less than 50%
Pathophysiology	Iron ions deposited intracellularly	Copper ions deposited in basement membranes
Clinical course if IOFB is not removed	Slow, relentless progression with loss of all vision	Variable, but may preserve reasonably good visual function

IOFB: intraocular foreign body
ERG: electroretinogram
RPE: retinal pigment epithelium

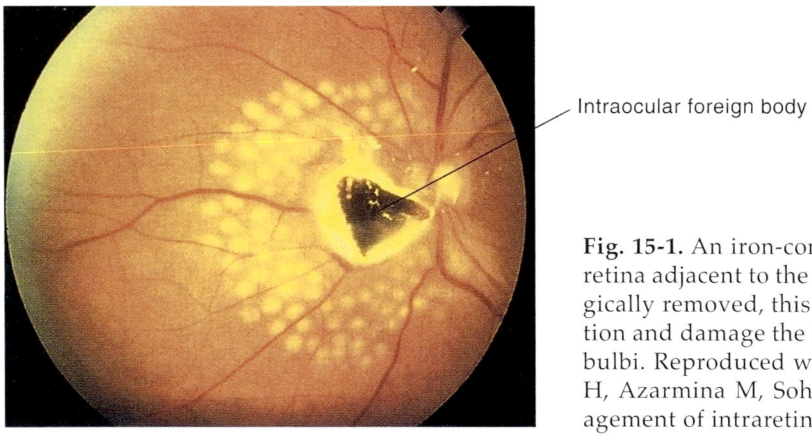

Fig. 15-1. An iron-containing foreign body is embedded in the retina adjacent to the nasal margin of the optic disc. Unless surgically removed, this foreign body will slowly undergo ionization and damage the ocular structures, as is typical of siderosis bulbi. Reproduced with permission from Ahmadieh H, Sajjadi H, Azarmina M, Soheleilian M, Baharivand N. Surgical management of intraretinal foreign bodies. *Retina*. 1994;14:398.

fined to the lens (which is avascular and has little metabolic activity) cause far less toxicity than comparable IOFBs situated in the posterior segment.

Mechanical factors notwithstanding, the single most important factor influencing the type and severity of metallosis is the metallic composition of the IOFB (Table 15-2). Metals with lower oxidation–reduction (redox) potentials are considered reactive and tend to undergo ion dissociation. They are more likely to cause tissue damage than metals with higher redox potentials.[2] Pure metals are more reactive than their alloys because the components that make up alloys, such as nickel and zinc, coat the dissociated ions and reduce their propensity for oxidation and, thus, tissue damage. Iron and copper have low redox potentials and therefore are reactive metals. In contrast, relatively inert IOFBs have high redox potentials (Exhibit 15-1).

Diagnosis and Location

As with any form of ocular trauma, when the patient has a penetrating injury to the eye the military ophthalmologist must adhere to a systematic approach, beginning with the history, followed by a thorough examination, and concluding with ancillary testing as indicated.

History

A comprehensive history is crucial with any injury. The history should be obtained from the patient and from anyone else who may have knowledge about the nature of the injury. Particular attention must be given to the circumstances of the trauma that might increase the risk of a metallic IOFB. A history of metal-on-metal contact, explosions, or firearm mechanisms necessitate a high index of suspicion. Whenever possible, it is helpful to obtain samples of the metals involved in the injuries to better evaluate the potential for short- and long-term ocular damage.

Ocular Examination

A thorough examination is performed in all cases of penetrating ocular injuries, with particular attention given to identifying direct signs of retained IOFBs. It is critical to carry out a fundus examination as soon as possible because the first look may be the best look. The view can rapidly deteriorate with the onset of cataract formation, inflammation, or diffusion of blood. The best evidence of an IOFB is direct visualization. But when the view is limited, indirect evidence of an IOFB may include a

TABLE 15-2

METALURGY OF INTRAOCULAR FOREIGN BODIES

Source	Metallic Composition
Shell (naval 5-in. and 155-mm artillery)	High-grade steel (98% iron, 1.7% copper, 0.2% manganese) with 99.5% copper rotation band
Bomb (2,000 lb, 1,000 lb, and 500 lb)	Grade 302/303 stainless steel (69% iron, 18% chromium, 9% nickel, manganese, and molybdenum) and lead-based paint
Cluster bomb unit	Grade 301 steel (69% iron, 19% nickel, 0.15% chromium), pyrotechnic zirconium, and plastic fins
Landmine	Aluminum alloy
Grenade	Zinc alloy case, grade 302 steel lever, barium chromate parts, and zirconium-nickel alloy parts
Bullet (rifle)	Brass or copper jacket, lead-tin alloy and steel core; brass jackets usually have pure copper rotating bands
Bullet (small-caliber)	Lead and lead–tin alloy (contains more lead than tin)
BB	Various manufacturers (brass, copper alloy, steel)
Pellet-gun pellet	Tin–lead alloy (contains more tin than lead)

For a complete detailed list of all military weapon components, access to the MIDAS database may be requested at http://www.dac.army.mil/TD/Midas/Index.htm.

EXHIBIT 15-1

REACTIVE AND NONREACTIVE COMPONENTS OF INTRAOCULAR FOREIGN BODIES

Nonreactive and Inert IOFBs	Reactive IOFBs
Gold	Copper
Platinum	Ferrous iron (Fe^{2+})*
Silver	Ferric iron (Fe^{3+})*
Tantalum	Lead†
Aluminum	Zinc†
Glass	Crystalline lens material
Plastic	Wood
Porcelain	Vegetable matter
Rubber	Cilia or hair
Talc	Bone
Gunpowder residue	
Stone	

*Ferrous iron is more toxic than ferric
†Usually well tolerated but can cause chronic nongranulomatous inflammatory reactions
IOFB: intraocular foreign body

corneal laceration, bubbles of air in the anterior or posterior segment, transillumination defects in the iris, discrete lenticular opacities, or wicks of vitreous hemorrhage not associated with diffuse bleeding.

Ancillary Studies

A variety of diagnostic modalities are available to assist in the evaluation of ocular trauma. Ancillary tests do not necessarily have to be obtained before primary wound closure. In situations where obtaining a diagnostic test will inordinately delay surgery, the test should be deferred until after surgery. Addressing potential IOFBs can be done as part of secondary surgical intervention in the days or weeks following initial repair. In military environments, the probability of a pure copper IOFB is so unlikely that urgent extraction of an IOFB is very rarely a consideration.

Plain film radiography and high-resolution CT scanning are considered the gold standards for evaluating an eye suspected of harboring an IOFB.[9,10] Although CT scans are generally preferable to plain film radiography for detecting and localizing IOFBs, plain films may be the only tool readily available in many military field environments, and plain film radiography is a very sensitive method for detecting metallic FBs larger than 2 mm.

Diagnostic ultrasonography can also be useful, although care should be taken prior to initial wound closure to minimize manipulation of the globe. There are documented cases in which diagnostic ultrasonography detected and localized an IOFB when even high-resolution CT scans missed the object.[10] Magnetic resonance imaging (MRI) is contraindicated when a ferromagnetic IOFB is suspected because of the potential for inducing additional damage from movement of the IOFB during the imaging procedure.

SIDEROSIS

Metallic IOFBs are most commonly made of iron alloys.[5] The group of characteristic clinical findings is called siderosis. All ferromagnetic IOFBs eventually cause some form of ocular damage if they are not removed. Toxic changes may be reversible in the early stages but will become irreversible after enough damage has occurred. Therefore, proper diagnosis and management are essential to preserve vision potential.

Ocular Findings

The ocular structures that are most commonly affected by siderosis are the iris and the lens; as a result, these structures also exhibit the most distinctive clinical changes. In time, however, virtually all structures of the eye can be affected in siderosis. The structures that are initially affected are usually those nearest the retained IOFB (see Figure 15-1). Later, ion dissociation and fluid movement damage more-remote structures.

Anterior Segment

Cornea. In rare cases, the stroma can develop a generalized rust-colored appearance, as can the endothelium. Corneal changes develop late in the clinical course, long after most other clinical findings have appeared.

Iris. Deposition of iron particles in the iris stroma causes a heterochromatic brownish discoloration in the affected eye (Figure 15-2). It is more readily apparent in blue and other lightly colored irides but an asymmetry can sometimes be detected in brown irides, with the affected eye appearing darker. In addition to their effects on iris color, iron particles can result in abnormal pupillary responses. The most common pupil abnormality is a middilated pupil that is minimally reactive to light.[5] Much less common is Adie's pupil, typified by light-near dissociation, segmental iris constriction, and supersensitivity to weak miotic drugs.[11] Pupil abnormalities can result from injury to muscle fibers, cholinergic neurons, or both. Both the heterochromia and pupil defects may be reversible following removal of the IOFB.

Lens. Early in the clinical course, brownish precipitates become apparent due to iron particles in

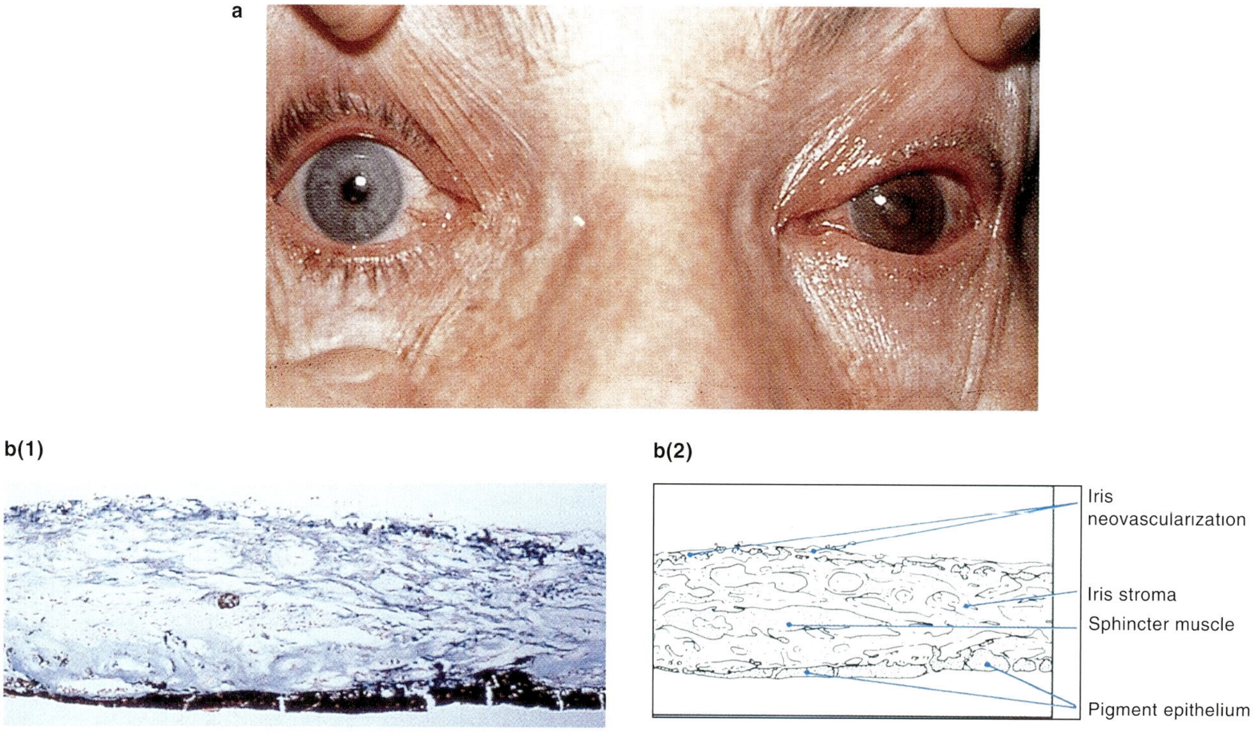

Fig. 15-2. (**a**) Iris heterochromia is seen in a patient with a retained ferromagnetic intraocular foreign body in the left eye. Iron particles deposited in the iris have caused the left eye to appear darker than the right eye. (**b**) Perls's stain imparts a blue color to iron and reveals the presence of diffuse iron deposition in the stroma and in the anterior layer of the iris pigment epithelium. Note the presence of iris neovascularization, a poor prognostic sign (there may be an increased risk of secondary glaucoma). Note that drawing b(2) is a schematic representation of photograph b(1), which is the actual photograph of the iris histopathological specimen. The labels in b(2) refer to the same structures in b(1). Reproduced with permission from Yanoff M, Fine BS. Surgical and nonsurgical trauma. In: *Ocular Pathology: A Color Atlas*. Philadelphia, Pa: JB Lippincott; 1988: Figures 5.36A and 5.36B.

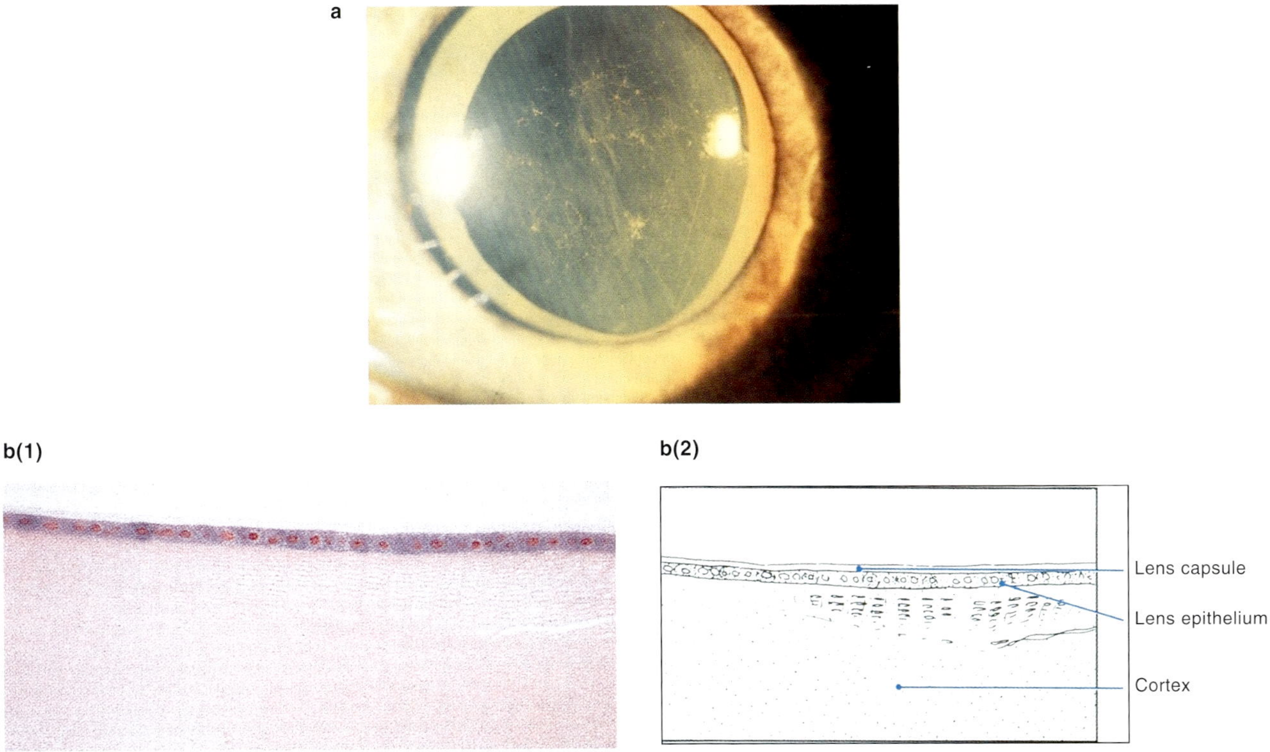

Fig. 15-3. (**a**) Anterior segment of a patient who underwent cataract extraction and posterior chamber lens implantation 5 years after penetrating ocular trauma with a retained ferromagnetic intraocular foreign body. Note the prominent rust-brown discoloration of the anterior lens capsule, which is due to iron deposition in the epithelial cells. The anterior vitreous demonstrates early fibrillar degeneration and mild opacification. (**b**) Perl's stain of the anterior lens demonstrates iron, as signified by the blue color, deposited in the epithelial cells. The lens capsule and cortex are normal. Note that drawing b(2) is a schematic representation of photograph b(1), which is the actual photograph of the histopathological specimen. The labels in b(2) refer to the same structures in b(1). Photograph a: Department of Ophthalmology, Naval Medical Center San Diego, San Diego, Calif. Views b(1) and b(2): Reproduced with permission from Yanoff M, Fine BS. Surgical and nonsurgical trauma. In: *Ocular Pathology: A Color Atlas*. Philadelphia, Pa: JB Lippincott; 1988: Figure 5.36D.

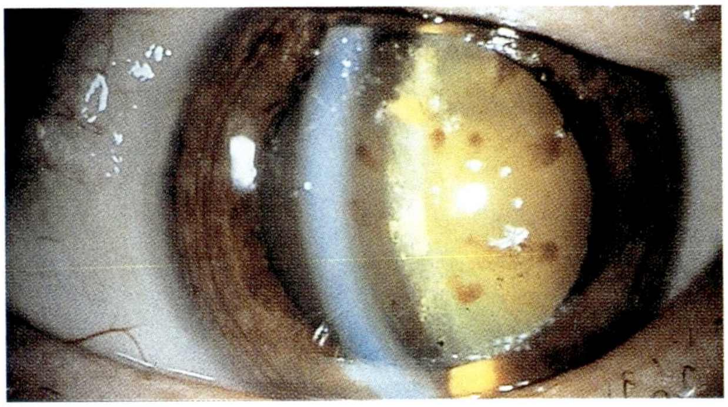

Fig. 15-4. A patient with long-standing hemorrhage in the eye. Iron deposition in the lens has caused a generalized cataract with patches of rust-brown discoloration. Hemosiderosis and siderosis are indistinguishable histologically. Reproduced with permission from Yanoff M, Fine BS. Surgical and nonsurgical trauma. In: *Ocular Pathology: A Color Atlas*. Philadelphia, Pa: JB Lippincott; 1988: Figure 5.36D.

the epithelial cells of the anterior lens capsule (Figure 15-3). Later, a nonspecific cataract develops with widespread yellowing of the lens cortex, mixed with large, rust-brown patches containing iron (Figure 15-4).

Trabecular Meshwork and Glaucoma. Gonioscopy rarely reveals distinct clinical findings of iron deposition, but histological studies have confirmed the presence of iron particles in the trabecular meshwork (Figure 15-5). Deposition of iron particles or secondary scarring of the trabecular meshwork can impede aqueous outflow, causing a secondary glaucoma. In some cases, the only clinical manifestation of siderosis may be glaucoma, which has been termed *subclinical siderosis secondary glaucoma.*[12] End-stage cases of secondary glaucoma may be associated with rubeosis irides, although the cause of angiogenesis has not been clearly established.[13]

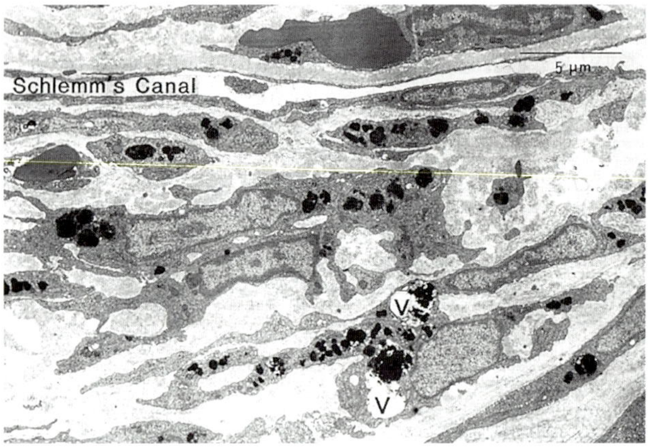

Fig. 15-5. The anterior chamber angle structures in a patient with siderosis demonstrate an open Schlemm's canal, but endothelial cells in the trabecular meshwork contain many siderosomes in their cytoplasm (dark, round granules). Some endothelial cells contain large cytoplasmic vacuoles (V). Reproduced with permission from Tawara A. Transformation and cytotoxicity of iron in siderosis bulbi. *Invest Ophthalmol Vis Sci.* 1986;27:235.

Posterior Segment

Retina. Iron deposition is first found in the cells of the retinal pigment epithelium (RPE) and the cells of Müller (Figure 15-6). This phenomenon results in a characteristic pigmentary degeneration of the RPE, which begins in the peripheral fundus and later extends to the posterior pole (Figure 15-7). The rate of progressive degeneration ranges from months to years. Later in the disease course, the RPE may disappear in widespread areas, the retina can take on an atrophic appearance, and gliosis may ensue in localized areas.[13]

Vitreous. The vitreous can take on a nonspecific, brownish discoloration and opacification. This effect is thought to be the result of iron interacting with hyaluronic acid, causing it to depolymerize. Additional factors influencing vitreous degeneration are unknown.

Electrophysiology Findings

The electroretinogram (ERG) is perhaps the most sensitive indicator of the early effects of siderosis and can demonstrate abnormalities even before clinical signs become apparent.[4,14] The time from initial injury until the onset of changes is apparent on ERG is variable, but it is usually at least several months. Because the peripheral retina is the first to develop clinical signs of degeneration, the ERG can detect abnormalities long before visual function becomes impaired. ERG may also be a valuable tool to measure progression of retinal damage over time in cases where surgical extraction of the IOFB is either deferred or not possible for whatever reason. In general, siderosis follows a continuously progressive detrimental course unless the IOFB is removed, and the ERG reflects the deterioration.

Sometimes, in the early stages of the disease, the ERG may reveal a so-called supernormal b-wave, which is defined as having an amplitude greater than 25% from baseline. The most common finding is a reduction in b-wave amplitudes. Later, progressive losses of amplitudes in both a- and b-waves

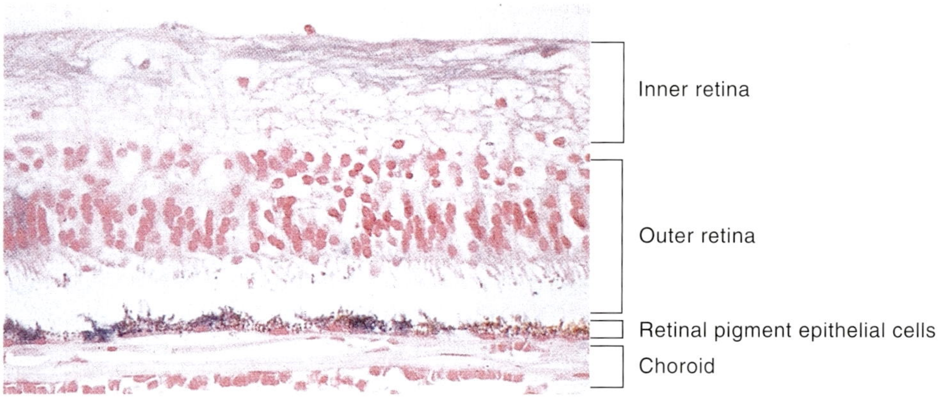

Fig. 15-6. Perls' stain demonstrates iron deposition in the retinal pigment epithelial cells and, to a lesser extent, in the retina. Note the prominent degeneration of the inner retina. Reproduced with permission from Yanoff M, Fine BS. Surgical and nonsurgical trauma. In: *Ocular Pathology: A Color Atlas.* Philadelphia, Pa: JB Lippincott; 1988: Figure 5.37C.

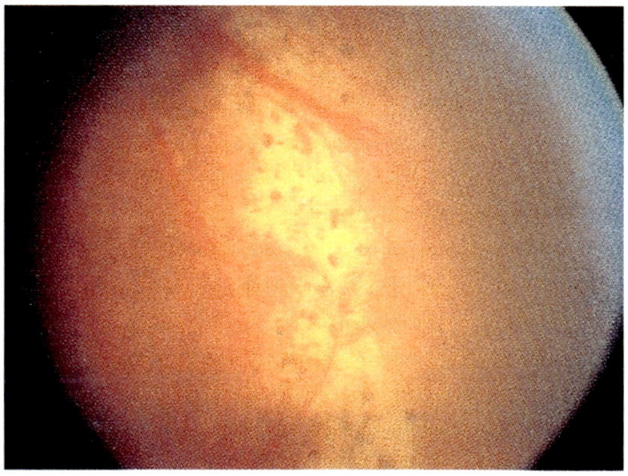

Fig. 15-7. Distinctive mottling of the pigment epithelium in the peripheral fundus is caused by a retained intraocular, iron-containing foreign body. Reproduced with permission from Yanoff M, Fine BS. Surgical and nonsurgical trauma. In: *Ocular Pathology: A Color Atlas.* Philadelphia, Pa: JB Lippincott; 1988: Figure 5.37B.

may occur (Figure 15-8), leading ultimately to flattening of the wave forms. ERG changes may be fully reversible if the IOFB is removed before a 50% reduction in amplitude occurs. When the amplitude is reduced by more than 50% from baseline, the changes are usually irreversible.[11]

Metal purity significantly influences the time course of ERG changes. Experimental studies with animals[4] demonstrated that pure iron particles decrease the ERG amplitude to a nonrecordable level in 100 days; in contrast, iron alloys containing 5% nickel had only a 50% ERG amplitude reduction at 100 days and required 240 days to cause an 80% reduction. These findings substantiate the observation that alloys cause less tissue damage than pure metals do.

Pathophysiology

Ferromagnetic IOFBs undergo electrolytic dissociation, resulting in gradual degradation of the FB and distribution of trivalent ferric ions throughout the eye. Following ion dissociation, the iron particles convert to ferric hydroxyphosphate and com-

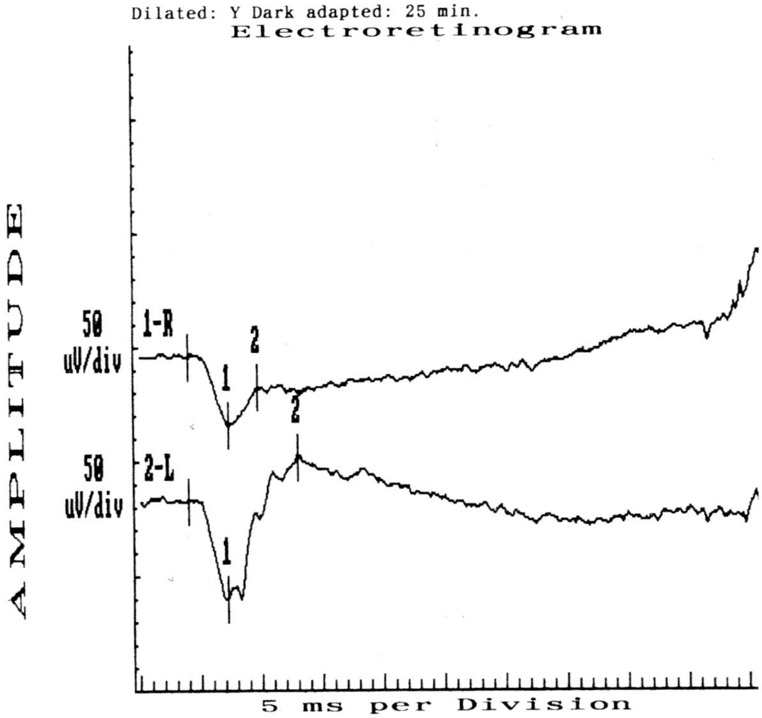

Fig. 15-8. A dark-adapted, bright-flash stimulus electroretinogram (ERG) from a patient with siderosis of the right eye (upper curve; lower curve represents the normal left eye) demonstrates reduction of nearly 75% in b-wave ("2" on ERG) amplitude and a reduction of approximately 25% in a-wave ("1" on ERG) amplitude. Electroretinogram: Department of Ophthalmology, Naval Medical Center San Diego, San Diego, Calif.

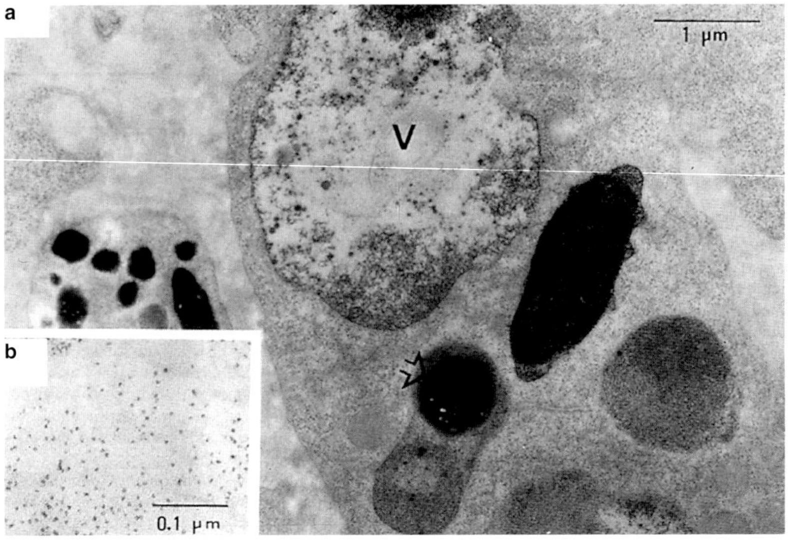

Fig. 15-9. (**a**) Fibroblasts and a melanocyte of the iris. There are numerous scattered ferritin particles and some siderosomes within the cytoplasm. A large vacuole (V) that contains ferritin particles and a siderosome (arrow) that includes both a pigment granule and ferritin particles are shown. Few ferritin particles are observed in the extracellular tissues (no stain, original magnification x 21,000). (**b**) A higher magnification of electron-dense particles within the vacuole. Typical square figures of the cores of ferritin are diffuse (no stain, original magnification x 150,000). Reproduced with permission from Tawara A. Transformation and cytotoxicity of iron in siderosis bulbi. *Invest Ophthalmol Vis Sci.* 1986;27:234.

bine with protein molecules known as apoferritin to form ferritin particles. Ferritin particles can be deposited intracellularly, where they can be found within the cytoplasm or occasionally within the cell nucleus. Ferritin particles can also be deposited extracellularly.[13]

Most of the intracellular ferritin particles are located in the cytoplasm, either as independent structures or in aggregate collections inside phagosome structures known as siderosomes (Figure 15-9).[15–17] Studies of the retina in siderosis using electron microscopy have demonstrated electron-opaque cores of ferritin, primarily in RPE cells and the cells of Müller (Figure 15-10).[15,16,18–21] Histologically, the findings of siderosis are indistinguishable from those of hemosiderosis, although the amount of iron is said to differ among cells in siderosis bulbi.[22,23] The reasons for this difference remain unknown.

Intracellular ferritin and siderosomes cause an interruption of normal cellular function and subsequent cell damage. The mechanism of damage relates to breakdown of lysosomes with the release of proteolytic enzymes, alterations in cell membrane permeability, and subsequent cellular degeneration and death.[13]

The distribution of ferritin particles among susceptible ocular structures varies, depending to a large extent on the resting location of the IOFB. Ferromagnetic IOFBs located in the posterior segment result in greater ferritin deposition in posterior structures such as the retina. In these circumstances, iron particles diffuse to adjacent structures. In con-

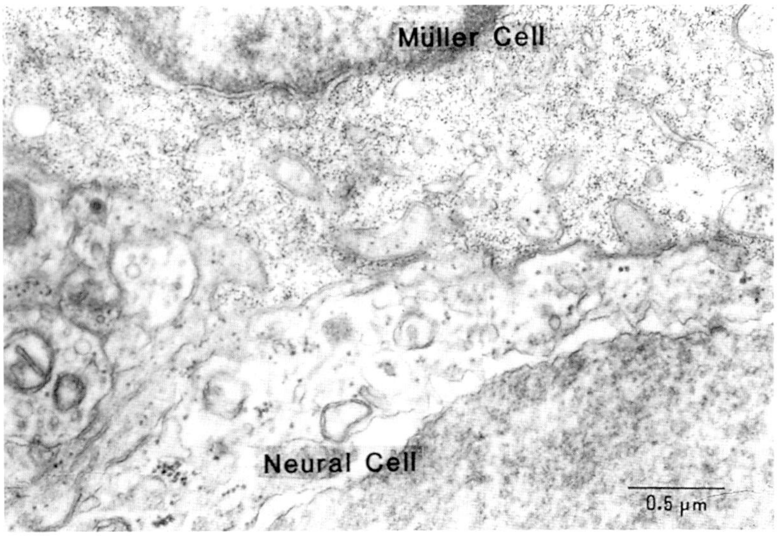

Fig. 15-10. A Müller cell (top) and a neural cell (bottom) are shown (no stain, original magnification x 38,000). There are numerous scattered ferritin particles in the Müller cell's cytoplasm but relatively few particles in the nucleus. There are also relatively few ferritin particles in the adjacent neural cell. Reproduced with permission from Tawara A. Transformation and cytotoxicity of iron in siderosis bulbi. *Invest Ophthalmol Vis Sci.* 1986;27:231.

trast, when an IOFB is located more anteriorly, iron particles disseminate via diffusion and the flow of aqueous humor.[13]

Clinical Course

Clinical observations and electrophysiological studies have conclusively demonstrated[14] that eyes with retained ferromagnetic IOFBs will undergo a slow, progressive, and unrelenting deterioration in visual function, resulting in the loss of all vision unless the IOFB is removed. When surgical intervention takes place before a 50% reduction in ERG amplitudes, much of the damage can be reversed.

Other forms of metallosis bulbi, such as chalcosis, do not have the same dismal prognosis as siderosis. The reason for this relates to differences in pathophysiology: siderosis results in intracellular ferritin and siderosome deposition with subsequent cellular death, whereas chalcosis is limited to deposition of iron particles in basement membranes. The pathophysiological mechanisms of cellular damage in chalcosis is not well understood, but the ensuing toxic effects associated with basement membrane deposition are far less significant than those due to intracellular iron deposition. The time course for cellular and visual dysfunction in siderosis varies, depending in part on the size and location of the IOFB and the purity of the iron. At the very least, the process requires several months before signs of the disease become manifest.

CHALCOSIS

IOFBs consisting of pure copper are extremely rare. Most copper-containing FBs are made of alloys such as brass or bronze. In the rare circumstance when an IOFB contains more than 85% copper, an acute and suppurative reaction develops that is clinically indistinguishable from fulminant infectious endophthalmitis. If not appropriately managed, this sterile endophthalmitis results in phthisis.[2,24] In contrast, chalcosis is a much milder condition that develops very slowly when IOFBs contain less than 85% copper. Brass is an alloy consisting of 68% copper, 30% zinc, and 2% iron. Zinc oxides coat the dissociated copper ions, rendering them less toxic to the tissues that absorb them. This composition is of particular relevance in military environments, because bullet casings or shells from firearms are typically made of brass (see Table 15-2).

Unlike those of iron, copper alloys are generally nonmagnetic. This distinction is significant when deciding on diagnostic imaging modalities and surgical extraction techniques.

Ocular Findings

The structures most commonly affected by chalcosis are the cornea, iris, lens, and macula. With the exception of macular involvement, the clinical characteristics of chalcosis are indistinguishable from those of hepatolenticular degeneration (Wilson's disease).

Anterior Segment

Cornea. The typical green-blue ring in the peripheral cornea, known as the Kayser-Fleischer ring, is a consequence of copper deposition in Descemet's membrane and the posterior stroma. The discoloration may often be segmental, most commonly affecting the superior and inferior cornea.[25] The nasal and temporal perilimbal regions may never develop discoloration, which could result in an observer's missing the Kayser-Fleischer ring unless the entire cornea is thoroughly examined.

Anterior Chamber and Iris. Bright, refractile particles may be seen circulating in the aqueous. As these particles settle and are taken up by the iris, heterochromia develops, with the affected iris exhibiting a greenish discoloration, in contrast to the brownish hue of the iris that develops in siderosis. The pupil may also be sluggish and minimally reactive; there have been no reports, however, of Adie's pupil in chalcosis.

Lens. The so-called sunflower cataract is pathognomonic of chalcosis (Figure 15-11). Copper ions are deposited in the anterior lens capsule basement membrane. When significant vitreous reaction is present, a nonspecific, posterior subcapsular cataract can also be seen.[25] The radial appearance of the anterior subcapsular cataract is related to the folds in the posterior surface of the iris. Movement of the iris with changes in pupillary aperture have a direct influence on the distribution of copper particles in the lens.[2]

Posterior Segment

Retina. In contradistinction to siderosis, most of the retinal changes in chalcosis are confined to the posterior pole. The peripheral retina generally appears normal, except for changes directly related

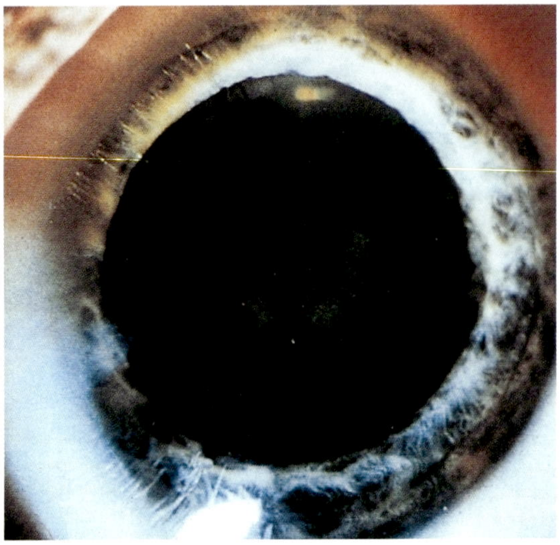

Fig. 15-11. Copper deposition in the anterior subcapsular regions of the lens in an eye with a retained intraocular foreign body has caused a sunflower cataract. Faint white circular area in the center of the photograph: sunflower cataract; yellow discoloration at the corneal limbus: Kayser-Fleischer ring of copper deposition; blue circular structure: iris. Reproduced with permission from Rosenthal AR, Marmor MF, Leuenberger P. Chalcosis: A study of natural history. *Ophthalmology.* 1979;86:1961.

to the initial injury itself. The most characteristic finding is the presence of glistening, refractile particles deposited in the macula and around vessels in the posterior pole, which may increase over time (Figure 15-12). These particles are located in the internal limiting membrane. In some cases, the entire internal limiting membrane of the macula appears to have a copper-colored sheen.[25]

Vitreous. The vitreous can undergo fibrillar degeneration, which is usually observed to some extent in all patients with chalcosis. Typically, these changes are most apparent in the anterior vitreous and consist of condensations of fibrils and cellular infiltrates that are sharply delineated from the rest of the vitreous[25] (Figure 15-13). Other changes may include a copper-colored opacification of the vitreous, as well as organization and strands adjacent to the IOFB. All of the vitreous changes may progressively worsen with time.

Electrophysiology Findings

As in patients with siderosis, patients with chalcosis may exhibit reduced b-wave amplitude on ERG. A supernormal b-wave has not been observed. An abnormal ERG eventually develops in all eyes with retained intravitreal copper FBs and precedes clinical findings in 50% of patients.[14] However, the ERG changes in chalcosis are much less severe than those seen in siderosis: very few patients with chal-

a

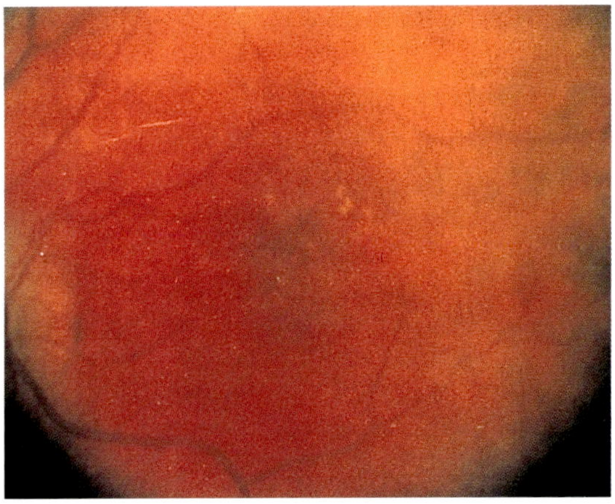

b

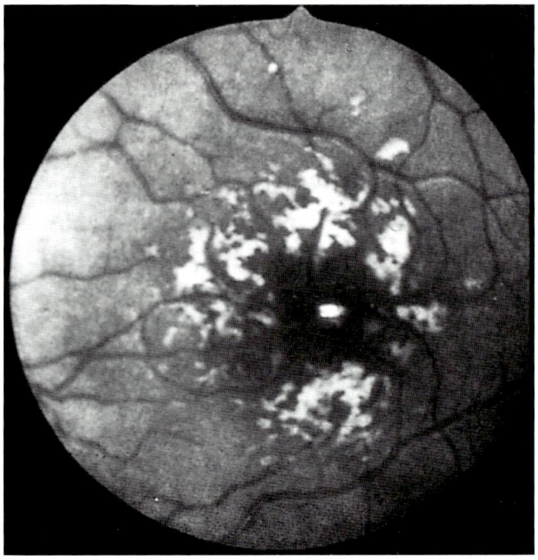

Fig. 15-12. (**a**) Early copper deposition within the internal limiting membrane of the macula results in brightly refractile particles. (**b**) A more advanced case of macular toxicity, characterized by extensive copper accumulation in the internal limiting membrane. Photograph a: Reproduced with permission from Rosenthal AR, Marmor MF, Leuenberger P. Chalcosis: A study of natural history. *Ophthalmology.* 1979;86:1961. Photograph b: Reproduced with permission from Delaney WV. Presumed ocular chalcosis: A reversible maculopathy. *Ann Ophthalmol.* 1975;7:378.

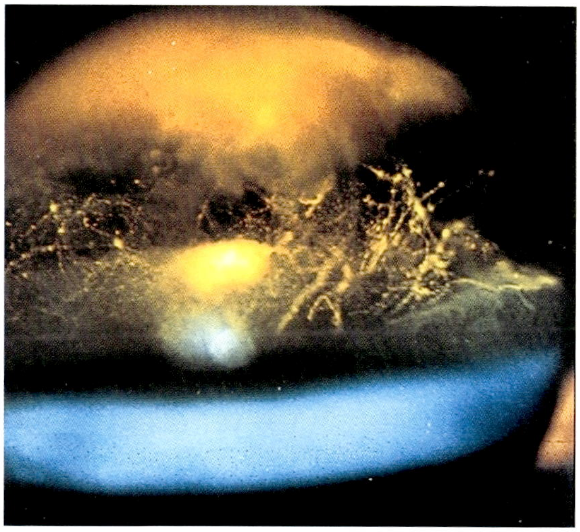

Fig. 15-13. Vitreous changes secondary to the presence of an intravitreal copper foreign body. A marked fibrillar degeneration and brownish tinge of the vitreous is apparent. Reproduced with permission from Rosenthal AR, Marmor MF, Leuenberger P. Chalcosis: A study of natural history. *Ophthalmology.* 1979;86:1962.

cosis experience more than a 50% reduction in b-wave amplitude. Moreover, after the ERG amplitudes fall to a certain level, they may remain stable without further deterioration for many years.[25] In addition to ERG observations in humans, electrophysiology studies[4] in rabbits have demonstrated that chalcosis causes far less damage than siderosis does. It is widely assumed that ERG changes of chalcosis are reversible, based on case reports of complete resolution of all clinical signs following removal of the instigating IOFB.[26] These case reports, the relatively benign nature of ERG changes in chalcosis, and the reversibility of ERG changes in siderosis after removal of ferromagnetic IOFBs all support the presumed ERG reversibility in chalcosis. However, no published case reports have actually documented reversibility.

Pathophysiology

Copper's interaction with intraocular fluids and tissues causes its ionization. Most copper ions become coated with zinc oxides, and this coating minimizes the potential for tissue toxicity. These coated ions have a propensity to be deposited on limiting membranes, in contrast to the tendency of iron particles to be distributed intracellularly. The most common ocular structures affected are Descemet's membrane, the anterior lens capsule, and the internal limiting membrane of the retina.[1,2]

As stated in the discussion of siderosis, the lack of intracellular deposits of toxic particles likely accounts for the more benign clinical course in chalcosis. In the rare case in which an IOFB contains more than 85% copper, the sterile endophthalmitis that develops is attributed to copper's chemotactic properties. The severe inflammatory response is characterized by abscess formation in the vitreous.[2,24,27]

Distribution of ions within the eye may be related to the standing electrical potential.[5] The cornea exhibits a positive charge relative to the optic nerve, which may induce ion distribution based on electrostatic forces. It is unclear why the macular region is selectively predisposed to copper deposition. Some observers[26] have speculated that it may be linked to the macula's higher metabolic rate as well as fluid movements in the eye. It is quite likely, however, that other factors are involved, because this theory fails to explain why siderosis initially affects the peripheral retina.

Vitreous opacification results from the degradation of hyaluronic acid, as is also seen in siderosis. Depolymerization of hyaluronic acid is associated with oxidation of ascorbic acid, and copper is known to accelerate the oxidation of ascorbic acid.

Clinical Course

The clinical course of chalcosis is variable but generally less severe than it is in siderosis, and chalcosis does not have a uniformly poor outcome. The extent of damage and visual impairment depends on several factors, including the size, alloy composition, and intraocular location of the IOFB, and adjacent tissue reaction. A retained copper-containing IOFB can be tolerated for years without serious toxicity to the retina or RPE.

One case series[25] reported on 10 patients with retained IOFBs of copper alloys who were followed from 4 months to 29 years; 9 of the 10 patients retained a final visual acuity of 20/60 or better. All 10 had clinical findings typical of chalcosis. IOFBs located in the vitreous were more likely to cause chalcosis, whereas in the anterior segment or the lens nucleus, small FBs could cause very few changes typical of this disease. Not all patients with chalcosis will maintain such a high degree of visual function. The two clinical findings that have the most deleterious impact on vision are (1) vitreous opacification and (2) macular toxicity.

The time for clinical signs of chalcosis to develop ranges from 4 months to 2 years.[25] Most of the ocular findings may resolve spontaneously if the IOFB dissolves, is spontaneously extruded, or is surgically removed.[28] In addition to the effects on visual acuity, abnormalities in color vision and visual field have been reported.[25] It is unclear, however, whether these findings are true sequelae of retinal dysfunction. It may be that they are the result of media changes, the effects of the initial trauma to ocular structures, or both.

MANAGEMENT

The goals in surgical management of penetrating IOFB injuries include optimal wound closure, restoration and preservation of ocular anatomy to the extent possible, prevention of secondary infection, and, in most cases, removal of the IOFB. Management of retained IOFBs was revolutionized in 1879 by the development of the Hirschberg hand-held electromagnet; its inventor used it to treat more than 100 patients. A landmark article[29] published in 1894 compared Hirschberg's series with another large series of electromagnetic IOFB extractions in 66 patients. Both series demonstrated excellent visual outcomes in nearly all anterior segment cases and outstanding results in 30% of posterior segment cases.

Some of the lessons learned nearly 100 years ago are still valid today:

- localize the metal as well as possible,
- remove metallic IOFBs early, and
- choose the extraction site and technique that minimize vitreous traction and collateral damage.

Modern advances in the management of these cases include the following:

- diagnostic imaging modalities that have improved IOFB localization,
- advent of vitreous surgery combined with wide-field intraoperative viewing systems,
- surgical instrumentation,
- improved magnets, and
- development and use of antibiotics to prevent and treat infections.

Results of modern vitreous surgery are such that approximately 33% of posterior segment IOFB cases recover visual acuity of 20/40 or better, 67% recover 20/200 or better, and 75% have ambulatory vision of 5/200 or better.[5,30–33] These results compare favorably with those pertaining to cases of penetrating ocular trauma without IOFBs. Discussions of current surgical techniques are found elsewhere in this textbook.

Prevention of metallosis is rarely a significant issue in the early, or primary, surgical management of ocular trauma. The only true indication for early removal of a metallic IOFB as part of the primary surgical procedure is when the object contains more than 85% copper or if there is a high probability of infection. Failure to intervene promptly in such cases is associated with a high risk of endophthalmitis and phthisis.[3,24] In all other forms of metallosis, the onset of clinical findings and toxicity generally requires at least several months and may be fully reversible even after delayed surgical intervention. Therefore, there is seldom an urgent indication to remove the IOFB.

The decision of when and whether to remove a metallic IOFB often becomes a side issue in the larger picture of managing ocular trauma. More times than not, removal of the IOFB is incorporated into the vitreoretinal surgery for treating more pressing indications, including

- the presence of a retinal tear or detachment,
- dense vitreous hemorrhage,
- prominent vitreous wicks following the path of an IOFB,
- significant lens disruption, and
- infection.

In the absence of other indications for surgery, determining when and if an IOFB should be removed assumes greater relevance. Inert IOFBs, particularly if they are small and not associated with other indications for surgery, may be reasonable to observe. Reactive metals, such as iron and copper alloys, however, deserve further consideration.

Siderosis

In general, there is seldom any dispute with the recommendation that all ferromagnetic IOFBs be removed to prevent the slow but relentless deterioration in visual function that occurs with siderosis. However, in certain circumstances, surgery might increase the risk of a poor visual outcome (eg, a deeply embedded IOFB in the posterior wall of the globe, or if the patient is reluctant to undergo a procedure). In one case series[3] of 84 eyes harboring iron-containing IOFBs, surgery was not performed in 8 eyes. When surgery is deferred for whatever reasons, observation for signs of siderosis onset and progression should be undertaken. The fact that the retinal changes affect the peripheral fundus before evolving to the macula enables the military ophthalmologist to monitor the patient with an added degree of comfort. Serial ERGs can be very useful in these circumstances. When reductions in b-wave amplitudes approach 50% of baseline, the option for surgery can be considered before further toxicity results in irreversible damage.

Chalcosis

In contrast to siderosis, no consensus exists around the timing and indications for surgery to remove copper-containing IOFBs, largely because the clinical course of chalcosis is more benign and self-limiting than it is for siderosis. Those who historically have favored a conservative approach recommend observation to determine if and when significant toxicity develops, usually in the form of vitreous opacification, advanced macular toxicity, or both.

Reports in the literature support the viewpoint that surgical intervention can be delayed in selected cases and may not always be necessary. In the case series[25] of 10 patients referred to previously, 7 patients maintained visual acuity of 20/40 or better for many years—even in the presence of sunflower cataracts and early maculopathy. Furthermore, case reports[28,34] have documented complete resolution of the clinical findings when the IOFB is either removed surgically or extrudes spontaneously as long as 15 years after the initial trauma.

With the advent of modern vitreoretinal surgical techniques, the ability to successfully intervene in IOFB cases and minimize iatrogenic complications has shifted current opinion more in favor of earlier surgical management—even before signs of chalcosis develop. Advocates[35] of surgical extraction of copper IOFBs refer to the same 10 patients[25] who were followed for up to 29 years and point out that only 2 had final visual acuity of 20/20. Furthermore, 6 of the 8 who had ERG testing demonstrated some degree of abnormality, and all 10 had vitreous degeneration to some extent. The authors[35] conclude that chalcosis is not completely benign and that it is not possible to accurately predict which cases will do well without intervention or for how long. Therefore, surgery is an appropriate consideration even when there are no other pressing indications for pars plana vitrectomy.

SUMMARY

Metallosis bulbi is the name of the condition in which retained metallic IOFBs damage ocular structures; the intraocular changes evolve slowly over months to years. Metallic FBs interact with surrounding tissues to undergo ionization, which is followed by distribution and uptake of liberated ions in various parts of the eye. Toxic effects of the ions result in characteristic clinical findings.

The two most common metals involved in ocular trauma are iron and copper. Iron-containing FBs cause a form of metallosis known as siderosis, and copper-containing FBs cause chalcosis. When a penetrating FB contains more than 85% copper, an acute and suppurative sterile endophthalmitis develops. The clinical findings most commonly seen in siderosis are

- iris heterochromia, with the affected eye having a rust-brown discoloration,
- diffuse cataract,
- RPE degeneration affecting the peripheral retina in the early stages before progressing to the posterior pole, and
- vitreous opacification.

Chalcosis, on the other hand, is characterized by

- the Kayser-Fleischer ring,
- iris heterochromia, with the affected eye having a greenish discoloration,
- a pathognomonic sunflower cataract,
- refractile precipitates in the macular region, and
- vitreous opacification.

Diagnostic modalities that are helpful in detecting metallic FBs include plain film radiography, CT scanning, ultrasonography, and electroretinograms. Electroretinograms often demonstrate reduction in b-wave amplitudes even before clinical signs become apparent. In general, the adverse affects on visual function are more severe in siderosis than chalcosis.

Unless the inciting FB is removed in siderosis, there will be progressive visual deterioration with loss of most vision. In chalcosis, in contrast, relatively good visual acuity may be preserved even in the presence of cataract and macular toxicity. The reason for the difference in prognosis relates to pathophysiology: siderosis is associated with deposition of iron ions intracellularly, whereas chalcosis results in copper ion deposition in basement membranes. Damage to ocular structures is far more extensive when the toxic products accumulate intracellularly.

Management of retained IOFBs must be considered within the context of other issues pertinent to surgical decision making. With the rare exception of copper-containing objects that are more than 85% pure, there is no need to incorporate removal of the FB in conjunction with primary wound closure. Very often, secondary surgical procedures are indicated in trauma cases, and removal of FBs is performed at that time. In the absence of any other indications for vitreoretinal surgery, inert IOFBs can be observed, but metallic iron and copper-containing objects should be removed. The early findings in metallosis may be reversible if the IOFB is removed prior to a 50% reduction in electroretinogram amplitudes, after which the damage may be permanent.

REFERENCES

1. Barry DR. Effects of retained intraocular foreign bodies. *Int Ophthalmol Clin.* 1968;8:153–170.

2. Duke-Elder S, MacFaul PA. The metallic corrosives. In: Chemical injuries. In: Duke-Elder S, MacFaul PA. *Non-Mechanical Injuries.* Part 2. In: *Injuries.* Vol 14. In: Duke-Elder S, ed. *System of Ophthalmology.* St Louis, Mo: Mosby–Year Book; 1972; § 3, Chap 11: 1089–1102.

3. Ahmadieh H, Sajjadi H, Azarmina M, Soheilian M, Baharivand N. Surgical management of intraretinal foreign bodies. *Retina.* 1994;14:397–403.

4. Knave B. The ERG and ophthalmological changes in experimental metallosis in the rabbit. *Acta Ophthalmol.* 1970;48:159–173.

5. De Bustros S. Posterior segment intraocular foreign bodies. In: Shingleton BJ, Hersh PS, Kenyon KR, eds. *Eye Trauma.* St Louis, Mo: Mosby–Year Book; 1991: Chap 21.

6. Percival SPB. A decade of intraocular foreign bodies. *Br J Ophthalmol.* 1972;56:454–461.

7. Brown IAR. Nature of injury. *Int Ophthalmol Clin.* 1968;8:147–152.

8. Virata SR, Kylstra JA, Peiffer RL. The ocular effects of intralenticular iron foreign bodies in rabbits. *Ophthalmic Surg.* 1995;26:142–144.

9. Sneed SR, Weingeist TA. Management of siderosis bulbi due to a retained iron containing intraocular foreign body. *Ophthalmology.* 1990;97:375–379.

10. Rubsamen PE, Cousins SW, Winward KE, Byrne SF. Diagnostic ultrasound and pars plana vitrectomy in penetrating ocular trauma. *Ophthalmology.* 1994;105:809–814.

11. Weiss MJ, Hoeldt AJ, Behrens M, Fisher K. Ocular siderosis diagnosis and management. *Retina.* 1997;17:105–108.

12. Shiar K, Ji SC, Sun XH. A clinical analysis of subclinical siderosis and secondary glaucoma. *Chung Hua Yen Ko Tsa Chih.* 1994;30:420–422.

13. Tawara A. Transformation and cytotoxicity of iron in siderosis bulbi. *Invest Ophthalmol Vis Sci.* 1986;27:226–236.

14. Knave B. Electroretinography in eyes with retained intraocular metallic foreign bodies: A clinical study. *Acta Ophthalmol (Suppl).* 1969;100:1–63.

15. Matsuo N, Hasegawa E. Histochemical and electron-microscopical studies on the retinal siderosis. *Acta Soc Ophthalmol Jap.* 1964;68:1702–1706.

16. Koshibu A. Ultrastructural studies of absorption of an experimentally produced subretinal hemorrhage, III: Absorption of erythrocyte breakdown products and retinal hemosiderosis at the late stage. *Nippon Ganka Gakkai Zasshi.* 1979;83:386–400.

17. Ghadially FN, Schneider RJ, Lalonde JMA. Haemosiderin deposits in the human cornea. *J Submicrosc Cytol.* 1981;13:455–464.

18. Farrant JL. An electron microscopic study of ferritin. *Biochim Biophys Acta.* 1954:13:569–573.

19. Richter GW. A study of hemosiderosis with the aid of electron microscopy. *J Exp Med.* 1957;106:203–206.

20. Richter GW. The cellular transformation of injected colloidal iron complexes into ferritin and hemosiderin in experimental animals. *J Exp Med.* 1959;109:197–200.

21. Kerr DNS, Muir AR. A demonstration of the structure and disposition of ferritin in the human liver cell. *J Ultrastruct Res.* 1960;2:313–217.

22. Cibis PA, Brown EB, Hong S. Ocular effects of systemic siderosis. *Am J Ophthalmol.* 1957:44(part 2):158–160.

23. Yanoff M, Fine BS. Surgical and nonsurgical trauma. In: *Biomedical Foundations of Ophthalmology.* Philadelphia, Pa: Harper & Row; 1982: Chap 6.

24. Rao NA, Tso MOM, Rosenthal R. Chalcosis in the human eye: A clinicopathologic study. *Arch Ophthalmol.* 1976;94:1379–1384.

25. Rosenthal AR, Marmor MF, Leuenberger P. Chalcosis: A study of natural history. *Ophthalmology.* 1979;86:1956–1972.

26. Delaney WV. Presumed ocular chalcosis: A reversible maculopathy. *Ann Ophthalmol.* 1975;7:378–380.

27. Rosenthal AR, Appleton B, Hopkins JL. Intraocular copper foreign bodies. *Am J Ophthalmol.* 1974;78:671–678.

28. Felder KS, Gottlieb F. Reversible chalcosis. *Ann Ophthalmol.* 1984;16:638–641.

29. Hildebrand H. Sixty-six magnet operations, with the successful extraction of particles of iron from the inferior of the eye in fifty-three cases. *Arch Ophthalmol.* 1894;23:167–171.

30. Benson WE, Machemer R. Severe perforating injuries treated with pars plana vitrectomy. *Am J Ophthalmol.* 1976;81:728–732.

31. Slusher MM, Sarin LK, Federman JL. Management of intraretinal foreign bodies. *Ophthalmology.* 1982;89:369–373.

32. Schock JP, Adams D. Long-term visual acuity results after penetrating and perforating ocular injuries. *Am J Ophthalmol.* 1985;100:714–718.

33. Williams DF, Mieler WF, Abrams GW, Lewis H. Results and prognostic factors in penetrating ocular injuries with retained intraocular foreign bodies. *Ophthalmology.* 1988;95:911–916.

34. Tulloh CG. Migration of intraocular foreign bodies. *Br J Ophthalmol.* 1956;40:173.

35. Michels RG. Discussion of presentation by Dr A. Ralph Rosenthal, et al. *Ophthalmology.* 1979;86:1970–1972.

Chapter 16

SYMPATHETIC OPHTHALMIA

THOMAS P. WARD, MD*

*Colonel, Medical Corps, US Army; Ophthalmology Residency Program Director, Ophthalmology Service, Walter Reed Army Medical Center, Washington, DC 20307-5001; Associate Professor of Surgery, Uniformed Services University of the Health Sciences, 4301 Jones Bridge Road, Bethesda, Maryland 20814-4799

INTRODUCTION

One of the most feared conditions in ophthalmology is sympathetic ophthalmia (SO), a condition in which, after one eye is injured, inflammation threatens blindness in both. Sir Stewart Duke-Elder probably gave the single most comprehensive description of this disease in 1966:

> Sympathetic ophthalmitis is a specific bilateral inflammation of the entire uveal tract of unknown etiology, characterized clinically by an insidious onset and a progressive course with exacerbations, and pathologically by a nodular or diffuse infiltration of the uveal tract with lymphocytes and epithelioid cells; it almost invariably follows a perforating wound involving uveal tissue.[1(pp558–559)]

SO, also known as sympathetic uveitis, is a rare, bilateral, granulomatous panuveitis that occurs after a penetrating injury to an eye. Following injury to an eye—a result of either surgery or accident—a variable period of time passes before a sight-threatening inflammation develops in *both* eyes. The injured eye is referred to as the *exciting* eye and the fellow eye as the *sympathizing* eye. The fact that injury to one eye can result in blindness of both has made SO of enormous concern to ophthalmologists. And because the highest recorded instances of this disease follow combat wounds, SO is of particular interest to military ophthalmic surgeons.

HISTORY

The concept of sympathetic inflammation is an ancient one; probably the first reference in the literature was in a note from Agathias in the anthology compiled from Constantius Cephalis (1000 CE [common era]): "the right eye when diseased often gives its suffering to the left."[1(p560)] The clinical disease was known to Hippocrates, and is also found in an old German textbook of ophthalmology.[1–3] Bartisch (1583) remarked that when one eye is injured "the other good eye is besides also in great danger."[1(p561)]

The modern history of the disease commences with the comprehensive clinical description of Mackenzie in 1840, who first termed the disease "sympathetic ophthalmia."[4] His report was supplemented 65 years later by the classic histopathological findings described by Fuchs.[5] In 1910, Elschnig was the first to propose the concept that SO was an autoimmune inflammatory disorder, possibly in response to uveal antigens.[6] Two well-known individuals were almost certainly victims of SO:

- Two years after an injury to one eye from a leather awl, Louis Braille, the French inventor of the Braille alphabet and teacher of the blind, experienced a gradual loss of vision in the other eye.[7]
- As a child, James Thurber, the American author and humorist, sustained a severe eye injury caused by an arrow during a game of William Tell, leaving him blind in one eye; eventually, "sympathetic ophthalmia overtook his other eye, leaving him totally blind amid his forties."[8]

Interestingly, SO was a condition well-known to veterinarians. Wardrop[9] drew attention to this fact in 1818:

> It is known among some farriers, that, if the eye first affected with this disease suppurates and sinks into the orbit, the disease does not attack the other eye, or subsides if it has commenced in it. Thus they have adopted a practice of destroying altogether the diseased eye, in order to save the other which is crudely done by putting lime between the eyelids, or thrusting a nail into the cavity of the eyeball, so as to excite violent inflammation and suppuration.[9(p139)]

The concept of inducing suppurative inflammation in an injured eye as a method of protecting the fellow eye became an accepted procedure in the treatment of human disease. Pre-Listerian surgeons intentionally produced a "beneficent" suppuration in a badly injured eye by passing a seton through it, believing that the purulent infection destroyed the factors responsible for the condition or prevented infection passing up the optic nerve by sealing the lymph spaces.[1] Prichard in 1851 was the first to practice enucleation as a therapeutic measure.[1] To this day, early removal of the injured eye remains the only sure way to prevent SO.

EPIDEMIOLOGY

Most cases of SO accompany perforating injuries of the globe in which uveal tissue, especially the ciliary body, is traumatized. Incarceration of uveal tissue has been a feature of nearly all cases (Figure 16-1).

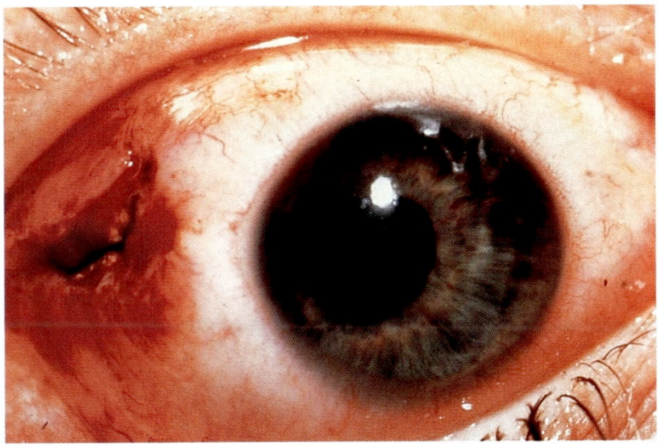

Fig. 16-1. An example of a penetrating eye injury from the Vietnam War. Note the dark uveal tissue emanating from the scleral laceration temporally. It is the exposure of uveal tissue to the conjunctival lymphatic system that is believed to be a major factor in the development of sympathetic ophthalmia. Photograph: Courtesy of Francis G. La Piana, MD, Colonel, Medical Corps, US Army (Ret), Ashton, Maryland.

Accidental wounds now account for about 65% of cases, and another 25% follow surgical wounds.[10] In 1972, Liddy and Stuart[11] reported an incidence of 0.19% following penetrating injury and 0.007% following intraocular surgery. SO occurs more often in children because of the high risk of accidental trauma. Elderly patients also appear to be at an increased risk of the disease because of the greater frequency of intraocular surgery in the aged. The disease does not appear to have a predilection for any race or for either gender, except that its incidence mirrors the increased incidence of ocular trauma in males.

The most common surgical procedures leading to SO include cataract extraction (particularly when complicated), iris surgery (including iridectomy), retinal detachment repair, and vitreoretinal surgery.[7,12–14] Surgical procedures complicated by the incarceration of the iris or the lens capsule in the wound are particularly prone to develop the condition. Other penetrating surgical procedures reported to have resulted in SO include paracentesis, cyclodialysis, and keratectomy, and the risk of SO increases when these surgical procedures are accompanied or followed by additional operations, particularly in the posterior segment of the eye.[15] The incidence of postvitrectomy SO has been estimated at 0.01%.[16] SO may occur after evisceration, probably as a result of remaining uveal tissue in the scleral emissary channels.[17]

Only very rarely has SO been diagnosed in cases where there was no perforating wound of the eye, and in many of these cases, the possibility of an occult globe rupture cannot be completely excluded. However, SO has been reported[18] following laser cyclocoagulation without apparent globe rupture. Occasionally, the disorder follows perforating corneal ulcers, ocular contusion without rupture of the globe, and intraocular malignancies.[19–21] SO has been diagnosed months after helium ion irradiation of a choroidal melanoma; however, a clinically inapparent scleral scar was detected on histopathological examination, possibly indicating an occult scleral rupture.[22]

The highest recorded incidences of SO have occurred during military conflict. In the American Civil War (1861–1865), 16% of all ocular injuries reportedly led to the development of SO. In the Franco–Prussian War (1870–1871), the reported prevalence of SO after ocular injuries was 55.5% among the Germans and 50% among the French. The disease was still relatively common in the Russo–Japanese War (1904–1905), during which it complicated 5% of eye injuries. In contrast, only rare cases of SO were reported in World Wars I and II, and none were reported in the Korean, Vietnam, and Persian Gulf wars.[1,3] Some of the earlier figures must be viewed with some skepticism: in the older literature in particular, SO probably was often confused with other forms of uveitis, and there were few, if any, specialized ophthalmologists among physicians in most wars before this century. Nevertheless, it is interesting and says much for the advances in eye care in the theater of operations that there has been such a dramatic decrease in the incidence of SO in the past century.

CLINICAL FEATURES

SO begins after a latent period following an injury to the eye. In general, 65% of SO cases occur 2 weeks to 2 months after injury, and 90% occur within the first year.[3,7] However, SO has been reported as early as 5 days after injury and as late as 66 years.[1,7] These figures become clinically important in the prevention of SO. Because the only known prevention is enucleation of the injured eye prior to the onset of the disorder, obviously such enucleation must be performed early. It is generally agreed that enucleation of an irreparably damaged eye should occur within 2 weeks of injury. Furthermore, although it may be assumed that the risk of SO is extremely small after 3 months, it may never reach zero. Any patient who has sustained a penetrating ocular injury should be considered to

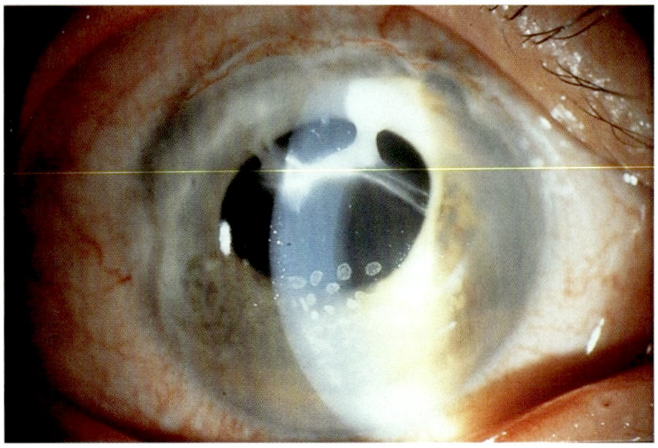

Fig. 16-2. An eye with sympathetic ophthalmia demonstrating the "mutton-fat" keratic precipitates characteristic of granulomatous intraocular inflammation. Scarring from the original injury is present in the superior cornea. Photograph: Courtesy of G. Foulks, MD, Chairman, Department of Ophthalmology, University of Pittsburgh Medical Center, Pittsburgh, Pa.

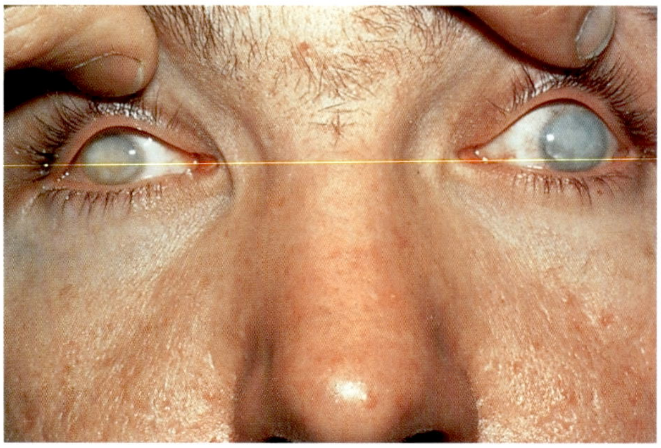

Fig. 16-3. Severe, bilateral granulomatous inflammation leading to loss of vision in both eyes. Note the shrunken appearance of the right eye indicating early phthisical changes. Photograph: Courtesy of G. Foulks, MD, Chairman, Department of Ophthalmology, University of Pittsburgh Medical Center, Pittsburgh, Pa.

be at lifelong risk, albeit very small, for the development of this disease.

The diagnosis, especially the early diagnosis, of SO is one of the most important in ophthalmology because prompt and aggressive therapy is required to save vision. The presenting symptoms of the disease include changes in accommodative amplitude, photophobia, and epiphora. Early signs on clinical examination include a low-grade, persistent uveitis associated with granulomatous ("mutton-fat") or small, white keratic precipitates (Figure 16-2). A diffuse thickening of the iris or iris nodules similar to that seen in sarcoidosis sometimes occurs. Posteriorly, small, yellow-white chorioretinal lesions (Dalen-Fuchs nodules), vitreous cells and haze, choroidal infiltration and thickening, retinal vascular sheathing, and disk edema may be seen. A similar clinical picture develops in the exciting eye and both eyes may proceed to blindness (Figure 16-3).

The presence of Dalen-Fuchs nodules is among the most classic findings in SO, so classic that they were once considered pathognomonic for the disorder. These nodules may occur anywhere in the fundus but are more common in the mid periphery.[3,23] They are yellowish white lesions, typically 60 to 700 μm (microns) in diameter, found in the subretinal space in at least one third of cases (Figure 16-4).[24] Dalen-Fuchs nodules are no longer considered pathognomonic for SO, as they have also been reported in other cases of granulomatous uveitis, such as sarcoidosis, tuberculosis, and the Vogt-Koyanagi-Harada syndrome (VKH).[24] Often, microscopic breaks occur in Bruch's membrane underneath the nodules.[25,26] These defects in Bruch's membrane may lead to the rare development of subretinal neovascularization.[27,28]

Systemic findings in SO are uncommon but possible. Vitiligo, poliosis, alopecia, dysacusis, and meningeal irritation—findings more commonly reported in the VKH syndrome—may be noted.[3,29] An

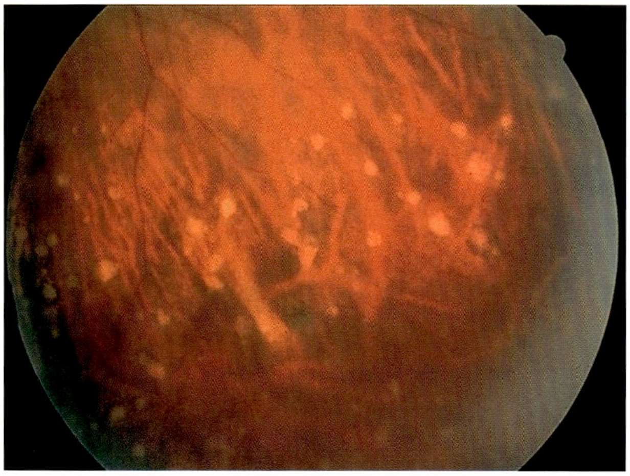

Fig. 16-4. The fundus of the eye of a patient with sympathetic ophthalmia. Note the characteristic yellowish white Dalen-Fuchs nodules in the mid periphery. These granulomatous lesions are found in at least one third of cases. Photograph: Courtesy of G. Foulks, MD, Chairman, Department of Ophthalmology, University of Pittsburgh Medical Center, Pittsburgh, Pa.

increased number of cells (mostly lymphocytes) in the cerebrospinal fluid can also be infrequently observed.[15] These similarities with the VKH syndrome suggest a possible relationship between the two diseases.

Fluorescein angiography seldom is necessary to establish the diagnosis of SO. There appear to be two types of abnormal fluorescence. The most frequently reported type is similar to that usually seen in VKH and consists of multiple sites of choroidal leakage with late coalescence of dye under serous retinal detachments. The sites of choroidal leakage correspond to the Dalen-Fuchs nodules observed clinically. The second, less-common angiographic appearance is similar to that seen in a number of other causes of posterior uveitis, such as acute posterior multifocal placoid pigment epitheliopathy. This form demonstrates lesions that (1) block the background choroidal fluorescence during the early phases and (2) stain late.[3,15,26,30]

SO runs a chronic course, with a marked tendency toward relapses, and the disease may culminate in a phthisical eye (or eyes) and blindness. Before the advent of corticosteroid therapy, the visual prognosis was extremely poor, with approximately 70% of affected eyes becoming permanently blind.[31] The more severe the inflammation, the poorer the prognosis; the earlier the diagnosis and more intensive the therapy, the better the outlook. Complications, including cataract, secondary glaucoma, exudative retinal detachment, choroidal scarring, and optic atrophy, are common in long-standing cases.

HISTOPATHOLOGY

The histopathological findings in SO, first described by Fuchs in 1905, consist of a diffuse, granulomatous uveitis with a massive lymphocytic infiltration and nests of macrophages, epithelioid cells, and multinucleated giant cells in both the exciting and the sympathizing eyes (Figures 16-5 and 16-6).[5] The inflammation is nonnecrotizing, and the epithelioid cells are often seen engulfing melanin pigment. The exciting eye differs from the sympathizing eye only by the evidence of and complications stemming from the preceding injury or surgical procedure. Nodules containing macrophages, epithelioid cells, and retinal pigment epithelial cells frequently occur between Bruch's membrane and the retinal pigment epithelium (ie, Dalen-Fuchs nodules; these are discussed in greater detail below). Eosinophils may be present in the uvea, especially in early cases.[7,32] The inflammatory process

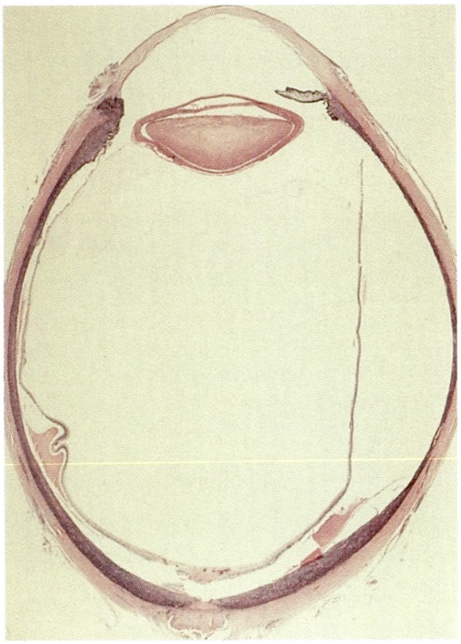

Fig. 16-5. This low-power photomicrograph demonstrates the diffuse uveal thickening secondary to inflammatory cells in a case of sympathetic ophthalmia (hematoxylin-eosin stain, original magnification x 1).

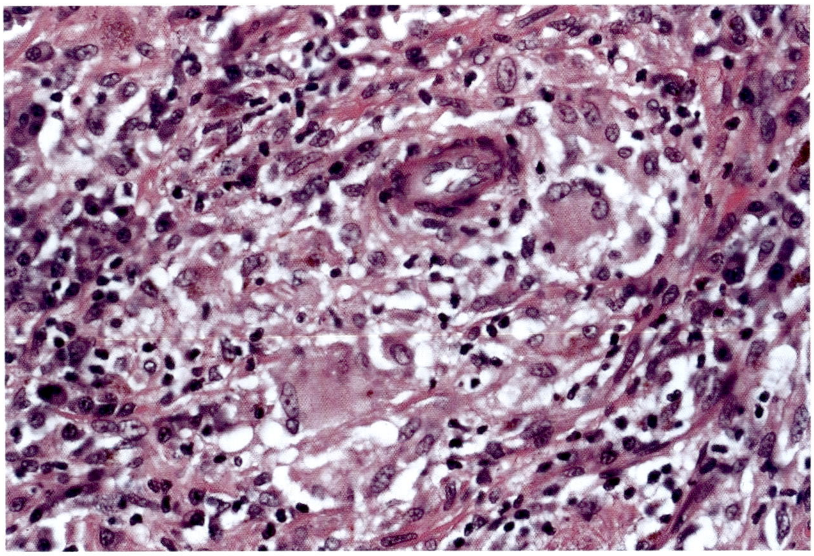

Fig. 16-6. Higher magnification of the uveal infiltrate demonstrating a chronic, granulomatous inflammation consisting of lymphocytes, epithelioid cells, and multinucleated giant cells. (hematoxylin-eosin stain, original magnification x 400).

classically spares the choriocapillaris and retina, and the posterior uvea is generally affected more than the anterior part. The pathological diagnosis depends mainly on the predominant T cell lymphocytic infiltration in the uvea, the early phagocytosis of pigment granules, and the presence of Dalen-Fuchs nodules.[33–35]

The uveal infiltrate consists predominantly of T cells, supporting the concept of a cell-mediated immune reaction (delayed hypersensitivity). Early in the disease, the majority of the T cells are of the helper/inducer subset, with less than 5% to 10% of the cells characterized as B cells, plasma cells, or monocytes.[35,36] In chronic cases, T cells of the suppressor/cytotoxic class predominate.[3,34,37] The change from predominantly helper/inducer T cells in acute disease to suppressor/cytotoxic T cells in the chronic phase is also seen in an animal model of SO, experimental autoimmune uveitis (EAU).[34]

A very specific histopathological finding in SO is that of Dalen-Fuchs nodules, which are clusters of epithelioid cells between the retinal pigment epithelium (RPE) and Bruch's membrane (Figure 16-7). These lesions are often pigmented, especially in chronic disease, and it used to be thought that the cells composing the nodule represented transformed RPE, forming a cagelike framework.[38,39] More recent studies have demonstrated that Dalen-Fuchs nodules are composed of a mixture of well-defined and closely packed epithelioid cells underlying a dome of RPE. Metaplastic cells from the RPE, lymphocytes, and giant cells may occasionally be found within the nodular structure.[7,24,34,35] In the late stages of SO, degenerated RPE can become an important component of the nodules.[3] Light- and electron-microscopic studies[25,26] reveal frequent breaks in Bruch's membrane underlying the nodules.

A zonal granulomatous reaction to the lens (phacoanaphylactic endophthalmitis, phacoantigenic uveitis, lens-induced uveitis) is often found in cases of SO (Figure 16-8). In one series it was found in 23% of 170 documented cases.[40] In a review of 100 cases of SO from the files of the Armed Forces Institute of Pathology, Washington, DC,[12] 14 cases were associated with phacoanaphylactic endophthalmitis (22% of the 46 eyes enucleated before 1950, compared with only 7% of the 54 eyes enucleated after 1950). This decline in the associated incidence of phacoanaphylactic endophthalmitis and SO has been demonstrated in several other reports. In a retrospective analysis[41] of 144 cases of phacoanaphylactic endophthalmitis from 1970 to 1988, only 4 cases (2.6%) of SO were diagnosed. In another series[42] of 105 cases of SO that spanned the years 1913 to 1978 and that contained 48 cases of phacoantigenic uveitis (46%), only 1 case of the 48 was detected after 1949. The authors of this latter study[42] attribute the decline in incidence to the introduction of corticosteroid therapy and the more-complete treatment that lens injuries currently receive.

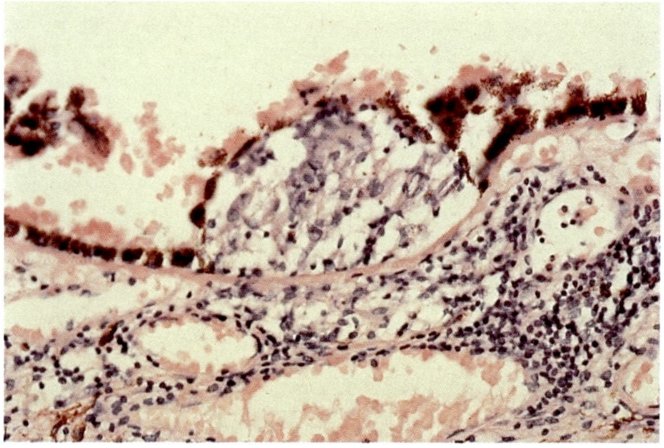

Fig. 16-7. High magnification of a Dalen-Fuchs nodule. This is a very specific histopathological finding in sympathetic ophthalmia, consisting of clusters of epithelioid cells between the retinal pigment epithelium (RPE) and Bruch's membrane (hematoxylin-eosin stain, original magnification x 800).

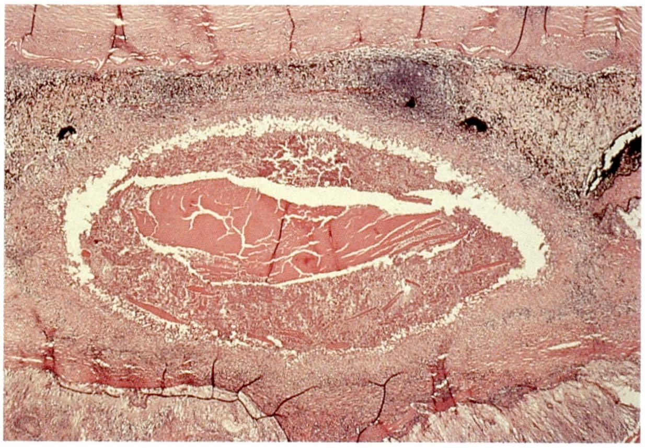

Fig. 16-8. A zonal granulomatous reaction to the lens (phacoanaphylactic endophthalmitis, phacoantigenic uveitis, lens-induced uveitis) is often found in sympathetic ophthalmia (hematoxylin-eosin stain, original magnification x 40).

PATHOGENESIS

Ever since SO was first described, physicians have speculated about a mechanism that could explain how an injury to one eye could result in inflammation of both. Writers in the 19th century hypothesized that the inflammation was propagated along the optic nerves and chiasm from one eye to the other; others suggested the trigeminal nerve as the route of transmission.[1]

Hypersensitivity Reaction Theories

That the disorder might represent a hypersensitivity reaction was first suggested in 1903, with uveal pigment proposed as the offending antigen.[6,43] The characteristic phagocytosis of melanin seen on histopathological examination would support a possible role for the pigment, but the experimental evidence for this is weak, and melanin generally is considered to be nonantigenic. However, investigators during the early 1990s described an insoluble uveal melanin preparation that can produce an inflammation limited to the uvea in immunized animals, and later workers reported that spontaneous recurrences of the inflammation occurred that were reminiscent of human SO.[3]

Uveal or retinal antigens other than melanin might be involved. Certainly the finding that uveal injury is an almost constant precursor to the development of SO makes the uvea a prime suspect. Uveal tissue alone is weakly antigenic, but its antigenicity can be increased with staphylococcal toxin or complete Freund's adjuvant.[44–47] Although this type of immunization produces a severe uveitis in guinea pigs and monkeys, it is nongranulomatous and does not resemble human SO. Antiuveal antibodies have been reported[48] in a high percentage of individuals with SO, and enhanced transformation of peripheral lymphocytes has been found[49] following exposure to homologous uveoretinal antigen. Others[44] consider the presence of circulating antibodies to uvea to merely represent a nonspecific result of tissue injury.

Evidence for Autoimmunity Role

There is persuasive evidence that clinical sympathetic ophthalmitis may represent an autoimmune response to antigens derived from the retinal photoreceptor layer.[50] Sera from patients with SO showed mild to moderate staining of the outer segments of the photoreceptors using an indirect immunoperoxidase technique.[51] Retinal extracts are highly antigenic and easily produce retinouveitis in experimental animals. Four of the potential retinal antigens are rhodopsin, retinal soluble antigen (S-antigen), interphotoreceptor retinoid binding protein, and recoverin.[3]

The most extensively studied of these has been S-antigen. EAU induced in animals by immunization with S-antigen is considered to be a model for the human ocular condition, resembling SO both clinically and in its response to therapy.[52–54] Cell-mediated immunity to the retinal S-antigen has been demonstrated in animals.[53] To date, however, circulating anti-S-antigen antibodies have not been detected in the sera of humans with SO.[51]

Specific epitopes of another retinal protein, interstitial retinoid binding protein (IRBP), are also capable of eliciting uveitis. Peptide fragments containing these epitopes, as well as IRBP itself, produce experimental autoimmune uveitis in Lewis rats.[55] Other recent immunohistochemical investigations suggest that SO is mediated by delayed T cell hypersensitivity directed at surface membrane antigens shared by photoreceptors, RPE cells, and choroidal melanocytes.[34] Interestingly, some of the antigens used to produce an experimental model of SO in animals (S-antigen, IRBP) also cause an inflammatory disease of the pineal gland. As yet no evidence has been reported for pineal gland involvement in human disease.[56]

The absence of lymphatics within the eye may play an important role in the pathogenesis of SO. Normally, intraocular antigens circulate to the blood and spleen, bypassing local lymph nodes, which may result in the induction of blocking antibodies or suppressor cells in the spleen. However, in cases of penetrating ocular trauma, these antigens drain directly into the regional lymph nodes, permitting the initiation of a cell-mediated immune response.[3,57] Thus, a key step in the development of SO may be the exposure of uveoretinal antigens to the conjunctival lymphatics. Simultaneously, bacteria (eg, *Propionibacterium acnes*), viruses, and other infectious agents can enter the eye through the wound, and this exposure might serve as an adjuvant to induce or up-regulate the inflammatory process.

Association With HLA Types

SO has been associated with certain human leukocyte antigen (HLA) types. For example, HLA-A11 has been reported[58] in patients with histopathologically proved SO; the relative risk in the disease group, compared with the control group, was 11. In another study[59] of the VKH syndrome and SO, strong associations of VKH with HLA-DR4 and HLA-DRw53 were found; the strongest associations observed were with HLA-DQw3. The small number of patients with SO in this latter study[59] precluded statistical analysis; nevertheless, similar HLA associations were noted. HLA class II loci (ie, HLA-DR, HLA-DQ, HLA-DP) appear to be especially important in immune responses mediated through T helper cells, because the surface molecules coded by these genes interact directly with antigen and with the T cell receptor in the regulation of immune responses.

Possible Role of Bacterial Antigens

Although the association with trauma, exposure of uveal tissue, and characteristic granulomatous inflammatory process is suggestive of a possible infective process, no confirmation of a causative organism has been reported to date. A causal role has been proposed for *Mycobacterium tuberculosis, Bacillus subtilis*, *Rickettsia*, and various viruses, and although infectious agents are sporadically isolated, none have fulfilled Koch's postulates.[60–62] In fact, it has long been known that SO rarely occurs in cases with endophthalmitis.[63] More likely, biological products (eg, a bacterial cell wall), which may be present in the wound, could act as immunostimulators and thereby up-regulate a local immune response. As has been noted above, although uveal tissue itself is only weakly antigenic, its antigenicity can be increased with staphylococcal toxin or complete Freund's adjuvant.[45–47]

It is tempting to hypothesize that the perforating ocular injury permits several events to take place. The first is that drainage of a uveal or a retinal antigen, or both, occurs through the conjunctival lymphatics, an event that does not occur under normal conditions. The second is that small amounts of adjuvant, such as bacterial cell wall or other immunostimulators, enter the eye through the perforation. These products then may upgrade profoundly the local immune response, causing it to bypass certain inherent suppressor mechanisms in genetically prone individuals. This phenomenon then leads to the inflammatory response that ultimately becomes the clinical entity recognized as SO.[64]

DIFFERENTIAL DIAGNOSIS

The major consideration in the differential diagnosis is VKH syndrome, a disease that has many features in common with sympathetic uveitis. Patients with the VKH syndrome have no history of trauma and typically have bilateral localized serous detachments of the retina, findings that are not typically seen in SO. VKH syndrome is also more prevalent in certain racial and ethnic groups. Despite these differences, the only clear distinctions between VKH and SO are (1) the history of trauma in SO and (2) the very rare occurrence of central nervous system symptoms and pigmentary changes in SO, findings that are often seen in VKH syndrome. In the typical case of SO, no laboratory studies are necessary for diagnosis. Should it be necessary to differentiate SO from VKH syndrome, a lumbar puncture should be performed early in the course of the disease. This reveals a pleocytosis in 84% of VKH cases, with mostly lymphocytes and monocytes present.[65]

Other causes of a bilateral, granulomatous panuveitis, such as sarcoidosis, pars planitis, and certain infections, are usually fairly easy to differentiate from SO on history and clinical examination. The association between SO and lens-induced uveitis has been mentioned above.[12,40,41] Either disease may occur alone, and both may be present in the same eye. This association is much greater than we would expect by chance alone and strengthens the hypothesis that lens-induced uveitis and SO are both immunological in nature. If lens-induced uveitis is present, then surgical removal of the lens or lens fragments should be considered.

TREATMENT

Enucleation

As stated above, the earliest method for the prevention of SO was to induce a suppurative inflammation in the injured eye. This treatment was well known to veterinary surgeons,[1,9,63] but for obvious reasons is not appropriate for humans. The classic method to prevent SO remains enucleation of the injured eye before the other eye develops disease. The role of enucleation was borrowed from veterinary surgery by Wardrop in 1818, put into clinical practice by Prichard in 1851, and fully established in ophthalmological routine as a measure of proven value by Critchett in 1863.[1] Enucleation of an injured eye within 2 weeks of injury almost always prevents the development of SO but is not an absolute preventive measure: SO does occasionally develop after enucleation. Of the 18 cases of SO from the Moorfields Eye Hospital, London, England, 1 (5.5%) occurred in a patient whose injured eye was enucleated before the onset of disease,[66] and of the 29 cases from the Armed Forces Institute of Pathology, 2 (6.9%) occurred after enucleation of the traumatized eyes.[67,3]

Evisceration is not an acceptable alternative to enucleation. SO can occur after evisceration, probably as a result of remaining uveal tissue in the scleral emissary channels. It would seem prudent not to perform eviscerations except perhaps in cases of endophthalmitis or in patients whose general condition is very poor, who thus may not be able to withstand the more-involved enucleation procedure.[17,68]

If there is reasonable doubt regarding the visual potential of an injured eye, then every effort should be made to preserve it. With aggressive immunosuppressive therapy, good vision may be retained in an exciting eye, sometimes better vision than in the sympathizing eye.[7] Careful microsurgical management of the wound, with prompt closure of all penetrating injuries, is an effective—although not absolute—measure for avoiding the development of SO. Uveal incarceration into the wound must be avoided.

Once definite signs of disease have started in the second eye, enucleation of the injured eye, except when it is blind or painful, is of little or no value and may be inadvisable. A review[69] of 257 cases of histopathologically proven SO indicated no benefit to the sympathizing eye from enucleation of the exciting eye, whether performed briefly before, concomitant with, or subsequent to the development of SO at various intervals following injury.

Some investigators,[42] however, have suggested that enucleation within 2 weeks after symptoms of SO have begun might improve the visual prognosis. Significantly fewer recurrences of inflammatory disease in patients who underwent early enucleation have been reported,[3] but there was no improvement in ultimate visual acuity. In a retrospective clinicopathological study[70] of 30 cases of SO, early enucleation of the exciting eye was associated with a benign clinical course: visual acuity better than 20/50 and fewer and milder relapses than eyes that underwent late enucleation. This remains a very controversial subject, with strong arguments for and against enucleation as a therapeutic measure.[70–73] It is probably advisable not to enucleate an eye with any visual potential. Enucleation should be reserved for those eyes with no light perception or perhaps with only bare light perception. There have been reports[74] of cases of sympathetic uveitis that showed sudden recovery of a sympathizing eye without enucleating the injured eye, even after a long period of unresponsiveness to corticosteroids.

Corticosteroids

Once SO has developed, the systemic therapy of first choice remains corticosteroids, and the inflammation usually responds rapidly. Corticosteroids have revolutionized the treatment of this disease. Before the use of corticosteroids the visual prognosis was generally poor, and approximately 70% of the eyes became permanently blind.[31] Now the prognosis is markedly better. Makley and Azar[75] found that 9 (64%) of 14 treated patients attained 20/60 vision or better, Lubin and colleagues[42] noted that 13 (72%) of 18 treated patients achieved 20/50 vision or better, and Reynard and colleagues[70] reported that 18 (82%) of 22 treated patients had 20/50 vision or better.

Large doses of corticosteroids should be given early in the course of the disease and continued for at least 6 months after apparent resolution of inflammation. In adults, oral doses as high as 100 to 200 mg of prednisone are suggested for the first week.[15] The initiating dose can be reduced by approximately 5 mg/wk—so long as the inflammatory activity remains controlled—to a maintenance dose of 5–10 mg/d.[7] Patients on systemic steroids require regular monitoring of their blood pressure and blood glucose levels. Infection needs to be ruled out before initiating systemic corticosteroids.

Although corticosteroids are very effective in the treatment of SO, they cannot prevent the development of the disease. Several reports[3,49,76] have demonstrated that SO may develop despite the use of systemic or topical corticosteroids.

Immunosuppressive Agents

In some patients, corticosteroid drugs alone are ineffective (which is unusual in SO), or too high a dose is necessary to achieve control (a more common problem). Additionally, medical problems and systemic or ophthalmological complications may prevent their protracted use by some patients, such as those with diabetes mellitus, uncontrolled glaucoma, or psychological problems. In these individuals, alternative treatment with immunosuppressive agents can effectively suppress inflammation, allowing a reduction of corticosteroid therapy to a nontoxic level.

The recommended agents are usually cyclosporin A (5 mg/kg/d) in patients younger than approximately 40 years or azathioprine (2 mg/kg/d in three divided doses) in older patients.[7,77] Because eyes with SO are usually infiltrated with numerous activated T cells, cyclosporine, a potent inhibitor of T cell function, can be a very effective therapeutic agent. The recommended dosages for a combination of cyclosporine and steroids are cyclosporin A (3–5 mg/kg/d) and prednisone (15–20 mg/d).[3,77] Renal function tests (eg, blood urea nitrogen, creatinine) should be monitored regularly in patients taking cyclosporine.

Other agents have been advocated for the treatment of intractable SO. Some authors[78,79] have advocated high-dose, short-term chlorambucil. Because chlorambucil is well absorbed from the gastrointestinal tract, it has the advantage of oral administration. With chlorambucil, corticosteroids can often be completely discontinued, whereas with cyclosporine they are often required, especially if the dose of cyclosporine needs to be decreased because of renal toxicity.[78] Methotrexate is another potentially useful drug and has the advantage of a weekly dosing schedule.[7]

IMPLICATIONS FOR MILITARY MEDICINE

Eye injuries will continue to be of major significance in combat. The incidence of eye injuries sustained by US forces has increased 18-fold since the Civil War, reaching 9% in the Vietnam War.[80] Conflicts since Vietnam have continued to demonstrate the increasing frequency of battlefield ocular injuries, reaching 13% of the patient volume at a major combat support hospital during the ground phase of the Persian Gulf War.[81] Therefore, soldiers are at continued risk for ocular injury and for subsequent development of SO. Prevention of eye injuries remains the best means to eliminate the risk of SO, and this fact lends further support to the argument for improved development, deployment, and use of eye armor.

Once a penetrating eye injury has occurred, however, trained ophthalmologists should promptly and meticulously close it. This procedure requires that ophthalmologists be present in the theater of operations, along with specialized equipment such as the operating microscope and microsurgical instruments. The dramatic decrease in the incidence of SO since the American Civil War—despite the overall increase in the incidence of ocular injuries—can be largely attributed to the advances in the management of traumatized eyes on the battlefield.

It must be stressed that enucleation should be considered only in those cases where the visual prognosis is nil and the eye is irreparable (Figure 16-9). Eyes with any potential vision should *not* be

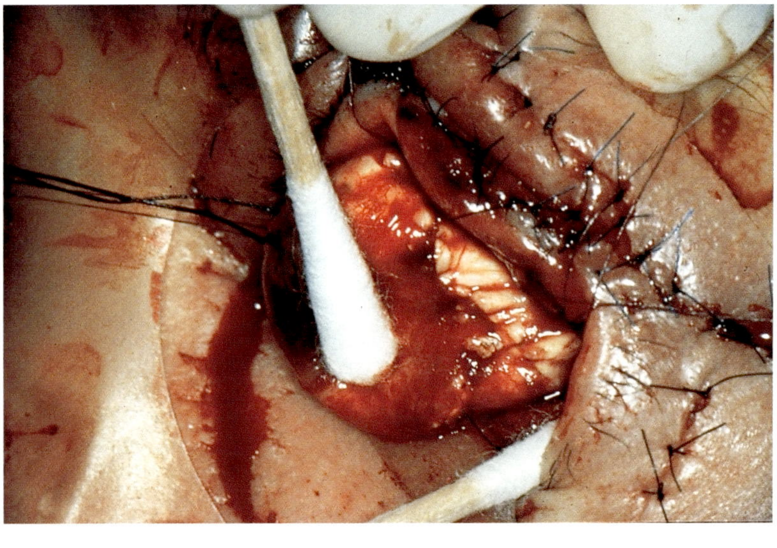

Fig. 16-9. This irreparably injured eye required enucleation to prevent the development of sympathetic ophthalmia. Such enucleations should be performed within 2 weeks of injury. This eye had no light perception (NLP) vision. Photograph: Courtesy of Francis G. La Piana, MD, Colonel, Medical Corps, US Army (Ret), Washington, DC.

enucleated. Enucleation, like the surgical care of penetrating eye injuries, also requires the presence of fully trained and competent ophthalmologists in the theater of operations. During the Vietnam War, a number of unnecessary enucleations occurred because the patients were managed by nonophthalmologists or by only partially trained ophthalmic surgeons.[82]

Careful follow-up should be afforded to all patients with penetrating eye injuries. The early signs and symptoms of SO must be carefully watched for, and, if the disease does develop, prompt and aggressive therapy must be initiated under the direction of an ophthalmologist.

SUMMARY

SO is a rare, bilateral, granulomatous uveitis, usually associated with a perforating eye injury. The exact cause is unknown, but it is believed to be related to an autoimmune response to retinal or uveal antigens or both. A severely injured eye with no prognosis for vision should be enucleated within 2 weeks of injury to prevent SO. The disease usually responds rapidly to corticosteroid therapy, but recalcitrant cases may require the addition of other immunosuppressive agents.

The highest incidence of SO has occurred in eyes injured on the battlefield; therefore, this disorder is of particular importance to military ophthalmologists, who should be present in the theater of operations. With modern microsurgical management of ocular injuries, the incidence of this disorder has dramatically decreased in the 20th century.

REFERENCES

1. Duke-Elder S, Perkins ES. *Diseases of the Uveal Tract*. Vol 9. In: Duke-Elder S, ed. *System of Ophthalmology*. Vol 9. London, England: Henry Kimpton; 1966: 558–559.

2. Albert DM, Diaz-Rohena R. A historical review of sympathetic ophthalmia and its epidemiology. *Surv Ophthalmol*. 1989;34:1–14.

3. Chan CC, Whitcup SM, Nussenblatt RB. Sympathetic ophthalmia and Vogt-Koyanagi-Harada syndrome. In: Albert DM; Jakobiec FM, eds. *Clinical Ophthalmology*. Philadelphia, Pa: WB Saunders; 1994: 1–5.

4. Mackenzie W. *A Practical Treatise on Disease of the Eye*. London, England: Longmans; 1840: 523–534.

5. Fuchs E. Über sympathisietende Entzündung (nebst Bemerkungen über seröse traumatische Iritis). *Graefes Arch Clin Exp Ophthalmol*. 1905;61:365–456.

6. Elschnig A. Studies on sympathetic ophthalmia, II: The antigenic effect of eye pigments. *Graefes Arch Clin Exp Opthalmol*. 1910;76:509–546.

7. Towler HMA, Lightman S. Sympathetic ophthalmia. *Int Ophthalmol Clin*. 1995;35:31–42.

8. Rosen MJ. *Tribute to a Genius*. 1999. Available at http://www.thurberhouse.org. Accessed Oct 2001.

9. Wardrop J. *Essays on the Morbid Anatomy of the Human Eye*. London, England: Constable; 1818: 139.

10. Foster CS. Ocular manifestations of immune disease. In: Garner A, Klintworth GK, eds. *Pathobiology of Ocular Disease: A Dynamic Approach*. New York, NY: Marcel Dekker; 1994: 172–174.

11. Liddy L, Stuart J. Sympathetic ophthalmia in Canada. *Can J Ophthalmol*. 1972;7:157–159.

12. Croxatto JO, Galentine P, Cupples HP, Harper D, Reader A, Zimmerman LE. Sympathetic ophthalmia after pars plana vitrectomy-lensectomy for endogenous bacterial endophthalmitis. *Am J Ophthalmol*. 1981;91:342–346.

13. Lakhanpal V, Dogra MR, Jacobson MS. Sympathetic ophthalmia associated with anterior chamber intraocular lens implantation. *Ann Ophthalmol*. 1991;23:139–143.

14. Lyons C, Tuft S, Lightman S. Sympathetic ophthalmia from inadvertent ocular perforation during conventional retinal detachment surgery. *Br J Ophthalmol*. 1997;81:612.

15. Goto H, Rao NA. Sympathetic ophthalmia and Vogt-Koyanagi-Harada syndrome. *Int Ophthalmol Clin*. 1990;30:279–85.

16. Gass JDM. Sympathetic ophthalmia following vitrectomy. *Am J Ophthalmol*. 1982;93:552–558.

17. Green WR, Maumenee AE, Sanders TW, Smith ME. Sympathetic uveitis following evisceration. *Trans Am Acad Ophthalmol Otolaryngol*. 1972;76:625–644.

18. Bechrakis NE, Müller-Stolzenburg NW, Helbig H, Foerster MH. Sympathetic ophthalmia following laser cyclocoagulation. *Arch Ophthalmol*. 1994;112:80–84.

19. Easom HA. Sympathetic ophthalmia associated with malignant melanoma. *Arch Ophthalmol*. 1963;70:786–790.

20. Riwchun MH, DeCoursey E. Sympathetic ophthalmia caused by non-perforating intraocular sarcoma. *Arch Ophthalmol*. 1941;25:848–858.

21. Joy HH. A survey of cases of sympathetic ophthalmia in New York State. *Arch Ophthalmol*. 1935;14:733–741.

22. Fries PD, Char DH, Crawford JB, Waterhouse W. Sympathetic ophthalmia complicating helium ion irradiation of a choroidal melanoma. *Arch Ophthalmol*. 1987;105:1561–1564.

23. Puliafito CA, Smith TR, Packer AJ, Albert DM. Ocular pathology for clinicians, II: Sympathetic uveitis. *Ophthalmology*. 1980;87:355–358.

24. Reynard M, Riffenburgh RS, Minckler DS. Morphological variation of Dalen-Fuchs nodules in sympathetic ophthalmia. *Br J Ophthalmol*. 1985;69:197–201.

25. Rao NA, Xu S, Font RL. Sympathetic ophthalmia: An immunohistochemical study of epithelioid and giant cells. *Ophthalmology*. 1985;92:1660–1662.

26. Sharp DC, Bell RA, Patterson E, Pinkerton RMH. Sympathetic ophthalmia: Histopathologic and fluorescein angiographic correlation. *Arch Ophthalmol*. 1984;102:232–235.

27. Carney MD, Tessler HH, Peyman GA, Goldberg MF, Williams DP. Sympathetic ophthalmia and subretinal neovascularization. *Ann Ophthalmol*. 1990;22:184–186.

28. Chew EY, Crawford J. Sympathetic ophthalmia and choroidal neovascularization. *Arch Ophthalmol*. 1988;106:1507–1508.

29. Rao NA, Marak GE Jr. Sympathetic ophthalmia simulating Vogt-Koyanagi-Harada's disease: A clinico-pathologic study of four cases. *Jpn J Ophthalmol*. 1983;27:506–511.

30. Segawa K, Matsuoka N. Sympathetic ophthalmia: A comparative fluorographic and electron microscopic study. *Jpn J Ophthalmol*. 1971;15:81–87.

31. Woods AC. *Endogenous Uveitis*. Baltimore, Md: Williams & Wilkins; 1956: 87–92.

32. Marak GE Jr, Font RL, Zimmerman LE. Histologic variations related to race in sympathetic ophthalmia. *Am J Ophthalmol*. 1974;78:935–938.

33. Chan CC, Nussenblatt RB, Fujikawa LS, et al. Sympathetic ophthalmia: Immunopathological findings. *Ophthalmology*. 1986;93:690–695.

34. Jakobiec FA, Marboe CC, Knowles DM II, et al. Human sympathetic ophthalmia: An analysis of the inflammatory infiltrate by hybridomamonoclonal antibodies, immunochemistry, and correlative electron microscopy. *Ophthalmology*. 1983;90:76–95.

35. Chan CC, BenEzra D, Rodrigues MM, et al. Immunohistochemistry and electron microscopy of choroidal infiltrates and Dalen-Fuchs nodules in sympathetic ophthalmia. *Ophthalmology*. 1985;92:580–590.

36. Kaplan HJ, Waldrep JC, Chan WC, Nicholson JKA, Wright JD. Human sympathetic ophthalmia: Immunologic analysis of the vitreous and uvea. *Arch Ophthalmol*. 1986;104:240–244.

37. Müller-Hermelink HK, Kraus-Mackiw E, Daus W. Early stage of human sympathetic ophthalmia: Histologic and immunopathologic findings. *Arch Ophthalmol*. 1984;102:1353–1357.

38. Font RL, Fine BS, Messmer E, Rowsey JF. Light and electron microscopic study of Dalen-Fuchs nodules in sympathetic ophthalmia. *Ophthalmology*. 1983;90:66–75.

39. Ishikawa T, Ikui H. The fine structure of the Dalen-Fuchs nodule in sympathetic ophthalmia, I: Changes in the pigment epithelial cells within the Dalen-Fuchs nodule. *Jpn J Ophthalmol*. 1972;16:254–265.

40. Blodi FC. Sympathetic uveitis as an allergic phenomenon. *Trans Am Acad Ophthalmol Otolaryngology*. 1959;63:642–649.

41. Thach AB, Marak GE, McLean IW, Green WR. Phacoanaphylactic endophthalmitis: A clinicopathologic review. *Int Ophthalmol*. 1991;15:271–279.

42. Lubin JR, Albert DM, Weinstein M. Sixty-five years of sympathetic ophthalmia: A clinicopathologic review of 105 cases (1913–1978). *Ophthalmology*. 1980;87:109–121.

43. Pusey B. Cytotoxins and sympathetic ophthalmia. *Arch Ophthalmol*. 1903;32:334–338.

44. Marak GE Jr, Tischler SM, Evans PY, Alepa FP. Pathogenesis of sympathetic ophthalmia. *Invest Ophthalmol*. 1971;10:162.

45. Lucic H. Sensitization of rabbits to uveal tissue by the synergic action of staphylotoxin. *Arch Ophthalmol*. 1939;22:359–369.

46. Collins RC. Experimental studies on sympathetic ophthalmia. *Am J Ophthalmol*. 1949;32:1687–1699.

47. Collins RC. Further experimental studies on sympathetic ophthalmia. *Am J Ophthalmol*. 1953;36:150–161.

48. Aronson SB. The role of non-specific tests in uveitis. In: Aronson SB, Gamble CN, Goodner ED, O'Connor GR, eds. *Clinical Methods of Uveitis*. St Louis, Mo: CV Mosby; 1968: 185–196.

49. Wong VG, Anderson R, O'Brien PJ. Sympathetic ophthalmia and lymphocyte transformation. *Am J Ophthalmol*. 1971;72:960–966.

50. Caspi RR. Basic mechanisms in immune-mediated uveitis disease. In: Lightman S, ed. *Immunology of Eye Diseases*. Dordrecht, The Netherlands: Kluwer Academic Publishers; 1989: 61–86.

51. Chan CC, Palestine AG, Nussenblatt RB, Roberge FG, Benezra D. Anti-retinal auto-antibodies in Vogt-Koyanagi-Harada syndrome, Behçet's disease, and sympathetic ophthalmia. *Ophthalmology*. 1985;92:1025–1028.

52. Wacker WB, Donoso LA, Kalsow CM, Yankeelov JA Jr, Organisciak DT. Experimental allergic uveitis: Isolation, characterization, and localization of a soluble uveitopathogenic antigen from bovine retina. *J Immunol*. 1977;119:1949–1958.

53. Nussenblatt RB, Kuwabara T, de Monasterio FM, Wacker WB. S-antigen uveitis in primates: A new model for human disease. *Arch Ophthalmol*. 1981;99:1090–1092.

54. Roberts AJ, Kasp E, Stanford M, Dumonde DC, Banga JP. Induction of experimental autoimmune uveoretinitis in Lewis rats with purified recombinant human retinal S-antigen fusion protein. *Eur J Immunol*. 1992; 22:951–956.

55. Sanui H, Redmond TM, Hu LH, et al. Synthetic peptides derived from IRBP induced EAU and EAP in Lewis rats. *Curr Eye Res.* 1988;7:727–735.

56. Kijlstra A, Hoekzema R, v.d. Lelij A, Doekes G, Rothova A. Humoral and cellular immune reaction against retinal antigens in clinical disease. *Curr Eye Res.* 1990;9(suppl):859.

57. Rao NA, Robin J, Hartmann D, Sweeney JA, Marak GE Jr. The role of the penetrating wound in the development of sympathetic ophthalmia: Experimental observations. *Arch Ophthalmol.* 1983;101:102–104.

58. Reynard M, Shulman IA, Azen SP, Minckler DS. Histocompatibility antigens in sympathetic ophthalmia. *Am J Ophthalmol.* 1983;95:216–221.

59. Davis JL, Mittal KK, Freidlin V, et al. HLA associations and ancestry in Vogt-Koyanagi-Harada disease and sympathetic ophthalmia. *Ophthalmology.* 1990;97:1137–1142.

60. Schlaegel TF Jr. *Essentials of Uveitis.* Boston, Mass: Little, Brown; 1969: 123–124.

61. Ikui H, Kimura K, Iwaki S. Electron microscopic study of ultrathin sections of sympathetic ophthalmia [preliminary report]. *Jpn J Ophthalmol.* 1958;2:13–20.

62. Ikui H, Kimura K, Nishio T, Furuyoshi Y. Etiology of sympathetic ophthalmia. *18th Int Cong Ophthal.* 1959;2:1285–1293.

63. Pusin SM, Green WR, Tasman W, Griffith WR, Rodriques M. Simultaneous bacterial endophthalmitis and sympathetic uveitis after retinal detachment surgery. *Am J Ophthalmol.* 1976;81:57–61.

64. Power WJ, Foster CS. Update on sympathetic ophthalmia. *Int Ophthalmol Clin.* 1995;35(1):127–137.

65. Ohno S, Minakawa R, Matsuda H. Clinical studies on Vogt-Koyanagi-Harada's disease. *Jpn J Ophthalmol.* 1988;32:334–343.

66. Hakin KN, Pearson RV, Lightman SL. Sympathetic ophthalmia: Visual results with modern imunosuppressive therapy. *Eye.* 1992;6(pt 5):453–455.

67. Shah DN, Piacentini MA, Burnier MN Jr, et al. Inflammatory cellular kinetics in sympathetic ophthalmia: A study of traumatized (exciting) eyes. *Ocul Immunol Inflamm.* 1993;1:255–262.

68. Ruedemann AD Jr. Sympathetic ophthalmia after evisceration. *Am J Ophthalmol.* 1964;57:770–790.

69. Winter FC. Sympathetic uveitis: A clinical and pathologic study of the visual result. *Am J Ophthalmol.* 1955;39:340–347.

70. Reynard M, Riffenburgh RS, Maes EF. Effect of corticosteroid treatment and enucleation on the visual prognosis of sympathetic ophthalmia. *Am J Ophthalmol.* 1983;96:290–294.

71. Lubin JR, Albert DM, Weinstein M. Reply to "Letter to the Editor." *Ophthalmology.* 1982;89:1291–1292.

72. Marak GE Jr. Recent advances in sympathetic ophthalmia. *Surv Ophthalmol.* 1979;24:141–156.

73. Jennings T, Tessler HH. Twenty cases of sympathetic ophthalmia. *Br J Ophthalmol.* 1989;73:140–145.

74. Kayazawa F. A case of sympathetic uveitis. *Ann Ophthalmol,* 1980;12:1106–1108.

75. Makley TA, Azar A. Sympathetic ophthalmia: A long term follow up. *Arch Ophthalmol.* 1978;96:257–262.

76. Mclean J. Steroid prophylaxis in sympathetic ophthalmia. *Am J Ophthalmol.* 1958;45:162–164.

77. Nussenblatt RB, Rodriques MM, Wacker WB, Cevario SJ, Salinas-Carmona MC, Gery I. Cyclosporin A: Inhibition of experimental autoimmune uveitis in Lewis rats. *J Clin Invest.* 1981;67:1228–1231.

78. Tessler HH, Jennings T. High-dose short-term chlorambucil for intractable sympathetic ophthalmia and Behçet's disease. *Br J Ophthalmol.* 1990;74:353–357.

79. Yang CS, Liu JH. Chlorambucil therapy in sympathetic ophthalmia. *Am J Ophthalmol.* 1995;119:482–488.

80. Wong TY, Seet MB, Ang CL. Eye injuries in twentieth century warfare: A historical perspective. *Surv Ophthalmol.* 1997;41:433–459.

81. Heier JS, Enzenauer RW, Wintermeyer SF, Delaney M, La Piana FG. Ocular injuries and diseases at a combat support hospital in support of Operations Desert Shield and Desert Storm. *Arch Ophthalmol.* 1993;111:795–798.

82. La Piana FG. Colonel, Medical Corps, US Army (Ret). Residency Program Director, Department of Ophthalmology, Washington Hospital Center, Washington, DC. Personal communication, May 1998.

Chapter 17

POSTTRAUMATIC ENDOPHTHALMITIS

CRAIG D. HARTRANFT, MD[*]; AND THADDEUS J. KROLICKI, MD[†]

Lieutenant Colonel, Medical Corps, US Army; Chief, Vitreoretinal Service, Madigan Army Medical Center, Tacoma, Washington 98431

†*Vitreoretinal Surgeon, Eye Clinic of Wisconsin, Wausau, Wisconsin 54403; formerly, Lieutenant Colonel, Medical Corps, US Army; Ophthalmology Service, Madigan Army Medical Center, Tacoma, Washington*

INTRODUCTION

Penetrating trauma to the globe (ie, a ruptured globe) is an ophthalmic challenge for many reasons. Few ophthalmologists see enough patients with this kind of injury to feel totally capable of handling them. Even surgeons who treat a large number of ruptured globes recognize that no two cases are exactly alike. Given this degree of variability in training and in case presentation, strategies for the repair of ruptured globes vary significantly. Endophthalmitis (ie, inflammation of the tissues within the eye) in the setting of trauma is another condition that the ophthalmologist sees infrequently; how the physician deals with penetrating trauma to the globe and resulting endophthalmitis can make the difference between salvaging vision or losing it to blindness or enucleation.

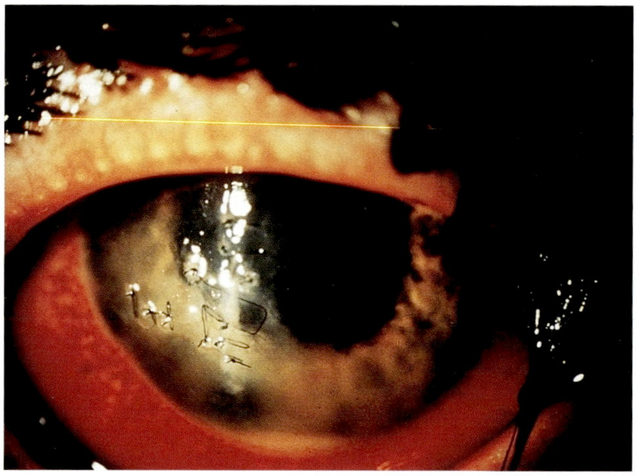

Fig. 17-1. Posttraumatic endophthalmitis with layered hypopyon. Photograph: Courtesy of Department of Ophthalmology, Madigan Army Medical Center, Tacoma, Wash.

Posttraumatic endophthalmitis (PTE) comprises one fourth of all culture-proven cases of endophthalmitis. It is estimated to develop in 2% to 11% of penetrating globe injuries.[1–5] When an intraocular foreign body (IOFB) is present, the potential for endophthalmitis increases; the reported incidence ranges from 4.7% to 15.0%.[6–9] Other risk factors include severe wounds, lens disruption, prolonged exposure of the intraocular contents to the environment, the setting in which the injury occurs, delays in diagnosis and treatment, advanced age of the patient, and compromised host immunity.[1,2,4,7]

PTE frequently carries a much poorer prognosis than postoperative endophthalmitis (POE) following planned surgery. Damage to ocular structures, including the cornea, lens, and retina, or infection with more virulent organisms tends to lessen the chance of visual recovery (Figure 17-1). The advent of improved microsurgical techniques and aggressive antimicrobial therapy have improved visual outcomes, but eyes with PTE still tend to fare poorly.[4,10]

The differences between PTE and POE are as profound as the differences between a number 64 Beaver blade and a machete, or an operating room and a barnyard. We ophthalmologists often extrapolate from our knowledge of POE when treating PTE, but the differences between the two must always be borne in mind. The differences begin with the vast differences in clinical setting. The uncontrolled environment that exists outside the operating room opens the door to many types of infectious organisms that are rarely if ever seen in POE. Contamination of a traumatic wound with soil or organic material is particularly likely, and such contamination is often associated with virulent organisms such as *Bacillus cereus* and *Fusarium solanae,* which are rarely encountered with POE. The likelihood of mixed infections is also much higher in the setting of trauma.

The difference between traumatic and planned surgical wounds is important both in terms of the greater exposure of intraocular contents to the environment with traumatic wounds and in the greater postoperative inflammation seen in these wounds. Inflammation and pain can mask the early signs and symptoms of PTE, making early diagnosis and treatment difficult. This delay in diagnosis and the accompanying damage to ocular structures contribute to a lower percentage of posttraumatic eyes recovering useful vision.[11]

MICROBIOLOGY

The profile of likely infecting organisms in PTE differs from that of POE in several ways. Exhibit 17-1 lists the causative organisms found most commonly in traumatic and postoperative endophthalmitis. *Staphylococcus* species are the most commonly isolated bacteria in both the traumatic and surgical environments. It is identified in up to 50% of posttraumatic cases and up to 47% of postoperative cases. The second most common organisms in the traumatic group are the *Bacillus* species, which typify the major difference between posttraumatic and postoperative endophthalmitis.

EXHIBIT 17-1

ORGANISMS MOST COMMONLY ISOLATED IN ENDOPHTHALMITIS

Posttraumatic Endophthalmitis (PTE)
- *Staphylococcus* species
- *Bacillus* species
- *Streptococcus* species
- Polymicroorganisms
- Gram-negative microorganisms
- Fungal species

Postoperative Endophthalmitis (POE)
- *Staphylococcus* species
- *Streptococcus* species
- Gram-negative microorganisms
- Polymicroorganisms
- *Bacillus* species
- Fungal species

Important references for the use of antibiotics in the treatment of endophthalmitis:

Barr CC. Prognostic factors in corneoscleral lacerations. *Arch Ophthalmol*. 1983;101:919–924.

Bohigian GM, Olk RJ. Factors associated with a poor visual result in endophthalmitis. *Am J Ophthalmol*. 1986;101:332–341.

Brinton GS, Topping TM, Hyndiuk RA, Aaberg TM, Reeser FH, Abrams GW. Posttraumatic endophthalmitis. *Arch Ophthalmol*. 1984;102:547–550.

Endophthalmitis Vitrectomy Study Group. Results of Endophthalmitis Vitrectomy Study: A randomized trial of immediate vitrectomy and of intravenous antibiotics for the treatment of postoperative bacterial endophthalmitis. *Arch Ophthalmol*. 1995;113:1479–1496.

Fisch A, Salvanet A, Prazuck T, et al. The French Collaborative Study Group on Endophthalmitis. Epidemiology of infective endophthalmitis in France. *Lancet*. 1991;338(8779):1373–1376.

Forster RK, Abbott RL, Gelender H. Management of infectious endophthalmitis. *Ophthalmology*. 1980;87:313–319.

Javitt JC, Vitale S, Canner JK, et al. National outcomes of cataract extraction: Endophthalmitis following inpatient surgery. *Arch Ophthalmol*. 1991;109:1085–1089.

Kent DG. Endophthalmitis in Auckland 1983–1991. *Aust N Z J Ophthalmol*. 1993;21:227–236.

Mieler WF, Glazer LC, Bennett SR, Han DP. Favorable outcome of traumatic endophthalmitis with associated retinal breaks or detachment. *Can J Ophthalmol*. 1992;27:348–352.

Nobe JR, Gomez DS, Liggett P, Smith RE, Robin JB. Post-traumatic and postoperative endophthalmitis: A comparison of visual outcomes. *Br J Ophthalmol*. 1987;71:614–617.

Parke DW II, Jones DB, Gentry LO. Endogenous endophthalmitis among patients with candidemia. *Ophthalmology*. 1982;89:789–796.

Parrish CM, O'Day DM. Traumatic endophthalmitis. *Int Ophthalmol Clin*. 1987;27(2):112–119.

Peyman GA, Daun M. Prophylaxis of endophthalmitis. *Ophthalmic Surg*. 1994;25:671–674.

Puliafito CA, Baker AS, Haaf J, Foster CS. Infectious endophthalmitis: Review of 36 cases. *Ophthalmology*. 1982;89:921–929.

Seal DV, Kirkness CM. Criteria for intravitreal antibiotics during surgical removal of intraocular foreign bodies. *Eye*. 1992;6:465–468.

Speaker MG, Milch FA, Shah MK, Eisner W, Kreiswirth BN. The role of external bacterial flora in the pathogenesis of acute postoperative endophthalmitis. *Ophthalmology*. 1991;98:639–649.

Thompson JT, Parver LM, Enger CL, Mieler WF, Liggett PE. Infectious endophthalmitis after penetrating injuries with retained intraocular foreign bodies. *Ophthalmology*. 1993;100:1468–1474.

Thompson WS, Rubsamen PE, Flynn HW Jr, Schiffman J, Cousins SW. Endophthalmitis after penetrating trauma: Risk factors and visual acuity outcomes. *Ophthalmology*. 1995;102:1696–1701.

Williams DF, Mieler WF, Abrams GW, Lewis H. Results and prognostic factors in penetrating ocular injuries with retained intraocular foreign bodies. *Ophthalmology*. 1988;95:911–916.

Wilson FM. Causes and prevention of endophthalmitis. *Int Ophthalmol Clin*. 1987;27(2):67–73.

B cereus infections are seen in only 3% of POE cases, but they are implicated in up to 46% of cases of PTE. *B cereus* is a highly virulent organism with the potential to devastate an eye in only a few hours (Figure 17-2); the destructive power of these infections is due to the ability of *B cereus* to produce enzymes and exotoxins that ravage the eye. Eyes can worsen visibly during the 1 to 2 hours it takes to get the patient to the operating room for diagnostic tap and antibiotic injections. The ophthalmologist, therefore, must be hypervigilant in watching for the development of *B cereus* endophthalmitis in traumatic cases. This diagnosis should especially be considered in cases where there is soil contamination of the wound, trauma occurring outdoors or in an agricultural environment, injuries which include IOFBs, and in the presence of constitutional symptoms such as fever, sweats, and an elevated white blood cell count.

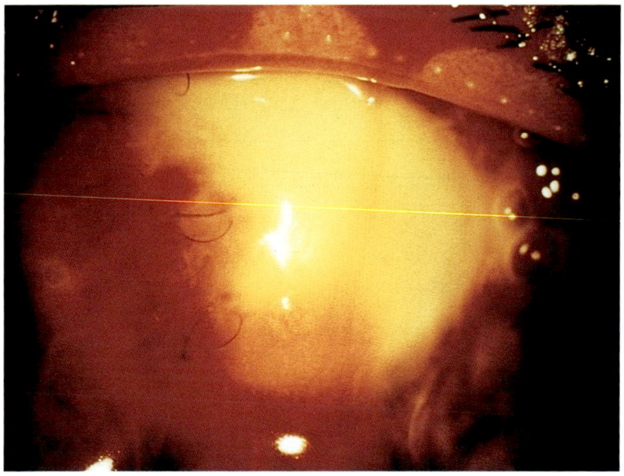

Fig. 17-2. Posttraumatic endophthalmitis caused by *Bacillus cereus.* Photograph: Courtesy of Department of Ophthalmology, Madigan Army Medical Center, Tacoma, Wash.

Additionally, PTE has a much higher incidence of mixed infections. These infections can be particularly difficult to treat, necessitating the use of two or more antibiotics with broad Gram-positive and Gram-negative coverage. Synergism between these drugs may also be particularly important in the setting of mixed infections.

MAKING THE DIAGNOSIS

The most critical aspect of treating endophthalmitis is making a timely diagnosis. The visual outcome, even the preservation of the globe, hinges on making the diagnosis with minimal delay. Because of the more virulent profile of infecting organisms and the possibility of mixed infection in PTE, the need for rapid diagnosis is especially urgent. Cases of PTE pose a greater diagnostic challenge than cases of POE because of the confounding variables presented by inflammation, pain, and swelling following trauma and its surgical repair.

Two important rules to follow to improve the chances of making an early diagnosis of PTE are

1. observe the patient closely, and
2. maintain a high index of suspicion.

Patients should be examined frequently during the initial postoperative period, looking for early signs and symptoms of endophthalmitis. Endophthalmitis occurs quickly, usually within 1 to 4 days following trauma.[2,10]

Purulent discharge, increasing anterior chamber or vitreous reaction, hypopyon, corneal edema, loss of a red reflex, lid edema, proptosis, and fever are signs that point toward the diagnosis of endophthalmitis. Increasing pain and photophobia out of proportion to the injury and visual loss are also worrisome. The examiner faces the challenge in these cases of differentiating normal, postreparative inflammation from the inflammation driven by infection.

Some signs of PTE are distinctive and point to particular invading organisms. A corneal ring abscess is particularly likely to signify a *B cereus* infection. Intraocular gas, although a sign of globe perforation, can also indicate an infection with gas-forming organisms, such as *Clostridium* species.

Ancillary testing can also be quite useful in establishing the diagnosis of PTE. First, cultures obtained at the time of the initial repair must be continuously reviewed. Any early evidence of growth coupled with mounting signs and symptoms of infection should prompt immediate treatment. Imaging (ultrasonography, plain film radiography, and computed tomography) can all be used to detect an occult IOFB, which can substantially increase the likelihood of PTE.

MANAGEMENT DURING THE PRIMARY REPAIR

Every repair of a traumatized eye requires endophthalmitis management. The details of the history are sought to determine the likelihood of infection. Is there a retained IOFB? How long has the eye been open? These questions and more are asked to help predict and prevent PTE.

At the time of repair, cultures and stains are prepared of the conjunctiva, wound, and of any tissue or debris removed from the eye. Initial Gram's and Giemsa stains (for bacteria) and Gomori's methenamine-silver stain (for fungal elements) should be performed. Chocolate and blood agar plates and thioglycolate broth should be inoculated and incubated at 37°C. Separate plates of blood and Sabouraud's agar should be prepared and incubated at 25°C. Alternatively, aqueous and vitreous samples can be inoculated directly into blood culture bottles.

Topical and subconjunctival antibiotics are used routinely for prophylaxis against PTE, and intravenous antibiotics are given for at least 72 hours. Quinolone may be administered orally if access to the operating room will be delayed and if intravenous antibiotics are not immediately available. These steps are a standard part of any repair of a ruptured globe.

The question of whether to use prophylactic intravitreal injections remains unanswered. In cases where the eye is violated by a grossly contaminated object, the decision to use intravitreal antibiotics at the time of initial repair—provided that the injections can be given safely and reliably into the vitreous cavity—is easy. In other cases where the likelihood of intraocular contamination is low, prophylactic antibiotics probably are not necessary. Unfortunately, most cases fall somewhere between these two extremes. In general, if the risk of infection is high and the posterior segment has been violated, then the use of prophylactic intravitreal antibiotics should be considered.

The use of subconjunctival steroids can be considered at the time of surgical repair of a ruptured globe. However, the use of systemic and intravitreal steroids should be avoided to reduce the chance of suppressing the immune system and the possibility of masking early signs and symptoms of infection.

MANAGEMENT AFTER INITIAL REPAIR

Following the initial repair, the patient must be monitored closely and frequently for the development of endophthalmitis. The ophthalmologist should take personal responsibility for checking all Gram stains. Cultures should be examined daily for growth. Any growth on the microbiological media in the presence of mounting signs or symptoms of PTE should be treated as an infection. Because PTE can rapidly cause overwhelming devastation, a high index of suspicion coupled with a low threshold for treatment is appropriate. If a diagnosis of endophthalmitis is a real possibility, anterior and posterior chamber taps with intravitreal antibiotic injections should be performed urgently. Hesitation leads to loss of vision and frequently loss of the eye. Both medical and surgical management aspects need to be considered.

Medical Considerations

Antibiotic Coverage

All cases of endophthalmitis, postoperative and posttraumatic, require broad-spectrum antibiotic coverage. Broad-spectrum coverage is especially important in PTE. Although 75% of postoperative endophthalmitis is caused by Gram-positive organisms, only 45% of PTE cases are attributable to Gram-positive organisms. Many drug regimens cover a wide range of Gram-positive and Gram-negative organisms, but only a few can be delivered in bactericidal doses without being toxic to the eye.

The currently recommended combination of drugs for intravitreal injection is vancomycin, 1 mg in a volume of 0.1 mL, and ceftazidime, 2.25 mg also delivered in 0.1 mL. Vancomycin is an excellent agent for Gram-positive coverage. The Endophthalmitis Vitrectomy Study[12] found that all Gram-positive organisms were sensitive to vancomycin. Ceftazidime is preferred for Gram-negative coverage because of the breadth of its effectiveness and low toxicity. Amikacin (0.4 mg) may be substituted for ceftazidime for Gram-negative coverage.

Choices of antibiotics for subconjunctival and topical administration should also be made to provide for broad coverage of Gram-positive and Gram-negative microorganisms. Vancomycin and clindamycin offer good Gram-positive coverage at doses of 25 mg, whereas ceftazidime (100 mg) gives good Gram-negative protection. Care must be taken not to introduce these agents inadvertently into the eye by either direct injection or injection in the area of a partially open wound. Topically, ciprofloxacin (0.3% hourly) or vancomycin (50 mg/mL) provides good coverage.

The use of systemic antibiotics in POE has not been proven beneficial.[12] However, most clinicians (including ourselves) recommend intravenous antibiotic coverage as prophylaxis. Prophylactic regimens against endophthalmitis in penetrating trauma without posterior segment involvement include both vancomycin (1 g, twice daily) and ceftazidime (1 g, three times daily) for at least 3 days. These antibiotics cross the blood–ocular barrier reasonably well and may reach therapeutic levels in the eye. Their entry into the eye is also aided by the weakening of the blood–ocular barrier that results from infection and trauma-induced inflammation. After 3 days of intravenous antibiotics, the patient (after discharge) is placed on 1 week of oral ciprofloxacin (500 mg, twice daily).

More aggressive treatment is warranted for treating PTE or providing prophylactic coverage in cases of penetrating trauma with contamination by dirt or vegetable matter, presence of an IOFB, or involvement of the posterior segment (Exhibit 17-2).[13]

Antifungal Treatment

Therapy for fungal PTE differs significantly from that of bacterial PTE. Unlike therapy for bacterial PTE, which is delivered at the time that specimens are collected, therapy for fungal endophthalmitis is *never* instituted unless (1) fungal elements are seen on stains from aqueous or vitreous specimens or (2) the cultures grow fungal species. Once the diagnosis is confirmed, intravitreal amphotericin-B (5 µg/0.1 mL) is given through the pars plana. Topical amphotericin-B drops (1.5 mg/mL) are given as frequently as every hour. Systemic amphotericin-B (0.25–1.00 mg/kg/d) is given intravenously in divided doses after consultation with an internist. Alternatively, fluconazole (100 mg orally, twice daily) can be administered for 2 to 4 weeks.[13]

EXHIBIT 17-2

ANTIBIOTIC RECOMMENDATIONS FOR POSTTRAUMATIC ENDOPHTHALMITIS

Use together for 3 d:
- Intravenous vancomycin, 1 g bid
- Intravenous ceftazidime, 1 g tid

Use for 1 wk after discharge:
- Oral ciprofloxacin, 500 mg bid

Use in combination:
- Intravitreal vancomycin (1 mg/0.1 mL); inject 0.1 mL through pars plana
- Intravitreal ceftazidime (2.25 mg/0.1 mL); inject 0.1 mL through pars plana

For injuries that run a high risk of contamination with *Bacillus* species:
- Intravitreal clindamycin (0.5 mg/0.1 mL); inject through pars plana

Use in combination:
- Subconjunctival cefazolin (100 mg) or vancomycin (25 mg)
- Subconjunctival ceftazidime (100 mg)

Use in alternation:
- Topical fortified cefazolin (50 mg/mL) or fortified vancomycin (50 mg/mL) every 1–2 h, alternating with ciprofloxacin (0.3%)

Source: Merbs SL, Abrams LS, Campochiaro PA. Endophthalmitis. In: MacCumber MW, ed. *Management of Ocular Injuries and Emergencies.* Philadelphia, Pa: Lippincott Williams & Wilkins; 1997: 280–281.

EXHIBIT 17-3

METHODS FOR OBTAINING INTRAOCULAR CULTURES AND DELIVERING INTRAVITREAL ANTIBIOTICS

Aqueous fluid culture from anterior chamber tap:

1. Apply topical anesthesia to cornea or administer a retrobulbar block.
2. Prepare surface of eye with 5% betadine solution.
3. Place a sterile lid speculum.
4. Use a 27- or 30-gauge needle on a tuberculin syringe to perform a paracentesis into the anterior chamber, and remove approximately 0.1 to 0.2 mL of aqueous fluid. Take care not to hit the lens in phakic eyes.

Vitreous fluid culture from vitreous tap:

1. Apply topical anesthesia to conjunctiva and administer either a subconjunctival or a retrobulbar injection of local anesthetic.
2. Prepare surface of eye with 5% betadine solution.
3. Place a sterile lid speculum.
4. Use a 22- to 25-gauge needle on a tuberculin syringe to perform a paracentesis through the pars plana 3 mm posterior to the limbus in pseudophakic eyes and 4 mm posterior to the limbus in phakic eyes. Remove approximately 0.1 to 0.2 mL of liquefied vitreous. Take care to direct the needle toward the optic nerve and not to advance it more than 1 cm.

Vitreous fluid culture from vitreous biopsy:

1. Apply topical anesthesia to conjunctiva and administer either a subconjunctival or retrobulbar injection of local anesthetic.
2. Prepare surface of eye with 5% betadine solution.
3. Place a sterile lid speculum.
4. Perform a limited peritomy before creating the larger sclerotomy 3 mm posterior to the limbus in pseudophakic eyes and 4 mm posterior to the limbus in phakic eyes. Use a supersharp knife for 23-gauge and smaller vitrectors, and a microvitreal retinal (MVR) blade for a standard 20-gauge vitreous cutter.
5. Use an unprimed vitreous cutter to obtain approximately 0.3 to 0.5 mL of undiluted vitreous. Aspirate the sample into a syringe.
6. Close the larger sclerotomy with 7-0 Vicryl, and reapproximate the conjunctiva with 6-0 plain gut. Smaller sclerotomies will seal without suturing.

Administration of intravitreal antibiotics through the pars plana:

1. Apply topical anesthesia to conjunctiva and administer either a subconjunctival or retrobulbar injection of local anesthetic.
2. Prepare the eye with 5% betadine solution.
3. Place a sterile lid speculum.
4. Using a 30-gauge needle on a tuberculin syringe, inject 0.1 mL of the antibiotic 3 mm posterior to the limbus in pseudophakic eyes and 4 mm posterior to the limbus in phakic eyes. Take care to direct the needle toward the optic nerve and not to advance it more than 1 cm. Use a separate needle and syringe for each antibiotic, which must be delivered through separate injections.
5. Check the intraocular pressure at this point. If it is elevated, an anterior chamber paracentesis may be required to normalize the pressure.

Source: Merbs SL, Abrams LS, Campochiaro PA. Endophthalmitis. In: MacCumber MW, ed. *Management of Ocular Injuries and Emergencies.* Philadelphia, Pa: Lippincott Williams & Wilkins; 1997: 279–280.

Antiinflammatory/Immunosuppressant Therapy

All patients who sustain penetrating eye trauma receive topical prednisolone acetate 1% (every 1–2 h) to decrease intraocular inflammation and atropine 1% (every 12 h) to provide cycloplegia. Patients who undergo surgical repair and receive intravitreal antibiotics are given subconjunctival dexamethasone (20 mg) at the end of the case.

Oral prednisone (1 mg/kg/d) may be administered to patients with PTE 24 hours after antibiotic therapy is initiated, provided the stains are negative for fungal elements.

Surgical Considerations

After the initial repair, aqueous and vitreous samples are obtained when the diagnosis of endophthalmitis is first seriously entertained. These samples may be obtained by needle aspiration, using a 27- or 30-gauge needle for the anterior chamber paracentesis and a 22- to 25-gauge needle for the pars plana tap (Exhibit 17-3).[13] Some clinicians recommend using a 23-gauge or smaller vitrector to obtain a vitreous biopsy.

What is less clear is when to perform a vitrectomy to retrieve a specimen and debride the eye. Several factors influence this decision, including

- integrity of the globe,
- visual acuity,
- the need for a large sample,
- the usefulness of vitreal debridement for reducing the infectious and inflammatory load, and
- the need for better dispersal of intravitreal antibiotics.

Owing to the difficulties inherent in any study of PTE, no clear or absolute guidelines have been developed to date with regard to the timing of this powerful treatment tool. However, if we extrapolate from the Endophthalmitis Vitrectomy Study,[12] any patient who develops PTE after initial repair of the injury should undergo vitrectomy if he or she only has light perception vision. Many vitreoretinal surgeons advocate performing vitrectomy and injecting intravitreal antibiotics even with vision better than light perception, especially if they are concerned that the eye might be infected with a virulent organism.

COURSE AFTER TREATMENT

After the diagnosis of PTE has been made and antibiotic therapy begun, much work remains. Cultures must be examined daily for evidence of growth, antimicrobial sensitivity tests must be checked, and the patient must be closely followed for signs of change. If the infection appears to be worsening, then the ophthalmologist, guided by microbiology reports, should consider repeating the injections or performing a vitrectomy within 48 hours of the diagnosis. Repeat cultures and Gram's stains are usually not performed at this point unless no organisms were isolated from the previous cultures.

A patient with good response to treatment will report diminished ocular pain within 24 to 48 hours. The amount of anterior segment inflammation and the height of the hypopyon seen at 24 to 48 hours after initiation of antibiotic therapy are less reliable signs to follow. In fact, both of these signs may initially worsen after injection of intravitreal antibiotics. The antibiotics kill the intraocular organisms, causing them to release toxins, which may temporarily increase anterior segment inflammation.

SUMMARY

PTE is one of the most devastating complications of the already-serious problem of globe rupture. Much progress has been made since the mid 1970s with advances in surgical technique and antibiotic therapies, but some aspects of this problem are as common today as they were in the 1950s. Delays in diagnosis are dangerous. The greater virulence of organisms associated with PTE, especially *B cereus*, diminishes the prognosis for recoverable vision. Also, traumatized eyes, especially when they are significantly disrupted, can have associated injuries to the cornea, lens, retina, and optic nerve. Severe damage to any of these structures can lessen the chance of obtaining useful vision from the eye.

REFERENCES

1. Boldt HC, Pulido JS, Blodi CF, Folk JC, Weingeist TA. Rural endophthalmitis. *Ophthalmology*. 1989;96:1722–1726.

2. Brinton GS, Topping TM, Hyndiuk RA, Aaberg TM, Reeser FH, Abrams GW. Posttraumatic endophthalmitis. *Arch Ophthalmol*. 1984;102:547–550.

3. Duch-Samper AM, Menezo JL, Hurtado-Sarrio M. Endophthalmitis following penetrating eye injuries. *Acta Ophthalmol Scand*. 1997;75:104–106.

4. Thompson WS, Rubsamen PE, Flynn HW Jr, Schiffman J, Cousins SW. Endophthalmitis after penetrating trauma: Risk factors and visual acuity outcomes. *Ophthalmology*. 1995;102:1696–1701.

5. Verbraeken H, Rysselaere M. Posttraumatic endophthalmitis. *Eur J Ophthalmol*. 1994;4:1–5.

6. Mittra RA, Mieler WF. Controversies in the management of open-globe injuries involving the posterior segment. *Surv Ophthalmol*. 1999;44:215–225.

7. Thompson JT, Parver LM, Enger CL, Mieler WF, Liggett PE. Infectious endophthalmitis after penetrating injuries with retained intraocular foreign bodies. *Ophthalmology*. 1993;100:1468–1474.

8. Behrens-Baumann W, Praetorius G. Intraocular foreign bodies: 297 consecutive cases. *Ophthalmologica*. 1989;198:84–88.

9. Williams DF, Mieler WF, Abrams GW, Lewis H. Results and prognostic factors in penetrating ocular injuries with retained intraocular foreign bodies. *Ophthalmology*. 1988;95:911–916.

10. Affeldt JC, Flynn HW, Forster RK, Mandelbaum S, Clarkson JG, Janus GD. Microbial endophthalmitis resulting from ocular trauma. *Ophthalmology*. 1987;94:407–413.

11. Nobe JR, Gomez DS, Liggett P, Smith RE, Robin JB. Post-traumatic and postoperative endophthalmitis: A comparison of visual outcomes. *Br J Ophthalmol*. 1987;71:614–617.

12. Endophthalmitis Vitrectomy Study Group. Results of Endophthalmitis Vitrectomy Study: A randomized trial of immediate vitrectomy and of intravenous antibiotics for the treatment of postoperative bacterial endophthalmitis. *Arch Ophthalmol*. 1995;113:1479–1496.

13. Merbs SL, Abrams LS, Campochiaro PA. Endoph thalmitis. In: MacCumber MW, ed. *Management of Ocular Injuries and Emergencies*. Philadelphia, Pa: Lippincott Williams & Wilkins; 1997: Chap 19.

Chapter 18

EYELID AND ADNEXAL INJURIES

KIMBERLY PEELE COCKERHAM, MD*

*Director, Ophthalmic Plastics, Orbital Disease and Neuro-Ophthalmology, Allegheny General Hospital, 420 East North Avenue, Pittsburgh, Pennsylvania 15212; Assistant Professor, Department of Ophthalmology, Drexel University College of Medicine, Philadelphia, Pennsylvania 19102; formerly, Major, Medical Corps, US Army; Director, Neuro-Ophthalmology, Orbital Disease, and Plastic Reconstruction, Department of Ophthalmology, Walter Reed Army Medical Center, Washington, DC

INTRODUCTION

Eyelid lacerations are a common emergency room challenge. The primary repair, which should be the definitive surgery, is too often performed by medical students or physicians without ophthalmological training.[1] Whether the setting is a civilian emergency room or a battlefield, ophthalmologists should be involved as early as possible. Inadequate repair can lead to ocular irritation, pain, and even loss of the eye in cases of severe eyelid dysfunction. A complete eye examination is essential before closing the wound to confirm the extent of injury—even if the wound appears deceptively simple. Fortunately, the eyelids are endowed with excellent blood supply, which allows direct closure under tension and creation of large flaps without the threat of necrosis.[1–7] By following three main guidelines, ophthalmologists can maximize the patient's functional and cosmetic outcome:

1. Perform careful anatomic repairs.
2. Preserve the maximum possible amount of tissue.
3. Make liberal use of advancement flaps, traction sutures, and postoperative skin grafts.

On the battlefield, eyelid lacerations and adnexal injuries are not considered true emergencies, and in triage settings, life-threatening and actual sight-threatening injuries (ie, open globes) should take precedence. Eyelid lacerations can be closed up to 72 hours after the injury without a great impact on functional or aesthetic outcome. Canalicular injury can also be delayed (up to 48 hours), allowing the all-important primary closure to be performed by an experienced ophthalmologist. All tissue should be preserved, and even obviously necrotic tissue or detached tissue should be preserved until definitive closure is performed. Eyelid lacerations should be irrigated with sterile saline whenever possible and patched for transport.

Future battlefield units may have tissue adhesive, or glue, at their disposal. Closure with this tissue glue appears to be a very time-efficient technique for laceration closure.[8] When battlefield conditions prohibit access to needed equipment, many innovations are possible. A sterile safety pin can serve as a punctal dilator and probe, or 4-0 nylon can be used as a lacrimal stent. Independent of conditions, however, principles of closure and tissue preservation always apply. Irrigation, patience, and a problem-solving outlook can often transform an ominous wound into an elegant functional closure.

HISTORY, EXAMINATION, AND ANCILLARY TESTING

A complete history of the wounding incident should be sought to determine the mechanism of injury and assess whether foreign bodies (FBs) might be present. The timing is also important; injuries that occurred more than 24 hours before the examination are at increased risk for infection and poor wound healing. Fortunately, the eyelids are well vascularized and thereby defy infection even with delayed closure. Most ophthalmologists primarily close eyelid lacerations up to 72 hours old; canalicular lacerations are best repaired within 48 hours.[5] The tetanus status of the patient should be addressed and appropriate antibiotic treatment initiated immediately.

Before addressing the eyelid injuries, best-corrected visual acuity must be documented, and a complete ocular examination should be performed wherever possible. The status of the pupil should be determined; the presence of anisocoria or an afferent pupillary defect should be quantitated. A slitlamp examination of the anterior segment and an indirect examination of the peripheral retina are ideal. *If in doubt, do no harm!* Always suspect an open globe in cases of proptosis, chemosis, low intraocular pressure, and decreased vision. Repair of eyelid and adnexal injuries should be delayed if an open globe is present or suspected. (The details of management of anterior and posterior segment trauma are addressed in Chapters 8–17 in this textbook.) The lacrimal gland, canaliculi, and the lacrimal sac should be specifically inspected to determine if occult injuries have occurred.

Examination of the eyelids and ocular adnexa should include documentation of the intrapalpebral fissure dimensions, levator function, and marginal reflex distance to confirm symmetry of the eyelid appearance and function. The upper eyelid should be gently everted to rule out FBs and to allow inspection of the palpebral lobe of the lacrimal gland.

Dye disappearance time allows initial assessment of lacrimal drainage integrity. Fluorescein strips or 2% fluorescein dye solution (Fluoress) is placed in the inferior cul-de-sac of both eyes. The dye should drain into the canaliculi and then the lacrimal sac within 5 minutes. Delay in this process may indicate canalicular, lacrimal sac, lacrimal duct, or nasal injuries. If the dye disappearance is delayed, further testing is indicated.

Classic Jones I and II testing is rarely performed. Instead, the puncta are inspected and gently dilated. If the patient is awake and cooperative, the nasal lacrimal system is irrigated with normal saline or Alcaine, a topical anesthetic. If a canaliculus is crushed proximal to the common canaliculus, clear irrigant will return with force from the puncta's being irrigated. If the canaliculi are blocked just distal to the level of the common canaliculus, clear irrigant will emerge from the opposite puncta. If a canalicular laceration is present, irrigation may well up in the medial wound or emerge from the site of disconnection.[9] Techniques for identifying the distal end of a canalicular laceration are discussed below in this chapter.

Further evaluation of the patient is essential if an FB, fracture, or deep orbital trauma is suspected. In ER or battlefield circumstances, plain film radiography may be used as a screening tool to identify large, metallic FBs or prominent fractures. Ultrasonography (A- and B-scans) is an effective tool for identifying intraocular or anterior orbital FBs but is not helpful for imaging the posterior orbit. Although computed tomography (CT) is excellent at identifying and localizing most FBs, magnetic resonance imaging (MRI) is superior at identifying subtle nonmetallic FBs.[10] However, if there is even a remote chance that metallic FBs are present and could be mobilized and cause damage if subjected to MRI, then CT is the study of choice.

If midfacial trauma is present in the setting of eyelid and canalicular disruption, an otolaryngologist should be involved to assess the extent of nasal injury. If the maxilla is extensively damaged, then an oral surgery consultation is also essential to allow simultaneous stabilization of the jaw. If a superior orbital fracture or cerebrospinal fluid leak is suspected, then neurosurgery consultation should be sought before any ophthalmic intervention.

SURGICAL MANAGEMENT OF EYELID LACERATIONS

The surgical approach is determined by the extent of injury. Once a complete ocular survey has confirmed that the globe is intact and that associated orbital fractures are unlikely, the eyelid laceration can be addressed. A thorough knowledge of eyelid and ocular adnexal anatomy is essential to avoid injury to vital structures and to maximize cosmetic outcome. It is important to keep in mind that tissue loss always appears more substantial because of tissue edema and contraction. Even dramatically disfigured eyelids can be repaired with careful reapproximation and knowledge of a few reconstruction options.[1–7,9]

There are four major types of eyelid lacerations:

1. superficial,
2. eyelid-margin involvement,
3. levator injury, and
4. complex tissue loss.

Anesthesia

Local infiltration anesthesia with a 50:50 mixture of 2% lidocaine (Xylocaine, mfg by AstraZeneca Pharmaceuticals LP, Wilmington, Delaware) with 1:200,000 epinephrine and 0.75% bupivacaine (Marcaine, mfg by Sanofi Winthrop Pharmaceuticals, New York, NY) and hyaluronidase (Wydase, mfg by Wyeth-Ayerst Pharmaceuticals, Philadelphia, Pa) is usually adequate for eyelid reconstruction. In more extensive injuries, regional nerve blocks may be additionally required. For regional anesthesia of lower lids, 1 mL of local anesthetic is injected into the infraorbital foramen located directly inferiorly to the supraorbital notch, 1 cm below the infraorbital rim. Blocking the supraorbital, supratrochlear, or lacrimal nerves blocks sensation to the upper eyelid.

Alternatively, the frontal and lacrimal nerve may be blocked by inserting a needle at the midpoint of the upper eyelid immediately below the orbital rim. A small amount of anesthetic (0.5 mL) is injected after the needle is advanced approximately 3 cm along the orbital roof. The medial canthus and lacrimal sac can be blocked by injecting the infratrochlear nerve, which lies immediately superior to the medial canthal tendon. In uncooperative adults or children, general anesthesia is usually necessary. If levator injury is suspected, a cooperative, lightly sedated patient enhances the prospects for postoperative symmetry.

Preoperative Preparation

Tetracaine ophthalmic drops are placed bilaterally, and corneal shells (rigid scleral protectors) are used whenever possible. The patient is prepped and draped in the usual fashion. Irrigation is then performed with normal saline. In the case of very contaminated wounds, irrigation with an antibiotic, such as bacitracin or cefazolin sodium (Ancef, mfg by GlaxoSmithKline, Research Triangle Park, NC), should also be performed. All visible debris or fragments should be removed manually. Traction suture placement is performed early to help with tissue retraction during the repair and left in place for postoperative traction.

Superficial Eyelid Lacerations

Even superficial eyelid lacerations should be irrigated with normal saline and the margins closed with 6-0 silk, plain gut, or nylon sutures. Sutures may be placed in a running or interrupted fashion. Care should be taken to evert skin edges to maximize the final cosmetic appearance of the wound (Figure 18-1). Horizontal or transverse lacerations should include both orbicularis and skin in the closure. The septum should never be closed. In the upper eyelid and the lateral lower eyelid, wound closure should be performed, whenever possible, parallel to horizontal skin tension lines. In the medial lower lid, horizontal defects should be closed in a vertical fashion to minimize vertical tension and subsequent development of ectropion (Figure 18-2).

When eyelid skin is missing, an advancement flap may be fashioned to allow a simple closure (Figure 18-3). Skin sutures should be removed in 3 to 5 days (plain gut sutures will dissolve within the same time). In the case of a vertical or multiple stellate laceration, the eyelid should be placed on traction for at least 7 to 10 days (Frost or reverse-Frost suture). This suture may be taped in place to allow monitoring of visual function.

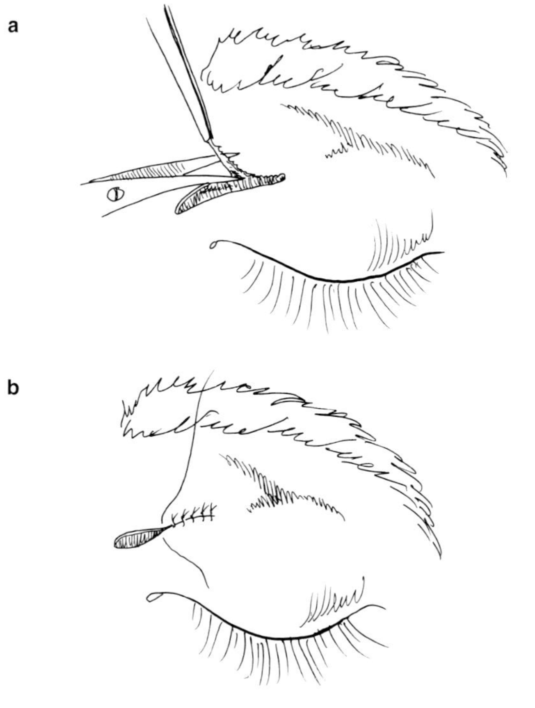

Fig. 18-1. Repair of a superficial laceration not involving the eyelid margin. (**a**) The eyelid laceration should be irrigated, carefully debrided, if necessary, and inspected to determine the depth and extent of the injury. Careful measurements of levator function should be performed. If a levator injury is suspected, exploration through an eyelid crease incision and repair is usually indicated. (**b**) Most superficial lacerations can be closed with a single-layer closure using interrupted or running 6-0 sutures (silk, plain gut, or nylon). Eyebrow lacerations, however, require a two-layer closure. The deep closure should be performed with a nonabsorbable suture such as 4-0 or 5-0 nylon and should relieve all tension on the wound edges. Drawing prepared for this textbook by Gary Wind, MD, Uniformed Services University of the Health Sciences, Bethesda, Md.

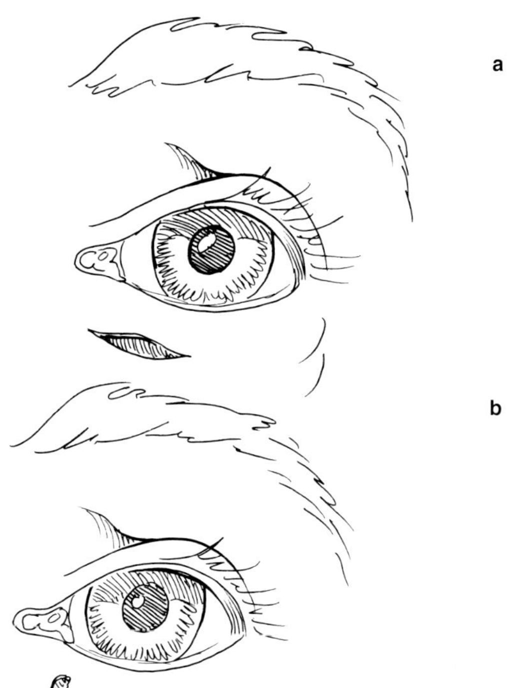

Fig. 18-2. Vertical closure of a medial horizontal defect. If the orientation of the laceration is horizontal and is located on the lower eyelid, reorientation of the wound closure to a vertical closure should be considered. (**a**) The eyelid should be placed on countertraction with a 4-0 nonabsorbable suture through the meibomian gland orifices. (**b**) Then, the laceration is closed vertically with 6-0 sutures. Drawing prepared for this textbook by Gary Wind, MD, Uniformed Services University of the Health Sciences, Bethesda, Md.

a

b

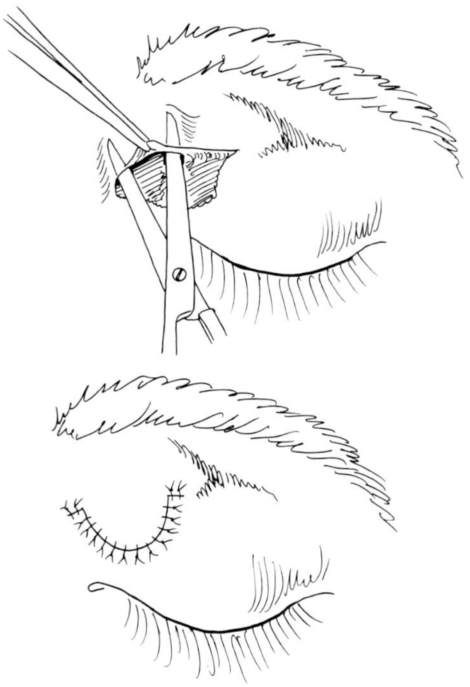

Fig. 18-3. If some tissue loss has occurred but the wound is superficial and does not involve the eyelid margin, an advancement flap can be fashioned. (**a**) The tissue that is to be advanced is generously undermined; Burrows operation to create triangles of skin may also be performed to augment the advancement. (**b**) The sutured wound is shown. If the tissue loss is greater, the remaining uncovered tissue may be allowed to granulate, or a skin graft may be performed. Drawing prepared for this textbook by Gary Wind, MD, Uniformed Services University of the Health Sciences, Bethesda, Md.

The use of cyanoacrylate tissue glue is an expedient way to close simple lacerations. It stabilizes the tissue, has an inherent antibacterial effect, and obviates the need for suture removal. Tissue glue can also help to augment the closure of necrotic or crushed tissues that are otherwise difficult to secure with sutures.[6] After irrigating the wound, hemostasis is achieved using monopolar or bipolar cautery. The wound must be dry to allow the tissue glue to create adequate adhesion. Forceps are then used to appose the edges of the laceration, and the tissue glue is applied sparingly by means of a tuberculin syringe fitted with a small-gauge needle to facilitate accurate application. Cyanoacrylate creates a strong bond for 3 to 5 days and then disintegrates spontaneously. Antibiotic ointment should not be applied because it accelerates breakdown of the glue.

Eyelid-Margin Involvement

Lacerations involving the eyelid margin require precise closure. Failure to appropriately approximate the edges results in eyelid notching. For tissue loss less than 25% of the total horizontal dimension of the eyelid, direct closure is usually possible (Figure 18-4). Primary closure is possible if the wound edges can be brought together with forceps. The wound is closed in the same fashion as for a standard pentagonal wedge. The eyelid margin is lined up using a 6-0 silk suture through the meibomian gland orifices.

A surgeon's knot is then thrown to confirm correct suture placement. If alignment is not ideal, the suture is removed and replaced to ensure approximation. If alignment is good, the knot is loosened and internal sutures of 5-0 or 6-0 chromic gut or polyglactin (Vicryl) are placed in the tarsus, sparing the conjunctiva and the skin. Care must be taken to avoid penetration of the conjunctiva to spare the cornea from irritation or even abrasion. The number of sutures placed is determined by the extent of the wound; the upper lid, with its more generous tarsus, usually requires at least three internal sutures. The skin is then closed using 6-0 silk, plain gut, or nylon. Additional 6-0 silk sutures are placed at the anterior (and in some cases, the posterior) eyelid margins, and all of the marginal sutures are left long and tethered under the anterior eyelid suture to avoid corneal contact. These sutures are then used to put tension on the wound so that healing will occur in an everted fashion to avoid lid notching and ectropion. Alternatively, an additional 4-0 suture (silk or nylon) may be placed just medial and lateral to the marginal sutures through the meibomian gland orifices, tied, and then left long to allow vertical tension (Figure 18-5). This measure is particularly helpful if the wound is under significant tension or the tissue is pulverized or necrotic.

Eyelid-margin sutures should remain in place for 7 to 10 days, whereas the skin sutures may be removed in 3 to 5 days. When irregular eyelid-margin deficits defy closure, a pentagonal wedge can be created using a scalpel, and then closed in a similar fashion (Table 18-1).

If the tissue volume loss exceeds 25%, then further measures are necessary; in the elderly, redundant skin may allow direct closure of wounds up to 50% tissue volume loss, but in younger patients a lateral canthotomy and cantholysis are necessary (Figure 18-6). If the tissue volume loss is between 25% and 50% in the upper lid (up to 75% in the

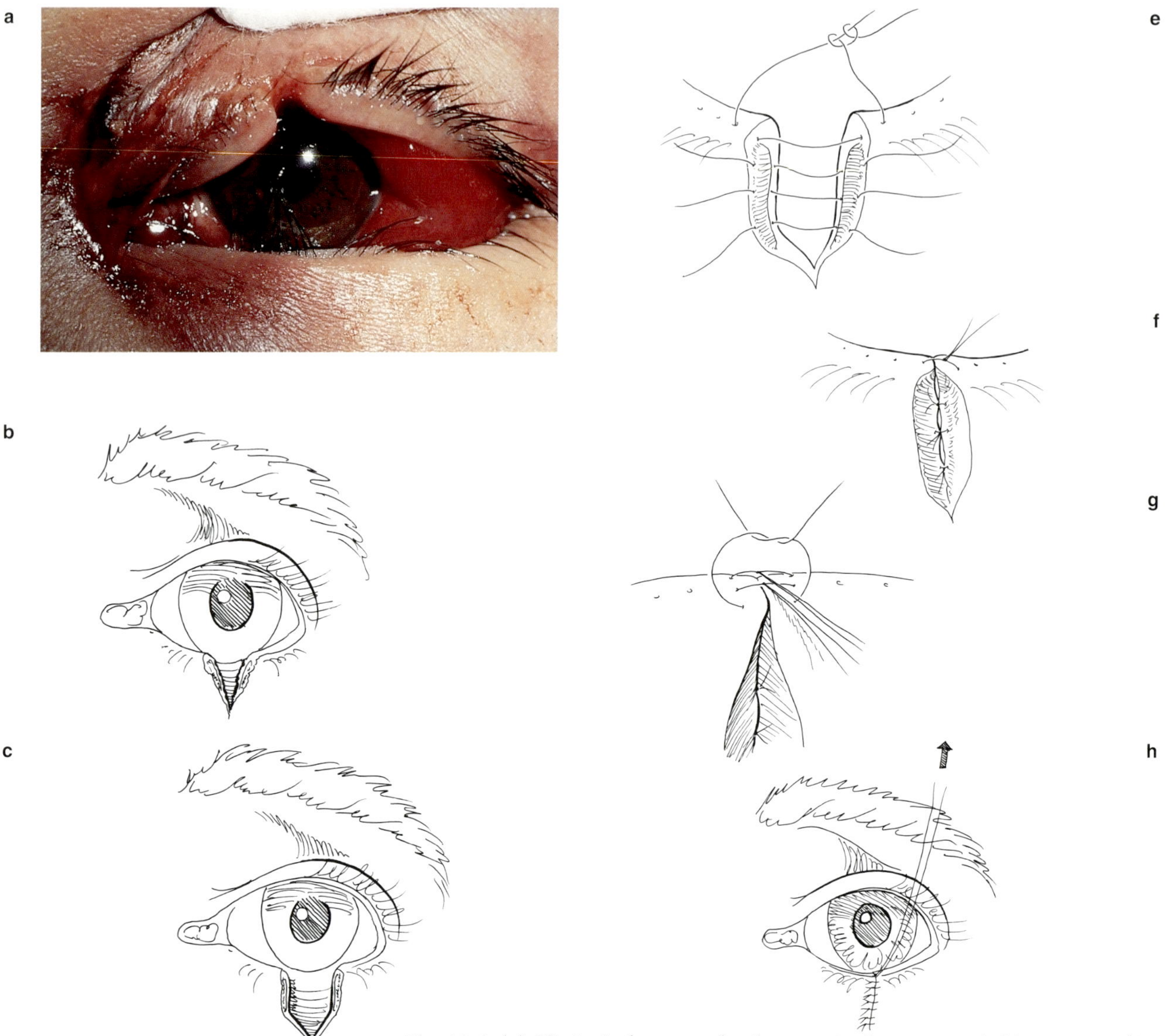

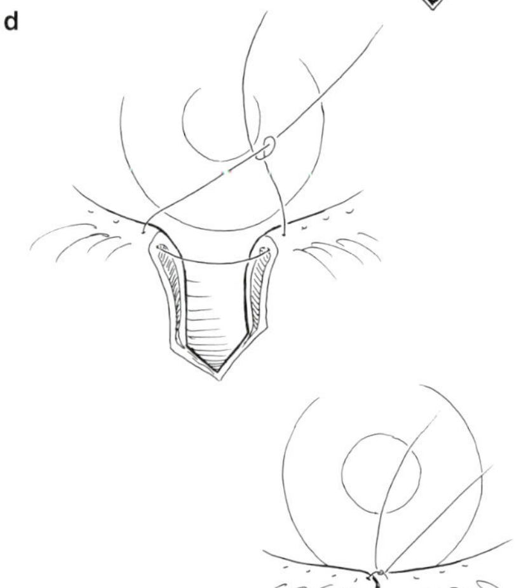

Fig. 18-4. (**a**) Clinical photograph of a marginal upper-eyelid laceration. (**b–h**) Repair of a marginal lower-eyelid laceration with less than 25% tissue loss. (**b**) An irregular laceration with tissue loss less than one fourth of the horizontal eyelid distance can usually be closed primarily. The technique is identical to the procedure used to close defects created after eyelid biopsy (pentagonal wedge closure). (**c**) The irregular traumatic laceration is freshened by creating a pentagonal wedge. (**d**) A 4-0 silk suture is placed in the eyelid margin (through the meibomian gland orifices 2 mm from the wound edges and 2 mm deep) and tied in a slipknot. Symmetrical suture placement is essential to obtain postoperative eyelid margin alignment. (**e**) The slipknot is loosened and approximately three absorbable 5-0 or 6-0 sutures are placed internally, encompassing the tarsal plate. (**f**) The skin and conjunctiva are not included in this internal closure. Anterior and posterior marginal sutures (6-0 silk) are then placed through the anterior and posterior eyelid margin. (**g**) The middle and posterior sutures are left long and tied under the anterior suture. (**h**) The skin is closed with 6-0 silk sutures, and the eyelid is placed on traction for at least 5 days. The skin sutures are removed 3 to 5 days later, and the marginal sutures are removed at 10 to 14 days postoperatively. Photograph: Courtesy of Department of Ophthalmology, Allegheny General Hospital, Pittsburgh, Pa. Drawings prepared for this textbook by Gary Wind, MD, Uniformed Services University of the Health Sciences, Bethesda, Md.

a

b

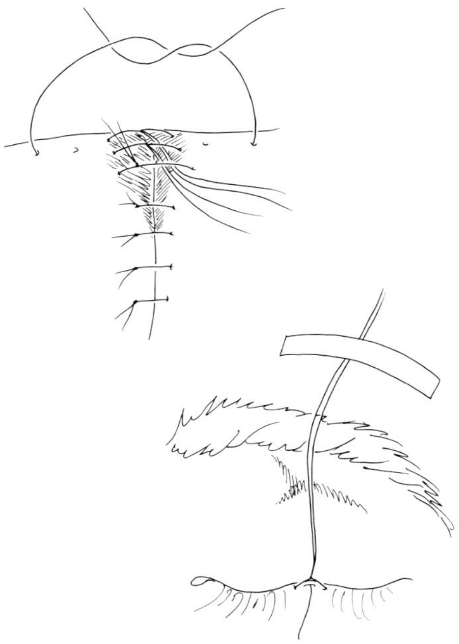

Fig. 18-5. Frost suture. (**a**) If the eyelid margin is macerated or necrotic, then an additional 4-0 nonabsorbable suture (eg, nylon) may be placed through the eyelid margin two to three meibomian gland orifices outside of the marginal silk suture placement. (**b**) The repaired laceration is placed under traction. Drawings prepared for this textbook by Gary Wind, MD, Uniformed Services University of the Health Sciences, Bethesda, Md.

TABLE 18-1

SUTURE RECOMMENDATIONS

Nature of Injury	Recommended Materials for Closure
Superficial Skin Laceration	6-0 plain gut, silk, nylon, or tissue glue
Eyelid Skin	
Margin	Three 6-0 silk in the margin
Tarsus	Two or three 5-0 or 6-0 Vicryl
Skin	6-0 silk or nylon
Eyebrow Injury	
Deep	Vertical mattress: 4-0 or 5-0 nylon or Vicryl
Skin	5-0 silk or nylon; tissue glue
Canalicular Injury	
Deep	8-0 or 9-0 nylon in tissue surrounding canaliculus
Skin	6-0 nylon
Medial Canthal Tendon Injury	
Medial resuspension to periorbita	4-0 nylon, Prolene, or wire
Skin	6-0 silk, nylon, or plain gut; tissue glue
Lateral Canthal Injury	
Lateral resuspension to periorbita	5-0 chromic gut, 4-0 Mersilene
Reconstruction of canthal angle	6-0 Vicryl internally; 6-0 silk externally
Skin	6-0 silk, nylon, or plain gut; tissue glue

a b c d e

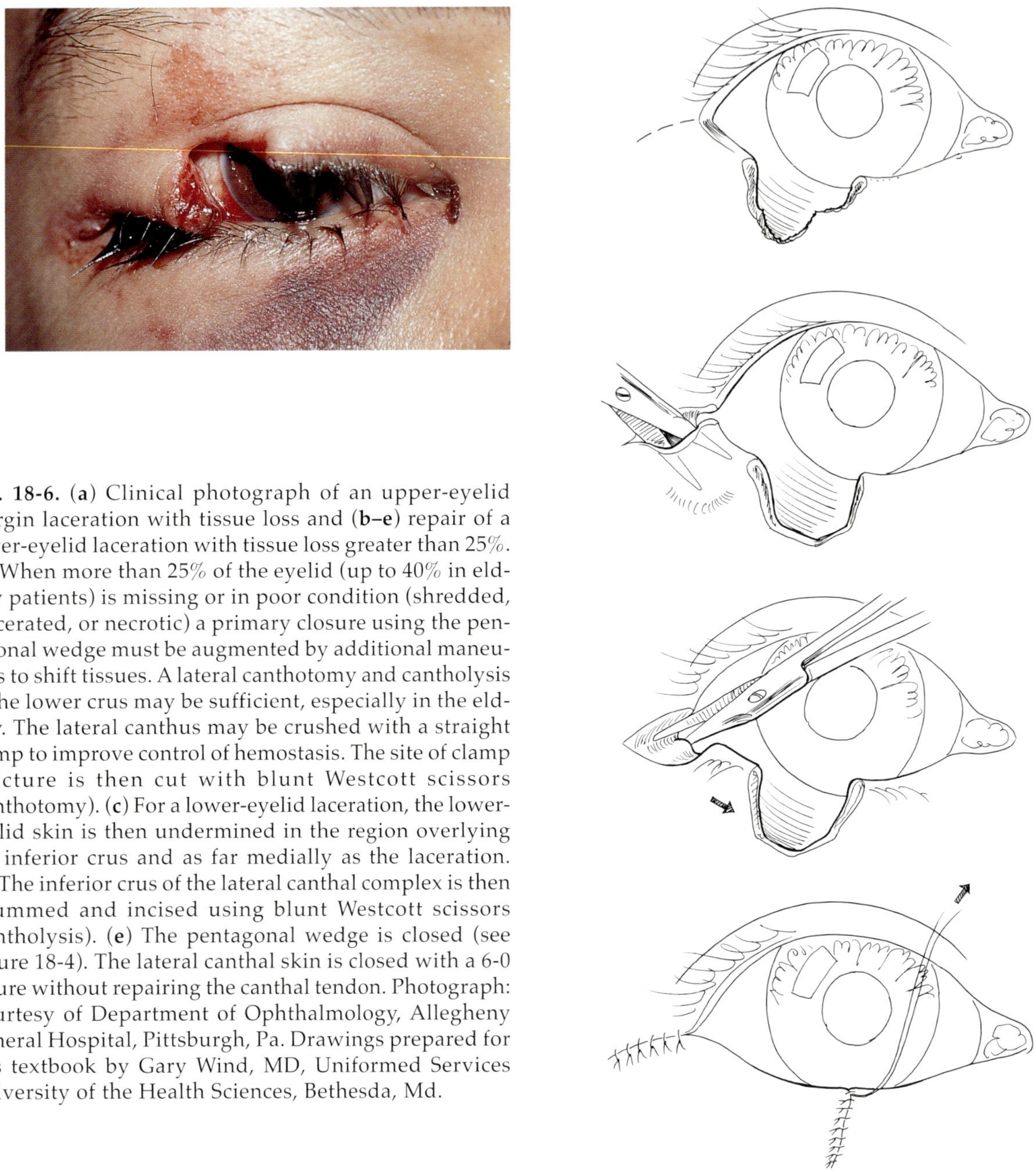

Fig. 18-6. (**a**) Clinical photograph of an upper-eyelid margin laceration with tissue loss and (**b–e**) repair of a lower-eyelid laceration with tissue loss greater than 25%. (**b**) When more than 25% of the eyelid (up to 40% in elderly patients) is missing or in poor condition (shredded, macerated, or necrotic) a primary closure using the pentagonal wedge must be augmented by additional maneuvers to shift tissues. A lateral canthotomy and cantholysis of the lower crus may be sufficient, especially in the elderly. The lateral canthus may be crushed with a straight clamp to improve control of hemostasis. The site of clamp stricture is then cut with blunt Westcott scissors (canthotomy). (**c**) For a lower-eyelid laceration, the lower-eyelid skin is then undermined in the region overlying the inferior crus and as far medially as the laceration. (**d**) The inferior crus of the lateral canthal complex is then strummed and incised using blunt Westcott scissors (cantholysis). (**e**) The pentagonal wedge is closed (see Figure 18-4). The lateral canthal skin is closed with a 6-0 suture without repairing the canthal tendon. Photograph: Courtesy of Department of Ophthalmology, Allegheny General Hospital, Pittsburgh, Pa. Drawings prepared for this textbook by Gary Wind, MD, Uniformed Services University of the Health Sciences, Bethesda, Md.

lower eyelid), then a Tenzel flap is necessary (Figure 18-7). The flap diameter should be twice the diameter of the defect, up to a flap size of 20 mm. Larger defects also require inferior crus cantholysis and release of the lateral septum and retractors. Both of these techniques mobilize lateral skin medially to allow closure of the wound under acceptable tension. If more than 50% of the upper eyelid or 75% of the lower eyelid is severely damaged or missing, then a larger flap or lid-sharing maneuver is required.[2,3]

If more than 50% of full-thickness lower eyelid is lost, a Hughes lid-sharing procedure is an excellent technique to provide the necessary posterior lamella support (Figure 18-8). The upper-lid conjunctiva and tarsus are mobilized from the upper eyelid and brought inferiorly to replace the posterior aspect of the lower eyelid. The anterior lamella (skin and orbicularis) may be provided as a free graft from the opposite upper eyelid, postauricular, or supraclavicular regions. The graft should be oversized by approximately 1 mm and secured with 6-0 silk.

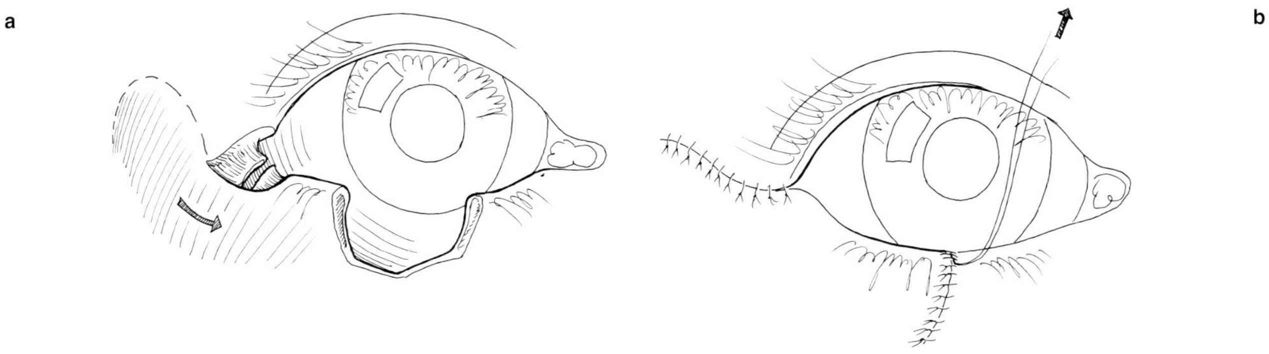

Fig. 18-7. Repair of a lower-eyelid laceration with tissue loss exceeding 50%. (**a**) If sufficient laxity is not present with the lateral canthotomy and cantholysis, then a Tenzel rotational flap is created, mobilizing tissue from the lateral upper lid for lower-lid laceration. (**b**) The final result after placement of skin sutures is shown. If primary closure of the eyelid margin is still not possible after these two procedures, then more-complex procedures—beyond the scope of most general ophthalmologists—are required. A Mustarde flap can be used to mobilize facial laxity to help with eyelid closure, or an eyelid-sharing technique from the opposite lid may be performed. Drawings prepared for this textbook by Gary Wind, MD, Uniformed Services University of the Health Sciences, Bethesda, Md.

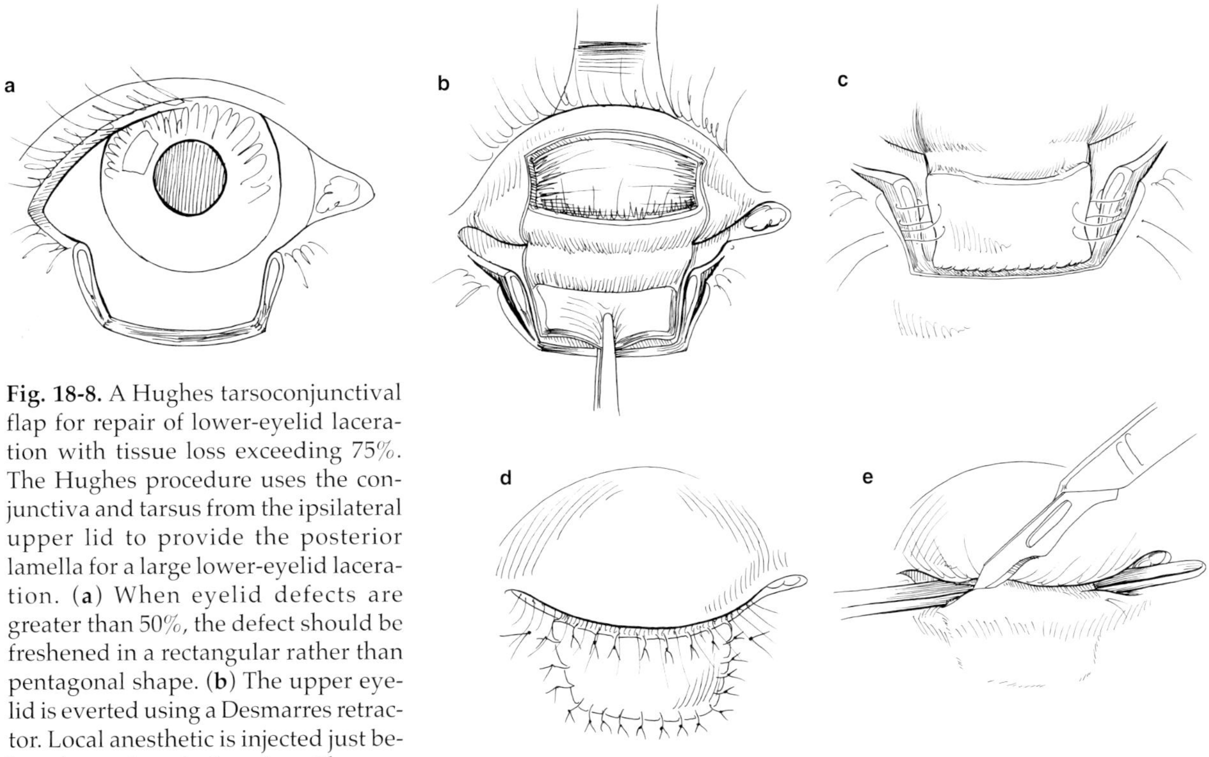

Fig. 18-8. A Hughes tarsoconjunctival flap for repair of lower-eyelid laceration with tissue loss exceeding 75%. The Hughes procedure uses the conjunctiva and tarsus from the ipsilateral upper lid to provide the posterior lamella for a large lower-eyelid laceration. (**a**) When eyelid defects are greater than 50%, the defect should be freshened in a rectangular rather than pentagonal shape. (**b**) The upper eyelid is everted using a Desmarres retractor. Local anesthetic is injected just below the conjunctival surface. The conjunctiva is incised 3 mm from and parallel to the eyelid border as the first step in the formation of a tarsoconjunctival flap. The conjunctiva and tarsus are then incised perpendicular to the original incision, creating a fornix-based flap. Sharp and blunt dissection are used to free the Müller's muscle from the flap. (**c**) The tarsus of the upper lid is sutured to the lower lid in a tongue-in-groove fashion using a 4-0 silk suture nasally and temporally. 7-0 Vicryl is then used to secure the tarsus to the conjunctiva inferiorly. (**d**) A skin graft from the contralateral upper eyelid, inferior advancement flap or a Tenzel flap may be used to replace the anterior lamella (skin and orbicularis). The skin graft pictured is best obtained from the contralateral—never the ipsilateral—upper eyelid and is secured with interrupted 6-0 silk sutures. If insufficient upper-eyelid skin is present, retroauricular or supraclavicular skin may be used as an alternative. (**e**) Six to 8 weeks after primary repair, the second-stage procedure should be performed. The tarsoconjunctival flap is incised approximately 1 mm above the intended upper-eyelid level. The globe should be protected with a malleable retractor or knife handle and the incision performed using a no. 15 Bard-Parker blade. This second-stage procedure should be performed 6 to 8 weeks after the primary repair. Drawings prepared for this textbook by Gary Wind, MD, Uniformed Services University of the Health Sciences, Bethesda, Md.

A bolster composed of cotton or a Telfa pad should be secured over the skin graft, using sutures that are left long for this purpose. The bolster and a pressure patch should be left in place for 5 days to minimize shrinkage or hypertrophic healing. Alternatively, a flap mobilized from excess lateral skin (Tenzel flap) may be used. If the defect is in the upper eyelid, the posterior lamella may be obtained from the contralateral upper-eyelid tarsus, or ear cartilage as a free graft. Other materials, such as donor sclera or preserved pericardium, have also been used with success.

If the posterior lamella is replaced with a graft, then the anterior lamella must be constructed from a medial- or lateral-based flap. The Cutler-Beard technique uses a full-thickness flap of lower-eyelid skin passed behind an intact bridge of lower-lid margin. Two grafts overlying one another are likely to fail because of inadequate blood supply. In the case of very large defects, a Mustarde flap, which mobilizes tissue from the cheek and lateral skin, should be performed (*a*) only by ophthalmologists with extensive experience or (*b*) with the help of a plastic surgeon. Inappropriate flap development can result in facial paralysis or flap necrosis (Exhibit 18-1).[2–7]

EXHIBIT 18-1

OPTIONS FOR REPAIR

Anterior Lamella (Skin, Orbicularis, Subcutaneous Tissue)

- Granulation < 5 mm (< 10 mm in medial canthal region)
- Primary closure: simple
- Advancement flap (with burrows triangles)
- Free skin graft: upper eyelid, retroauricular, and supraclavicular
- Tenzel semicircular flap
- Cutler-Beard tunnel flap (upper-eyelid reconstruction)
- Mustarde flap

Posterior Lamella (Conjunctiva, Tarsus)

- Free tarsal graft
- Hughes tarsoconjunctival graft (lower-eyelid reconstruction)
- Hard palate (lower eyelid only)
- Donor sclera
- Preserved pericardium
- Ear cartilage
- Nasal septum

Levator Injury

If posttraumatic ptosis is noted or if orbital fat is present in the wound, then a deeper laceration should be suspected. Ptosis may due to a levator laceration or penetration, edema, hemorrhage, or nerve injury. Careful exploration allows inspection of the levator muscle and can rule out deeply imbedded FBs (Figure 18-9). If the levator aponeurosis is injured, then primary repair should be performed whenever possible.

Familiarity with the layers of the eyelid is essential; the levator lies deep to the preaponeurotic fat, orbital septum, orbicularis, and skin. Therefore, if fat presents in the wound, then the orbital septum has been violated and a levator injury is very likely. The technique of reapproximating the levator is similar to the techniques utilized in levator aponeurosis resection for ptosis. If the laceration size limits visualization of the levator, then a skin-crease incision can be performed to improve exposure. The overlying orbicularis is excised, and the septum is identified and incised, allowing visualization of the preaponeurotic fat. The fat is carefully elevated from the levator aponeurosis, and any defects or regions of dehiscence are identified.

Two complementary techniques may aid in the assessment of eyelid anatomy, especially in the challenging traumatized wound. The surgeon may grasp the levator and have the patient look up and down; these eye movements create tension and confirm that the levator is the tissue being grasped. Alternatively, the surgeon may grasp and pull downward on the presumed septum; resistance should be noted because the septum is attached to the superior orbital rim. If lacerated, the levator can be repaired utilizing 6-0 silk or Vicryl. If completely disinserted, it can be reattached utilizing two or three double-armed sutures allowing approximation to the tarsus. Be careful to avoid inclusion of the septum in wound closure; the septum should not be closed. Surgical repair of ptosis should be performed in an awake patient, if possible, to allow matching of the eyelid level to the normal side.[7,9]

Complex Eyelid Injuries

More-complex eyelid lacerations require problem-solving techniques similar to those required by a jigsaw puzzle. Although initially, tissue loss may appear to be extensive, when the corners are

a

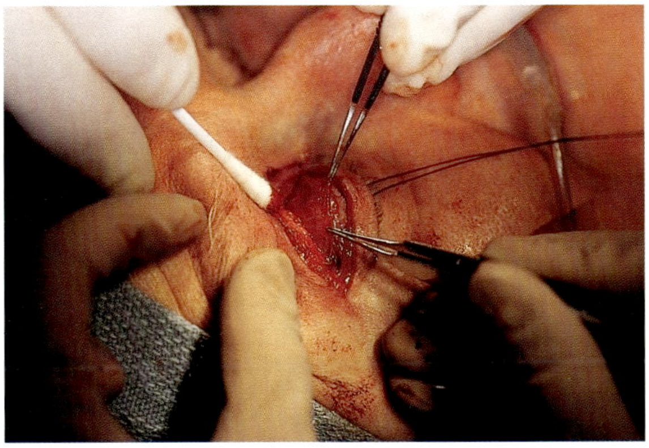

b c d e

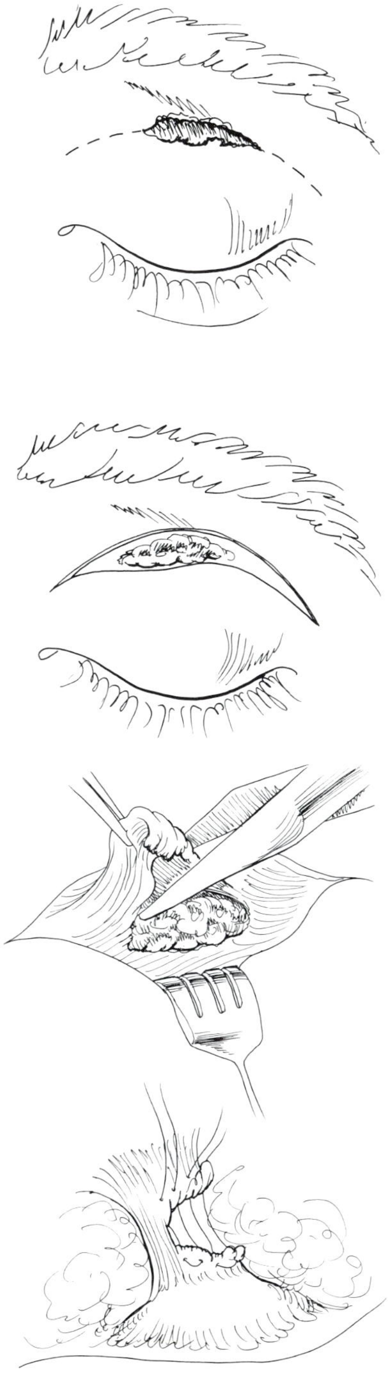

Fig. 18-9. (**a**) The clinical photograph demonstrates an intraoperative view of the levator as seen during exploration and repair of the levator complex. (**b–e**) The drawings depict repair of eyelid laceration involving the levator. (**b**) The eyelid laceration is inspected and fat is visible in the wound. On examination, the patient cannot elevate the eyelid (complete ptosis). (**c**) The eyelid laceration is extended along the eyelid crease to allow maximum exposure. (**d**) The orbicularis is removed overlying the septum superiorly. The levator, septum, and preaponeurotic fat are identified. The levator is freed from the septum using cotton-tipped applicators and light, blunt dissection. (**e**) The edge of the levator is identified and reattached to the tarsus with two or three double armed sutures (6-0 silk or Vicryl). The goal is to reestablish the preoperative position of the levator. In the case of complete dehiscence, the levator may have been ripped along the entire insertion and retracted posteriorly requiring additional dissection to identify the anterior edge of levator aponeurosis. If significant portions of the levator are missing or destroyed, primary levator advancement may be indicated. Photograph: Courtesy of Department of Ophthalmology, Allegheny General Hospital, Pittsburgh, Pa. Drawings prepared for this textbook by Gary Wind, MD, Uniformed Services University of the Health Sciences, Bethesda, Md.

reapproximated, the true extent of tissue loss may be much less. Every attempt should be made to accomplish complete closure; 6-0 silk, plain gut, or nylon sutures are placed in an interrupted fashion and should remain for 3 to 5 days. Certain suture techniques, such as the far-near–near-far technique, help relieve superficial wound tension.

Allowing small, superficial defects to heal by secondary intention can result in acceptable cosmesis if they are very small (< 5 mm) or located in the medial canthal region and less than 1 cm in diameter. Eyelid-margin involvement or extensive tissue loss, however, mandate primary repair.[3,5,7] Skin grafting or large flap advancements should be performed in the acute setting only when severe corneal exposure is present. Complex cases are best delayed if possible so that the primary repair can be performed by experienced, subspecialty-trained ophthalmologists.

Total Avulsion

In the case of total avulsion, the amputated tissue should be retrieved from the injury scene, wrapped in moistened Telfa padding, and carefully preserved on ice during transport. The avulsed tissue should be soaked in a diluted antibiotic prior to reattachment. If necrosis is present, debridement should be minimal and not prohibit wound closure. The avulsed tissue should be secured in an anatomically correct location using a layered closure. If the tarsus is involved, it should be closed in a fashion analogous to the pentagonal wedge described above. Avulsed eyelid tissue that is carefully handled and reattached appropriately has a good chance of surviving and providing adequate function and cosmesis.[3,5,7,9,10]

SURGICAL MANAGEMENT OF ADNEXAL INJURIES

Eyebrow and canalicular injuries commonly occur in association with eyelid lacerations. Injury to the medial canthal ligament frequently accompanies medial lacerations. Lateral canthal lacerations and lacrimal gland and sac injuries are more unusual.

Eyebrow Injuries

The eyebrow may be lacerated in isolation or in continuation with an eyelid injury. The skin in the eyebrow region is thicker than in the eyelid and requires at least a two-layer closure. The deep closure should result in skin approximation. A gap before skin closure will result in an unacceptable postoperative incisional width. Sutures such as 4-0 or 5-0 nylon or Vicryl are often used in a buried, interrupted fashion (eg, vertical mattress technique). The skin is then closed with interrupted or running 6-0 gut, silk, or nylon sutures or with tissue glue.[3]

Canalicular Injuries

Although direct injuries to the lacrimal gland and lacrimal sac are rare because each lies within its own fossa, injuries to the canaliculi are common. Blunt injuries can result in contusions or posttraumatic stenosis of these tiny structures. More commonly, however, a laceration of the medial aspect of the upper or lower eyelid disrupts the continuity of one of the canaliculi (Figure 18-10). Dog bites are a common cause of such injuries, especially in children.[11] A fist striking the cheek can also disrupt the canaliculi. In such cases, the temporal swelling can mislead even the most prudent examiner. Finally, on occasion, a well-intentioned surgeon can cause injury to these delicate structures while repairing an adjacent injury. To avoid this kind of inadvertent iatrogenic injury, the canaliculus should be dilated and a probe placed while adjacent lacerations are repaired. Suspicion and inspection are keys to the identification and early repair of canalicular injuries. Although most ophthalmologists feel comfortable repairing a wide variety of eyelid lacerations, repair of the canaliculi prompts concern in even the most skilled retinal or anterior segment surgeon.[5,7,8,11–15]

The management of canalicular lacerations is controversial. Recommendations in the literature range from observation (if only one canaliculus is injured) to canalicular repair with intubation of the upper and lower systems. Although epiphora is not a guaranteed outcome if an injured canaliculus goes unaddressed, repair should be attempted if possible. Repair can be delayed for 48 hours without affecting the outcome.

Surgical repair begins with identification and dilation of the puncta and probing of the proximal aspect of the injured canaliculus. Magnification is essential, although repair is possible using loupes; a microscope is often necessary. Using magnification, inspection of the correct region (posterior to the medial eyelid stump, adjacent to the caruncle)

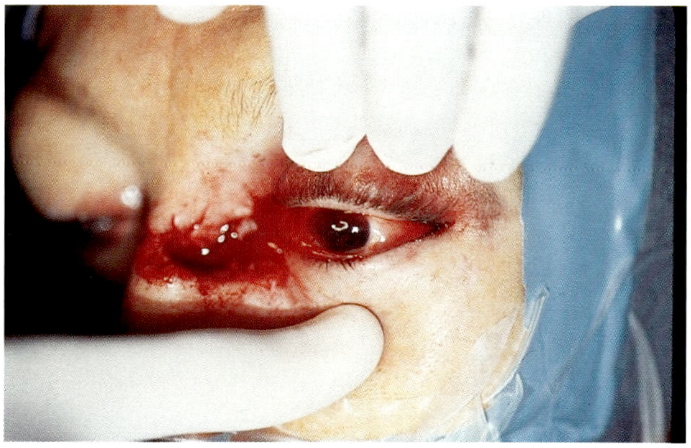

Fig. 18-10. A medial laceration with suspected canalicular injury. All lacerations that extend medial to the puncta should be explored to determine the status of the canaliculi and the medial canthal tendon. Photograph: Courtesy of Department of Ophthalmology, Allegheny General Hospital, Pittsburgh, Pa.

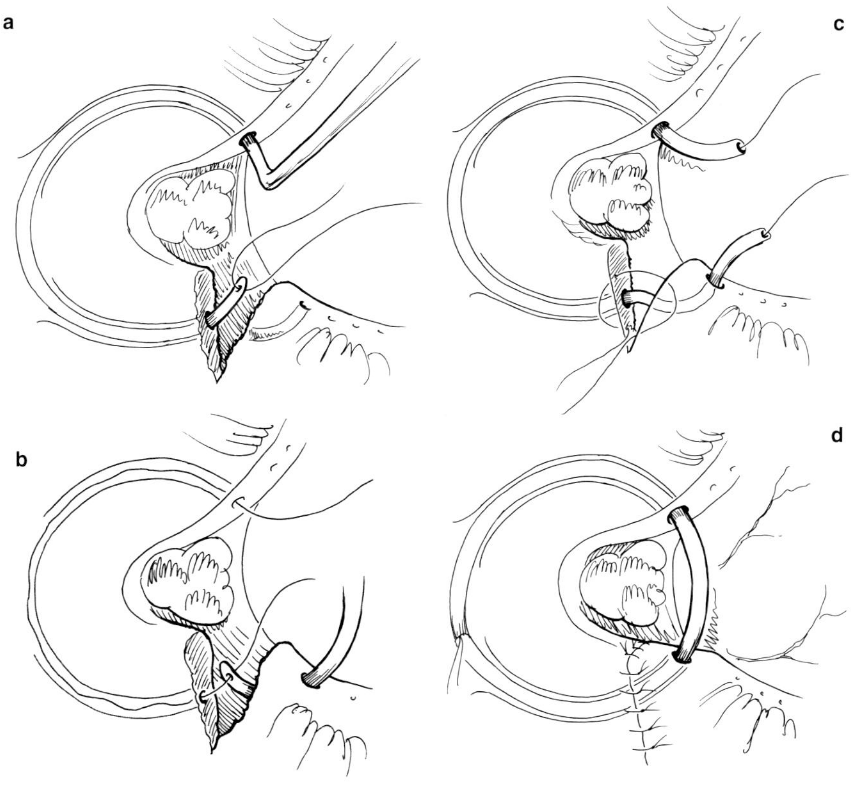

Fig. 18-11. Pigtail probe technique for distal canalicular identification. (**a**) The pigtail is inserted through the uninvolved upper punctum and then passed through the common canaliculus and out the medial end of the lower canalicular laceration. 6-0 nylon suture is then threaded through the eyelet on the end of the pigtail probe so the probe can be carefully pulled back through the common canaliculus and out the intact canalicular system. (**b**) The pigtail probe is then inserted through the proximal canalicular edge so that it passes from the punctum into the wound. The eyelet is threaded with the same 6-0 suture and pulled through the punctum. The 6-0 suture now traverses the entire canalicular system. Silicone tubing is then threaded over the 6-0 suture, completing the intubation of the canalicular system (15–20 mm of silicone tubing is necessary). (**c**) The canalicular laceration is then repaired. A single-suture technique is a good alternative to the multiple-suture technique. The single 7-0 Vicryl suture is placed in a horizontal mattress fashion. The goal is to align the tissues surrounding the canaliculus; direct repair of the canaliculus is not necessary. (**d**) Following the laceration repair, the 6-0 suture is tied such that the ends of the silicone tube are approximated and the section of silicone tube containing the knot positioned in the common canaliculus. The silicone tube should not be long enough to contact the cornea or short enough to "cheesewire," or cut, through the puncta. Drawings prepared for this textbook by Gary Wind, MD, Uniformed Services University of the Health Sciences, Bethesda, Md. NOTE: the normal angulations of the canaliculi have been simplified for these illustrations.

may reveal the white, round, rolled edges of the cut medial end. Additional measures are frequently required to identify the cut end amid the tissue edema and distortion. Normal saline, with or without 2% fluorescein, may be irrigated from the uninjured puncta and visualized as it exits the detached distal end of the injured canaliculus. Methylene blue is not recommended because once applied, it stains the entire field.

If the distal end of the canaliculus cannot be located, a pigtail probe may be used (Figure 18-11). The occasional lacrimal surgeon should be very careful; if used in the wrong way, the pigtail probe can damage the lacrimal sac and uninvolved canaliculus. The pigtail probe should be used with a very delicate touch and abandoned immediately if smooth passage does not occur the first time. Once the pigtail probe is appropriately inserted, silicone tubing can be cannulated over a 6-0 polypropylene suture and the knot rotated so that it lies within the lacrimal sac. The soft tissues surrounding the injured canaliculus are approximated using 8-0 or 9-0 nylon suture. Nonreactive suture (eg, nylon) is preferred to avoid inflammation and potential secondary stricture of the canaliculus, which are associated with dissolution of absorbable sutures.

The canaliculus itself does *not* require repair. A variety of monocanalicular stents are available but have not been found to be superior to stenting the entire system with standard silicone tubes (ie, Crawford, Donahue, or Jackson tubes). Although monocanalicular stents are often easier to place, the proximal end is secured to the skin or inferior cul-de-sac, which promotes premature tube dislocation (Figure 18-12). Table 18-2 lists an array of equipment for canalicular diagnosis repair and suggests some field-expedient substitutes.

Recanalization of mucosal surfaces is rapid, yet how long the tubes should remain in place is debated (2 wk[2,3] to 6 mo[10,12]). If the patient is not both-

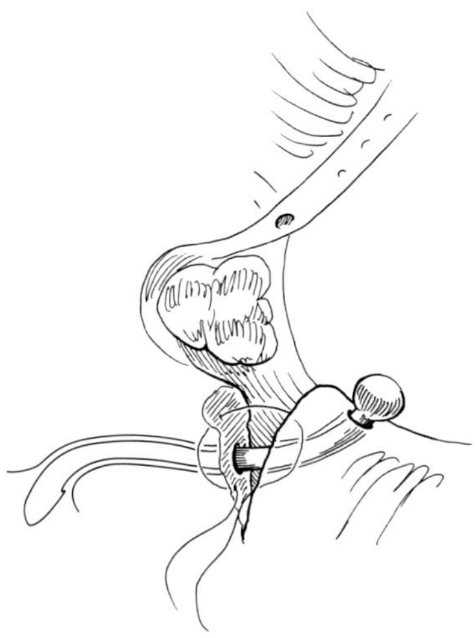

Fig. 18-12. Monocanalicular stent placement. If the distal end of the canalicular laceration is easily identified, a monocanalicular stent can be slipped in place, and then the canalicular laceration can be repaired (see Figure 18-11). Drawing prepared for this textbook by Gary Wind, MD, Uniformed Services University of the Health Sciences, Bethesda, Md.

TABLE 18-2

EQUIPMENT REQUIRED FOR CANALICULAR REPAIR

Traditional	Improvisations
Punctal Dilator	Safety pin
Lacrimal Probes (Bowman no. 00, 1, 2)	Paper clip
Canalicular Irrigation Cannula	25-gauge needle with the tip filed flat
Canalicular Stents	4-0 nylon suture
Veirs Rod (Ethicon, Inc*)	—
Johnson Wire Stent (Karl Storz Industrial Endoscopy*)	—
Silicone Tubing (Dow Corning Corp*)	—
Mini Monoka (FCI, Inc*)	—

*Distributor

ered by the tubes, a 6-month course is ideal in severely traumatized cases.

Medial Canthal Injuries

Medial canthal disruption or significant medial skin defects can occur in isolation or in conjunction with canalicular lacerations. If the posterior limb of the medial canthus is disrupted, rounding occurs and telecanthus typically develops. Reapproximation of the canthal tendon to the periosteum overlying the posterior lacrimal crest may be accomplished with 4-0 monofilament suture (eg, nylon) on a small, reverse-cutting needle but more often requires screws or plates for definitive repair.

Overcorrection is the goal in the immediate postoperative period; the medial punctum should be pulled 1 to 2 mm medial to its normal position and be markedly inverted. Care must be taken to maintain the natural position of the medial canthus 2 mm lower than the lateral canthus. Tissue loss in the region of the medial canthus can be managed effectively with granulation, a graft, or a glabellar flap. In the case of medial canthal injury, the canaliculus should be repaired first, the tendon should then be reattached (with special attention to its posterior aspect), and, finally, skin or eyelid-margin lacerations should be addressed. The conjunctiva does not require repair, but the plica semilunaris and caruncle should be reconstructed with buried, interrupted, 6-0 plain gut sutures to achieve better cosmesis.[2,3,5]

Lateral Canthal Injuries

Lateral canthal injuries require deep repair to preserve the shape and position of the eyelid. If the lateral canthus has been entirely disrupted, care should be taken to identify the superior and inferior crus, resuspend the inferior crus to the periorbita, and reform the lateral canthal angle. The suspension is very similar to a lateral tarsal strip procedure. The inferior crus is resuspended to the periorbita using a 4-0 polyester or 5-0 chromic suture. If no periorbita remains, a miniplate may be placed along the lateral orbital margin and 4-0 or 5-0 nylon sutures used to attach the lateral canthus.

The superior and inferior crus should be internally (6-0 Vicryl) and externally (6-0 silk or nylon) secured to one another to recreate the normal sharp angle of the lateral canthus. The skin can be closed in an interrupted or running fashion with 6-0 silk, nylon, gut, or tissue glue. If inferior eyelid trauma is also present, a temporary lateral tarsorrhaphy or a Frost suture should be placed for upward traction and prevention of postoperative ectropion or eyelid retraction.

Lacrimal Sac and Lacrimal Gland Injuries

Lacrimal sac and duct injuries tend to accompany midfacial injuries that fracture the lacrimal or ethmoid bones or both. These injuries are very difficult to identify in the acute setting, and primary repair is not typically an issue. Dacryocystorhinostomy (DCR) or conjunctivo-dacryocystorhinostomy (C-DCR) with Pyrex (Jones) tube placement may be necessary at a later time.[7,9]

Injury to the lacrimal gland may be confused with fat presenting in the wound. In any lateral eyelid injury, fat prolapse should be assumed to be lacrimal gland tissue until proven otherwise. The levator aponeurosis provides the anatomical separation between the palpebral and orbital lobes of the lacrimal gland. Orbital fat tends to have a yellow-white appearance, whereas lacrimal gland is more flesh- or pink-colored. In traumatic wounds, these color distinctions may be blurred because of contamination, edema, and blood. Suspected lacrimal gland tissue should be replaced into its fossa and the overlying skin defect closed, as described above in the Superficial Eyelid Lacerations section.[4,7]

POSTOPERATIVE WOUND CARE

Postoperative wound care should include daily cleaning of crusting with cotton-tipped applicators and hydrogen peroxide whenever possible. Topical antibiotic ointment (erythromycin or bacitracin) should be applied at least daily. In the case of delayed closure, an oral antibiotic with broad-spectrum coverage should be prescribed. The eyelids are very well vascularized and heal well despite delayed closure or even complete avulsion.

Minimizing contraction during the healing of the wound is very important. Countertraction with a suture (Frost or reverse Frost) through the eyelid margin (preferably using 4-0 nylon or silk) should be placed in all traumatic eyelid injuries. The more significant the eyelid deficit, the longer the eyelid should be left on traction. Skin grafts should be pressure-patched for at least 5 days, and longer for larger defects. Plastic tape can be used to exert upward traction on the malar fat pad and minimize the effects of gravity. Frost sutures, pressure patching, and unweighting of the cheek should be combined in complex eyelid injuries.

SUMMARY

Injuries to the eyelids and ocular adnexa are very common in civilian and battlefield settings. These injuries are often accompanied by intracranial or facial injuries, so stabilization of the patient and attention to the classic ABCs (airway, breathing, and circulation) of trauma care are crucial. If midfacial injuries are present, relying on a team of expert otolaryngologists, oromaxillofacial surgeons, and, occasionally, neurosurgeons maximizes the patient's functional and cosmetic outcome.

Eyelid and ocular adnexal injuries are also commonly associated with injury to other aspects of the globe and orbit. A complete history and ophthalmic examination are always indicated prior to intervention. CT scans should be performed if FBs or fractures are suspected. All wounds should be carefully irrigated and all but very severely necrotic tissue preserved.

Primary closure of the eyelid defect should be performed within 72 hours; canalicular laceration repair should be performed within 48 hours. Completely avulsed tissue should be soaked in antibiotic solution and used for repair whenever possible. If primary closure is not possible, then a combination of skin grafts, lid-sharing techniques, and flaps is necessary. The types of suture or canalicular stenting material are far less important than a meticulous primary closure that respects eyelid and adnexal anatomy. Finally, liberal use of traction sutures, pressure patches, and taping minimizes the effects of gravity and maximizes the cosmetic outcome.

REFERENCES

1. Nash EA, Margo CE. Patterns of emergency department visits for disorders of the eye and ocular adnexa. *Arch Ophthalmol*. 1998;116:1222–1226.

2. Flanagan JC, Mazzoli RA, Bigham WJ. Reconstruction of the lower eyelid. In: Stewart WB, ed. *Surgery of the Eyelid, Orbit and Lacrimal System*. Vol 2. Monograph 8. San Francisco, Calif: American Academy of Ophthalmology; 1994: Chap 20.

3. Nunery WR. Reconstruction of the upper eyelid. In: Stewart WB, ed. *Surgery of the Eyelid, Orbit and Lacrimal System*, Vol 2. Monograph 8. San Francisco, Calif: American Academy of Ophthalmology; 1994: Chap 21.

4. Green JP, Charonis GC, Goldberg RA. Eyelid trauma and reconstruction techniques. In: Yanoff M, Duker JS, eds. *Ophthalmology*. London, England: Mosby; 1999: Chap 13.

5. Goldberg RA. Orbital and adnexal trauma. *Curr Opin Ophthalmol*. 1992;3:686–694.

6. Kersten RC, Kulwin DR. Reconstruction of periocular soft tissue defects. In: Naugle TC, ed. *Diagnosis and Management of Oculoplastic and Orbital Disorders*. New York, NY: Kugler Publications; 1995: 145–158.

7. American Academy of Ophthalmology. Orbit, eyelids and lacrimal system. In: Kersten RC, ed. *Basic and Clinical Science Course*. San Francisco, Calif: American Academy of Ophthalmology; 1997–1998: 138–141.

8. Veloudios A, Kratky V, Heathcote JG, Lee M, Hurwitz JJ, Kazdan MS. Cyanoacrylate tissue adhesive in blepharoplasty. *Ophthal Plast Reconstr Surg*. 1996;12:89–97.

9. Marrone AC. Eyelid and canalicular trauma. In: Stevenson CM, ed. *Ophthalmic Plastic, Reconstructive and Orbital Surgery*. Newton, Mass: Butterworth-Heinemann; 1997: Chap 7.

10. Specht CS, Varga JH, Halali MM, Edelstein JP. Orbitocranial wooden foreign body diagnosed by magnetic resonance imaging: Dry wood can be isodense with air and orbital fat by computed tomography. *Surv Ophthalmol*. 1992;36:341–344.

11. Slonim CB. Dog bite–induced canalicular lacerations: A review of 17 cases. *Ophthal Plast Reconstr Surg*. 1996;12:218–222.

12. Kennedy RH, May J, Dailey J, Flanagan JC. Canalicular laceration: An 11-year epidemiologic and clinical study. *Ophthal Plast Reconstr Surg*. 1990;6:46–53.

13. Reifler DM. Management of canalicular laceration. *Surv Ophthalmol*. 1991;36:113–132.

14. Herman DC, Bartley GB, Walker RC. The treatment of animal bite injuries of the eye and ocular adnexa. *Ophthal Plast Reconstr Surg*. 1987;3:237–241.

15. Hawes MJ, Segrest DR. Effectiveness of bicanalicular silicone intubation in the repair of canalicular lacerations. *Ophthal Plast Reconstr Surg*. 1985;1:185–190.

Chapter 19

MANAGEMENT OF EYELID BURNS

JOHN D. NG, MD*; AND DAVID E. E. HOLCK, MD†

*Assistant Professor of Ophthalmology, Division of Oculoplastics, Orbit, Lacrimal, and Reconstructive Surgery, Casey Eye Institute, Oregon Health and Sciences University, Portland, Oregon 97201; formerly, Lieutenant Colonel, Medical Corps, Flight Surgeon, US Army; Director, Oculoplastic, Orbital and Reconstructive Surgery Service, Brooke Army Medical Center, Fort Sam Houston, Texas
†Lieutenant Colonel, US Air Force, Medical Corps; Flight Surgeon; Director, Oculoplastic, Orbital and Reconstructive Surgery Service, Wilford Hall Medical Center, Lackland Air Force Base, Texas 78236-5300

INTRODUCTION

Ocular and eyelid involvement in facial burns are common in both military and civilian settings. More than two thirds of burns involving the face may include the eye or periocular area. Moreover, reviews from major burn centers demonstrate that up to 15% of *all* patients treated for burn wounds have burns involving the ocular and periocular region.[1–4] Most patients in civilian burn centers suffer flame burn injuries.[3,4] Frequent ocular injuries seen as a result of facial burns include lid burns, contracture leading to ectropion (outward turning of the eyelids), and lagophthalmos (inability to close the eyelids), conjunctival burns, conjunctivitis, foreign bodies (FBs), corneal burns, abrasions, and perforations. Because of the life-threatening nature of severe burn injuries to the face and the associated massive swelling, ocular injuries may not be noticed early and treatment may be delayed.[1,5–7] Appropriate early intervention can have a significant effect on the final outcome for the burn patient.

Burns to the eyelids may be caused by thermal (especially flame or flash burns), electrical, chemical, or ionizing radiation sources. The severity of burns depends on the intensity of the burning agent (both the quantity of heat generated or transmitted by the burning agent, and the concentration and amount of the burning agent), the duration of exposure, and the body's response.[2,8,9] Thermal injuries are the most frequent cause of ocular and periocular burn injuries. Liquid thermal burns vary in severity depending on the substance. The temperature of noncombustible liquids, like water, is usually less than 70°C on contact, and such liquids dissipate rapidly from the initial contact area, thereby causing only superficial damage. On the other hand, the temperature of combustible liquids, like gasoline, at contact is usually greater than 100°C, and these liquids tend to be more viscous and may ignite clothing. Therefore, the damage is more localized but often deeper. Most injuries seen with flash burns involve the eyelids and are superficial[10] because of the ocular protective mechanisms: rapid reflex closure of the eyelids, abrupt head movements, and elevation of the globe with eyelid closure (Bell's phenomenon).

Burns resulting from electrical injury are unique because the underlying tissue destruction may be much more extensive than the superficial skin injury. Therefore, a high index of suspicion for deep injury is required, even in seemingly minor electrical burns.[11,12]

Injuries from acids result in coagulative necrosis, which acts as a buffer against deeper tissue penetration. Alkali burns penetrate much deeper because of tissue saponification and, hence, are associated with greater injury. In the field environment, ionizing radiation injury may occur from exposure to nuclear weapons or radioactive munitions. In most mild-to-moderate exposures, radiation burn damage is delayed until vasculopathy develops. Additionally, long-term, cancer-inducing effects may result.

The history of injury can provide vital clues regarding the nature, extent, and initial therapy for the burn patient.[9,10] Life-threatening systemic injuries must be addressed before beginning eye care. In the acute evaluation of facial, neck, and periocular burns, the medical caregiver must be keenly suspicious of a coexisting inhalational burn injury. Inhaled toxic gases that are incomplete products of combustion may directly damage the lower respiratory tract. Evidence of carbonized sputum in a patient who otherwise appears well but who has had thermal exposure should alert the caregiver to the likelihood of significant airway injury. Airway obstruction may worsen a few hours after presentation because of increasing airway edema. Inhaled hot air can damage the mucous membranes of the mouth and upper respiratory tract. And burn injury to the neck or chest may also contribute to respiratory difficulty.

On the battlefield, evaluation and treatment of burns to the eyes and eyelids are tailored according to the echelon level at which the injury occurs and the medical expertise available. Appropriate securing of the airway may be lifesaving in the acute stages before soft-tissue swelling has occurred. Careful monitoring of fluid replacement is mandatory in this period.[7,8] Adherence to Advanced Trauma Life Support (ATLS) and Advanced Cardiac Life Support (ACLS) protocols is critical.[13] Tetanus immunization status should be evaluated and treated accordingly.[7]

TYPES AND DEGREES OF EYELID BURNS

Burns are usually categorized in two ways: by etiology (type of burn) and by amount of tissue damage (degree of injury). Etiologically, an eyelid burn is any injury to the eyelid skin due to exposure to heat, a caustic chemical, electricity, or ionizing radiation. Eyelid burns due to thermal expo-

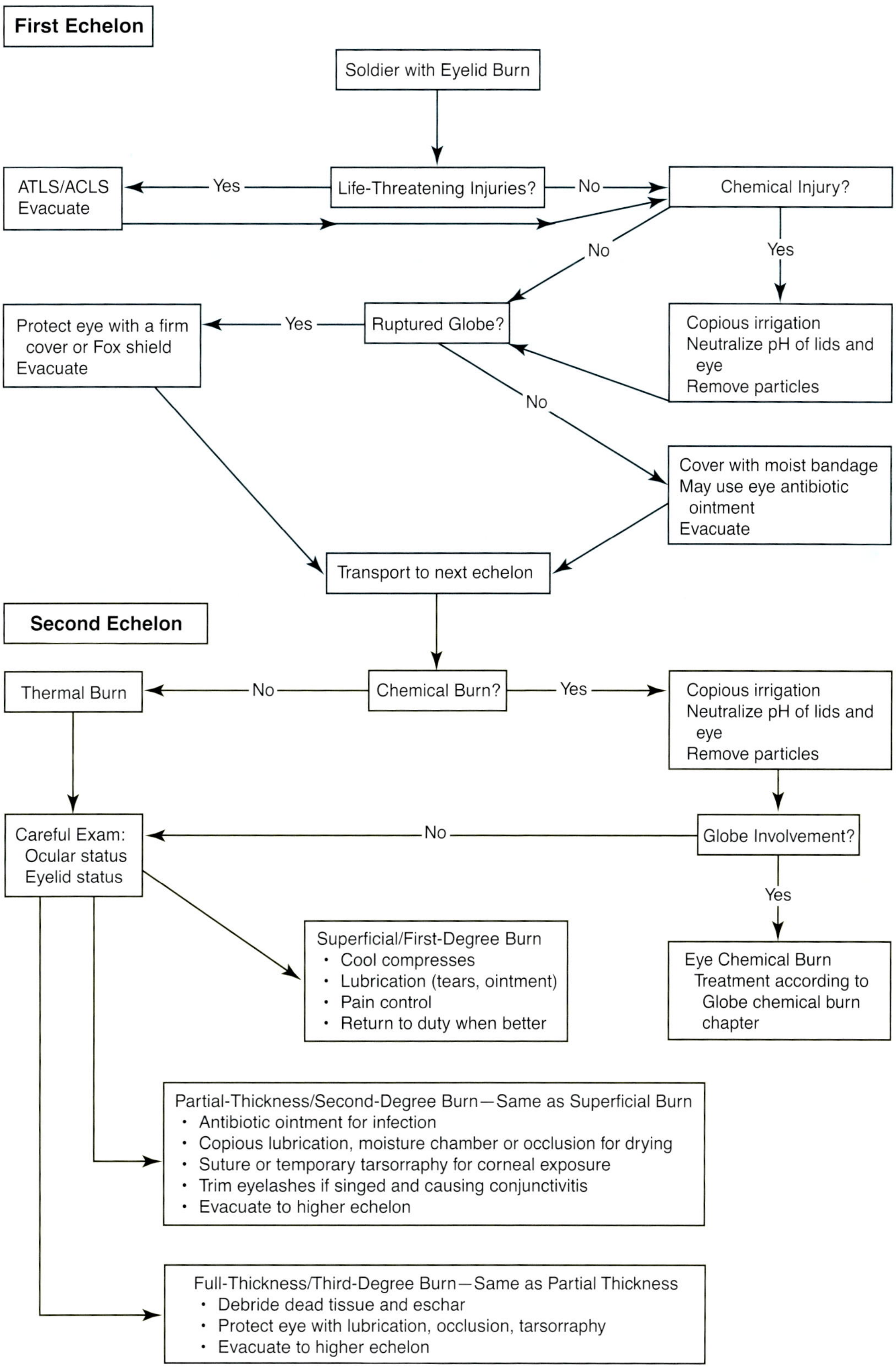

ATLS: Advanced Trauma Life Support (American College of Surgeons)
ACLS: Advanced Cardiac Life Support (American Heart Association)

Fig. 19-1. Flow chart for acute management of eyelid burns.

sure are the most common and account for 96%[8] of all burns. Thermal burns can occur from blast injuries, incendiary munitions, or from direct exposure to flames or hot liquids and gases. Typically, flash burns are more superficial than flame burns, because of the short exposure time common with flash burns.[8,9,13,14]

Chemical burns are usually caused by contact with an acid or alkali compound. A burn injury from direct current may be caused by lightning strikes, whereas one from alternating current usually occurs during contact with high voltage. Low-voltage electrical exposure rarely causes a burn injury. Ionizing radiation burns may be secondary to therapeutic exposure, accidental exposure, or the use of nuclear weapons. Except for high-dose exposure, deep-tissue radiation burn damage is usually delayed until radiation-induced vasculopathy develops 6 months to 2 years after exposure. On the other hand, deep-tissue burn damage from chemical, electrical, or thermal injury is immediate.[9]

In the theater of operations, evaluation and treatment of eyelid burns should focus on protecting the eye by diagnosing the extent of damage, intervening rapidly to prevent further damage to the eyes and eyelids, returning soldiers with mild injury to duty quickly, and stabilizing soldiers with more-serious eyelid damage for evacuation and definitive care (Figure 19-1).

As with any other burn injury, eyelid burns are classified as first-, second-, or third-degree in severity. In 1994, however, to better describe their pathology, they were also classified as superficial, partial-thickness, and full-thickness burns.[12] First-degree (superficial) eyelid burns involve the epidermis only. Erythema and edema are characteristic. The skin remains intact; however, there may be some degree of skin shrinkage. A first-degree burn can be likened to a mild-to-moderate sunburn (Figure 19-2). First-degree burns are self-limited and heal spontaneously.

Second-degree (partial-thickness) burns involve the epidermis and part of the dermis. In second-degree burns, the skin often shrinks and blisters. The blisters may break open, causing weeping and crusting of serous fluid. Open blisters with serous exudate provide a significant opportunity for bacterial infections. Second-degree burns are more painful than first-degree burns because sensory nerve terminals have been injured and exposed (Figure 19-3). Second-degree burns often heal spontaneously but with some contracture and superficial scarring.

Third-degree (full-thickness) burns are the most serious. The epidermis is completely destroyed, and the injury involves the entire dermis and part or all of the subcutaneous tissue. Charring and loss of skin characterize third-degree burns. The skin of-

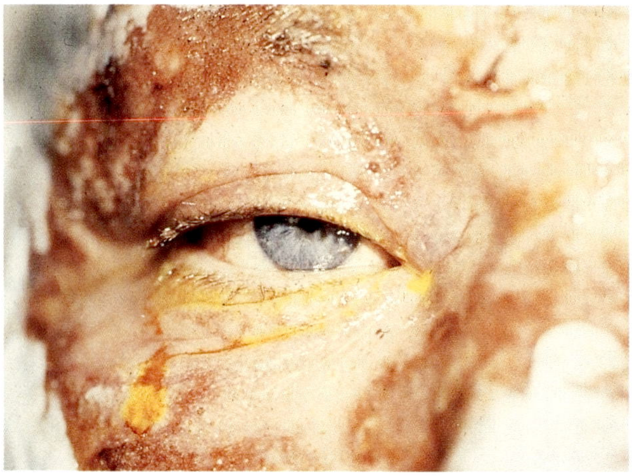

Fig. 19-2. First-degree eyelid burn. Note erythema and mild edema of the upper eyelid along the pretarsal and preseptal skin. There is no loss of epidermis, but there are areas of second-degree burns near the eyebrow.

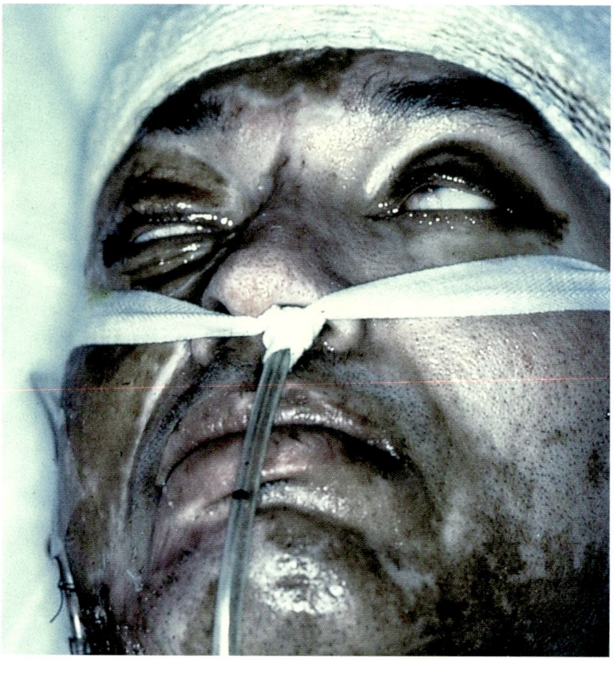

Fig. 19-3. Second-degree eyelid burn of both upper eyelids. Injury involves epidermal loss and is more painful than a first-degree burn. Blisters and oozing of serous fluid may be present, and lid contraction may occur. Photograph: Courtesy of Department of Ophthalmology, Wilford Hall Medical Center, Lackland Air Force Base, Tex.

ten appears carbonized, white-brown, and waxy. The carbonized, dry eschar provides a nidus for infection and requires frequent debridement. Areas of third-degree burns are painless because of damage to sensory nerves; however, tissue surrounding the burn may be painful due to lesser degrees of burn injury.

Third-degree burns of the eyelids usually imply full-thickness injury, as the lids are approximately 2 mm thick and have very little subcutaneous tissue (Figure 19-4). Lids with severe second-degree and third-degree burns are commonly accompanied by significant burn injury to the surrounding tissues, including the face, forehead, scalp, ears, mouth, neck, and torso. This involvement implies a high risk for life-threatening injuries and damage to the most common sources for skin grafts for eyelid reconstruction.

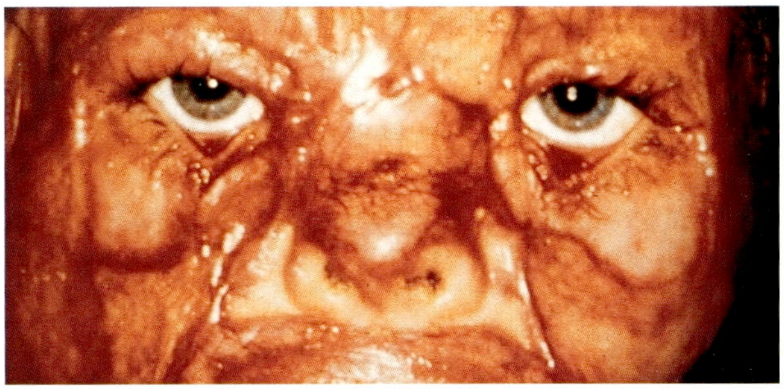

Fig. 19-4. Third-degree eyelid burn of the right upper eyelid. Injury involves full-thickness skin. Charring and white-brown waxy consistency is often present. Third-degree burns usually are not painful. Tissue is damaged, and contraction and lagophthalmos are usually present. Photograph: Courtesy of Department of Ophthalmology, Wilford Hall Medical Center, Lackland Air Force Base, Tex.

EYELID BURN INJURIES, HEALING, AND COMPLICATIONS

When tissue is exposed to a burn injury, the area of injury often resembles a bull's-eye target, with the severity of injury decreasing from the center to the periphery. In a third-degree burn, the central area is *the zone of coagulation,* where tissue is destroyed and no longer viable, hence its characteristic white, leathery appearance.

The area just peripheral to the center is the *zone of stasis,* which temporarily has decreased vascularity but can recover barring further injury. The zone of stasis can be divided into a superficial zone and a deeper zone. The superficial zone demonstrates early stasis because it sustains greater injury and becomes ischemic within 2 hours, owing to vasoconstriction and platelet aggregation with thrombosis. The deeper zone shows delayed stasis with ischemia beginning between 4 to 24 hours after the injury. If cared for properly, hair follicle epithelial cells remain viable and will repopulate and migrate.

The third and most peripheral area is the *zone of hyperemia.* Vascular structures remain intact and the area blanches on pressure. There is no cell death, only edema and erythema.[11] Second-degree burns do not have a zone of coagulation but do have varying degrees of zones of stasis and hyperemia. First-degree burns demonstrate zones of hyperemia only.

First-Degree Burns

Superficial burns are commonly caused by sunburn, ultraviolet ray exposure, and short-duration flash burns. They are dry burns with edema and no blistering. Erythema and pain are common. Histologically, superficial burns only involve epidermal layers. Healing occurs in 3 to 7 days, accompanied by superficial peeling. There is no scar formation although discoloration may develop.

Second-Degree Burns

Mild (superficial) partial-thickness burns are commonly caused by immersion scalds of short exposure. The wounds blister, weep, and form moist blebs. There is intense erythema, significant pain, and temperature sensitivity. Histologically, epidermis and some papillary dermis are involved. Healing occurs within 7 to 21 days without grafting and with little or no scarring. Pigmentary changes, however, are common.

Moderate (deeper) partial-thickness burns are commonly caused by immersion scalds of longer duration and flame injury. Blisters are large and thick-walled; they increase in size. The skin appears mottled white and pink to cherry-red. Histologically, the epidermis, papillary dermis, and reticular dermis are involved. Some subcutaneous involvement may occur. Healing occurs in 21 to 35 days in uncomplicated cases. If infection or reinjury occurs, the wound may convert to a full-thickness injury.

Severe partial-thickness burns have a propensity to develop hypertrophic scars and to convert to full-thickness injuries.

Third-Degree Burns

Full-thickness burns are usually caused by

chemical, electrical, flame, and scald injuries. The skin appears dry, leathery, nonpliable, and there may be charring, eschar, and significant avascularity. There is little or no pain; the hair in the affected area pulls out easily. Histologically, the wound includes the subcutaneous tissue and may include fascia, muscle, tendon, and bone. In a small lesion, healing from the leading edge of the wound may occur over several weeks. In larger lesions, grafting is necessary; otherwise, healing takes many months.[12]

Healing Process

Reepithelialization of wounds occurs from epithelium located at wound edges and skin appendages, such as hair follicles, sebaceous glands, sweat glands, and their ducts. For large areas, granulation tissue must first bridge the wound before epithelialization can occur. Contraction occurs in second- and third-degree wounds and aids in restoring epithelial continuity; however, contraction often distorts the functioning of the eyelids.[15]

Complications of Eyelid Burns

The eyelids serve several functions. They protract, or close, to protect the eye from wind-borne dirt and debris and the drying effects of the environment. The eyelids retract, or open, to provide an unimpeded visual axis for seeing. The eyelids contain glands that secrete the aqueous (accessory glands of Krause and Wolfring) and lipid (meibomian glands) portions of tears. They also blink to spread the tear film evenly over the eye, which is crucial for visual clarity. The lacrimal drainage system begins in the eyelids as the lacrimal puncta and continues as the canaliculi, lacrimal sac, and the lacrimal duct, which empties beneath the inferior turbinate in the nose. The lids act as a lacrimal pump to remove the tears from the ocular surface and drain them into the nose. Burn injuries to the eyelids can compromise one or all of these functions and cause visual debilitation.

Eyelids that cannot close put the soldier at risk of sustaining corneal FBs, abrasions, and ulcers that cause significant pain, impairment, and possible loss of the eye. Eyelids that cannot open because of burns may leave the soldier essentially blind and ineffective in the battlefield. A blinded soldier also requires the help and time of another soldier to assist him or her to safety.

An injured or scarred lacrimal drainage system anywhere along its length may cause epiphora (a wet, tearing eye due to abnormal drainage of tears), which interferes with visual clarity. An abnormal tear pump mechanism can also leave the soldier with epiphora.

Therefore, treatment of eyelid burns is a vital component in caring for warfare injuries. Effective treatment of minor injuries allows the soldier to return to duty with minimal delay. Significant eyelid burns, which are likely to develop any or all of these complications, require proper evaluation and management to protect the eye and limit damage to injured structures. Early evacuation of severely burned patients is required to minimize consumption of resources in the theater of operations and to maintain the best prognosis possible for the soldier.

EVALUATION AND TREATMENT OF EYELID BURNS

Casualties with eyelid burns often have concomitant facial, neck, and upper torso burns (see Figure 19-1). Airway compromise should always be considered. Therefore, immediate evaluation and treatment should follow the ATLS[16] and ACLS[17] protocols.

1st Echelon

If a casualty might have a chemical burn to the eyes, then the eyes and eyelids should be thoroughly rinsed with sterile water or saline. Rapidly irrigating the offending chemical and returning the ocular tear film pH to normal can significantly decrease morbidity and improve visual outcome. The rinse may require several liters of fluid and should be done as soon as possible after the chemical injury. If sterile water or saline is not available, then any neutral, relatively clean liquid will suffice until sterile solutions are available. Particulate matter must be gently rinsed out because it may contain chemical reagents and cause further damage.

Once copiously irrigated and debrided of foreign material, the lids should be covered with a moist bandage, if possible. First-degree burns may need only to be rinsed clean. Bandaging for second- or third-degree burns is desirable, if available.[1,2,13,14] Antibiotic eye ointment (eg, bacitracin, gentamycin) may be used with bandaging. If neither ointment nor bandage is available, the wound should be kept moist to decrease tissue necrosis and eschar formation. Desiccation of a burn wound can increase ischemia in the zones of stasis where partial vascular compromise exists.[12]

If an open globe injury is suspected, then bandaging of lid burns is contraindicated and a protective shield should be placed over the orbital rim to prevent pressure on the eye (Figure 19-5). Direct pressure on an open globe will increase the ocular injury, may expel intraocular contents, and can cause irreversible damage to an otherwise salvageable eye.

2nd Echelon

If a chemical burn is suspected, the eyes should be copiously flushed with normal saline solution to remove any residual chemicals and particulate matter, and treatment should be initiated as described in Chapter 7, Chemical Injuries of the Eye. Additionally, the eyelids and periocular tissue should be rinsed of all chemicals in a similar manner. The remainder of the evaluation is the same as for radiation, electrical, and thermal burns[13] (described below).

Evaluation of the Eyes

The initial 2nd-echelon evaluation determines the status of the eyes. The ocular examination must be performed as soon as possible, because the eyelids often swell shut after an eyelid burn injury. Swollen eyelids and pain associated with first- and second-degree burns often render a delayed examination extremely difficult and possibly hazardous to the injured eye. A complete history is needed to direct the examination and to determine chronic management. The mechanism of injury should be elicited. Specifically, was the burn due to a blast injury or to thermal, chemical, electrical, or radiation exposure?

Initial Visual Acuity. Visual acuity is measured with a standard eye chart or near-vision acuity card. If these are not available, any reading material may be used. The vision must be clearly documented for baseline examinations. If an eye chart is not available, it is sufficient to describe that the patient was able to read fine or large print at reading distance. If the patient cannot see clearly enough to read, the examiner should determine if he or she can count fingers, see hand motion, or detect light in that order. Any measurement should be accurately recorded.

Status of the Conjunctiva (Ocular Mucous Membranes). The examiner should check for lacerations or loss of mucosal surface from blast or burn injury. Injury to the conjunctiva can cause a dry eye due to damage to the tear-producing glands: the accessory aqueous-producing glands of Krause and Wolfring, the mucosal goblet cells, the lipid-producing tarsal meibomian glands, and the ducts of the main aqueous-producing lacrimal gland. A dry eye is at significant risk of ulceration and perforation, especially if the eyelids are damaged and incapable of protecting the ocular surface. Deepithelialization of both the palpebral (lid) conjunctiva and the bulbar (ocular) conjunctiva can cause symblepharon formation (scarring between these two surfaces). Immobile eyelids and a tethered globe may result.

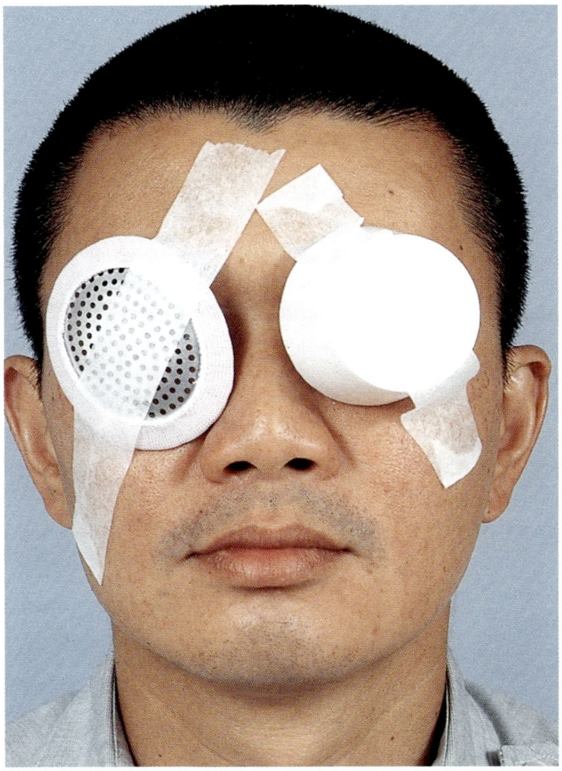

Fig. 19-5. Eye shields. A Fox shield (left) and a modified disposable cup (right). Either may be used to protect the potentially ruptured eye from direct pressure. The shield or cup is placed over the eye with the rim of the shield resting on the bony prominence of the orbital rim. No pressure should be placed on the eyelids or eye itself. The shield is secured in place with a piece of tape.

Status of the Cornea. The examiner should check for lacerations, abrasions, and burn injuries to the cornea and sclera. Corneal and scleral lacerations must be emergently repaired. Corneal abrasions must be treated with lubrication and topical antibiotics to prevent infection and ulceration that can lead to perforation. Ischemia due to coagulation of limbal vessels can lead to corneal breakdown. If ischemia is noted, the examiner should follow the protocol in the corneal burn section.

Anterior Chamber. The examiner should check for a collapsed chamber or hyphema, which can indicate an open globe or significant blunt trauma from a blast injury. Hyphema may lead to increased intraocular pressure, traumatic glaucoma, and corneal blood staining, which can cause significant ocular morbidity.

Shape of the Eye. In difficult cases in which the ocular examination is severely limited because of other severe injuries, the examiner should determine if gross eye deformity is present to rule out a ruptured globe. Ruptured globes should be immediately referred for surgical treatment. If an open globe injury is suspected, treatment should follow the protocol for penetrating injuries. In the interim, the eye should be protected with an eye shield (see Figure 19-5).

Evaluation and Treatment of the Eyelids

Once the eyes have been examined and treated accordingly, the eyelids should be examined. The extent and degree of the eyelid burns are determined, and facial burns adjacent to the eyelids must be noted as well, because contraction of tissue can be transmitted to the eyelids, causing restriction and decreased function. The initial appearance of burned tissue can be deceiving; the extent of damage tends to delineate itself over the next several days. Specifically, severe partial-thickness burns must be aggressively cared for to limit damage and prevent progression to full-thickness injury due to progressive ischemia. The life- and sight-threatening burn wound complication that medical officers must vigilantly guard against is bacterial infections; the organisms most commonly implicated in burn infections include *Streptococcus, Staphylococcus, Pseudomonas,* and *Proteus* species, and *Escherichia coli*. Burn wounds should be kept clean and moist. Dry eschar increases the likelihood of secondary infection. The examiner must also be alert to several signs that may indicate other impending complications (Table 19-1).

Initial 2nd-echelon treatment involves removing any residual chemicals or foreign bodies, as described above, and protection of the eye and eyelids. Burn injuries to the eyelids are often complicated by decreased tear production from damage to lacrimal, conjunctival, and eyelid glands, all of which contribute to tear production (Figure 19-6). As previously mentioned, decreased tearing increases the risk of corneal drying, abrasions, ulcers, and perforations. Additionally, the burn-injured eyelid is often less mobile and may not

TABLE 19-1

EYELID BURNS: SIGNS OF POSSIBLE COMPLICATIONS

Sign Observed	Possible Complication
Loss of eyelid tissue, causing exposure of the eye and cornea (exposure keratopathy)	Tissue loss requires immediate attention and protection of the eye.
Shrinkage of eyelid tissue with lagophthalmos, causing exposure of the eye	Mild lagophthalmos in an alert patient may be asymptomatic, but burn injuries in an unconscious patient can remove the eye's protective mechanisms (eg, tear production, blink reflex, Bell's phenomenon, and corneal tactile sensitivity) and place the eye in jeopardy. Mild symptoms of exposure can be treated with lubricating drops and ointment. More severe lagophthalmos requires aggressive lubrication and ocular surface protection. In the obtunded patient, even mild lagophthalmos can be devastating because the patient's blink reflex is absent, and there is suppression of the Bell's phenomenon. Loss of Bell's phenomenon increases the risk of corneal drying of the exposed surface.
Loss of eyebrows or lashes in an otherwise normal-looking eyelid	Finding suggests thermal damage, which may result in delayed complications of lid contraction, tissue loss, and corneal exposure. Patients with singed lashes should be observed over the first week to check for delayed effects of thermal damage. These patients may also complain of foreign body sensation, which may be due to lash particles falling onto the ocular surface.

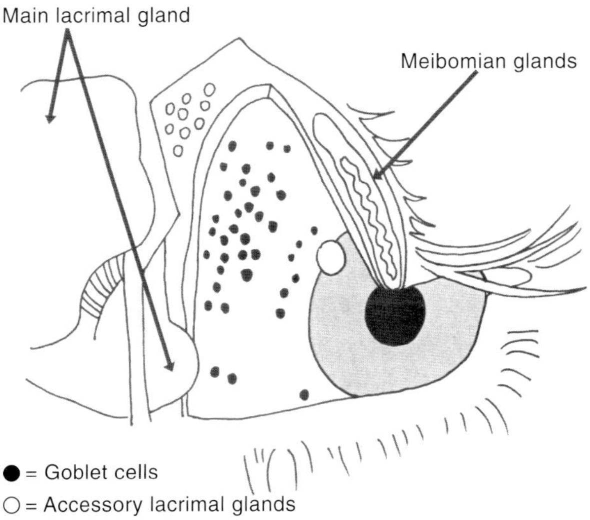

Fig. 19-6. Tear production system. The diagram shows the glands responsible for production of the aqueous and sebaceous components of tears. Any or all of these glands can be damaged by thermal, electrical, chemical, or radiation burns. Drawing: Courtesy of Department of Medical Illustrations, Brooke Army Medical Center, Fort Sam Houston, Tex.

protect the eye sufficiently. Debris in the battlefield can further increase the risk of secondary ocular injury.

Treatment at the 2nd echelon also depends on the type and extent of the burn, and the anatomical structures affected. Chemical injuries should be irrigated copiously (at least 2 L) with normal saline or water. The pH of the injured eye should be checked using pH testing strips to ensure that ocular surface neutrality is attained. When neutral, the patient should be rechecked periodically to verify that no continual damage is occurring by missed particles or chemicals.

Mild first-degree burns with no eyelid contraction or corneal exposure may be treated with topical ophthalmic antibiotic ointment (eg, erythromycin) and cool compresses. Artificial tears may be helpful for mild ocular irritation. Assuming no other injuries, the soldier may be returned to duty. The soldier should be informed of the possibility that a mild second-degree burn might manifest itself in a few days, and that mild pigmentary changes of the skin might also occur.

Significant first-degree burns that cause the eyelids to swell and droop over the pupils (a mechanical ptosis) may require several days of cool compresses, pain control, and topical antibiotic or lubricating ophthalmic ointment. Once the soldier can open his or her eyelids and see, he or she may be returned to duty.

Second- and third-degree burns should be treated similarly to first-degree burns, but they are at greater risk of Gram-negative bacterial infections. Application of gentamycin or tobramycin ointment may be indicated. However, care must be taken to watch for a toxic keratopathy (seen as diffuse staining of the cornea with fluorescein stain under a cobalt-blue light), which may develop with prolonged use of gentamycin and tobramycin. For deeper wounds, wet to dry physiological saline dressings should be used and systemic antibiotics initiated if infection is suspected. The saline dressings are used to decrease formation of dry coagulum (scabbing), which is a nidus for infection, and to decrease progression of ischemia in the zone of stasis.[13,18,19]

Eyelids with second- and third-degree burns often contract and cause some lagophthalmos, and if that happens, the soldier should be evacuated to the 3rd echelon for medical care. If significant exposure of the cornea is evident or if there is lagophthalmos with corneal drying and an epithelial defect, aggressive treatment is required to prevent corneal ulceration or perforation. The first line of treatment is frequent application of ophthalmic antibiotic ointment (at least six times daily). If antibiotic ointment is not available, then a nonmedicated lubricating ophthalmic ointment (eg, Refresh PM, mfg by Allergan, Inc, Irvine, Calif) or even soft, moist saline dressings can be used.

If ointment alone is not effective or if there is insufficient staffing to maintain that regimen, then a moisture chamber or cellophane occlusion should be placed over the antibiotic-ointment-lubricated eye (Figure 19-7). The moisture chamber—acting like a greenhouse—keeps the moisture from evaporating from the surface of the eye. The chamber and the cellophane also keep out foreign material and help maintain a more physiological local temperature. Patients with significant facial and head burns may not tolerate moisture chambers, and if there is periocular skin loss or excessive weeping of serous fluid, a bubble chamber may not stay in place. In these settings, the cellophane patch may be the best alternative.

If the moisture chamber is not available or is ineffective, a temporary tarsorrhaphy suture should be placed (Figure 19-8). A suture tarsorrhaphy is created by passing a double-armed 5-0 suture though a bolster (small piece of foam, rubber, or plastic) and through the lower lid just inferior to the lashes. The needles are passed out through the lower-lid gray line and into the upper-lid gray line.

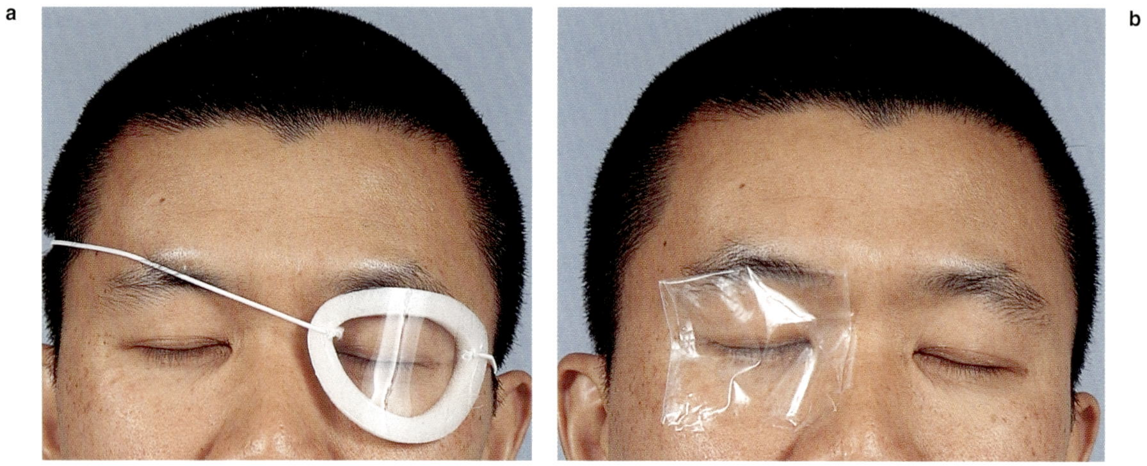

Fig. 19-7. Occlusive moisture dressings. (**a**) A moisture chamber (mfg by Wilson Ophthalmic Corp, Mustang, Okla). (**b**) A cellophane occlusive dressing. Both types of dressing require frequent application of lubricating ointment and act like greenhouses to keep the eye surface moisturized.

The sutures are then passed out the upper-lid skin above the lashes and through another bolster before the suture ends are tied. The sutures may be tied in a bow to facilitate periodic examinations of the ocular surface. The bolster reduces the incidence of sutures "cheesewiring," or cutting through, the eyelid tissues.

It is important to realize that suture tarsorrhaphy is a temporary measure and will not prevent cicatricial changes to the eyelid. Additionally, a suture tarsorrhaphy may be associated with eyelid margin irregularities. In severe contracture, the lids may pull through the tarsorrhaphy suture, which results in a cheesewire laceration of the eyelid. Surgical marginal tarsorrhaphies are not often used because the lid margin anatomy is destroyed, making reconstruction more difficult.

If singed lashes are present, consider cutting the lashes with scissors coated with antibiotic ointment. This will prevent debris from falling into the conjunctival cul-de-sac and irritating the cornea and mucous membranes.[18,19]

3rd Echelon

A patient with eyelid burns should be evaluated by an ophthalmologist at the 3rd echelon. By this time, any acid or alkali burn should have been diagnosed and acutely treated, otherwise severe progressive damage would have occurred. In-depth examination of the eye and periocular structures is essential. Ocular injuries must always be ruled out first. Definitive subacute and chronic eyelid treatment is then provided.[5]

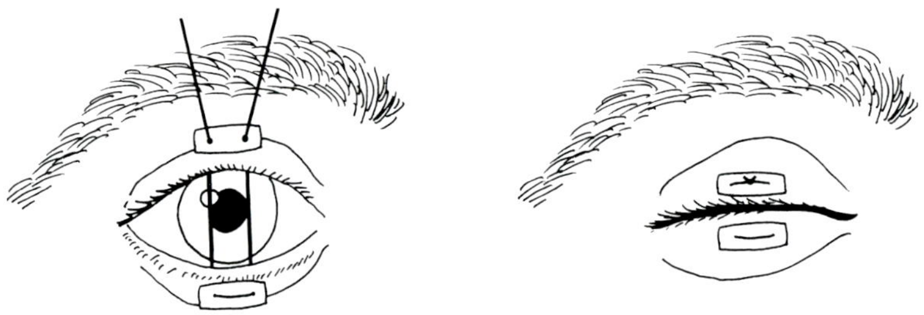

Fig. 19-8. Suture tarsorrhaphy. A double-armed 4-0 suture (silk, nylon, or Vicryl) is passed through a foam or rubber bolster (cut from a surgical drain) and through the eyelid skin 4 mm inferior to the eyelashes. The sutures exit the lower lid through the gray line (middle portion of the lid margin). Both ends are then passed through the gray line of the upper lid and out through the skin about 4 mm above the upper lash line. The sutures are passed through another bolster and tied securely to pull the eyelids closed. Several such sutures may be placed along the length of the lid to achieve maximum corneal protection. The bolster reduces the risk of the suture cheesewiring through the injured eyelid tissue. Caution is necessary to avoid suture contact with the globe. Drawing: Courtesy of Department of Medical Illustrations, Brooke Army Medical Center, Fort Sam Houston, Tex.

Evaluation

The components of the 3rd-echelon eye and eyelid examination are similar to but more extensive than those of the eye and periocular examination at the 2nd echelon. Examinations at the 3rd echelon are conducted by medical officers, some of whom may be trained and certified ophthalmologists.

Visual Acuity. Best corrected visual acuity should be obtained and, if abnormal, correlated with clinical findings to explain the deficit. Results should be compared to the initial visual acuity to determine prognosis and course of the injury. Decreased visual acuity can be due to multiple etiologies, including lid deformities, dry eyes, epiphora, corneal irregularities and scars, anterior chamber hyphema or inflammation, iris damage, cataract, vitreous hemorrhage, retinal injuries, and optic nerve injuries.

Pupil Examination. The pupil examination is performed to determine if significant blunt trauma or blast injury may have damaged the anterior visual pathway, as an afferent pupillary defect (APD) or Marcus-Gunn pupil would suggest. APD is detected by having the patient focus on an object in the distance to prevent accommodative miosis (pupil constriction at near). In a darkened environment, a penlight is shined directly through the pupil of one eye, and the pupil constriction is observed. The light is then immediately shined in the opposite eye, and pupil constriction is observed. If one pupil constricts more sluggishly than the other, does not constrict at all, or actually dilates when the light is brought from the opposite eye, then the more-sluggish pupil is abnormal and is determined to have an APD. Anisocoria (asymmetrical pupils) can be due to a variety of causes including trauma to the iris root, iris sphincter damage, or iris ischemia due to thermal-induced hypovascularity. Intracranial injury may also cause anisocoria from a third–cranial nerve palsy.

Ocular and Lid Motility. The eyes should be examined carefully for motility to rule out orbital or neurological injury. The lid motility is examined as well to determine whether there is mechanical or neurological dysfunction due to burn or blast injury. For example, a ptotic lid with poor mobility can be caused by mechanical restriction from lid edema or burn scarring, or it could be due to a third-nerve palsy stemming from increased intracranial pressure from a related head injury.

Complete Slitlamp Examination. A thorough slitlamp examination is performed. Eyelid margins are examined for damage to the meibomian glands, puncta, and canaliculi. The conjunctiva is examined for lacerations and abrasions that can signal a penetrating globe injury or potential symblepharon formation (contracted conjunctival scarring between the eyelid and eyeball conjunctiva). The cornea is also examined for lacerations, abrasions, limbal ischemia (seen as a white, noninjected border between the sclera and cornea), and FBs. The anterior chamber is examined for FBs, hyphema (blood in the anterior chamber), angle recession (seen as a deeper than normal anterior chamber angle between the iris root and the cornea), and inflammation (seen as haziness in the anterior chamber). Significant anterior chamber "flare" out of proportion to anterior chamber "cell" may signal ischemia ("flare" and "cell" pertain to the gradation of anterior chamber inflammation). The iris is examined for sphincter tears or lacerations. The lens is examined for dislocation, subluxation, or traumatic or ischemic cataract.

Eyelashes. Singed lashes and eyebrow hairs may indicate thermal damage, which may manifest itself over several days. Therefore, patients with singed lashes should be observed. If an FB sensation is due to lash particles on the eye, the lashes should be trimmed and lubricated with ointment.

Eyelids. The degree and extent of burns must be determined to evaluate globe coverage, motility, lagophthalmos (amount of exposure on eyelid closure), ectropion (outward turning of the eyelid margin), entropion (inward turning of the eyelid margin, often with lashes rubbing against the cornea). Children have thin skin and, therefore, experience greater depth of burn with increased scarring and disfigurement.[20]

Face. Look for adjacent burns, which may contract and pull on the eyelids causing ectropion, retraction or lagophthalmos, and exposure keratopathy. Also, note whether the usual donor sites for skin graft (upper eyelids and retroauricular, periclavicular, and inner arm areas) are involved.

Intraocular Pressure. Monitor intraocular pressure (IOP) for elevation or hypotony. Elevated IOP may indicate traumatic glaucoma due to anterior chamber angle injury or traumatic cataract. Low IOP may signal occult globe rupture, choroidal or retinal detachment, or anterior segment ischemia.

Posterior Segment (Fundus) Examination. The posterior segment should be evaluated for inflammation, FBs, retinal detachment, chorioretinal injuries, and optic nerve injuries.

Treatment

Treatment at the 3rd echelon should include copious irrigation of chemical burns if this was not adequately done at lower echelons. Examine the eyes and remove any remaining chemical particles from the conjunctiva and eyelids. Then, proceed according to the protocol for chemical ocular injuries (Chapter 7, Chemical Injuries of the Eye). Once stable, the eyelids should be treated as indicated in the sections that follow.

First-Degree Burns. Because first-degree burns are self-limited and heal well, these superficial burns are seen at the 3rd echelon only because the patient has other injuries. Treatment includes applying cool compresses and providing analgesics as needed. Occasionally mild, transient lagophthalmos and corneal exposure occur and are treated with artificial tears and ointment for lubrication.

More-severe exposure in an obtunded patient may require a moisture chamber (see Figure 19-7). Numerous moisture chambers are commercially available. Some are self-adhesive and are applied much like an elastic bandage. However, the adhesive irritates some patients' skin, and, if the periocular area is lubricated for adjacent burns, this type of moisture chamber does not stay in place well.

Another common type of moisture chamber has an elastic band and is worn like a pirate patch. This system works well if an adhesive chamber irritates the skin or if periocular lubrication is present. The drawbacks to the pirate patch moisture chamber are that the elastic can irritate injured scalp and head skin and when patients turn in their sleep, they can dislodge the patch. More commonly, patients have a mechanical ptosis due to lid edema rather than lagophthalmos. Mechanical ptosis actually protects the eye from exposure, especially in unconscious patients.

Second-Degree Burns. Cicatricial changes usually accompany second-degree or partial-thickness burns. If the patient is awake, corneal and conjunctival exposure and drying should be treated with artificial tears. Ophthalmic lubricants or an ophthalmic antibiotic ointment (if a corneal epithelial defect is present) should be used six or more times per day for an unconscious patient. If drying is severe, the following measures should be considered:

- moisture chambers over the eyes;
- cellophane, ocular-occlusive dressings (applied six times per day); and
- temporary suture tarsorrhaphies (see Figures 19-7 and 19-8).

The cellophane occlusive dressing can be made by cutting a square of cellophane wrap to a size that will completely cover an eye and reach the orbital rims on all sides. The cellophane is kept in place by the adhesive effect of the topical eye ointment. This dressing has the advantage of not irritating the periocular skin because there is no glue adhesive. It also avoids pressure irritation because it has no elastic band. The cellophane dressing stays in place even if the patient moves in bed. If the lids are completely missing, it allows the patient to have some vision while providing barrier protection.

The temporary suture tarsorrhaphy may be necessary if excessive lagophthalmos allows significant corneal drying. The tarsorrhaphy temporarily sews the eyelids closed (see 2nd-Echelon Treatment, above).

If the lacrimal system is involved, nasolacrimal system intubation with silicone tubing should be considered to prevent cicatrization and future nasolacrimal system obstruction and epiphora (Figures 19-9 and 19-10). The tubing is left in place for 3 to 9 months, until the cicatrizing changes of the lid have stopped, or until the patient is unable to tolerate the tubes once initial healing has occurred. If well tolerated, the silicone stents may be left in longer, keeping in mind that burn-scar remodeling continues even past the 1-year mark. Monocanalicular intubation may be more beneficial than a bicanalicular tube, as the bicanalicular tube may cause cheesewiring of the canaliculi as the lid tissue contracts and places excess traction on the canaliculi.

Third-Degree Burns. Aggressive treatment is warranted for third-degree, or full-thickness, burns of the eyelids. Frequent lubrication is essential. Severe cicatrizing ectropion with unresponsive corneal drying should undergo surgical relaxing incisions of the burn scars (Figure 19-11). When the lids are significantly immobilized because of contraction, the skin and underlying scar tissue must be sharply transected to allow the lids to protract over the globe.

If a temporary suture tarsorrhaphy does not hold, then Frost sutures should be placed to keep the lids closed and on traction (Figure 19-12). A Frost suture is created much like a suture tarsorrhaphy. Both ends of a double-armed suture are passed through a bolster and through the lid like a tarsorrhaphy suture. However, instead of passing them through the opposite lid, the trailing ends are taped to the forehead (for the lower lid) or to the cheek (for the upper lid). Again, caution is needed to verify (1) that the suture is correctly passed through the tar-

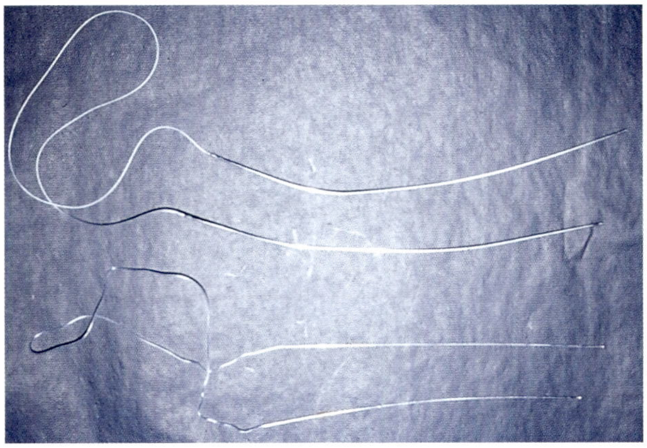

Fig. 19-9. Silicone stents. Shown are two types of silicone stents, which may be passed through the nasolacrimal system to prevent cicatricial closure and obstruction. A Guibor tube (top) may be retrieved with a grooved director. A Crawford tube with an olive-tipped introducer (bottom) is retrieved by a Crawford hook (similar to a small crochet hook).

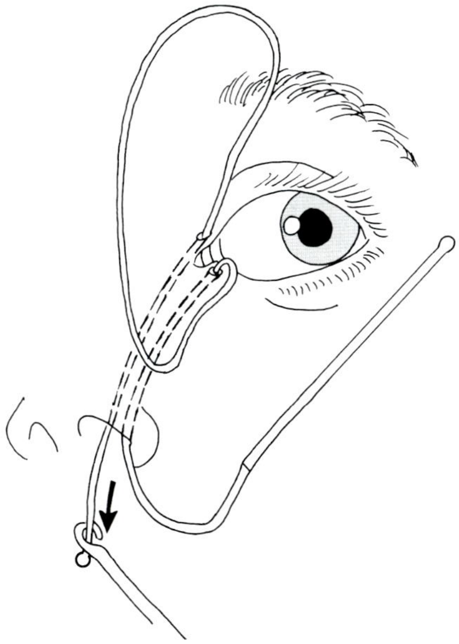

Fig. 19-10. Intubating the nasolacrimal system. The figures show passage of the silicone stents through the vertical and horizontal canaliculi into the nasolacrimal sac and down into the nose through the nasolacrimal duct (a closed loop). The tube is retrieved below the inferior turbinate with a Crawford hook.

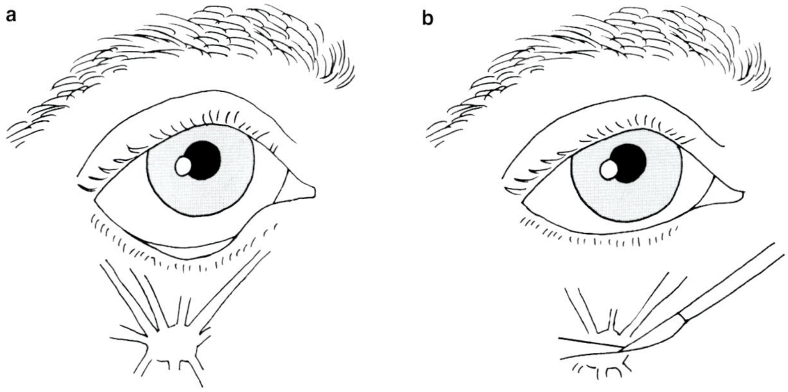

Fig. 19-11. Relaxing incision. The cicatrix (**a**) of the lower eyelid (**b**) is incised with a scalpel blade to release the retraction and ectropion.

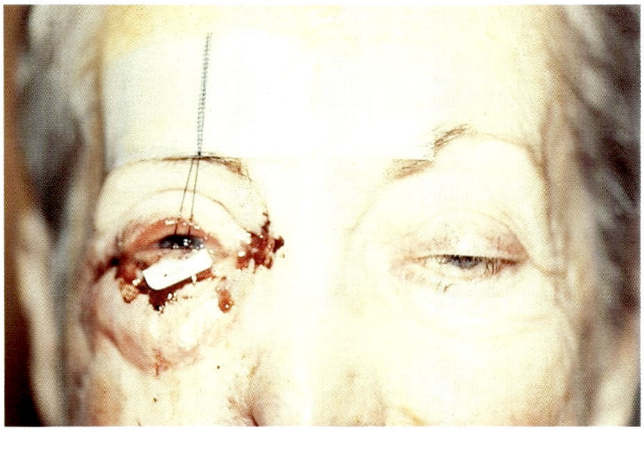

Fig. 19-12. A Frost suture is used to put the eyelid on traction, prevent recurrence of retraction, and to allow the eyelid to cover the eye. A Frost suture is placed by passing a double-armed suture (4-0) through the wound and out through the lower eyelid gray line. The suture is pulled up and secured to the forehead with benzoin and plastic tape.

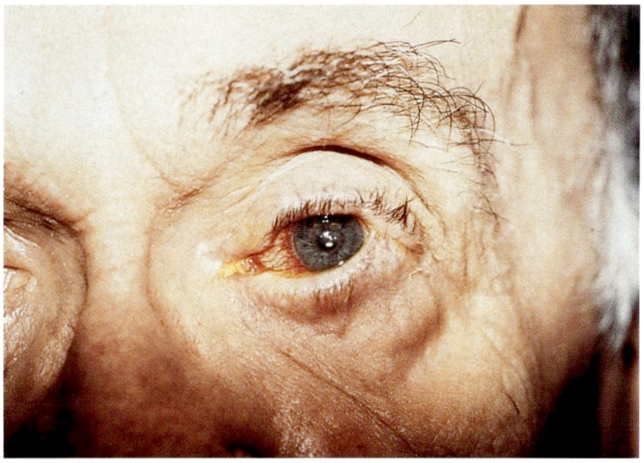

Fig. 19-13. A non-margin-sharing tarsorrhaphy preserves the integrity of the eyelid margin. A scalpel blade is used to incise the upper eyelid conjunctiva and the superior 4 mm of tarsus. Vertical incisions are made with fine scissors, and the shade-like pedicle of tissue is sewn into the upper conjunctiva of the lower lid with 6-0 Vicryl. This technique provides support of the lower eyelid and coverage of the cornea.

sal plate—the thick, fibrous, connective tissue condensation at the lid margin—for adequate fixation and (2) that no suture contacts the globe. It is often difficult to adequately secure the trailing ends of the sutures because of periocular burns and the application of lubricants to the patient's skin.

If necessary before evacuation, non-margin-sharing temporary tarsorrhaphies may be considered (Figure 19-13). (Margin-sharing tarsorrhaphies are not commonly used because they distort the lid margins, making any subsequent reconstruction even more difficult.) Before the technique for non-margin-sharing tarsorrhaphies is outlined, a cross-sectional review of the normal lid anatomy is indicated. The layers of the eyelid going from superficial to deep at the level of the tarsal plate are as follows: eyelid skin, orbicularis oculi muscle, distal end of the levator aponeurosis, tarsus, and conjunctiva. Above the tarsal plate, the layers are as follows: eyelid skin, orbicularis oculi muscle, orbital septum, preaponeurotic orbital fat, levator aponeurosis, Müller's muscle, and conjunctiva. In the lower eyelid, the eyelid retractor components are less well developed. The equivalent of the levator aponeurosis is the capsulopalpebral fascia, and the Müller's muscle equivalent is the inferior tarsal muscle. Otherwise, the layers at and below the level of the tarsus in the lower lid are similar to those of the upper eyelid.

The non-margin-sharing tarsorrhaphy is created by everting the upper eyelid and incising the conjunctiva and tarsus approximately 4 mm above the lid margin. Vertical incisions are made in the conjunctiva and Müller's muscle. The pedicle is then undermined in a plane between Müller's muscle and the levator aponeurosis. Once this is accomplished, the lower lid is horizontally incised on the mucosal side about 2 mm below the lid margin in a length corresponding to that of the upper-lid pedicle flap. The tarsoconjunctival flap from the upper lid is sewn into the lower-lid incision using 6-0 Vicryl (polyglactin) suture.

The non-margin-sharing tarsorrhaphy provides excellent globe coverage in patients with lagophthalmos from significant eyelid burns. This procedure does not distort the lid margin and is created from posterior lamellar lid tissue, which is less often involved in burn injuries. Therefore, secondary reconstruction is less difficult, and reversal of the procedure only requires transection of the flap where it comes off the upper lid and recession of the Müller-conjunctival pedicle to prevent eyelid retraction.

Patients with extensive second-degree burns (lagophthalmos and corneal drying not responding to the use of tears) and third-degree burns of the eyelids should be stabilized, have their globes protected, and be evacuated to the continental United States (CONUS) for definitive care. Patients with these burns usually also have extensive injuries or burns on other body areas, which alone would require evacuation.

Burns of the conjunctiva (ocular mucous membranes) inevitably lead to scarring and contracture and, if not treated early, to symblepharon formation (adhesions between the mucous membranes of the eyelids and the globe). Symblepharon formation is frequently seen with chemical injuries. Necrotic tissue must be removed and a symblepharon ring, spacer, or even a large therapeutic contact lens should be placed to minimize adhesion formation. The eyes should be evaluated at least twice daily, and any early symblepharon should be lysed with a glass rod or a moistened cotton-tipped applicator. Copious lubricating eye ointment should be used to prevent drying and for patient comfort. Antibiotic ointment should be strongly considered, given the risk of infections in burn wounds.

Evaluation and Treatment in the Continental United States

Evaluation in CONUS of patients with eyelid burns should first focus on the status of the eyes. The following must be ruled out: a ruptured globe;

intraocular injury; or ocular surface injury due to the burn itself, exposure, drying, and corneal infection, which may have occurred during the evacuation process. If any of these injuries is noted, appropriate treatment algorithms should be followed as described above.

Once the eye is determined to be healthy, or when the ocular injuries are stabilized, evaluation should focus on the status of the eyelids. Globe protection, eyelid function, and cosmetic appearance should be considered in that order of priority.

Needed interventions are carried out by the fully trained and experienced military ophthalmologists, who will be found at CONUS hospitals.

Evaluation

The CONUS evaluation, when completed, should contain the answers to the following questions:

- How much and to what degree are the eyelids burned?
- How much of the eyelids remain and which parts are missing?
- Is the eyelid ectropic, entropic, or retracted?
- Is the canalicular system involved or destroyed?
- What is the status of the tear film, and which component has been affected?
- What is the status of the globe's protective mucosal covering?
- How does the eyelid look relative to a normal eyelid?

Extent and Degree of Burns. Reassessment is crucial to determine proper short-term and long-term treatment and prognosis. Superficial and mild partial-thickness burns can often be conservatively managed. Severe partial- and full-thickness burns require significant immediate attention. Burns previously billed as partial thickness may have progressed during transit to full-thickness injuries because of infection, desiccation, or less-than-adequate interim care owing to wartime constraints.

Status of Remaining Eyelids. The anatomical status of the eyelids should be evaluated to plan for reconstruction. A systematic approach should be used to evaluate the status of the anterior, middle, and posterior lamellae. The eyelids should be evaluated for their protraction, retraction, tear pump function, and cosmetic appearance. Loss of anterior lamella requires reconstruction with full-thickness skin grafts or rotational or transposition skin and muscle flaps. Posterior lamella loss calls for mucous membrane grafting and, if tarsal support is lost, a tarsal substitute such as hard palate mucosal grafts, donor sclera, and other autologous or synthetic materials. In burn patients, the posterior lamella is involved when injury extends through the anterior lid structures. Therefore, in most instances, full-thickness lid loss is present and more-complex procedures combining vascularized pedicle flaps for one lamella and free grafts for the other lamella are required. Loss of the middle lamella (septum) usually causes scarring and restricted lid movement; reconstruction for this problem involves releasing the scar and placing a "spacer" to decrease additional scarring.

Diminished protraction (lid closure) is caused by mechanical restriction, damage to the orbicularis oculi muscle, or injury to the seventh cranial nerve because of adjacent trauma. Inability to close the eyelids (lagophthalmos) can be mild to severe and should be treated accordingly as previously discussed.

Diminished retraction (lid opening) causes ptosis. Mild ptosis may be asymptomatic but more-significant ptosis can decrease vision if the lid obscures the pupil and interferes with the visual axis. Therefore, persistent ptosis should be repaired for visual rehabilitation.

Proper closure and anatomical position of the eyelid are responsible for tear removal. Abnormalities can cause epiphora (tears running out of the eye onto the cheek). Tests such as the dye disappearance test and the Jones 1 and 2 tests and visual inspection should be performed to evaluate the status of the tear pump.

The dye disappearance test, a diagnostic test of tear pumping and drainage, is performed by instilling fluorescein dye into the eyes and watching for its removal under cobalt-blue lighting. The patient is allowed to blink normally but should not wipe the eyes. At 5 minutes, almost all of the dye should be removed from the eye. If dye is still present, a delayed clearance problem exists. Asymmetry of remaining dye indicates a unilateral (ie, a worse) problem in the eye with the most dye. Tears running down the cheek may indicate a tear pump problem. An abnormal dye disappearance test may be due to an abnormal tear pump, insufficient tear production to wash out the dye, an obstruction or malposition of the puncta, or a blockage of the canalicular–nasolacrimal system.

The Jones 1 test, the second diagnostic test of tear drainage, is performed by instilling fluorescein dye in the eyes, as was done in the dye disappearance test. In the Jones 1 test, a cotton-tipped applicator is placed under the inferior turbinate to detect dye. If dye is present on the cotton-tipped applicator, tears are cleared normally. If no dye is detected, however, either the tear pump is malfunctioning or the canalicular–nasolacrimal drainage system is blocked. Although the Jones 1 test is a physiological test of tear drainage, no dye may be detected in about a third to half the patients with normally functioning drainage apparatuses.

The Jones 2 test, the last of the tests of tear drainage, is performed after an abnormal (no dye detected) Jones 1 test. After the Jones 1 test, residual dye is irrigated from the conjunctival cul-de-sac. Then clear saline is irrigated through the canaliculi while an attempt is made to detect dye beneath the inferior turbinate. If no fluid is recovered from the nose after irrigation, then a blocked drainage system is present. If clear fluid is detected, then the tear pump is malfunctioning and is unable to pump dye into the lacrimal sac; because fluid is recovered, however, the drainage system is anatomically patent. On the other hand, if dye enters the nose with irrigation, then the tear pump functions to push dye into the tear sac, although the drainage system might be functionally or partially blocked. Finally, if the lower eyelid seems lax or there is punctal ectropion, the tear pump may not be functioning well.

Position of the Eyelids at Rest. Is the eyelid ectropic, entropic, or retracted? In addition to the dynamic lid position and function discussed above, the static position of the eyelids at rest should be determined.

An ectropic lid may cause exposure keratitis, epiphora, FB sensation, and blurry vision. Ectropion in burn patients is usually cicatricial, either from direct lid involvement or transferal of traction from adjacent tissue such as a cheek burn. Treatment is aimed at releasing the traction and replacing the lost tissue.

On the other hand, an entropic lid is generally more worrisome than an ectropic one because the sequelae occur more rapidly. An entropic lid can cause a mechanical keratitis from lashes or keratinized lid skin rubbing against the cornea, which can cause significant corneal injury if not immediately addressed. Entropion in burn patients may be due to conjunctival scarring, although this is less common in thermal than in chemical burns. A patient with preexisting lid laxity may have spastic entropion due to ocular irritation after a burn injury. Treatment is aimed at relieving the irritation and breaking the cycle of spasm.

Eyelid retraction in burn patients is usually due to scarring and is treated much like an ectropion.

Condition of the Canalicular System. Is the canalicular system involved or destroyed? Inspection of the canalicular system of the eyelids often reveals that the punctum is closed or ectropic due to scarring. If ectropic and permanent, surgical correction may be necessary. If the punctum is closed, it can be surgically opened with a punctal dilator or sharply cut with a scalpel or Wescott scissors.

If the puncta appear normal and if epiphora is present, the cause should be determined using the dye disappearance test and Jones 1 and 2 tests (described above). Additionally, the canaliculi should be irrigated with physiological saline solution in a 3-mL syringe and a blunt 23-gauge cannula. If fluid reaches the nose, then the lacrimal drainage system is open. If fluid does not reach the nose but instead drains out the opposite punctum (ie, out the upper when the lower punctum is irrigated), then a nasolacrimal duct obstruction is probably present. However, if fluid does not reach the nose but drains out the same punctum that is being irrigated, then the canaliculus being irrigated is obstructed. Note that this is similar to the Jones 2 test discussed previously.

Nasolacrimal duct obstruction is uncommon in burn patients unless severe facial burns around the nose involving the bone are present, or if the patient has a midfacial injury from a blast. If a nasolacrimal duct is obstructed, the patient may need a dacryocystorhinostomy (DCR). In this procedure, an osteotomy is created in the lacrimal sac fossa and a direct connection is made between the lacrimal sac and the nasal cavity. A DCR can be performed endoscopically through the nose or externally through a Lynch skin incision in the medial canthal area. To promote mucosal epithelialization of the bypass tract, anterior and posterior mucosal flaps can be created from the lacrimal sac and nasal mucosa, which are sutured together. Additionally, a silicone stent is usually placed through the canaliculi and through the osteotomy and into the nose to reduce cicatricial closure of the mucosal bypass tract. The stents are removed once healing is relatively complete, usually at about 3 months postoperatively.

Canalicular obstruction or destruction is more common with eyelid burns. If the burn injury is mild (superficial), simple canalicular intubation as previously discussed may be adequate. If severe (partial- or full-thickness), however, canalicular reconstruction is very difficult, owing to scar formation, and the patient may eventually require a conjunctivodacryocystorhinostomy (C-DCR) with a Jones tube. In this procedure, an external Lynch incision is made, much like that in a DCR. An osteotomy at the lacrimal sac fossa is created with rongeur forceps. A no. 69 Beaver blade is passed through the conjunctiva just lateral to the caruncle and into the lid through the osteotomy and into the nasal cavity. A Pyrex Jones tube is then passed through this tract into the nose and secured into place with a suture at the lid margin. The Lynch incision is closed in two layers, and the Jones tube fixation suture is removed in 7 to 10 days. The Jones tube bypasses the entire blocked canalicular system and allows the tear lake to drain directly into the nose by means of gravity and capillary action.

Status of the Tear Film. Which components have been affected? The tear film should be evaluated for its quantity and quality because eyelid burns can alter all components. The meibomian glands at the lid margin can be damaged, reducing the sebaceous (lipid) layer of the tear film; this causes decreased lid lubrication and increased tear evaporation. If the conjunctiva is significantly involved, then the accessory glands of Krause and Wolfring or even the main lacrimal gland could be injured. If this is the case, the aqueous component of the tear film would be diminished, resulting in significant keratitis sicca (see Figure 19-6). Likewise, because the mucous layer of the tear film is made by conjunctival goblet cells, conjunctival injury can cause poor corneal wetting if the inner mucous tear film layer is compromised or missing.

Assessment of the tear film is done mainly with Schirmer's tests, tear break-up time, direct visualization, and, in some medical centers, chemical analysis and impression cytology. Schirmer strips—standardized strips of filter paper—are placed in the inferior conjunctival cul-de-sac and draped over the lower eyelid. The Schirmer 1 test measures basal and reflex tear production. It involves putting the strips onto an unanesthetized eye. The amount of strip wetting is measured in millimeters after 5 minutes (normal = ≥ 15 mm). The Schirmer 2 test measures reflex tear production. It involves placing the strips onto the eye after topical anesthetic is applied. The inferior turbinate is then irritated with a cotton-tipped applicator, and the amount of wetting is measured (normal = > 10 mm). The basal tear secretion test is a variant of the Schirmer tests, in which the strips of filter paper are placed into the anesthetized eye after excess tears have gently been removed with a cotton-tipped applicator. The amount of wetting is measured after 5 minutes (normal = ≥ 10 mm). Care must be taken when drying the surface of residual tears, as excess vigor may stimulate reflex tearing.

The Schirmer tests and the basal tear secretion test measure the aqueous component of the tear film. Tear break-up time, on the other hand, measures the stability of the tear film on the surface of the eye. Nonanesthetic fluorescein dye (usually from moistened fluorescein strips) is placed onto the ocular surface. While at the slitlamp and under cobalt-blue light, the patient is first asked to close his or her eyes, then to open them and resist blinking. The observer then counts the number of seconds before the tear film breaks up on the ocular surface, which, under the blue light, is seen as a dark spot appearing in the uniform green fluid layer on the cornea. The tear film should normally be stable for 15 seconds. Early break-up implies either instability of the tear film because of an insufficient sebaceous layer, allowing early evaporation, or poor wetting because of an insufficient mucous layer on the cornea. Topical anesthetics should not be used in this test, as they alter the test results.

Tear composition analysis and impression cytology are advanced techniques that will not be discussed here. Nevertheless, ophthalmologists can appreciate that a significant alteration in any of the tear components could cause ocular surface disease, patient discomfort, and visual degradation.

Status of the Mucosal Covering. What is the status of the globe's protective covering? As stated earlier, burn injury involving the conjunctiva may result in symblepharon and the globe's being fixed to the eyelids. Careful examination is required to reduce the amount of symblepharon formation and to plan for replacing a mucous membrane layer on the globe and eyelids.

Comparison With a Normal Lid. How does the eyelid look relative to a normal eyelid? Once the functional and ocular protective status of the lids has been evaluated and addressed, then attention can be directed to eyelid aesthetics. Common concerns include skin texture, lash loss, hypertrophic scars, lid and canthal angle positions, medial canthal webbing, and eyebrow hair loss.

Treatment

Treatment in CONUS includes all the lower-echelon treatments described. These procedures are often repeated once the patient has arrived in a CONUS hospital because of persistence of the signs or worsening of the condition. An oculoplastic surgeon should be consulted to perform definitive reconstruction or emergent reconstruction of a severely burned eyelid. Definitive delayed reconstructive surgery should occur no earlier than 3 months after the initial injury. If surgery can be delayed longer (up to 1 year), the outcome of reconstruction may be improved, as postoperative cicatricial changes are reduced by then and better revascularization of the injured tissue will have occurred. However, visual rehabilitation often necessitates earlier repair.

Reconstruction of the burned eyelids should focus first on protecting the eye (protraction), then on visual function (retraction to clear the visual axis), and finally, for the patient's psychological well-being, on cosmetic appearance. Multiple procedures are available to deal with the complex nature of the cicatrized eyelid and are beyond the scope of this book. However, for a basic understanding of what procedures are available, a brief description of selected procedures is provided.

Treatment modalities in CONUS hospitals include conservative treatment to allow scar relaxation and maturation; restoration of lost eyelid tissue; and correction of eyelid and canthal malpositions, disorders of eyelid retraction and protraction, trichiasis, disorders of the mucosal lining of the eyelid, and abnormalities of the tear drainage system.

Conservative Treatment. In eyelid burn patients, if the eyes are well-protected and visual function is adequate, then definitive repair should be delayed up to 1 year, if possible. Cutaneous and subcutaneous burn scars are slow to mature, and maximum natural relaxation of scar tissue is desired prior to surgery. Scar relaxation may be expedited by manual massage, use of topical vitamin E or cocoa butter, and constant, long-term pressure to the wound area using custom-fitted masks made of silicone, Flexan, or plastic, all of which can be manufactured by Uvex or Jobst.[13] Pressure splints placed directly on the eyelids are impractical because they interfere with vision and put pressure on the eye. However, lid malpositions due to adjacent tissue scarring (eg, on the cheek) respond very well to custom-fitted pressure splints. Given the slow process of rehabilitation to give the patient a sense of progress toward recuperation, it is often helpful to engage him or her as much as possible in massage and stretching regimens.

Once the cicatrix has maximally relaxed, or if more-immediate intervention is required to protect the eyes or allow the patient to see, surgical rehabilitation should proceed in an organized, stepwise fashion. The patient should be well-informed about the long road to recovery and the need for multiple operations and revisions.

Restoration of Eyelid Skin. Loss of eyelid skin is treated with skin grafts or, if undamaged eyelid tissue is available, transposition flaps. Cultured autogenous skin[21] and alloplastic material are available for use[22] in patients without an adequate skin source (Exhibit 19-1). The most commonly used free-graft sources for the eyelids include the upper eyelid skin from the normal contralateral lid (if

EXHIBIT 19-1

SKIN GRAFTS FOR RESTORATION OF LOST EYELID TISSUE

Autologous grafts:

In the absence of an adequate skin source, a few of the patient's own skin cells may be sent for culture. Unfortunately, the process of growing human skin is time-consuming and expensive, and even in light of the screening and processing methods used, a concern regarding disease transmission accompanies all grafts—even when the donor and the recipient are the same person.

Alloplastic grafts:

Alloderm (LifeCell Corp, The Woodlands, Tex) is an acellular, nonimmunogenic dermal grafting material that can be used in place of skin. Because it is made from an inert substance, the graft lacks epidermal cells, and the graft recipient's skin cells must migrate onto the biological bed for resurfacing. The process may be even slower if the adjacent tissue also suffered thermal damage.

Allografts:

As an alternative, nonimmunogenic allografts can be used. Apligraf (Novartis Pharmaceuticals Corporation, East Hanover, NJ) is harvested from neonatal foreskin, which is then processed to make it nonimmunogenic. This material, being human in origin, has intact epithelium; therefore, the graft may heal faster.

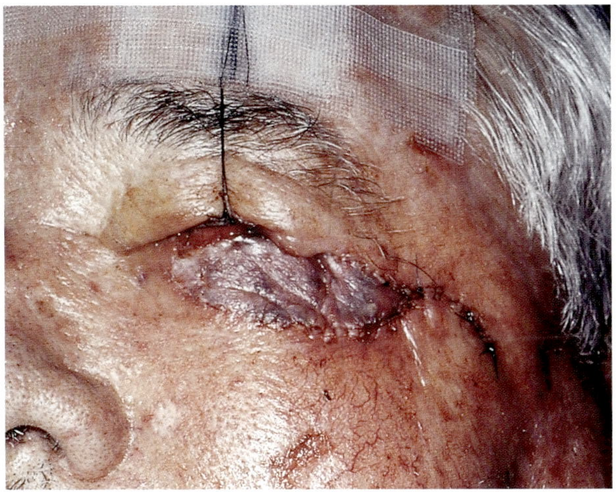

Fig. 19-14. This photograph depicts a full-thickness skin graft to an eyelid defect to correct cicatricial ectropion. The skin graft may be taken from the upper eyelid, the retroauricular or periclavicular areas, or the inner arm or inner thigh. Thin, pliable, hairless skin is preferred. The skin-grafted lid is then put on traction with a Frost suture, and a pressure dressing is placed over the graft for 1 week to prevent hematoma formation below the graft.

present), retroauricular skin, supraclavicular and infraclavicular skin, upper inner arm (volar surface) skin, and inner thigh skin[20,23] (Figure 19-14). Grabosch and colleagues[22] reported successful use of prepuce skin for the eyelid in severely burned patients.

Successful skin graft healing requires a relatively healthy vascular bed. In patients with partial-thickness or localized full-thickness burns, the posterior lamella of the eyelid may be intact, with blood supplied by the palpebral conjunctiva and Müller's muscle. In such cases, the eyelid scar is incised, or a lid crease incision can be performed and the deeper cicatrix released, until the eyelid is mobile and has full excursion. The lid is then put on traction with a double-armed 4-0 suture through the lid margin. The defect is measured, and an oversized graft (usually one-and-a-half to two times the size of the defect) is also measured and then harvested from an appropriate donor site. Care should be taken to keep the graft as thin as possible for optimal function and cosmesis. In some instances, a thick, partial-thickness skin graft (0.4 to 0.5 mm in depth) harvested with a dermatome may give good results with comparatively little contracture.[22–24] The graft is then sewn into place with 6-0 fast-absorbing gut sutures. The traction suture is put on traction and taped into place (on the forehead or cheek, if possible) to keep the graft on stretch and decrease contraction. Antibiotic ointment, a nonadhesive dressing, and a pressure patch or bolster splint are placed on the graft and secured with tape to prevent hematoma under the graft, which might increase the likelihood of graft failure. The patch and the traction suture are removed in approximately 5 days.

In defects that are smaller or that require a vascularized skin source, transposition flaps (eg, from the upper to the lower eyelid with the pedicle based laterally) may be useful. However, the skin adjacent to the burn wound is often damaged as well, and so these transposition skin flaps are not used often. In the medial canthal area, a midline glabellar or median forehead flap may be used for reconstruction.

When there is full-thickness loss of eyelid tissue, both posterior and anterior lamellae require reconstruction. Surgical repair necessitates having at least one vascularized lamella. In burns severe enough to destroy the entire eyelid, it is unlikely that there is adequate adjacent well-vascularized skin, especially for the upper eyelid. Therefore, most reconstruction of the upper eyelid utilizes posterior lamella pedicle flaps with anterior lamella free grafts (described above). If the cheek and face skin are not compromised, a Mustarde flap with a mucosal membrane graft (eg, from the hard palate) can be used to reconstruct the lower eyelid. Otherwise, a posterior pedicle flap must be used as well.

The most common techniques for large, full-thickness reconstruction of the lower eyelid include the modified Hughes tarsoconjunctival flap, the Hewes laterally based tarsoconjunctival flap, and the Mustarde flap. In the modified Hughes procedure (Figure 19-15), the upper eyelid is everted over a Desmarres retractor, and a Beaver blade is used to incise the conjunctiva and tarsus approximately 5 mm above the lid margin for the length of the lower-lid defect to be filled. The dissection is carried out superiorly in a plane between Müller's muscle and the levator aponeurosis. The conjunctiva is incised vertically in a superior direction. The flap is then brought down into the lower eyelid defect and sewn into place with 6-0 Vicryl sutures. A full-thickness skin graft or comparable material is harvested, placed on the pedicle flap, and sewn into place with 6-0 fast-absorbing gut suture.

The wound is dressed in much the same way as a skin graft. The reconstruction is allowed to heal for approximately 6 to 8 weeks, sometimes longer, depending on the vascular status of the burned area. Once healed, the pedicle is transected where it joins

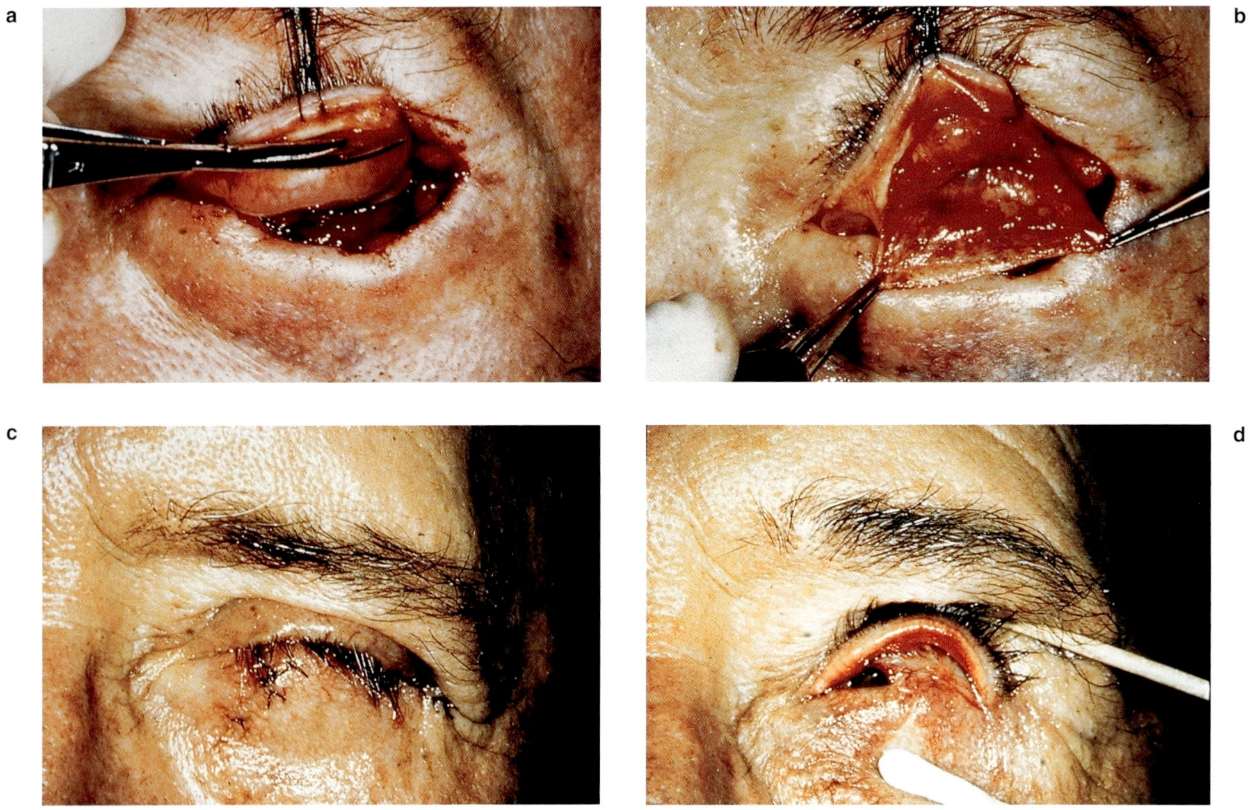

Fig. 19-15. The Hughes tarsoconjunctival advancement flap for the reconstruction of the lower eyelid is a staged procedure, requiring the globe to be covered for 6 weeks. The pedicle is then transected and the lid margin is reconstructed. (**a**) The lower eyelid defect is shown. The tarsoconjunctival flap is being developed. (**b**) The tarsoconjunctival flap is brought down into the lower lid defect. (**c**) Redundant lower eyelid skin is brought over the tarsoconjunctival flap, as in this case, or a full-thickness skin graft can be placed over the mucosal flap. (**d**) The well-healed pedicle can be transected. The lower lid margin can then be reformed.

the upper eyelid and separated into anterior and posterior lamellae. Excess skin is excised, and the mucosa is draped over the lid edge, extending over the lid margin. It is then sewn in place with 6-0 fast-absorbing gut. The mucosa exposed to the environment eventually becomes keratinized. The conjunctiva and Müller's muscle may need recession if the upper lid is retracted after transection of the pedicle flap.

The Hewes flap is similar to the modified Hughes except that it is a laterally based tarsal conjunctival flap with a free skin graft. Because the flap is based at the lateral canthus, the flap does not obstruct the palpebral fissure. Therefore, it is a single-stage procedure.

The Mustarde flap requires an extensive undermining of skin from the lateral lower lid extending to the preauricular area and inferiorly toward the angle of the jaw. The skin flap is then rotated superomedially and sewn into place with deep 5-0 or 4-0 Vicryl sutures and 6-0 fast-absorbing gut or nylon sutures. The posterior lamella is recreated with mucous membrane and often a rigid material to act as a tarsal substitute (eg, banked sclera, high-density porous polyethylene [Medpor, mfg by Porex Surgical Inc, College Park, Ga], nasal septal cartilage, and auricular cartilage). These materials usually require a mucous membrane covering, such as buccal mucosa. Alternatively, hard palate grafts or Alloderm (mentioned above) may be used for the posterior lamella without requiring mucous membrane grafting.

The most common techniques used for large, full-thickness upper eyelid reconstruction include the Cutler-Beard procedure, the glabellar flap, and the laterally based transposition flap from the suprabrow area. The Cutler-Beard procedure (Figure 19-16) involves incising the lower eyelid full thickness below the tarsus (approximately 6 mm) and extending the width of the upper-lid defect. The incision is extended directly inferiorly at each end of the

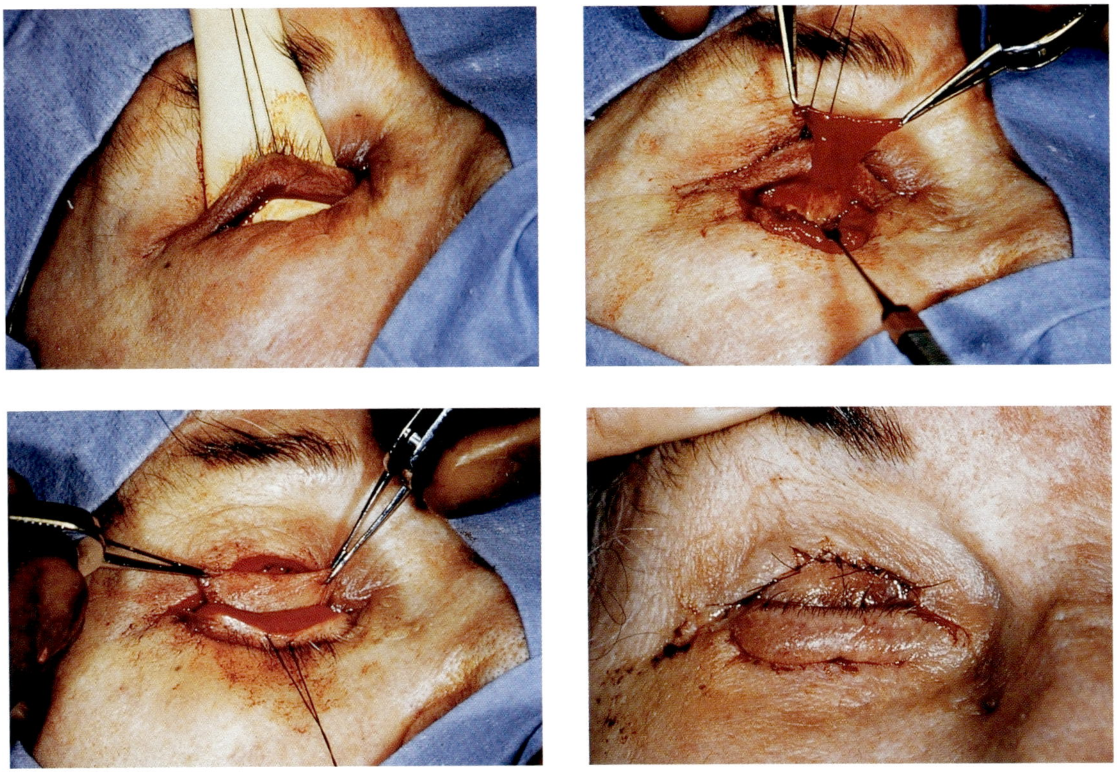

Fig. 19-16. The Cutler-Beard advancement flap for the reconstruction of the upper eyelid is also a staged procedure. (**a**) In this photograph, the upper-lid defect is partially covered by the lid plate. A full-thickness incision is made across the lower eyelid, as shown. (**b**) The conjunctival flap is advanced superiorly. (**c**) The conjunctival flap is sewn into the upper-lid defect, and the skin flap is similarly brought underneath the lower-lid margin bridge and into the upper-lid defect. A tarsal substitute, such as sclera, may be placed between the two lamellae. (**d**) The defect is repaired. The pedicle is transected after 6 weeks, and the upper-lid margin is reconstructed.

horizontal incision so that the full-thickness pedicle can be brought behind the bridging lid margin of the lower lid and into the upper eyelid defect. The lamellae of the pedicle are separated and a tarsal substitute (such as those for the Mustarde flap, above) is sewn between the two lamellae at the level of the superior tarsus. The pedicle is then sewn into the defect in multiple layers with 6-0 Vicryl sutures. The tarsal substitute is sewn edge to edge with any remaining upper-lid tarsus. The skin is closed in the usual fashion.

The glabellar flap is essentially a medially based transposition flap that is brought down from the midline of the forehead and across the upper lid to fill in the defect. The blood supply is based off the supratrochlear vessels. This flap mainly supplies anterior lamella and, if used for full-thickness defects, a mucous membrane graft must be used to line the defect, and a tarsal substitute is required to give the lid rigidity. Unlike in the lower eyelid, a graft of hard palate tissue does not work well in the upper lid because the graft tends to irritate the corneal surface with lid excursions. The temporally based transposition flap has a less well-defined blood supply and, therefore, may not be as useful in cases of complete loss of the upper eyelid.

In cases of full-thickness loss of both upper and lower eyelids on the same side, reconstruction is extremely difficult. The main goal, however, is to protect the globe. In these (albeit rare) cases, we have mobilized forniceal and bulbar conjunctiva from the upper and lower fornices and sewn them together. This provides a mucosal covering for the cornea. The exposed, nonepithelialized surface of the mobilized conjunctiva is covered with skin grafts. A small opening in the conjunctiva may be left centrally and the edge of the mucosa sewn to a corresponding opening in the skin graft. The opening provides a small aperture for vision and for monitoring of the corneal status.

Eyelid Malpositions. Cicatricial ectropion is the most common eyelid malposition caused by eyelid burns. The ectropion may stem from direct eyelid tissue scarring or from transmission of contracture from adjacent tissue (eg, cheek or forehead). Treatment is aimed at releasing the tension on the eyelid, preferably at the site of scarring.

Eyelid cicatricial ectropion is caused by shortening or scarring of the anterior lamella. The main treatment is relaxation of the scar tissue. If the scar is small and damage to surrounding tissue is minimal, the scar can be incised with Z-plasties to reduce the tension on the lid by changing the vector of pull. Unfortunately, in burn patients, the surrounding tissue is often injured, and simple Z-plasty scar relaxation is not adequate to correct the ectropion.

Similarly, advancement or rotational skin–muscle flaps from adjacent sites may be used to fill in the tissue shortage after the scar is released. In cases of significant adjacent tissue loss or burn injury, free grafting is often needed.[25] The free graft of choice is full-thickness skin graft from the upper lid, retroauricular area, periclavicular area, inner arm, or inner thigh where the skin is thin and hairless. If these areas are not available, thick split-thickness skin grafts from hairless areas may be harvested with a dermatome set between 0.4 and 0.5 mm thickness. Alternatively, Alloderm or Apligraf (see above) may be used. After grafting, the lid should be placed on stretch and a pressure patch placed as described above.

In less severe cases of contracture or in cases with deeper scarring, a subperiosteal midface elevation or suborbicularis oculi fat elevation (the SOOF lift) may relieve enough vertically oriented tension from the lower face to correct the eyelid ectropion (Figure 19-17). The SOOF lift is accomplished through either a lower-lid infraciliary or transconjunctival approach to the inferior orbital rim. Once the rim is reached, the periosteum is incised just inferior to the orbital rim, and a subperiosteal dissection is carried out toward the gingival sulcus. The infraorbital neurovascular bundle is left intact. The lower-face periosteum may be released to give further elevation. The deeper facial tissue is suspended with 4-0 nylon sutures to the periosteum at the inferior orbital rim and the lower lateral rim. Alternatively, small suture fixation holes may be drilled at the orbital rim for attachment. The transconjunctival incision may be closed with 6-0 fast-absorbing gut suture, and the lateral canthal tendon is resuspended to the lateral orbital rim at a more elevated position in anticipation of future contraction. If an infraciliary incision is used, the anterior lamella may be augmented with a skin graft as well.

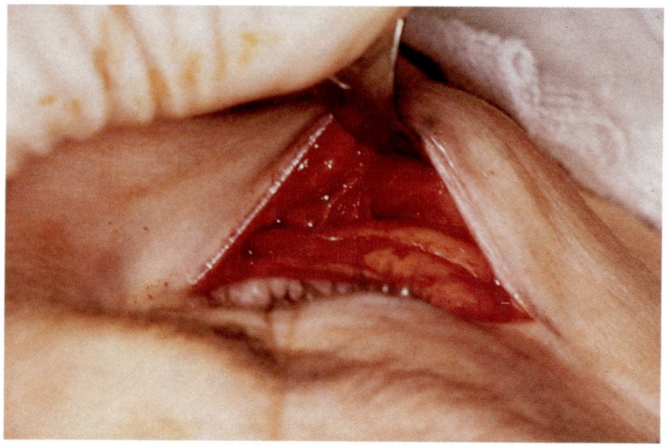

Fig. 19-17. Midface lifting procedure used to release and recess the midface soft tissue. A subperiosteal plane is dissected along the anterior surface of the maxilla. Care is taken to avoid injuring the infraorbital neurovascular bundle, as shown in the photo to the left of the retractor. This procedure facilitates lid elevation and ocular coverage using available skin and soft tissue, possibly circumventing the need for a skin graft.

If additional coverage of the medial globe is required because of medial lid retraction, a medial lid margin adhesion procedure may be performed by deepithelializing the canalicular portion of the eyelid margin and suturing it together using 6-0 Vicryl sutures (Figure 19-18). Care must be used to avoid damaging the canalicular system. Bowman lacrimal probes may be passed into the canaliculi during the procedure as a guide to avoid damaging the canaliculi.

Entropion is less commonly found in burn patients unless there has been a chemical burn to the conjunctival surface. Otherwise, entropion occurs in burn patients only if mild senile entropion is already present. If underlying lower-lid laxity, overriding orbicularis, or retractor dehiscence are present, then irritation from a burn injury or lash debris may cause a spastic entropion. Spastic entropion can be treated by removing the offending cause (eg, an FB) and providing copious lubrication to break the spastic lid closure cycle. Quickert–Rathburn sutures may be helpful to overcome this problem. They are performed by passing double-armed sutures (eg, 4-0 chromic) through the inferior conjunctival fornix, full-thickness through the lid, and exiting just under the lashes. Several such sutures may be used across the eyelid to evert it.

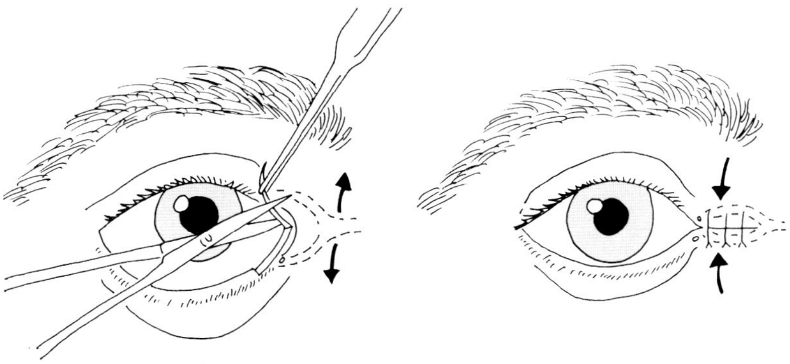

Fig. 19-18. A medial canthal lid margin adhesion procedure performed to maximize globe protection. Care is taken to avoid injury to the canalicular system. Drawing: Courtesy of Department of Medical Illustrations, Brooke Army Medical Center, Fort Sam Houston, Tex.

More severe cases of senile entropion require lower-lid tightening (Figure 19-19), reattachment of the lower-lid retractor to the inferior tarsal border, and occasional debulking of the overriding preseptal orbicularis muscle.

In case of cicatricial entropion, the posterior lamella needs lengthening with mucous membrane grafts, tarsal substitutes, or both, as described above. It is important to repair entropion, because the in-turned lashes can irritate and damage the corneal surface.

Canthal Malpositions. Burn scars may cause displacement of the medial and lateral canthal tendons from their normal positions. They may be dragged in any direction and usually are displaced away from the globe, interfering with proper globe apposition and tear pump function. Repair of canthal malposition is similar to repair of eyelid malposition. Scar relaxation is required and tissue augmentation may be accomplished with transposition or free grafts. Additionally, the medial canthus is often subject to webbing, and the canthal tendons often need resuspension to their proper anatomical positions.

Canthal webbing is usually addressed by incising and relaxing the scarred tissue. Combinations of Z, Y-V and W-plasties are often required. If eyelid tissue is in very short supply, glabellar flaps or skin grafts may be used to augment the medial canthus, and laterally based flaps and skin grafts may be used for the lateral canthus. If the medial canthal tendon is displaced, it must be resuspended to the posterior lacrimal crest so the lid is apposed to the globe. Similarly, the lateral canthus must be suspended to approximate the lateral lid to the globe (see Figure 19-19).

The medial canthal tendon can be isolated through a skin incision along a medial canthal lid fold or incised scar. The tendon is resuspended to the periosteum with a permanent suture. If this is not secure, a suture hole may be drilled into the lacrimal crest from which to suspend the tendon. Screws, plates, and anchors are available for suspension; however, the bone in the medial canthal area is often thin and cannot support this hardware. In severe cases, transnasal wiring may be required for telecanthus repair.

The lateral canthal tendon can be resuspended with a lateral tarsal strip procedure to the periosteum at the lateral orbital tubercle. If the tendon is damaged, a lateral rim periosteal flap can be mobilized for lateral lid attachment. Also, the tendon may be directly secured to the lateral rim with a drill hole for the permanent suture.

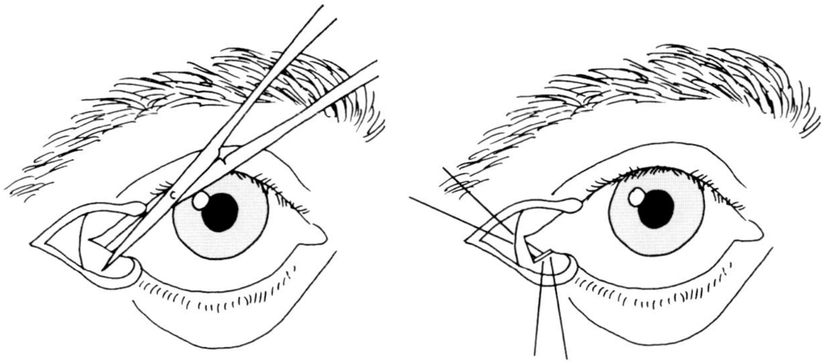

Fig. 19-19. A horizontal lid-tightening procedure similar to a lateral tarsal strip is performed to prevent eyelid laxity and maximize globe protection. Drawing: Courtesy of Department of Medical Illustrations, Brooke Army Medical Center, Fort Sam Houston, Tex.

Disorders of Eyelid Retraction. For the upper eyelid, the eyelid retractors consist of the levator palpebrae and its aponeurosis and Müller's muscle; for the lower eyelid, the retractors are the capsulopalpebral fascia and the inferior tarsal muscle. Proper retractor function, especially of the upper lid, is required for good visual function. Upper retractor dysfunction results in ptosis or a droopy lid, which may block the visual axis. Lower retractor dysfunction may result in a higher-than-normal lid position, or reverse ptosis; however, this does not usually interfere with the visual axis and is less of a concern. Indeed, in a burn patient, a slightly elevated lower lid may help protect the eye from exposure.

Upper-lid ptosis is not very common in burn patients unless the levator aponeurosis has been damaged or the tissue was injured from a blast. In early stages of burn injury, ptosis may be mechanical from swelling. In the chronic stages, however, persistent ptosis is more likely due to middle lamella scarring or retractor damage. The amount of the defect (in this case, ptosis and levator function) will guide intervention. Additionally, forced generations of eyelid closures (isometric contractions of the lids) should be performed if cicatricial restriction of lid excursion is suspected.

If the ptosis is primarily due to scarring, then surgical release of the scar may be required. Intraoperative assessment for multiple causes is usually required; any new findings should be addressed at the time. Once the scar is released, ptosis may still be present because of dehiscence of the levator aponeurosis, which requires repair. In general, ptotic lids with good levator function respond well to aponeurotic surgery, those with moderate excursion may do well with levator muscle surgery, and those with poor function require frontalis slings. Detailed description of ptosis surgery is available in any oculoplastic textbook. Furthermore, a burn patient is more prone to dry eye problems, and a conservative approach to ptosis repair is warranted—especially when function is moderate to poor—because the indicated procedures usually cause some degree of lagophthalmos.

Disorders of Eyelid Protraction. The orbicularis oculi muscle forms part of the anterior lamella of the eyelids and is, therefore, commonly injured in eyelid burns. The orbicularis oculi muscle forms the main protractor muscle. As stated earlier, proper eyelid closure is needed for eye protection, distribution of the tear film, and tear pumping. In most eyelid burns, inability to close the eyes is due to (1) cicatricial eyelid retraction or (2) ectropion due to anterior, posterior, or middle lamella scarring. When the scar is released, the lids often are able to close normally.

In more-severe burns with damage to the orbicularis muscle, eyelid protraction may still be hampered despite release of all cicatricial processes. In such instances, the weak or absent orbicularis muscle requires adjunctive support. Surgical procedures can be aimed at static or dynamic eyelid closure.

Static eyelid closure procedures decrease the palpebral fissure, giving greater protection to the eye and decreasing the distance that a weakened orbicularis muscle would have to move the lid for full closure. These procedures include those described for correcting cicatricial ectropion/retraction (eg, skin grafting, SOOF lift) (see Figures 19-14 and 19-17). The lateral canthal tendon may also be supraplaced, and the lower lid can be supported with semirigid spacers such as hard palate mucosa (Figure 19-20), sclera, ear or septal cartilage, Alloderm, or Medpor. Additionally, tarsorrhaphies may be done both laterally and medially (avoiding the canalicular system) to add further support and lid closure (see Figure 19-18).

a

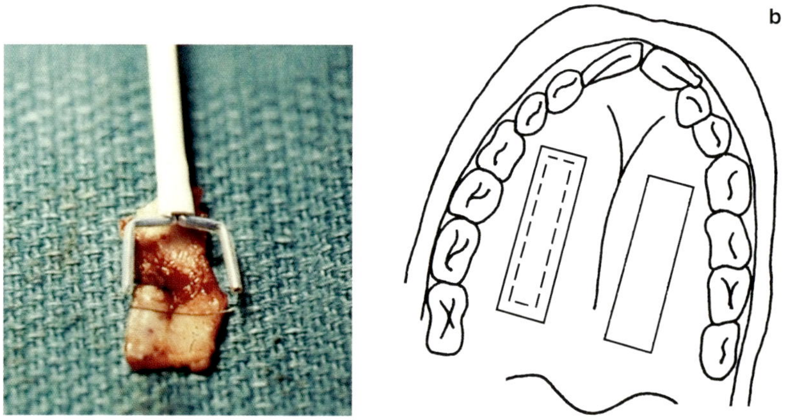

b

Fig. 19-20. (**a**) Mucosa from the patient's hard palate has been harvested with a radiofrequency mucotome unit for mucosal lengthening of the eyelid. (**b**) Schematic diagram of the hard palate mucosa donor site. Drawing: Courtesy of Department of Medical Illustrations, Brooke Army Medical Center, Fort Sam Houston, Tex.

Dynamic eyelid closure is achieved with placement of either upper-lid gold weights or palpebral springs. The upper-lid gold weight allows gravity to pull the eyelid down when the levator palpebrae is relaxed. The gold weight is placed in a supratarsal position and fixed with permanent sutures. The location is accessed through a standard blepharoplasty incision with dissection carried down to the anterior surface of the tarsal plate. Palpebral springs are similarly placed. They fit into the upper and lower eyelids and close spontaneously when the levator is relaxed. With prolonged use, ptosis from dehiscence of the levator aponeurosis may occur. More-advanced techniques have been tried in patients with facial nerve palsy using temporalis muscle transfers and exogenous nerve stimulation; this information is available in textbooks on facial plastic and head and neck reconstruction and therefore will not be further discussed here.

Trichiasis. Eventually, trichiasis (inwardly directed lashes) causes significant damage to the cornea and to visual function. In the early stages, until the burn injury matures, copious lubrication and selective forceps epilation are adequate. In the chronic stage, however, definitive treatment is indicated. If there are only a few offending lashes, they may be permanently destroyed using electrolysis units or a monopolar cautery with a fine needle tip directed at the lash bulbs. Argon laser at a slitlamp can be used to ablate the lash bulbs in an anesthetized lid.

If a group of lashes are localized in one area, then a full-thickness wedge resection can be used to remove them. The wedge resection can also be used to remove a section of distorted lid margin, if needed, to protect the eye from irritation (Figure 19-21). However, this may not be the best option in thermally damaged eyelids with tissue loss. Cryotherapy is also useful in eliminating lash bulbs. Less damage to adjacent tissue occurs when the lid is split into anterior and posterior lamellae at the gray line and the lash follicles are selectively frozen. In severe burns, the anterior lamella can be recessed away from the lid margin and an intervening buccal mucosal membrane graft can be placed with or without meticulous extirpation or excision of all the offending lashes.

Disorders of the Mucosal Lining. In burn patients, abnormalities of the mucosal lining include symblepharon, eyelid posterior lamella cicatrization or tissue loss, and bulbar (eyeball) conjunctiva loss. Definitive repair of symblepharon varies according to severity. Mild symblepharon may simply be surgically lysed. Moderate symblepharon may require mucosal rearrangement after lysing. Rearrangement can be accomplished with multiple Z-plasties and rotational or transposition conjunctival flaps to reduce tension between the bulbar and the palpebral conjunctivae.

More-severe cases have insufficient conjunctival tissue, and mucosal membrane grafting is required. Autogenous mucosal membrane sources (discussed above) include buccal or lip mucosa and hard palate mucosa (which is usually reserved for the lower eyelid to give it vertical support). Once the symblepharon is lysed, the defect is filled with mucous membrane graft tissue. The buccal mucosal graft can be harvested freehand with a scalpel and Wescott scissors, and then cauterized for hemostasis. The graft is sewn into place with 7-0 Vicryl or

a b

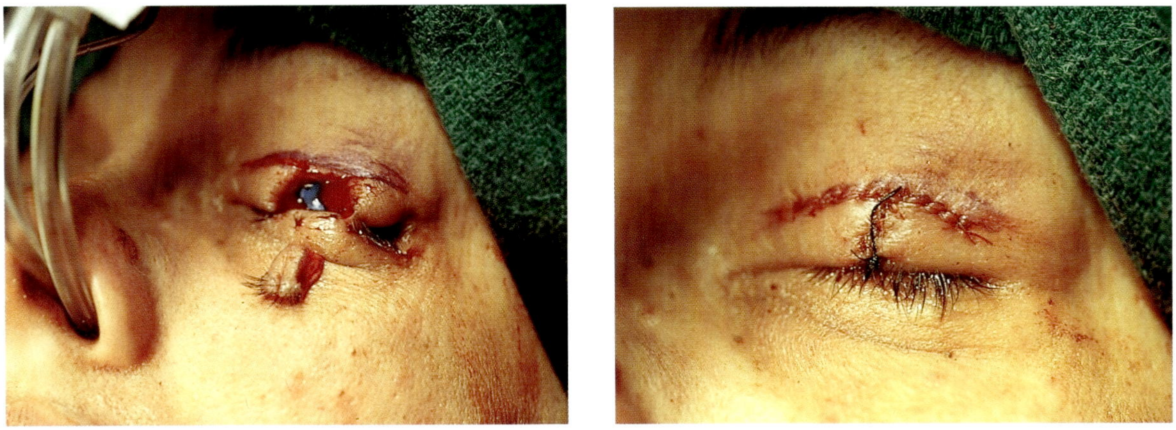

Fig. 19-21. (**a**) A pentagonal wedge resection permits (**b**) reformation of a smooth eyelid contour and removal of trichiatic lashes to restore normal tear pump mechanisms and to avoid ocular irritation.

6-0 fast-absorbing gut sutures. Occasionally, a symblepharon ring (ie, a plastic or silicone conformer ring to prevent conjunctival fornix contraction) must be placed until the mucosa heals in place. Alternatively, double-armed fornix reconstructive sutures placed full thickness through the fornix and out through the eyelid skin may be used to hold the mucosal grafts in place. Full-thickness buccal mucosal grafts work well on the eyelid but are too thick for the ocular surface. A mucotome, used to harvest ultrathin mucosal membrane, may be also be used for bulbar conjunctival replacement. An ultrathin graft avoids the erythematous appearance of full-thickness mucosa on the globe.

Repair of eyelid posterior lamella loss was discussed above. Repairing posterior lamellae addressed release of the scar, replacement of mucosal surfaces, and use of tarsal plate substitutes (see Figure 19-20). Bulbar conjunctival loss may occasionally heal spontaneously, provided there is no palpebral mucosa loss that would cause adhesions and symblepharon. In most cases, grafting is required. Bulbar mucosa can be replaced with autogenous bulbar conjunctiva from an uninjured site or opposite eye. If unavailable, ultrathin buccal mucosal membrane is a good alternative. Shimazaki and colleagues[26] reported the use of amniotic membrane transplantation for ocular surface reconstruction in patients with chemical and thermal burns.

Tear Drainage System Abnormalities. In burn patients, the most common abnormalities of the tear drainage system involve the puncta, canaliculi, and tear sac, owing to the burn injury itself and scar formation involving the eyelids. It is very uncommon for the nasolacrimal duct to be involved because it is protected by the bony nasolacrimal canal. In cases of blast injury or severe burns to the midface involving the facial bones, an injury to the nasolacrimal duct may occur. Malpositions of the eyelid (see earlier discussion) can affect the tear pumping mechanism even though normal tear drainage system components are present. Problems directly involving the puncta, canaliculi, lacrimal sac, and nasolacrimal duct are addressed here.

Punctal stenosis or occlusion from scarring is common in eyelid burns. Mild stenosis can be addressed with sequential punctal dilation with or without placement of a punctal stent. If the stricture is localized to the punctum, a punctal plug may suffice as a stent. If the punctum is occluded or if the stenosis is refractory to dilation, then the punctum may be surgically opened with a supersharp blade, sickle knife, or sharp-tipped Wescott scissors. To prevent reocclusion, a stent may be placed or a two-snip procedure performed. The two-snip procedure is performed by placing one blade of a sharp Wescott scissors into the punctum and the other onto the mucosal surface of the lid. The punctal orifice is then cut on the mucosal side of the lid. This process is repeated just medial or lateral to the initial incision so that a V-shaped wedge of the vertical canalicular wall on the mucosal side of the lid is excised, creating a large, posteriorly placed punctum.

Canalicular stenosis can be addressed with sequential dilation by passing Bowman lacrimal probes of increasing size. Once adequate dilation is achieved, the drainage system must be intubated with Crawford tubes or similar stents to prevent restenosis. Additionally, the canaliculi may be dilated with a balloon catheter such as the LacriCATH (mfg by Atrion Medical, Birmingham, Ala). Once dilated, intubation is still required and should be left in place for 6 to 12 months. If a canaliculus is obstructed and the obstruction is focal and distal to the medial canthus, then the obstructed section can be excised and the canalicular portion of the lid margin primarily repaired over an intubated canalicular system. If the obstruction is focal but close to the medial canthus, then a Bowman probe can be forced through the obstruction and into the sac.

Alternatively, a holmium (Ho) laser with an intracanalicular probe can be used to ablate the obstruction. The canalicular system is then intubated with the hope that mucosal epithelium will migrate toward the center—from normal canalicular mucosa along the stent toward the lacrimal sac and vice versa. Ophthalmologists should note that the success of procedures decreases whenever surgical insult occurs adjacent to tissue damage. If canalicular obstruction persists or is more-severe, then the entire canalicular system must be bypassed via a C-DCR (described above).

If scarring or strictures are mild, then injured lacrimal sacs may be amenable to simple intubation of the lacrimal drainage system with or without balloon dilation. If more-severe, the sac must be surgically explored with an external skin approach and a DCR or C-DCR may be required to restore tear drainage.

Finally, obstruction of the nasolacrimal duct may be partial or complete. Partial obstruction may respond to balloon catheter dilation and intubation along with an antibiotic and steroid regimen to reduce postoperative scarring from inflammation and bacterial colonization. For complete or refractory partial obstructions, a DCR with intubation should be performed.

SUMMARY

Management of eyelid burns—first-degree, or superficial; second-degree, or partial-thickness; and third-degree, or full-thickness—occurs at all echelons of care, from battalion aid stations at the 1st echelon to medical centers in CONUS. At each level of care, the burns—whether acute, subacute, or chronic—receive echelon-appropriate evaluation and treatment before the casualty is transported to the next rearward echelon, where greater medical expertise is available. At the 1st echelon, emergent care focuses on lifesaving ATLS and ACLS principles and techniques and the immediate treatment of chemical burns. Urgent care focuses on diagnosing ruptured globes and ocular injuries and limiting the extent of thermal burn injuries. Management at higher echelons, where military ophthalmologists are found, always includes repeating the steps from the lower echelons, not only to avoid the possibility of misdiagnosis and incomplete treatment of burns but also because the full extent of eyelid burn wounds sometimes manifests over time.

Acute and subacute management focuses on protecting the eye and its visual potential and on limiting the extent of the damage that has occurred to the eyelids and surrounding tissue. Long-term management involves critical evaluation of the injured eyelid in terms of its functional components, malpositions, protraction, and retraction. Scar maturation followed by definitive surgical reconstruction occur in CONUS, where eye protection, then visual function, and finally cosmetic appearance are addressed.

At each echelon, casualties are reevaluated for evacuation, which is necessary for two reasons: (1) diminished vision makes the soldier nonfunctional on the battlefield, and (2) extensive burns to the eyelids are usually accompanied by serious injury to the rest of the body, including the respiratory passages. In general, only patients with first-degree and very mild second-degree burns are kept at the lower echelons and returned to duty, and soldiers with second- or third-degree burns to the eyelids are evacuated back to CONUS.

REFERENCES

1. Stern JD, Godfarb IW, Slater H. Ophthalmological complications as a manifestation of burn injury. *Burns*. 1996;22:135–136.

2. Kulwin DR. Thermal, chemical, and radiation burns. In: Steward WB, ed. *Surgery of the Eyelid, Orbit and Lacrimal System.* Vol 1. San Francisco, Calif: American Academy of Ophthalmology; 1993: Chap 12.

3. Guy RJ, Baldwin J, Kwedar S, Law EJ. Three years' experience in a regional burn center with burns of the eyes and eyelids. *Ophthalmic Surg*. 1982;13:383–386.

4. Still JM, Law EJ, Belcher KE, Moses KC, Gleitsmann KY. Experience with burns of the eyes and lids in a regional burn unit. *J Burn Care Rehabil.* 1995;16:248–252.

5. Karesh JW. The evaluation and management of eyelid trauma. In: Tasman W, Jaeger EA, eds. *Clinical Ophthalmology*. Vol 5. Philadelphia, Pa: Lippincott-Raven; 1996: Chap 75.

6. Astori IP, Muller MJ, Pegg SP. Cicatricial postburn ectropion and exposure keratitis. *Burns*. 1998;24:64–67.

7. Stern AL, Pamel GJ, Benedetto LG. Physical and chemical injuries of the eyes and eyelids. *Dermatol Clin*. 1992;10:785–791.

8. Edlich RF, Nichter LS, Morgan RF, Persing JA, Van Meter CH, Kenney JG. Burns of the head and neck. *Otolaryngol Clin North Am*. 1984;17:361–388.

9. Cepela MA, Kulwin DR. Adnexal burns. In: Nesi FA, Lisman RD, Levine MR, eds. *Smith's Ophthalmic Plastic and Reconstructive Surgery*. 2nd ed. St Louis, Mo: Mosby; 1998: Chap 6.

10. Kalish E, Stiebel-Kalish H, Wolf Y, Robinpour M, Hauben DJ. Scorched eyelashes: Do we treat them right? *Burns*. 1998;24:173–175.

11. Nose K, Isshiki N, Kusumoto K. Reconstruction of both eyelids following electrical burn. *Plast Reconstr Surg.* 1991;88:878–881.

12. Johnson C. Pathologic manifestation of burn injury. In: Richard RL, Staly MJ, eds. *Burn Care and Rehabilitation: Principles and Practice.* Philadelphia, Pa: FA Davis Co; 1994: Chap 3.

13. Kulwin DR. Treatment of periorbital burns. *Adv Ophthalmol Plast Reconstr Surg.* 1988;7:167–169.

14. Frank DH, Wachtel T, Frank HA. The early treatment and reconstruction of eyelid burns. *J Trauma.* 1983; 23:874–877.

15. Garber PF, MacDonald D, Beyer-Machule CK. Management of trauma to the eyelids. In: Della Rocca RC, Nesi FA, Lisman RD, eds. *Ophthalmic Plastic and Reconstructive Surgery.* St Louis, Mo: Mosby; 1987.

16. Committee on Trauma, American College of Surgeons. *Advanced Trauma Life Support Program for Physicians: Instructor Manual.* 5th ed. Chicago, Ill: American College of Surgeons; 1997.

17. Cummins RO. *Advanced Cardiac Life Support: ACLS Provider Manual.* Dallas, Tex: American Heart Association; 2001.

18. Trojan HJ. Treatment of burns of the eye and adnexa. *Trop Doct.* 1980;10:59–61.

19. Burns CL, Chylack LT. Thermal burns: The management of thermal burns of the lids and globes. *Ann Ophthalmol.* 1979;11:1358–1368.

20. Neale HW, Billmire DA, Carey JP. Reconstruction following head and neck burns. *Clin Plast Surg.* 1986; 13:119–136.

21. Gallico GG III, O'Connor NE, Compton CC, Kehinde O, Green H. Permanent coverage of large burn wounds with autologous cultured human epithelium. *N Engl J Med.* 1984;311:448–51.

22. Grabosch A, Weyer F, Gruhl L, Brink JC. Repair of the upper eyelid by means of the prepuce after severe burn. *Ann Plast Surg.* 1991;26:427–430.

23. Shore JW, McCord CD, Popham JK. Surgery of the eyelids. In: Tasman W, Jaeger EA, eds. *Clinical Ophthalmology.* Vol 5. Philadelphia, Pa: Lippincott-Raven; 1996: Chap 78.

24. Huang TT, Blackwell SJ, Lewis SR. Burn injuries of the eyelids. *Clin Plast Surg.* 1978;5:571–581.

25. Kobus K. Late repair of facial burns. *Ann Plast Surg.* 1980;5:191–204.

26. Shimazaki J, Yang HY, Tsubota K. Amniotic membrane transplantation for ocular surface reconstruction in patients with chemical and thermal burns. *Ophthalmology.* 1997;104:2068–2076.

Chapter 20

ORBITAL TRAUMA

ROBERT A. MAZZOLI, MD[*]; DARRYL J. AINBINDER, MD[†]; AND ELIZABETH A. HANSEN, MD[‡]

[*]*Colonel, Medical Corps, US Army; Chief and Chairman of Ophthalmology, Director, Ophthalmic Plastic, Reconstructive and Orbital Surgery, Madigan Army Medical Center, Tacoma, Washington 98431-5000; Clinical Associate Professor of Surgery (Ophthalmology), Uniformed Services University of the Health Sciences, 4301 Jones Bridge Road, Bethesda, Maryland 20814-4799*

[†]*Lieutenant Colonel, Medical Corps, US Army; Director, Ophthalmic Oncology and Pathology, and Staff, Ophthalmic Plastic, Reconstructive, and Orbital Surgery, Madigan Army Medical Center, Tacoma, Washington 98431-5000*

[‡]*Colonel, Medical Corps, US Army; Director, Comprehensive Ophthalmology, Madigan Army Medical Center, Tacoma, Washington 98431-5000; Clinical Assistant Professor of Surgery (Ophthalmology), Uniformed Services University of the Health Sciences, 4301 Jones Bridge Road, Bethesda, Maryland 20814-4799*

INTRODUCTION

Because of the number of structures present in a relatively small space, the management of orbital trauma demands exacting evaluation. Appropriate management requires in-depth knowledge of anatomical structures and their surgical relations. Additionally, because the energies causing orbital trauma are often much greater than those that cause purely ocular trauma, adjacent nonocular structures (eg, nose, paranasal sinuses, midface and jaw, brain) are commonly injured as well (Figures 20-1 and 20-2). Because of this, extensive orbital trauma is often best managed by a multidisciplinary team, on which ophthalmology must be represented. Typical head-and-neck trauma teams include representatives from neurosurgery, otorhinolaryngology (ear, nose, and throat [ENT]), plastic surgery, and oromaxillofacial surgery (OMFS).

In most wartime scenarios—and certainly in many peacetime situations—the general ophthalmologist may be called on to assist or direct the management of orbital trauma, either as a member of a head-and-neck trauma team in the event of complex injury, or as the primary physician in the event of isolated globe or adnexal injury. Extended

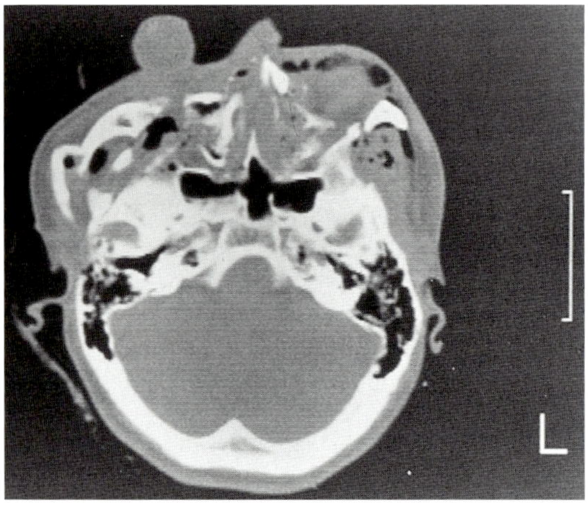

Fig. 20-1. An unrestrained passenger in a motor vehicle accident hit the dashboard and windshield with his face and head. The urgent computed tomography scan demonstrates traumatic enucleation / avulsion of the right eye and massive disruption of the naso-orbital-ethmoid region, as well as bilateral fractures of the zygomaticomaxillary complex. Such high-energy injuries almost always involve multiple anatomical areas and demand multidisciplinary team management. With emergent intervention, the patient survived this dramatic injury.

a

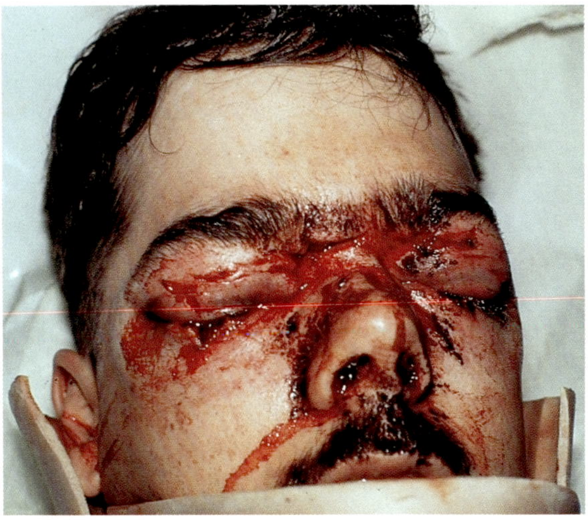

b

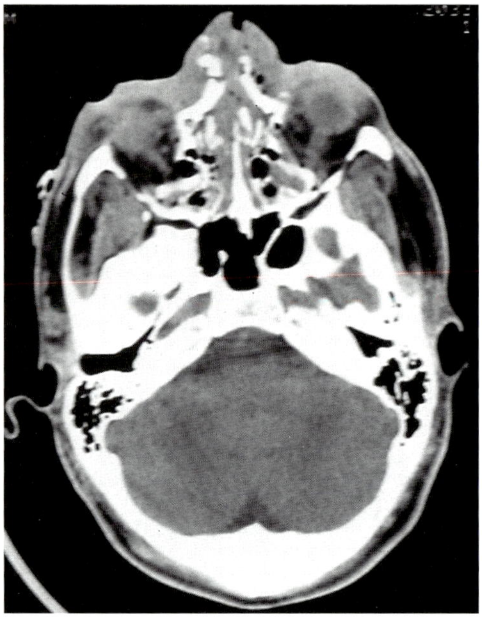

Fig. 20-2. (**a**) A 24-year-old man was attempting to secure a shipping pallet with a tie-down chain when the chain broke and recoiled into his midface. He arrived in the emergency department, and an ophthalmologist was called to evaluate his eyes and orbits. The patient was alert and oriented, and his airway was not compromised. Fortunately, his eyes were not involved. (**b**) The computed tomography scan shows massive naso-orbital-ethmoid disruption, which required open reduction and internal fixation. Such injuries require multispecialty cooperation in evaluation, management, and surgical planning to ensure the maximal functional and surgical outcome. In these cases, early surgery generally leads to the best result.

training in ophthalmic plastic and reconstructive surgery may be an unavailable luxury; nevertheless, the ophthalmologist must take an active role in the evaluation and management of all orbital injuries. Although many other specialists can offer experience in the repair of bony orbital injuries, no other physician can evaluate the globe and its adnexa as expertly as an ophthalmologist can.

ORBITAL ANATOMY AND MIDFACIAL BUTTRESSES

Orbital Soft Tissues

An extended discussion of orbital soft-tissue anatomy is beyond the scope of this chapter. Suffice it to say that the orbit contains fat, muscles, nerves, blood vessels, and above all, the globe (Figure 20-3). The single most important structure within the orbit is the eye. Beyond all else, the ophthalmologist's primary concern—the raison d'être—must be the evaluation, restoration, and preservation of the globe's integrity. Orbital concerns must *always* be secondary to the eye and vision. In current practice, whether in peacetime or combat, it is inexcusable and indefensible to overlook or forego evaluation of the eye of a patient who has suffered orbital trauma. For this reason, it is incumbent on any physician—regardless of specialty—who is evaluating an orbital injury to seek the expertise, advice, and assistance of an ophthalmologist (Figure 20-4).

The orbit has a rich vascular supply, with arterial contributions from both the internal and the external carotid circulations. The venous circulation, as part of the valveless head-and-neck system, is particularly fragile and susceptible to both direct and indirect trauma, such as remote pressure changes as may be caused by sudden decompression, Valsalva pressure, strangulation, or chest compression (Figure 20-5). Consequently, hemorrhage within the orbit is a near-constant companion to

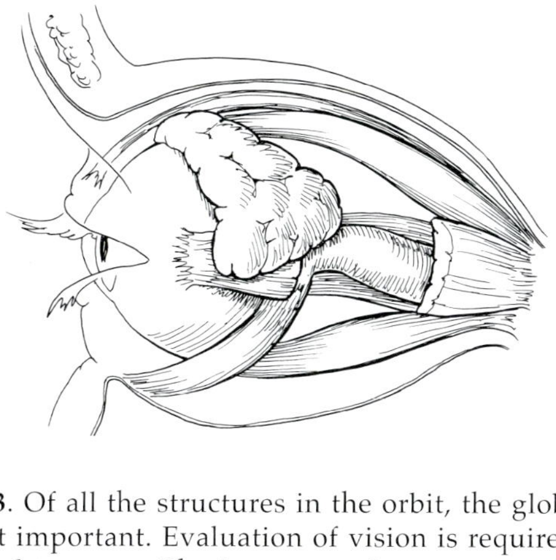

Fig. 20-3. Of all the structures in the orbit, the globe is the most important. Evaluation of vision is required in all orbital traumas. The intramuscular septum, which connects the extraocular muscles, subdivides the orbital compartments into the intraconal and extraconal spaces. Drawing prepared for this textbook by Gary Wind, MD, Uniformed Services University of the Health Sciences, Bethesda, Md.

a

b

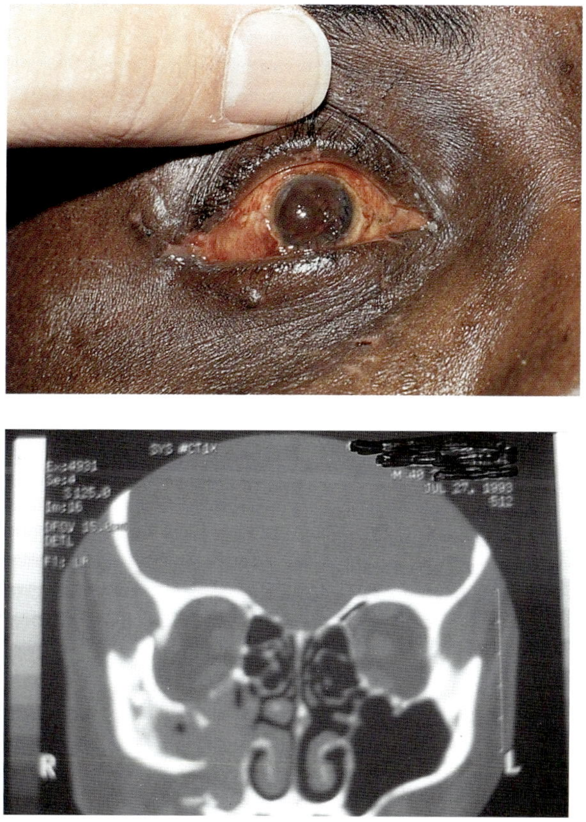

Fig. 20-4. Primary and emergency medical personnel must be acutely aware that facial injuries often affect both the eye and orbit. Likewise, the ophthalmologist evaluating an ocular injury must keep in mind the possibility of concomitant orbital injury. While evaluation and repair of the eye must always take priority over orbital and adnexal injuries, these injuries may require attention nonetheless. (**a**) This 40-year-old man was struck over the right cheek with a glass bottle, which shattered, resulting in the large corneoscleral and lid lacerations. The globe and lid were repaired before the patient was transferred for further treatment, but unfortunately, the eye remained blind. (**b**) A computed tomography scan demonstrates a concomitant right zygomaticomaxillary complex fracture, which was repaired by open reduction and internal fixation before enucleation.

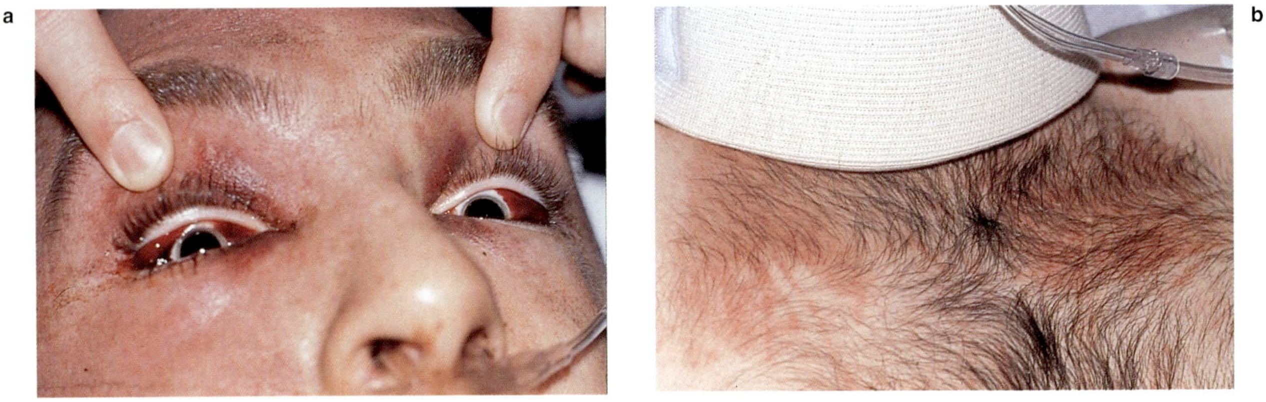

Fig. 20-5. Orbital hemorrhage after chest compression. Increased central venous pressure impedes venous return from the head and neck, often resulting in orbital hemorrhage. (**a**) This patient, an infantry soldier, was engaged in night training maneuvers when an armored personnel carrier rolled through his unit's area and directly over him. Because it had been raining heavily and the ground was especially soft, he survived the accident, suffering intracerebral hemorrhage, other internal injuries, a fractured pelvis, and avulsion of the right brachial plexus nerve roots. Amazingly, the only ocular damage was the bilateral subconjunctival hemorrhages, which are evident in this clinical photograph. (**b**) The thoracic contusion sustained by the patient.

orbital trauma, especially penetrating trauma.

Because the orbit is confined by a dense periorbita (periosteum) surrounded by four bony walls, the orbital contents can decompress in only one direction—anteriorly—and even that is limited by the fibrous orbital septum and canthal structures. Bleeding into this confined space can quickly lead to devastating ocular and orbital consequences. Hemorrhage may occur either within the orbit proper or in the subperiosteal space and can result from either blunt or penetrating trauma, or from remote barotrauma. It may also mask the presence of an orbital foreign body

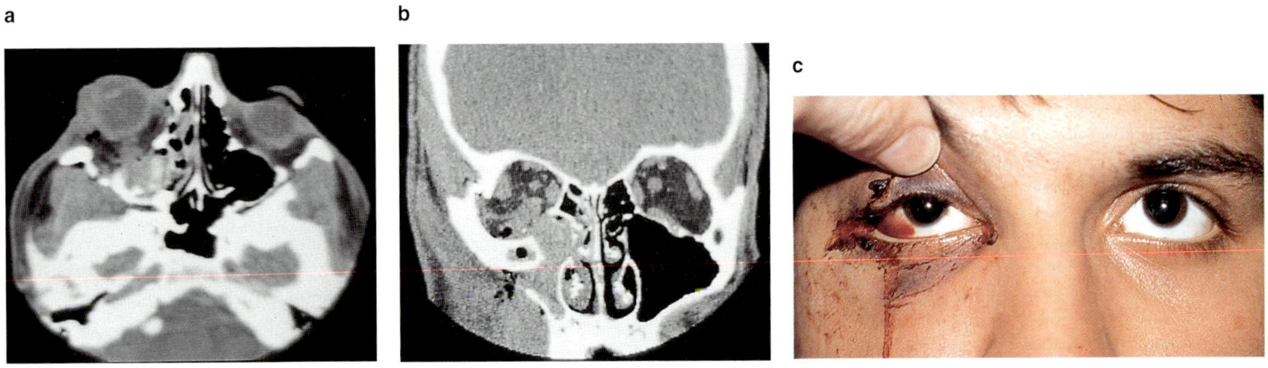

Fig. 20-6. Late orbital hemorrhage and vision loss. When this 20-year-old man first presented to the emergency department after a fistfight, his visual acuity and motility were "normal." However, over the ensuing 20 minutes, the patient complained of decreased vision in the right eye, increased proptosis, limited motility, and pain. (**a**) An emergent computed tomography (CT) scan revealed a large right zygomaticomaxillary complex fracture with sinus opacification secondary to marked hemorrhage. Significant proptosis is evident, as are adnexal soft-tissue swelling and orbital emphysema. Ophthalmologic examination revealed vision of 20/100 with an afferent pupillary defect, tense proptosis, and an intraocular pressure of 44. Immediate canthotomy and cantholysis resulted in return of 20/70 vision, resolution of proptosis, and reduction of intraocular pressure to 26. (**b**) A follow-up CT scan made 2 hours later shows the hemorrhage extending into the inferior orbital soft tissues, although it does not appear to significantly involve the remainder of the intraorbital soft tissues. The amount of sinus clot was sufficient to prevent further drainage of hemorrhage, resulting in increased orbital pressure. (**c**) The same patient 2 days after presentation. The canthotomy and cantholysis are easily seen. Vision was 20/20. He subsequently underwent open reduction and internal fixation and did well.

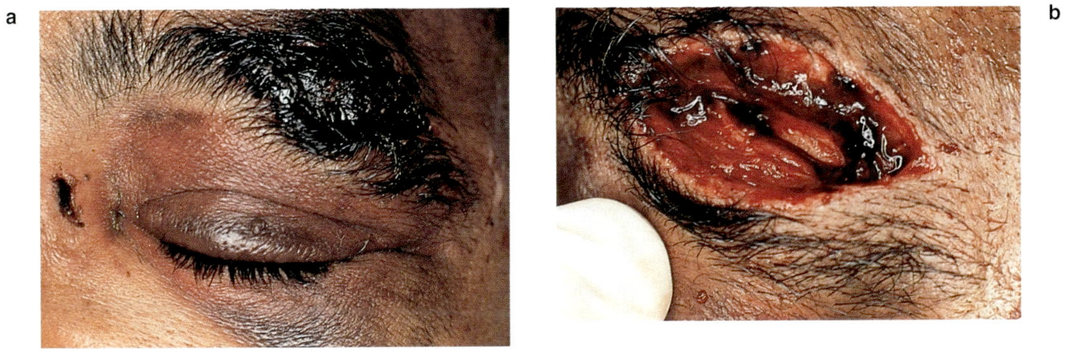

Fig. 20-7. (**a**) This patient was involved in a motor vehicle accident and suffered a brow laceration. At initial evaluation in the emergency department, the laceration was believed to be minor, having self-sealed with coagulum. It was not explored or sutured, but was patched and the patient was referred for routine evaluation the next day. (**b**) After debridement, the true depth of the wound was revealed, which extended to the periosteum, with underlying bony fracture.

(FB). Therefore, orbital hemorrhage always requires prompt evaluation. Additionally, because active bleeding can continue long after the initial injury, vision must be followed vigilantly, even after the initial presentation (Figure 20-6). More will be said about the evaluation and management of orbital hemorrhage later in this chapter.

Ophthalmologists should always maintain a high index of suspicion for occult penetrating trauma. By the time the patient presents for evaluation, many apparently minor lacerations will have reapproximated and sealed with serum, coagulum, and clot. Often, however, these lacerations disguise retained FBs (such as slivers of windshield glass) or deep injury and may be much more significant than they first appeared (Figures 20-7 and 20-8).[1] Lid and facial lacerations should, therefore, be meticulously cleaned, explored, and debrided of FBs, and lid lacerations, especially, should be thoroughly inspected to rule out full-thickness involvement and

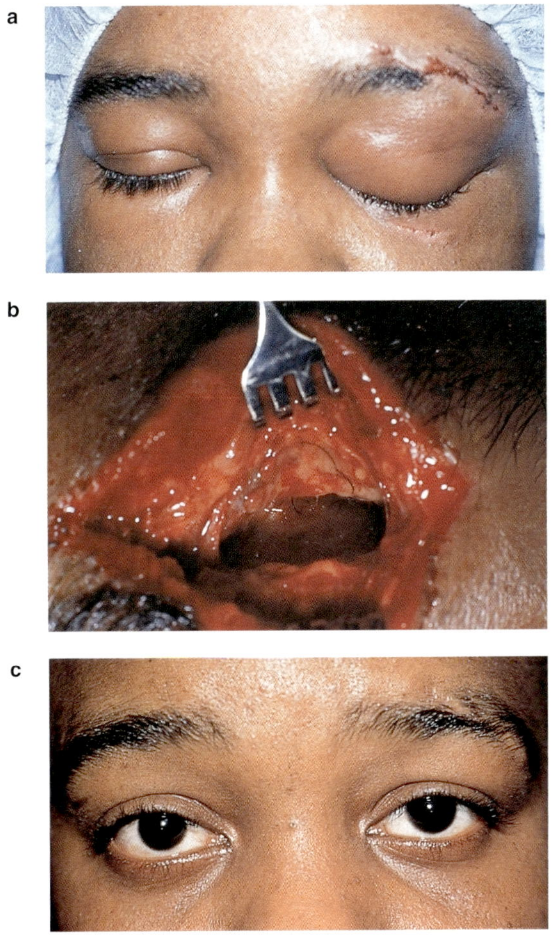

Fig. 20-8. Unexplored brow laceration. This left brow laceration resulted from a rock thrown during a bar fight. When the patient presented to the emergency department, the wound was felt to be of limited depth and therefore was irrigated and sutured. (**a**) Over the ensuing week, increasing brow pain and lid swelling that were unresponsive to oral antibiotics prompted referral to the ophthalmology clinic, where a tender, fluctuant pocket was palpated at the brow. (**b**) The wound was reopened and explored, revealing approximately 20 retained brow hairs. Only sterile reactive fluid was drained. Full exploration, however, revealed that the wound extended to the periosteum. The wound was debrided, irrigated, and reclosed over a drain. The patient subsequently did well. (**c**) The same patient 7 months later.

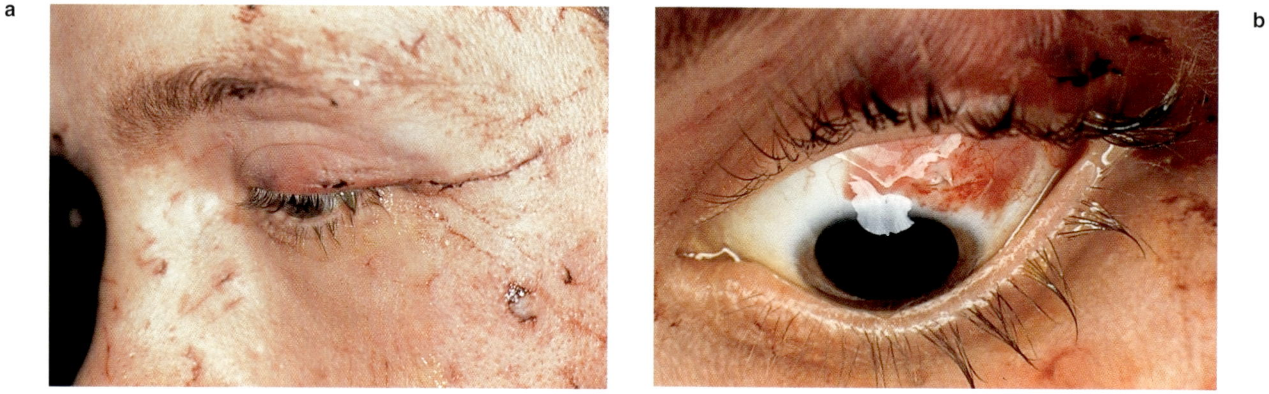

Fig. 20-9. Unsuspected globe trauma. (**a**) This patient was involved in a motor vehicle accident with multiple, apparently superficial, facial lacerations from windshield glass slivers. The lacerations were primarily debrided and sutured in the emergency department, and the patient was referred to the eye clinic the following day for routine evaluation of the lid lacerations. Visual acuity was noted to be 20/50. Many lacerations still harbored glass slivers. (**b**) Thorough examination disclosed an undetected scleral laceration and vitreous hemorrhage. Lid puncture wounds can be seen laterally. No intraocular foreign body was found on surgical exploration. The globe was repaired and the patient's vision returned to 20/20.

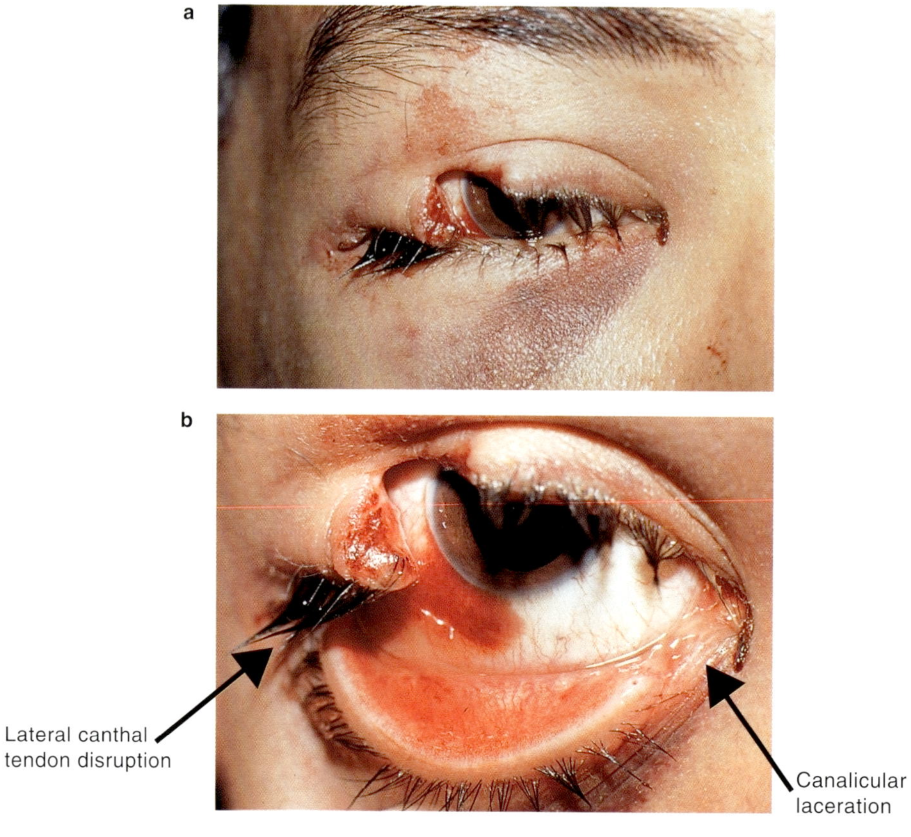

Fig. 20-10. Unrecognized adjacent injury. Canalicular trauma should always be suspected in lid trauma. (**a**) This man was struck with brass knuckles and was referred for treatment of the upper lid laceration. Close inspection of the medial canthus shows the lid to be misleadingly well apposed, with only a small hemorrhagic coagulum implying any injury to the structure. (**b**) A complete examination revealed concomitant—and previously unrecognized—complete disruptions of the lower canaliculus and lateral canthal tendon.

a b

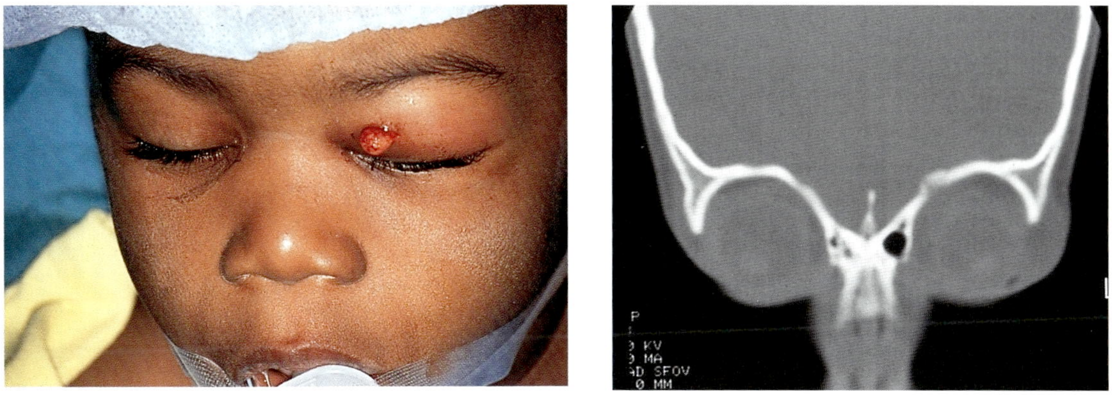

Fig. 20-11. Unsuspected orbital injury. Herniated or visible orbital fat is prima facie evidence of orbital injury, the extent of which is never known on presentation. (**a**) This 2-year-old boy fell on a pencil while running. The patient was alert, oriented, and normally playful during the examination, the only abnormality discovered being the lid laceration and herniating orbital fat. (**b**) A computed tomography scan demonstrated intracranial puncture of the orbital roof. Fortunately, no treatment was needed other than debridement and closure of the lid wound. Similar injuries can also harbor retained foreign bodies.

unsuspected globe injury or canalicular damage (Figures 20-9 and 20-10). Because the orbital fat lies behind the orbital septum, visible orbital fat is an ominous sign, by definition disclosing an orbital injury, and should provoke extended examination with computed tomography (CT), magnetic resonance imaging (MRI), or both (Figure 20-11).

Orbital Bony Anatomy

Seven bones come together to make up the four walls of the bony orbital socket, which takes the shape of a quadrangular pyramid. The orbit is lined with periosteum (the periorbita), which is densely adherent at the orbital rim, the optic canal, and orbital fissures. The periorbita is relatively loosely adherent along the plates of the bony walls, creating a potential space for the accumulation of subperiosteal fluid and blood. None of the bony plates are especially thick, and all can easily be fractured. The orbital floor and medial wall, being adjacent to sinus air spaces, are especially vulnerable to hydrostatic and mechanical buckling forces. Although the bone of the medial wall (the lamina papyracea) is physically thinner than that of the orbital floor, the honeycombed arrangement of the underlying ethmoid air cells gives the medial wall a significant structural advantage over the floor, which is obliged to sit over the cavernously empty maxillary sinus (Figure 20-12). Consequently, the most frequently fractured wall is the floor, not the medial wall. The roof and the lateral wall, on the other hand, being veritably sandwiched between soft tissues (brain and orbit on the roof, temporalis muscle and orbit on the lateral wall), are more substantially cushioned against fractures. Therefore, fracture of either of these walls is indicative of significant traumatic energy.[1–4]

Midfacial Buttresses

The orbital rim, which is arranged as a quadrilateral spiral and is significantly thicker than the remainder of the bony walls (see Figure 20-12), is an essential component of the midfacial buttress system. Unfortunately, the concept of midfacial buttresses is one that is not widely addressed in the general ophthalmic literature. Nonetheless, it is the vernacular among the other services that may be consulting ophthalmology in cases of extensive trauma (ie, ENT, plastic and craniofacial surgery, OMFS, or neurosurgery).[5] Because the orbital rim is integral to the buttresses, the evaluation and repair of rim fractures necessitates that ophthalmologists have at least a cursory knowledge of this concept.[5,6]

The buttresses are to the face what I-beams, girders, studs, and joists are to buildings: they provide the major structural support on which all the other walls, floors, roofs, and ceilings are hung. They maintain the facial skeleton in three dimensions: vertical height, horizontal width, and anteroposterior projection (Table 20-1).

Some areas of the orbital and facial bones are substantially thicker than the bony plates that extend from them (eg, the superior rim vs the orbital roof, or the inferior rim vs the anterior maxillary face and the orbital floor; see Figure 20-12). With-

a b

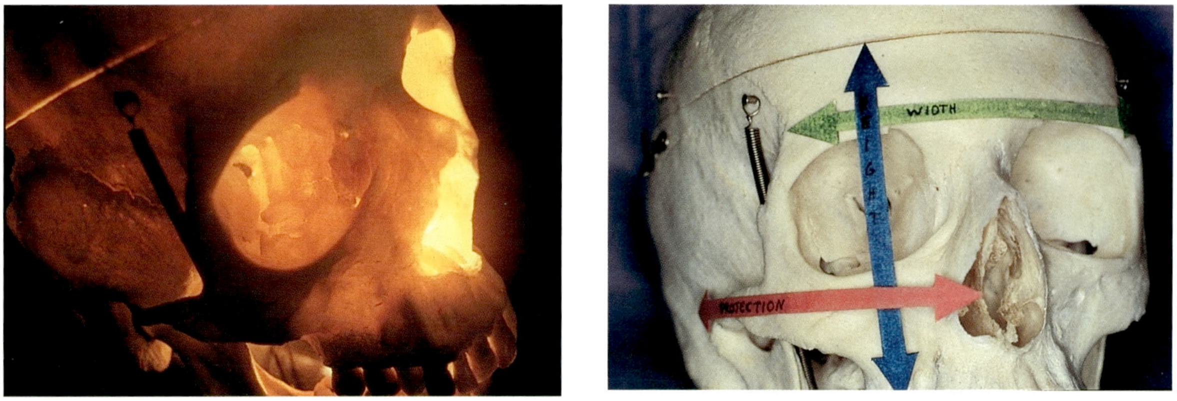

Fig. 20-12. (**a**) The bones of the orbital walls are all very thin, as this transilluminated skull demonstrates. The corrugated ethmoid air cells are clearly visible. These give the medial wall substantially increased strength, compared with the floor, which physically is thicker. The roof and lateral orbital walls are thin, as well. The midfacial buttresses are seen as noticeably thicker areas of bone, much thicker than the orbital plates. The buttresses provide a stable, rigid framework for the face and skull, and they maintain facial width, height, and projection. The areas of the orbital rim, the zygomaticomaxillary complex buttress, and the nasomaxillary buttress are clearly identifiable. (**b**) The integrity of these buttresses is essential in maintaining the three-dimensional facial framework.

out these areas of bony reinforcement, the thinner facial plates alone would not be strong enough to counter the muscular forces of the facial muscles—let alone the dynamic contractile forces of posttraumatic cicatricial changes—and the face would collapse in a large, unstable heap. For example, imagine a house of cards; it might be able to stand up weakly on its own, but it cannot handle much stress (Figure 20-13). In fact, if the buttresses are intact, loss of all the adjacent walls would not significantly alter the three-dimensional size of the face, just as a house or building remains stable and identifiable with only its frame intact even if all the plasterboard and plywood walls have been removed. The reverse, as stated before, is not true: if all the plasterboard and plywood are intact but the studs and weight-bearing walls (ie, the buttresses) are buckled, the building will not be stable (Figure 20-14).

This is not to say that the loss of the thinner bony plates is inconsequential. On the contrary, loss of an orbital wall may have significant functional and cosmetic sequelae, even if the rim is completely intact. Loss of the orbital floor causes, for example, hypo-ophthalmia, enophthalmos, and diplopia and requires surgical repair (just as a hole in the floor of a third-floor office has to be repaired lest the furniture fall through it into the second-floor office below). The point is that if the girders of the building are buckled, repairing only the hole in the floor does little for the ultimate stability of the building; the buttresses must be stabilized first.

Because the buttresses are two-dimensional plates instead of simple bars, they actually have some structural strength in two directions (eg, the ethmoid plate of the medial wall supports not only height but also projection). Consequently, aligning the horizontal and vertical buttresses ensures projection. Some authors believe that the most important determinant in ensuring projection is reestablishment of accurate facial width, the key structure being the zygomatic arch.[4]

TABLE 20-1

MIDFACIAL BUTTRESSES

Dimension	Buttress
Vertical (height)	Zygomaticomaxillary complex (key element)
	Nasomaxillary
	Pterygomaxillary
	Fronto-ethmoid-vomer
Horizontal (width)	Superior rim
	Inferior rim
	Zygomatic arch (key element)
	Maxillary alveolus and palate
Anteroposterior (projection)	Zygomatic arch
	Maxillary alveolus
	Fronto-ethmoid-vomer

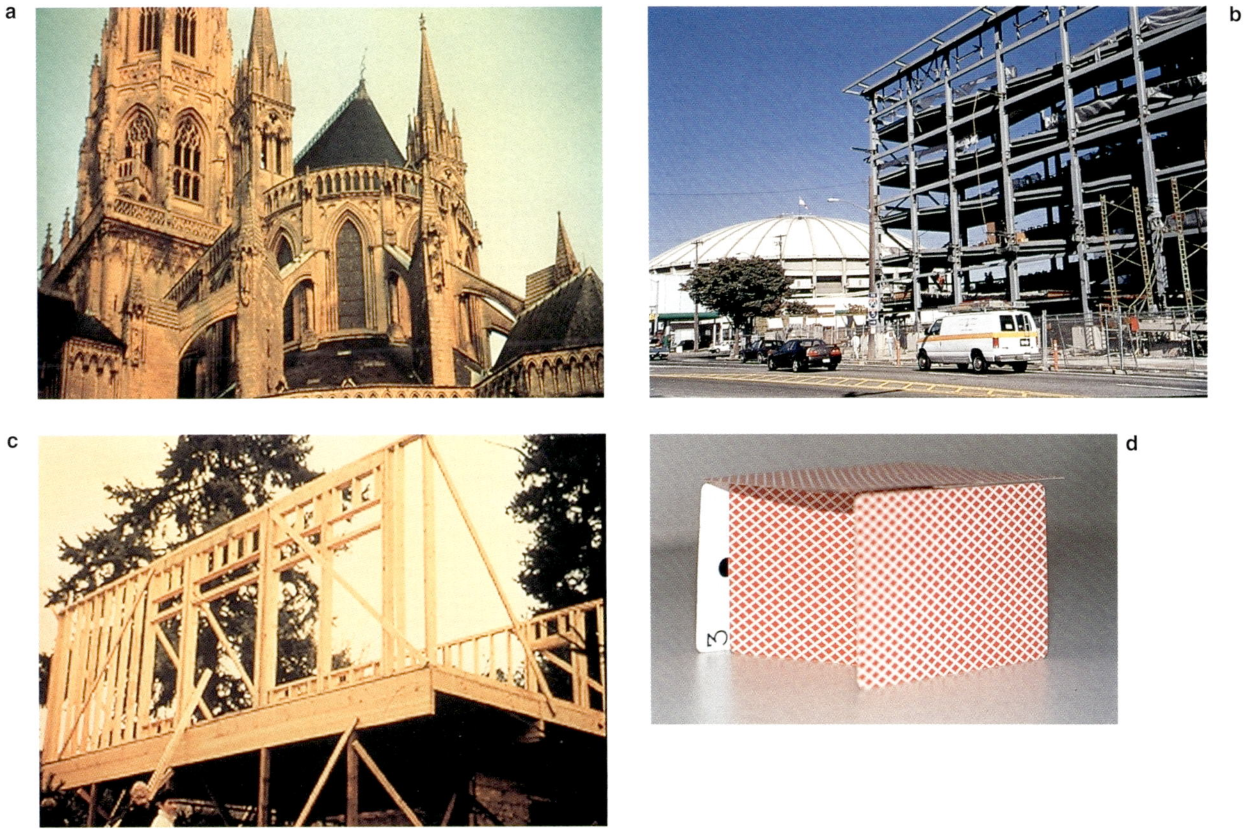

Fig. 20-13. Architectural buttresses help maintain three-dimensional structural stability. Without architectural buttresses—such as (**a**) the external flying buttresses of the Cathedral of Notre Dame, Bayeau, France, or (**b**) the internal buttresses of such modern structures as Seattle's Safeco Field and Kingdome, or (**c**) the studs and joists of modern housing—structures would have little strength against three-dimensional forces and would have the stability of (**d**) a house of cards.

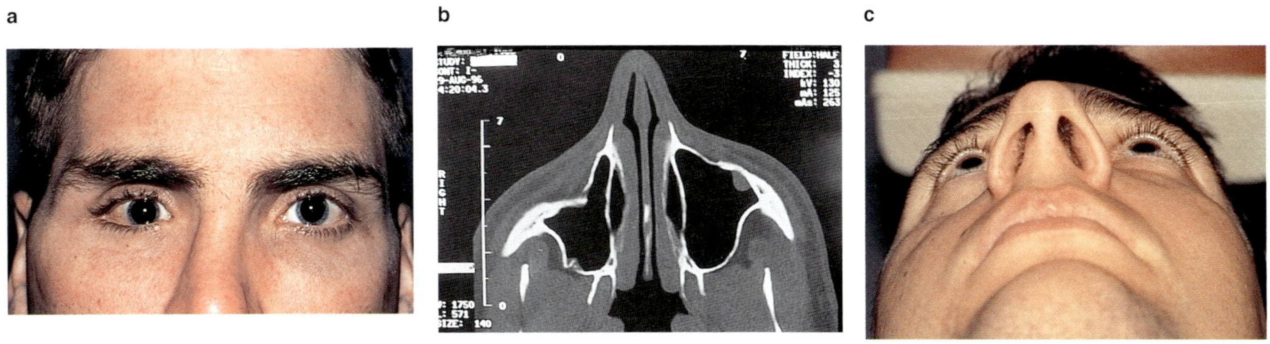

Fig. 20-14. Reconstitution of the midfacial buttresses after trauma is essential for maintaining proper facial projection. (**a**) A patient who suffered multiple midfacial fractures, including a zygomaticomaxillary complex fracture, after a parachute fall. Failure to reestablish proper articulation of the midfacial buttresses resulted in long-term orbital enlargement, increased facial width, malar flattening, and significant facial distortion. Despite frank right hypoglobus, the patient did not complain of symptomatic diplopia. (**b**) This computed tomography scan is of a different patient, who suffered a zygomaticomaxillary complex fracture in a car accident. (**c**) Three years later, this patient exhibits persistent malar flattening and significant enophthalmos as a result of insufficient reduction and poor alignment of the midfacial buttresses. Late repair of such deformities is difficult, because secondary soft-tissue contracture and fibrosis resist bony repositioning.

IMAGING

Although imaging for trauma is the subject of Chapter 4, Imaging of Ocular and Adnexal Trauma, some thoughts on orbital applications are nonetheless appropriate here. Imaging is always indicated in orbital trauma, and whether the ophthalmologist is looking for intraorbital foreign bodies (IOFBs), soft-tissue integrity, or bony fractures, the various imaging modalities—CT, MRI, and even plain film radiography—can provide significant information.

Computed Tomography

Currently, the most useful information for evaluating and managing orbital trauma is gained with CT. It provides the best visualization of bony integrity, gives reasonably good soft-tissue detail, and discloses many FBs, especially metallic ones. Many other FBs, however, such as those composed of glass, vegetable material, wood, and plastic, are poorly detected. Although CT scanners are currently deployed with many field hospitals, they are not universally available at all operational medical units. Nevertheless, CT is currently the imaging modality of choice for most orbital trauma.[7,8]

In general, a noncontrast protocol of 3-mm slices in both axial and true coronal planes gives sufficient information to manage most traumas. Certain conditions or circumstances warrant modification of this protocol. If true coronal views are not possible (eg, if the patient has a cervical spine injury), thin-slice (1.0–2.0 mm) axial studies give enough

a b c d

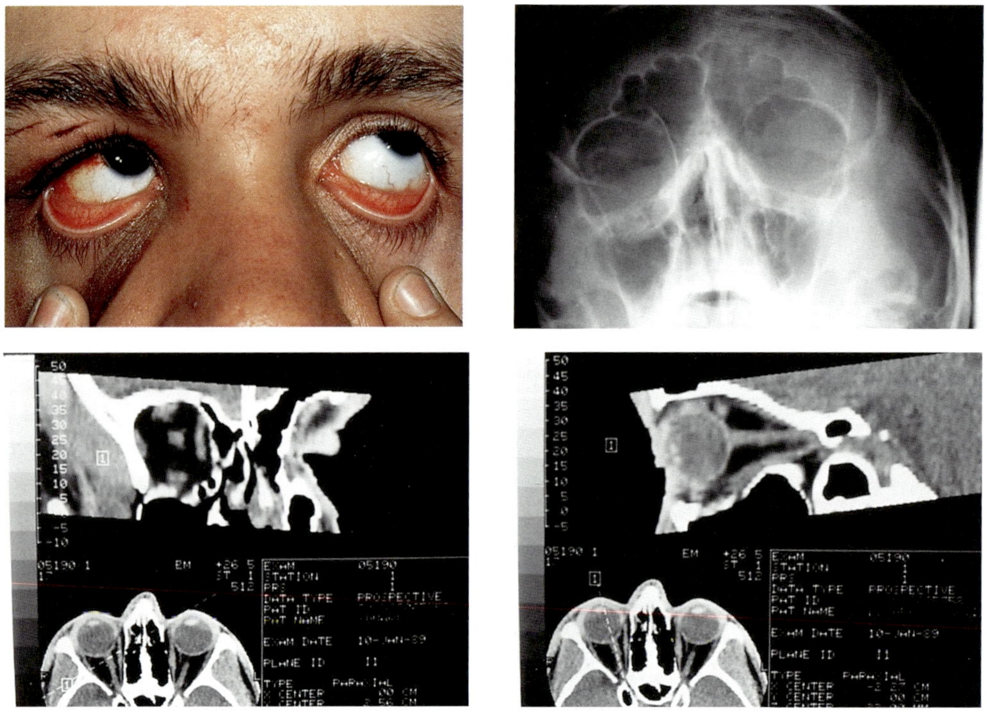

Fig. 20-15. Imaging: blowout fracture. (**a**) This 19-year-old man was the victim of an assault. The visual acuity was 20/20 in both eyes, but he complained of symptomatic diplopia in all fields of gaze, worst in upward left gaze. (**b**) A plain film radiograph (Waters's view) shows depression of the right orbital floor, but no gross herniation of orbital tissues into the maxillary sinus (the "tear drop" sign) is seen. (**c**) A coronal computed tomography (CT) scan, however, clearly demonstrates a large fracture of the medial orbital floor, with suggestion of perimuscular soft tissue entrapment. (**d**) Sagittal reconstruction localizes the fracture to the antero-middle floor and again shows soft-tissue entrapment. Note: Views c and d are reformatted views, as evidenced by the step artifacts of reconstruction and lack of metal scatter artifact from dental fillings. However, better detail is usually attained by direct coronal views. If reconstructed views are needed, initially obtaining the thinnest slices (1.5–2.0 mm) maximizes the quality of the reconstruction. Helical CT techniques produce excellent multiplanar reconstructions.

detail to allow reformatting into acceptable coronal views (Figure 20-15). If the ophthalmologist is looking specifically for optic canal trauma, 1.0–1.5-mm axial views give the best information (Figure 20-16). Thicker slices (eg, 3.0-mm) give adequate information for managing most facial traumas, but they are more prone to volume-averaging-induced artifacts that can mask subtle but significant detail and are, therefore, inadequate for complete evaluation of the canal. Because head or brain CTs are oriented differently from orbital views, slices of 5-mm thickness are unreliable when evaluating the orbital apex and should not be used. The patient is better served by the ophthalmologist's ordering the appropriate study at the outset than by his or her trying to "interpolate" a substandard study. If optic canal trauma or traumatic optic neuropathy is suspected, it behooves the ophthalmologist (or the emergency department physician) to convey the need for thin-slice orbital scans to the radiologist as soon as possible, so that the patient will not have to make multiple and unnecessary trips to the scanner.

Remembering that the skull does not reach adult size until about age 16 years, acquiring 3-mm slices on a child's orbit is akin to getting 5-mm slices on an adult. Volume-averaging makes discrimination of fine detail very difficult in such thick slices. Therefore, in children younger than 12 to 13 years of age, 1.0- to 2.0-mm slices generally yield the most useful information (helical, or spiral, scanners now make this easy).

When planning reformatted views, obtaining the thinnest scans possible maximizes the quality of the reconstructed views. Remember, however, that the quality of any reformatted view is degraded by metal artifacts and signal-averaging (Figure 20-17). On the other hand, when the patient has extensive dental fillings or prior metal facial plating, then reformatted coronal views from thin-slice axial views often eliminate the metal-scatter artifact of direct coronal views. Nevertheless, direct coronal views generally give more reliable information than reformatted views (see Figures 20-15 and 20-16).

Although three-dimensional images of orbital and facial trauma make impressive lecture slides, such reconstruction is associated with unacceptable levels of signal degradation and artifact, which limits its usefulness in acute trauma management. Currently (2002), three-dimensional reconstruction adds little relevant information and is of little use in acute orbital trauma, although it is useful in many peacetime situations (eg, management of craniofacial and synostotic syndromes). But because spiral scan techniques now allow the rapid acquisition of thin, seamless slices, three-dimensional formatting may become more applicable in acute trauma management (Figure 20-18).[7,8] Occasionally, sagittal reconstruction is worthwhile (see Figures 20-15 and 20-17).

Recent advances in CT technology have decreased both the amount of radiation delivered and the time required for scanning. Spiral scanning allows rapid studies and therefore is useful in many situations (eg, acute chest and head trauma, vascular imaging, and when scanning children). Spiral techniques permit reconstructed views of exceptional quality. Such refinements in image quality will likely continue as software and hardware improve.[7]

Unfortunately, CT is not without its drawbacks. What it contributes in bony detail is often lost in soft-tissue resolution. Many FBs are isodense with bone, hemorrhage, fat, and inflammation and are therefore very difficult to detect. Metal artifacts—from dental fillings, metal plates, wires, or other FBs—can induce such destructive interference that a high-quality scan may not be obtainable (Figure 20-19). Although the patient and the CT gantry can be repositioned so that most of the X-ray beams avoid the metal, the resulting orientations and cross-sections are often so atypical or unusual that they are difficult to interpret—even by physicians accustomed to unusual scans (Figure 20-20).

Spiral scans, while dramatically decreasing the scan time, may do so at the expense of decreasing the life of the X-ray tube. Because the beam is turned on from the beginning of the spiral to the end, it can get much hotter than it does during a conventional scan, during which the tube cools between slices. Of course, spiral scanning is merely a CT technique; it can be performed as needed and then the machine can be returned to its conventional usage. Nonetheless, helical techniques can dramatically increase X-ray tube maintenance and decrease the expected tube life. Consequently, spiral scans should be ordered only if conventional scans are unacceptable.

Many of these drawbacks are compounded in the field environment. Although mobile, the equipment is heavy, bulky, and expensive. Replacement parts can be difficult to obtain during combat operations, when the scanner is most needed. In addition, the scanner might be located in a separate trailer or van within the field hospital, which can lead to difficulties in patient transportation and flow (Figure 20-21). Despite significant advances in decreasing

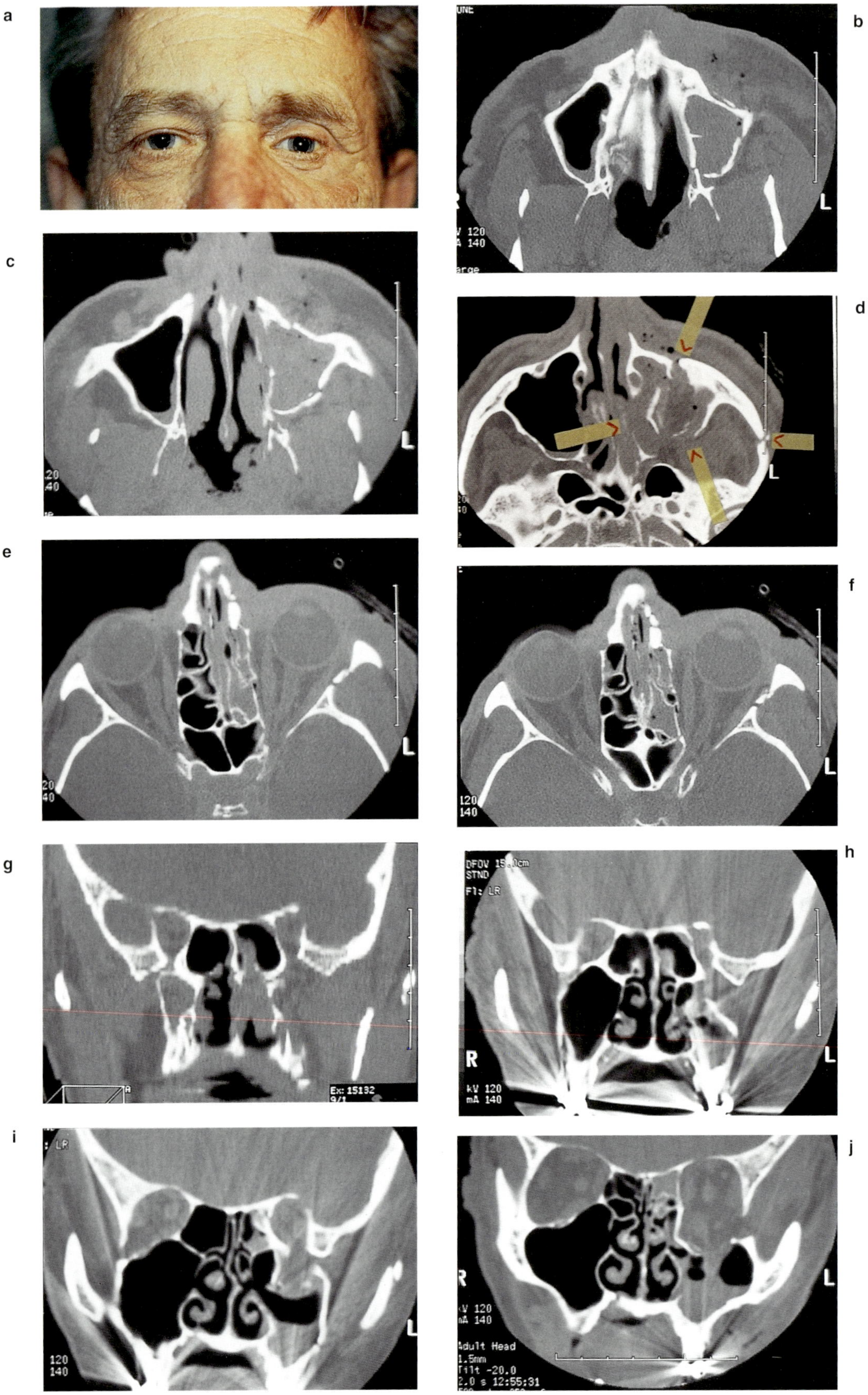
a
b
c
d
e
f
g
h
i
j
DFOV 15.0cm
STND
kV 120
mA 140
Ex: 15132
Adult Head
1.5mm
Tilt -20.0
2.0 s 12:55:31

k

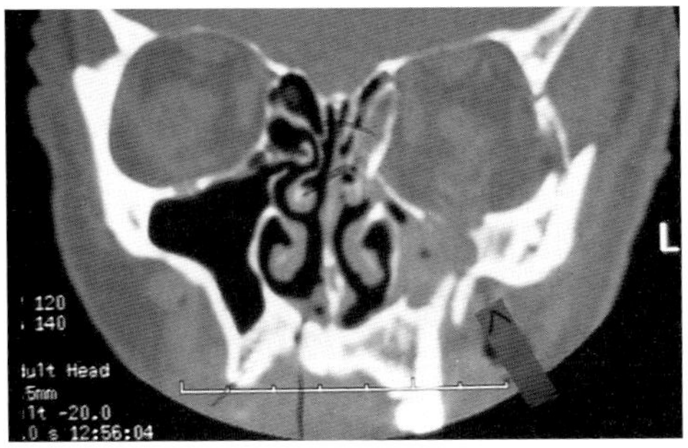

Fig. 20-16. Multilevel facial trauma and traumatic optic neuropathy. (**a**) A spooked horse trampled the chest and face of this 63-year-old patient, who is shown here 4 months postoperatively. Amazingly, he did not lose consciousness and was able to make his own way to the emergency department, where he reported decreased vision in the left eye. Visual acuity was 20/30 in the right eye and 20/70 in the left eye, with subjective red color desaturation and an afferent pupillary defect. He also had restrictive diplopia in 10° upgaze. There was significant point tenderness over the zygomaticomaxillary (ZM) suture, the zygomaticofrontal (ZF) suture, the zygomaticomaxillary complex (ZMC) buttress, and the zygomatic arch (ZA) suture. Trismus, malocclusion, and clinically evident enophthalmos were noted. The optic nerves were flat and without pallor. (**b**) A thin-slice (1.5-mm) axial computed tomography (CT) scan showed multilevel facial fractures, including fracture of the right hard palate and maxillary plate and (**c**) left ZMC. Disruption of the left pterygoid plate classifies this as a "unilateral" Le Fort I fracture. (**d**) A higher slice demonstrates displaced fractures of the inferior rim, the medial and posterior maxillary walls, and the ZA (arrows). Coupled with the fractures of the anterior and medial maxillary walls and pterygoid, involvement of the nasal rim in the area of the nasolacrimal duct constitutes a Le Fort II fracture.

(**e**) A midorbital view shows comminuted nasal and left medial wall fractures, as well as minimally displaced fractures of the left lateral wall. This constitutes a Le Fort III fracture as well as a naso-orbital-ethmoid (NOE) fracture. Because of the complexity of many modern facial fractures, the Le Fort classification often inadequately describes the true extent of the injury. Consequently, many trauma surgeons forego attempting to categorize fractures under this system and opt instead for a simple description of the structures involved. Also evident is a small fracture of the posterior ethmoid-sphenoid plate at the left orbital apex, in the region of the superior orbital fissure and optic canal. This image—just below the optic canal—shows a small bony fragment that displaces the medial rectus but does not appear to directly encroach into the canal. (**f**) This adjoining image shows the optic canal well, almost in its entirety. The bony canal does not appear fractured or physically compromised but may, nonetheless, harbor an invisible, nondisplaced hairline fracture. When evaluating a patient with potential traumatic optic neuropathy, thin-slice images, such as these 1.5-mm views, give the best detail of the optic canal. Similarly, direct, true coronal films are more discriminating than reconstructed views. (**g**) A coronal view at approximately the same level of the orbital apex, reconstructed from the 1.5-mm axial study, shows the step artifact characteristic of reconstructions but no metal scatter artifact from prior dental work. No fracture is convincingly demonstrated in this image. (**h**) On the other hand, this image of the area of the optic canal taken 5 days later is a true coronal view, as evidenced by the smoother bone and tissue contours and dental artifact. A nondisplaced fracture of the posterior ethmoid is clearly seen here. (**i**) This coronal CT scan also shows the extent of the floor fracture, extending posteriorly to the area of the inferior orbital fissure. Complete reduction of all herniating orbital tissues in this region is extremely difficult, and puts the optic nerve at risk from surgical compression and manipulation.

(**j**) More anterior views show the marked disruption of the left floor, with herniation of the orbital tissues into the maxillary sinus below. Rounding of the inferior rectus muscle indicates disruption of the periorbital septae, which keeps the muscle in its naturally elliptical shape (compare with the right eye). Such large fractures require a substantial and rigid plate that can be cantilevered over the maxillary sinus to support the orbital tissues. Many times, the floor plate will have to be secured to the orbital rim. Current options for the plate material include calvarial bone, iliac bone, channeled and unchanneled porous polyethylene sheets, and titanium mesh plates.

(**k**) This image clearly shows the disruption of the left ZMC buttress (arrow) and separation of the ZF suture. It also shows the degree of collapse of the medial orbital wall, floor, and nasolacrimal duct, in the area of the maxillary osteomeatal complex. Disruption of the right maxillary alveolus (grease pencil marks) and dislocation of the base of the nasal septum are also evident. The patient was treated for traumatic optic neuropathy with "megadose" corticosteroids (methylprednisolone 30 mg/kg intravenous loading dose, followed by 15 mg/kg every 6 h for 48 h), with rapid visual improvement to 20/25. Five months later, a trace afferent pupillary defect was still present in the patient's left eye, red desaturation remained slightly diminished, and visual fields showed a slight enlargement of the blind spot. Facial fractures were surgically reduced within 1 week of injury, requiring use of multiple titanium fixation plates. The floor was reconstructed with a porous polyethylene sheet. Residual enophthalmos is evident (see view "a"), but the patient has full ocular motility. Despite a significant amount of left hypoophthalmia, because the hypoglobus is purely vertical with retention of parallel visual axes, the patient does not suffer diplopia. In general, surgical repair of facial fractures can be postponed for 7 to 10 days. However, large fractures such as these should be repaired as soon as is feasible, taking into account such factors as acute swelling and patient stability.

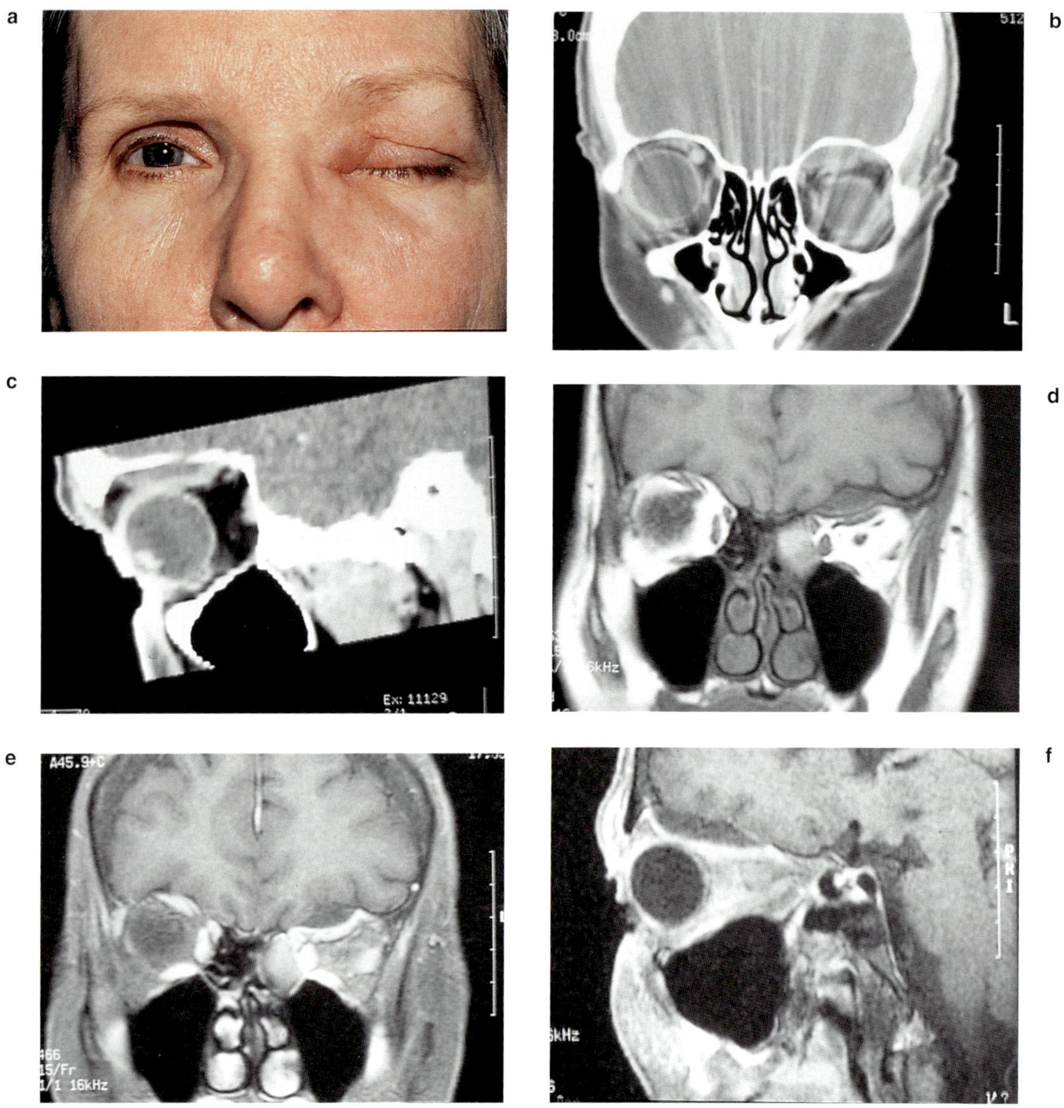

Fig. 20-17. Subperiosteal hemorrhage. (**a**) This patient, a 54-year-old woman, complained of spontaneous orbital fullness and pressure in the left eye. She denied trauma, Valsalva pressure, or metabolic disorder. Examination revealed ptosis, proptosis, hypoglobus, and mild limitation of supraduction. (**b**) This coronal computed tomography (CT) scan demonstrates a homogeneous, biconvex mass along the roof. A thin separation between the levator/superior rectus complex and the mass is suggested but is not conclusive. Notice the dental artifact, which indicates a true (not a reformatted) coronal scan. (**c**) This sagittal CT reformation shows the lenticular mass limited by the periosteum. Notice the lack of dental metal scatter and the step artifact, which is characteristic of reconstructions. A lytic bony defect is seen just above the mass. Despite being reconstructed from thin-slice primary studies, whether this defect is real or merely a reconstruction artifact is difficult to tell here. Such dilemmas are inherent limitations of reformatted views. (**d**) This coronal T1 magnetic resonance imaging (MRI) scan shows a bright, fat–tissue separation between the darker signals of the superior muscle complex and the periosteum, localizing this process to the subperiosteal space. (**e**) Coronal T2 MRI and (**f**) sagittal fat-suppressed T1 MRI images demonstrate a mildly heterogeneous signal from the mass, which is consistent with subperiosteal hemorrhage (SPH). No bony defect of the roof is seen on the sagittal MRI, but the periosteal attachments are once more clearly evident. The patient underwent superior orbitotomy, with evacuation of a liquefied SPH, and did well subsequently.

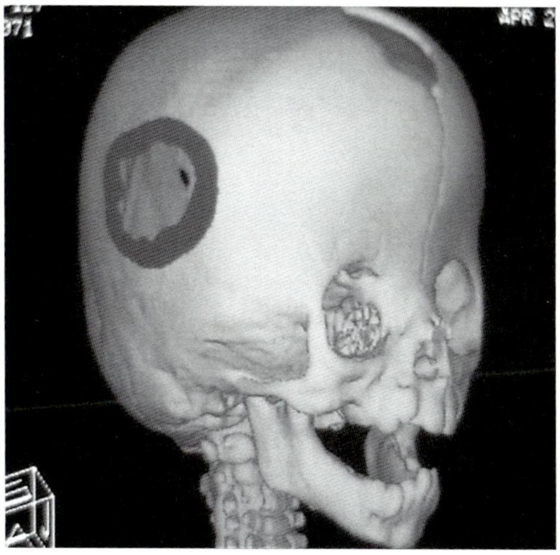

Fig. 20-18. Three-dimensional (3-D) reconstruction is rarely useful in acute trauma because of unacceptable signal dropout and artifact. Nonetheless, it is quite useful in craniofacial evaluation and surgical planning. This 3-D computed tomography (CT) scan clearly shows complete bicoronal craniosynostosis and significant metopic suture narrowing. The anterior fontanel is large. The lateral bony defect laterally is artifactual. Notice the amount of signal void and dropout in the interior orbit. Such artifact makes 3-D reconstructions unreliable in acute trauma.

a b c

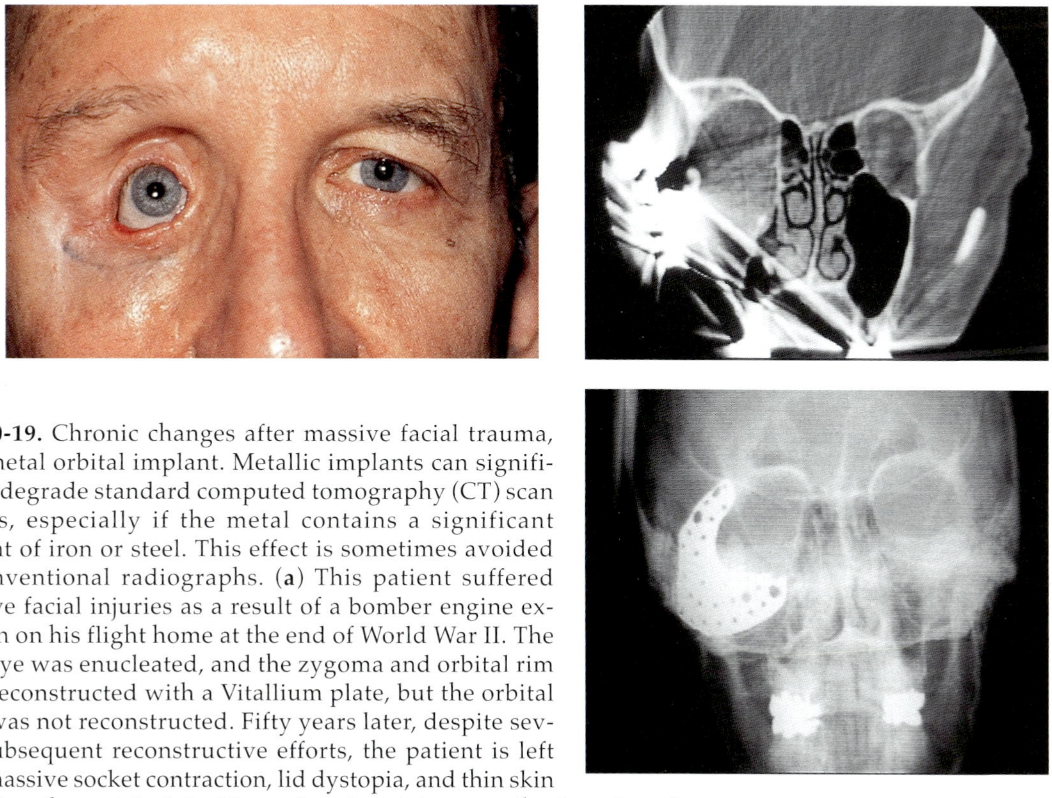

Fig. 20-19. Chronic changes after massive facial trauma, with metal orbital implant. Metallic implants can significantly degrade standard computed tomography (CT) scan images, especially if the metal contains a significant amount of iron or steel. This effect is sometimes avoided by conventional radiographs. (**a**) This patient suffered massive facial injuries as a result of a bomber engine explosion on his flight home at the end of World War II. The right eye was enucleated, and the zygoma and orbital rim were reconstructed with a Vitallium plate, but the orbital floor was not reconstructed. Fifty years later, despite several subsequent reconstructive efforts, the patient is left with massive socket contraction, lid dystopia, and thin skin overlying the metal plate. He can barely retain a prosthesis and prefers not to wear one.

(**b**) The CT scan shows the extent of the orbital disruption, with massively enlarged orbital volume and missing lateral orbital wall. Unfortunately, the Vitallium plate and dental work artifact degrade the signal so significantly that other details are obscured. Trying to mentally reconstruct an image of the metal plate from the fragmented images of the CT scan is exceedingly difficult. (**c**) On the other hand, a plain film radiograph, posteroanterior view, clearly demonstrates the shape, contour, detail, and position of the plate and the dental work. It does not, of course, adequately demonstrate the orbital soft tissues. Orbital reconstruction of such cases is frustrating for both the patient and the surgeon, as the contracted tissues resist advancement, and poor tissue vascularity leads to surgical failure.

a b c d

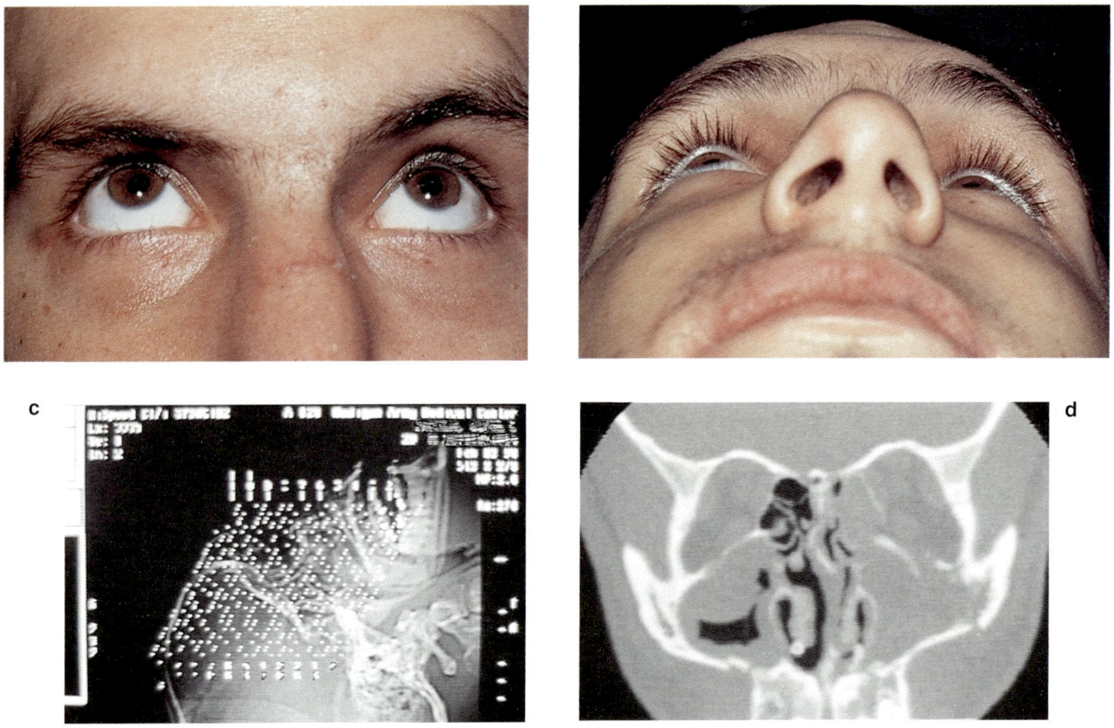

Fig. 20-20. (**a**) During night training maneuvers, this 20-year-old Army Ranger prematurely exited a helicopter 40 feet off the ground and suffered significant head, facial, back, and extremity trauma. After being stabilized at a local hospital, he was evacuated for further evaluation and treatment. On presentation at the medical treatment facility, the patient's ocular examination was surprisingly unremarkable. Large fractures are often nearly asymptomatic, as the bony fragments are either too comminuted or too displaced to cause entrapment. In such cases, the ophthalmologist must have a high index of suspicion, based on associated symptoms. The patient denied diplopia in any field of gaze, including up-gaze, and demonstrated full, unrestricted ocular motility. On close questioning, however, he admitted to sensory dysesthesia over cranial nerve V_2 bilaterally as well as mild trismus. He denied malocclusion. He had significant point tenderness over the zygomaticomaxillary and the zygomaticofrontal sutures as well as over the zygomaticomaxillary complex (ZMC) buttress. (**b**) The left maxilla was significantly depressed.

(**c**) Because of the cervical spine injury, the patient could not be properly positioned, nor could the CT gantry be fully tilted for true coronal scan. This figure shows the image plane. (**d**) The off-axis orbital scan resulted in this atypical image. The angulation is such that the midposterior orbit is seen in the same frame as the maxillary alveolus, the midmaxillary sinus, the zygomatic body, and the ZMC buttress. Compare the orbital contour in these images with those seen in Figures 20-31, 20-40, 20-43, and 20-44. Images such as these are often difficult to interpret. Nevertheless, the image reveals bilateral ZMC fractures and a large, left-floor blowout fracture. Note the rounding of the left inferior rectus, denoting disruption of the periorbita. Also noted are fractures of the maxillary alveolus and nasal septum. The patient underwent an open reduction and internal fixation of his panfacial fractures and did well.

the time required to obtain a scan, CT can nonetheless be slower than conventional radiography. The inability to properly position a casualty with multiple wounds may limit or degrade the study, either in peacetime or in wartime. When considering a mass casualty environment, CT assets may require prioritization, especially when theater evacuation policies are taken into account. Because it is computer dependent, any failure of the support software has an immediate and profound impact on the quality of care delivered, and remedying such problems in the field or under combat conditions is not as easy as during peacetime.

Like any other highly technical equipment, CT requires a skilled operating technician to ensure its proper function and maintenance as well as to provide acceptable studies. CT technicians can often double as general radiology technicians, but the reverse is not necessarily true. Continued operation in the dusty, dirty, hectic environment of the combat zone can be expected to take a toll not only on the physical equipment but also on the CT personnel.

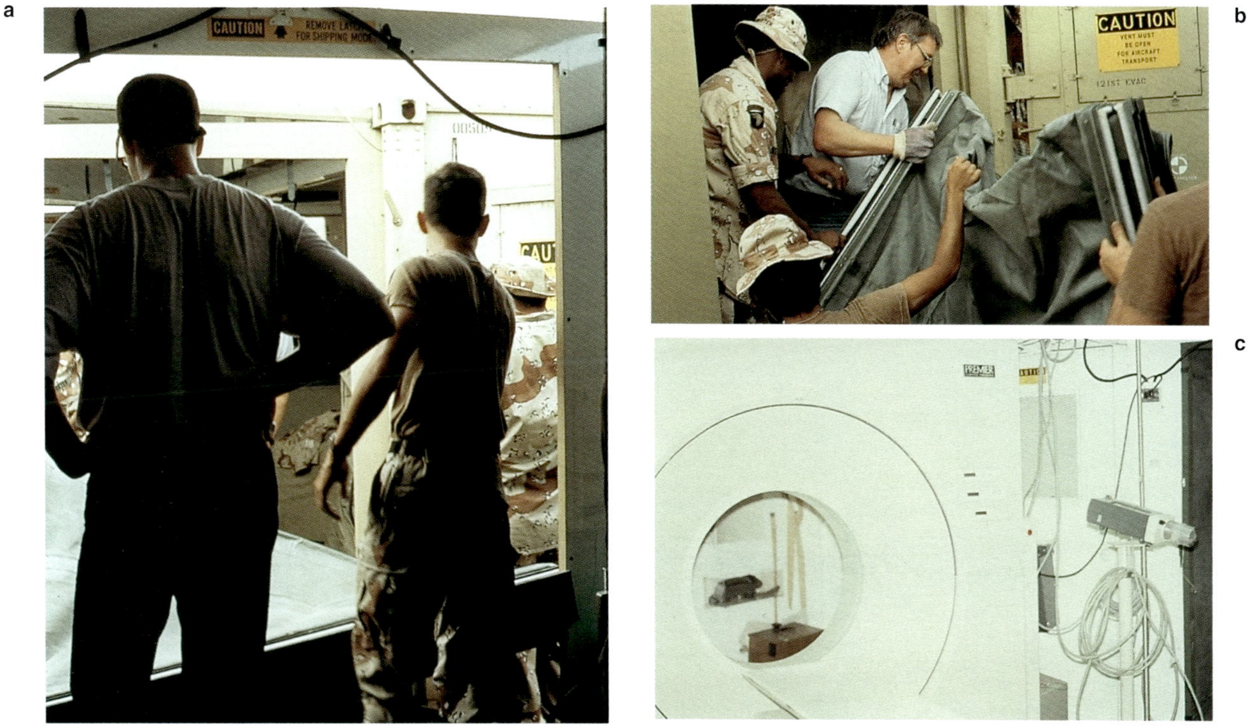

Fig. 20-21. Field computed tomography (CT) scanner. Typically, military ophthalmologists will be deployed to medical units with field CT capability. Physical constraints such as (**a, b**) narrow doorways may impede rapid patient movement and CT evaluation of all traumas in the combat zone. (**c**) Field scanners such as this one, which was deployed to Somalia during Operation Restore Hope (1992–1993), provide fully functional, sophisticated imaging capability.

Magnetic Resonance Imaging

MRI gives excellent soft-tissue detail but suffers in bony resolution. Consequently, its application in orbital trauma is as an adjunctive study rather than the primary imaging modality. It is excellent for revealing many orbital FBs, especially dry wood (green or wet wood may be invisible) and materials that contain little water (few free protons).[9,10] MRI offers the significant advantage of direct multiplanar image formatting (ie, axial, coronal, and sagittal views are generated by one pass through the scanner without the patient's having to be repositioned). However, because of its inherent reliance on strong magnetic fields, MRI cannot be used without first excluding the possibility of metallic FBs via either CT or plain film radiography. Because of the high likelihood of wounds caused by metallic fragments, this consideration applies regardless of which body part is the focus of the study: abdominal wounds cannot be imaged by MRI if there is the possibility of head-and-neck metallic fragments; likewise, a head/orbital injury cannot be imaged if there are other, more peripheral, metallic fragments. MRI is very useful in identifying blood and its breakdown products, and it can help differentiate structures that are homogeneously dense on CT. It is also extremely useful in delineating whether a process is occurring in the subperiosteal space or within the orbit proper (Figure 20-22; also see Figure 20-17).

The advent of MRI brought the anticipation that it would soon supplant CT as the principal imaging modality for all orbital applications, but to date (2002) such has not been the case. MRI is still significantly limited in its ability to identify foreign materials such as glass, plastic, and wet wood. Spatial resolution also remains a limitation, as the thickness of MRI slices still cannot equal the resolution of thin-slice CT. Additionally, because of the way MRI information is obtained, MRI "slices" cannot be overlapped as they are in CT images (eg, spiral-scan slices are seamless, or continuously overlapped), and as a result, some gaps between MRI images always exist. Orbital surface-coil techniques significantly enhance signal detail, but the equip-

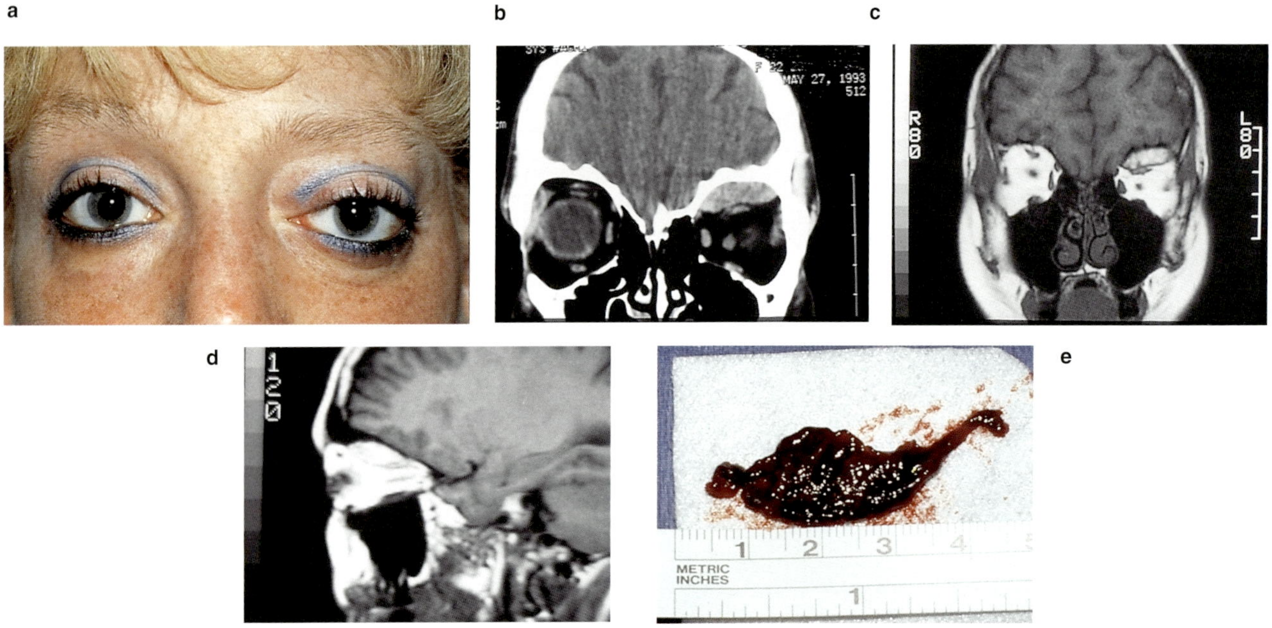

Fig. 20-22. (**a**) This 24-year-old woman complained of acute proptosis in the left eye and diplopia after vomiting. (**b**) Inferior globe displacement implies a superior orbital process, which is confirmed by a coronal computed tomography (CT) scan. Close inspection reveals a fat-density stripe separating the biconvex mass from the levator/superior rectus complex. This finding is virtually pathognomonic for a subperiosteal process. (**c**) A coronal T1 magnetic resonance imaging (MRI) scan verifies the subperiosteal location. A bright fat stripe is interposed between the superior muscle complex and the dark periosteal signal. The mass is noted to be of heterogeneously mixed intensity. (**d**) A sagittal T1 MRI scan demonstrates the subperiosteal nature of the mass. The periosteal attachments—at the internal orbital rim anteriorly and frontosphenoidal suture posteriorly—limit the mass size. This lenticular appearance is characteristic of subperiosteal hemorrhage (SPH). The patient was initially observed conservatively, as many SPHs will resolve spontaneously. However, the proptosis increased approximately 2 weeks after presentation, and repeat CT demonstrated near doubling of the mass size. (**e**) The patient underwent superior orbitotomy and evacuation of the mass, which was found to be an organized hematoma. Such a well-organized SPH can become chronic and precipitate rebleeding, bone destruction, and conversion to a cholesterol granuloma.

ment needed is not universally available. Consequently, most orbital MRI scans are performed with head coils only.

Although MRI has certainly earned its place alongside CT in peacetime orbital trauma management, one of the greatest current limitations to the use of MRI for orbital trauma in the combat theater is the physical size of the magnet and the strength of the magnetic field generated. Magnets of 0.5 tesla (T) may be sufficient for general-purpose imaging, but orbital imaging demands magnet strengths of 1.5 T. The stronger the field strength, the better the resolution and detail. Most magnets of this strength are located in fixed facilities; mobile scanners use weaker magnets. As the magnet field strength increases, so too does the requirement for cooling the magnet. Again, the physical demands of space and technology—the magnet cannot simply be turned off and on—may limit the ready mobility of the larger scanners that are needed for orbital application.

Many considerations compound the impracticality of urgent MRI, especially in a combat environment. Metal objects cannot be brought into the immediate area of the magnet; consequently, the scanner may have to be located away from the rest of the field hospital and away from other metal objects (eg, motor pool, weapons room). Combat and medical personnel must remove any metallic personal items, such as load-bearing-equipment, weapons, identification tags, and the like. If the patient is intubated and reliant on ventilator support, the ventilator must be nonmagnetic. Positioning an intubated patient inside the scanner poses its own difficulties. Additionally, all of the technical and personnel concerns mentioned for CT are applicable for MRI.

MRI has other drawbacks as well. In contrast to the X-ray images obtained by CT, the images created by MRI are derived from radio signals emitted by the relaxation of radio-excited atoms (usually hydrogen). The inherent weakness of these signals dictates that the receiving antennas be placed very close to the "transmitter" (ie, the patient). This requirement explains the claustrophobic environment of the MRI scanner and the surface coils. In such close confines, physical motion easily creates radio-signal artifact and degradation. To counter the claustrophobia, "open" scanners that do not completely enclose the patient have been developed. Unfortunately, the larger opening decreases the field strength of the magnet below that needed for acceptable orbital scans.

Perhaps the single most formidable impediment to MRI in the acute trauma setting is the time required for scans. CT scan times have been dramatically reduced (especially with the advent of helical scanners), but despite improvements in software, MRI techniques still dictate long periods of immobility inside a claustrophobic enclosure. Although imaging protocols have advanced materially beyond the traditional T1 and T2 images, the length of scan times still depends on excitation times, repetition times, echo times, and the number of images needed. This generally means that trauma patients are reasonable candidates for MRI only if they are—or after they have become—medically stable. When considered in the setting of trying to deliver trauma care urgently, MRI is still relegated to the role of an adjunct study. Improved software and scanning techniques may be able to decrease scan times, but until then, MRI will continue to have a limited role in acute trauma management.

Conventional (Plain Film) Radiography

Plain film radiography may be the Model T of imaging: it is not fancy or glamorous, it is cheap and somewhat clunky, but in a pinch, it is better than nothing. It shows bones adequately but is poor for visualizing soft tissues. It shows metallic FBs well and quickly, but most other types of FBs are missed or lost in overlying shadows. Given the increased reliance on CT and MRI, the fine art of reading plain films for orbital trauma is being lost. However, plain film radiography is still the cheapest of all the modalities, and the equipment is technologically unsophisticated, ubiquitous, has known performance characteristics, and is easy to set up, move, and maintain.

Occasionally, plain film radiography actually gives a better image of an FB than CT does (see Figure 20-19), especially in the presence of large metal FBs, which induce considerable metallic scatter on CT (Figures 20-23 through 20-25). In this setting, plain films are often a valuable adjunct to CT. Bone-free dental films or hypocycloidal tomograms can also be used when looking for small, metallic FBs. The biggest drawbacks of plain film are its very poor demonstration of tissue relationships and detail, the small number of images, and the inability

a

b

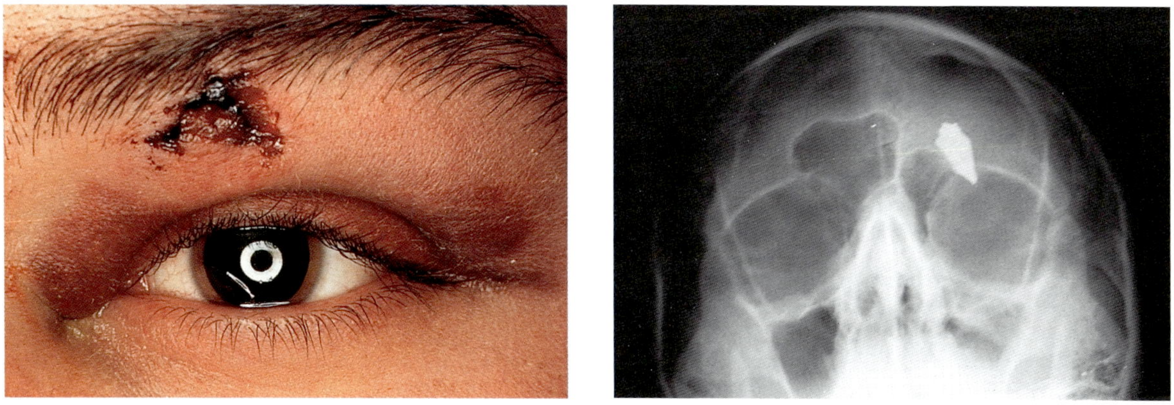

Fig. 20-23. Many orbital foreign bodies (FBs) are the result of easily identified events. (**a**) This 21-year-old soldier was standing next to a campfire during a field exercise. Other soldiers had thrown unexpended M-16 blank ammunition into the fire. After one explosion, the patient felt an object strike his left brow (see Figure 20-24). In addition to the obvious lid laceration, examination showed corneal contusion and edema but no other globe trauma. (**b**) A plain film radiograph (Waters's view) showed a large metal orbital FB in the anterior orbit. Plain film is useful for demonstrating the number, shape, and size of such foreign bodies but is insufficient for determining ocular penetration. Because of its anterior location, this FB was removed without complication. In general, however, metallic FBs—especially those in the deep orbit—should be left alone.

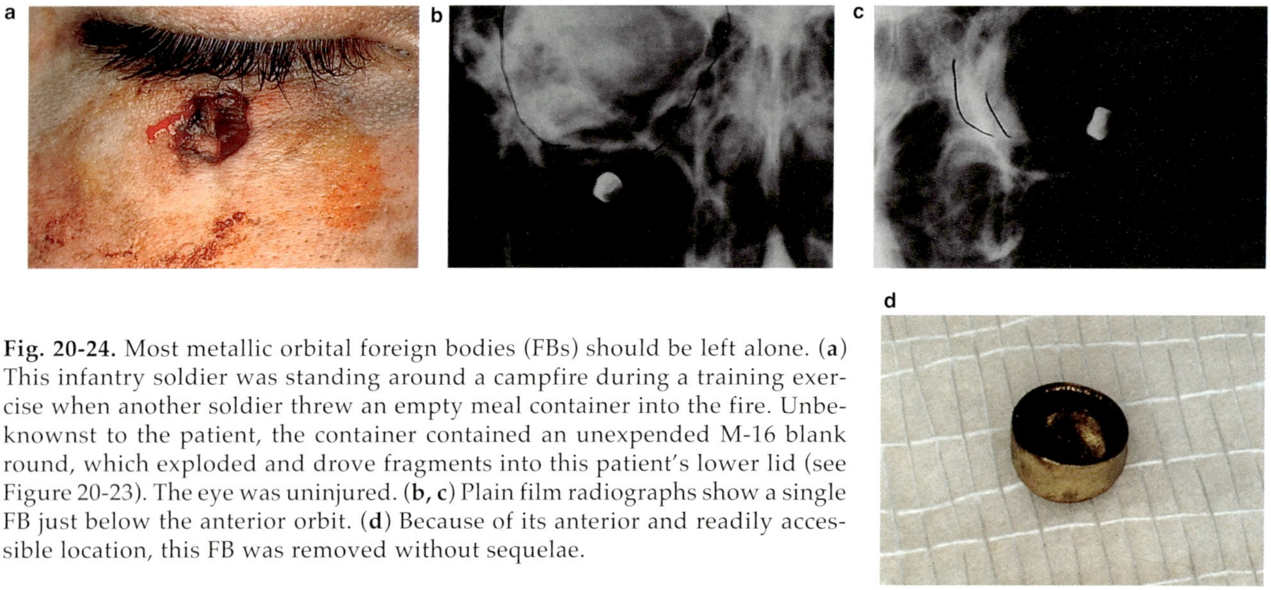

Fig. 20-24. Most metallic orbital foreign bodies (FBs) should be left alone. (a) This infantry soldier was standing around a campfire during a training exercise when another soldier threw an empty meal container into the fire. Unbeknownst to the patient, the container contained an unexpended M-16 blank round, which exploded and drove fragments into this patient's lower lid (see Figure 20-23). The eye was uninjured. (b, c) Plain film radiographs show a single FB just below the anterior orbit. (d) Because of its anterior and readily accessible location, this FB was removed without sequelae.

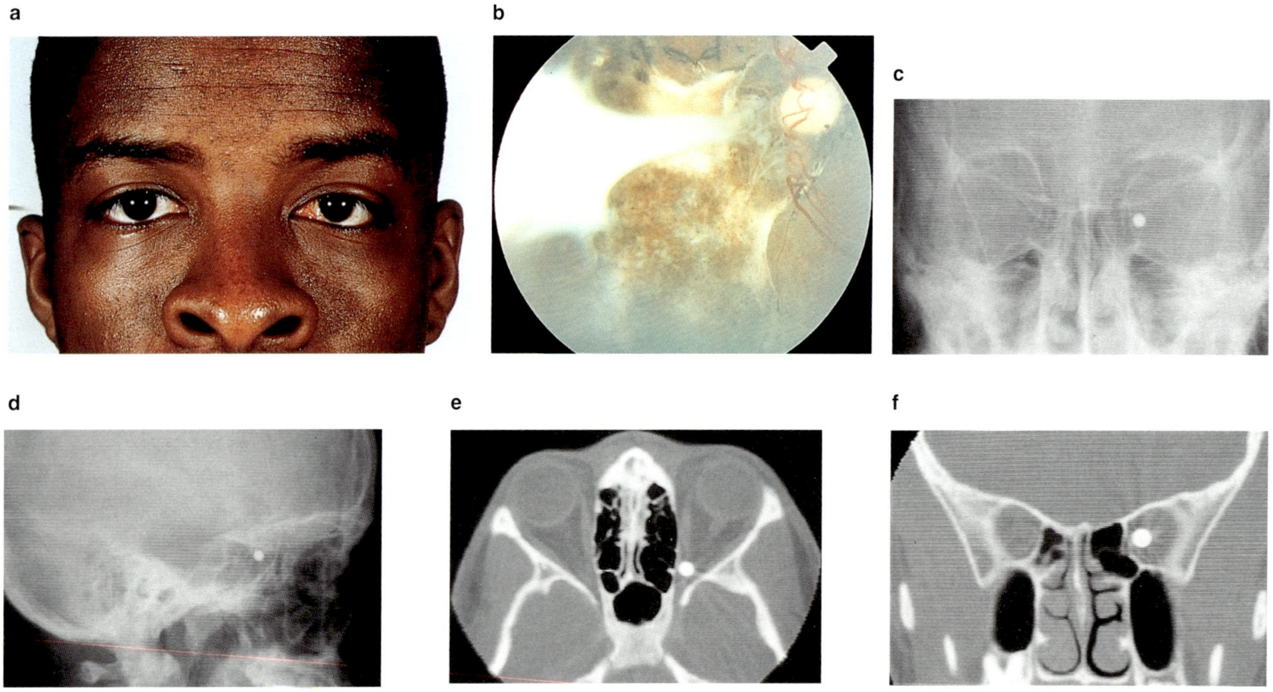

Fig. 20-25. Forgotten orbital foreign body (FB). Most injuries that produce orbital FBs could have been prevented had any kind of spectacle lens been worn. BB guns and air rifles, in particular, are common causes of orbital FBs. Ocular damage and loss of vision in these cases is usually severe but occasionally is surprisingly minimal. (a) This 23-year-old soldier presented with diplopia and 20/20 vision in both eyes but with (b) intraocular evidence of chronic retinitis sclopetaria and optic nerve pallor in the left eye, although he denied previous ocular trauma. (c, d) Plain film radiographs show a spherical, metallic FB—a BB—at the orbital apex. When shown the radiographs, the patient vaguely recalled having been struck by a BB as a child but denied receiving any medical treatment. Notice how well the plain film radiographs show the shape and character of the FB but how poorly they demonstrate tissue relationships. Before the advent of computed tomography (CT), localization of this FB would have been performed via Sweet or Comberg techniques. (e, f) The CT scans show the BB lodged at the orbital apex between the left medial rectus and optic nerve, in the region of the superior orbital fissure. In contrast to the plain film radiographs, the CTs show significant metal scatter artifact but excellent tissue relationships. FBs such as these are best managed by simple observation. This patient eventually developed progressive visual field loss and gaze-evoked amaurosis, prompting craniotomy and removal of the BB. Fortunately, he retained 20/20 vision and the visual field loss reversed. Photographs d and e: Reproduced from Otto DS, Nixon KL, Mazzoli RA, et al. Chorioretinitis sclopetaria from BB ex memoria. *Ophthalmic Surg Lasers*. 2001;32:152–155.

for computer manipulation. Therefore, its uses in the planning and management of significant orbital trauma are severely limited. Nonetheless, some cursory knowledge of plain film techniques (such as Comberg's or Sweet's localization of IOFBs) and of which plain film views give the most information (Waters's and Caldwell's views for the orbital floor, medial wall, and rims) can serve more than historical interest—especially during combat, when both the CT and MRI scanners are no longer functioning.[11]

ORBITAL HEMORRHAGE

As stated previously, hemorrhage almost constantly accompanies orbital trauma. Hemorrhage can occur in three locations: the intraconal space, the extraconal space, and the subperiosteal space (Figure 20-26). Retrobulbar hemorrhage can be a devastating occurrence, leading to blindness quickly after the trauma if not addressed promptly and completely. Consequently, vision *must* be checked as soon as possible after the injury. But because bleeding can continue or resume long after the initial injury, vision must be vigilantly followed, even after the initial evaluation. Although orbital fracture (especially floor or medial wall fracture) might be assumed to allow automatic decompression of orbital hemorrhage into the adjacent sinus, in fact, clotting of the blood within the sinus can effectively prevent drainage of recurrent bleeding and therefore lead to renewed visual danger.

Treatment requires prompt evacuation and decompression of the space in which the hemorrhage has occurred. Medical treatments, such as large doses of intravenous corticosteroids or osmotics (such as mannitol), can aid in the management of hemorrhage, but immediate surgical decompression of the orbit remains the mainstay of treatment. Immediate canthotomy and cantholysis can be sight-saving and can be performed without anesthesia if urgently needed. This releases the soft-tissue tether of the lids, which restricts passive anterior decompression and allows the globe to proptose as needed. On sufficient release, the surgeon feels the lower lid swing away freely, the orbit should become less tense, and blood should escape freely. Occasionally, however, no fluid escapes, even after the lid has been well detached. This can occur if the hemorrhage is sequestered in the intraconal space or if the hemorrhage is subperiosteal. If no blood escapes and the orbit remains tense, then the deep intraconal orbit should be opened so that the hemorrhagic pocket is decompressed. This procedure is best performed with blunt tenotomy scissors positioned in the inferolateral quadrant (between the lateral and the inferior rectus muscles) and directed posteriorly. With blunt dissection, the scissors are opened widely until the intermuscular septum is opened, orbital fat prolapses, and blood drains. If no relief of orbital tension ensues, the hemorrhage may be located in the subperiosteal space.

Subperiosteal hemorrhage (SPH) occurs most commonly on the orbital roof, but it can occur along any bony wall (see Figures 20-17 and 20-22). It can be caused by direct blunt trauma to the orbit (eg, fist strike) or other head traumas (eg, extension of subgaleal hematomas of the forehead and skull). SPH has also been reported as a consequence of metabolic diseases such as sickle cell anemia and

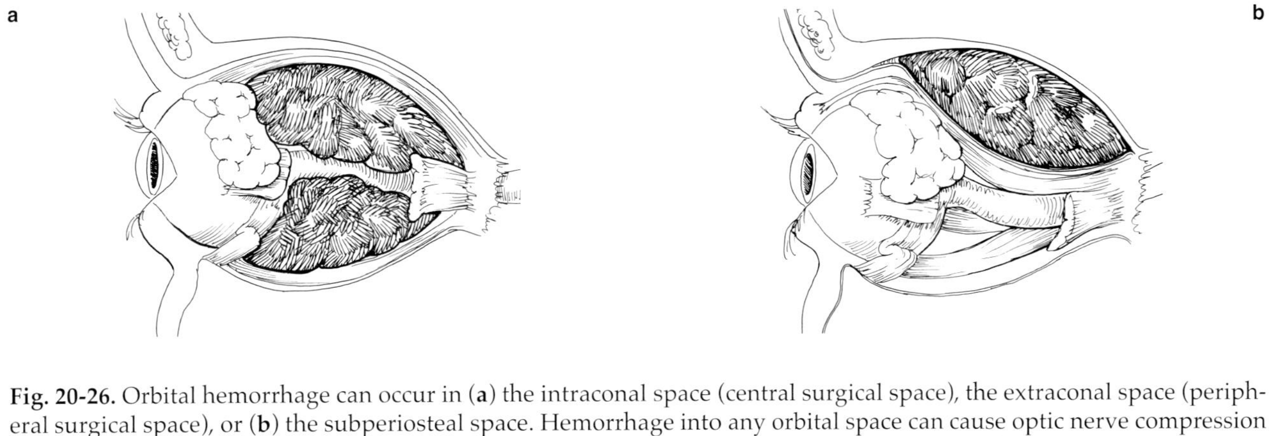

Fig. 20-26. Orbital hemorrhage can occur in (**a**) the intraconal space (central surgical space), the extraconal space (peripheral surgical space), or (**b**) the subperiosteal space. Hemorrhage into any orbital space can cause optic nerve compression and loss of vision. Patients with orbital hemorrhage must be evacuated promptly if vision is threatened. Drawings prepared for this textbook by Gary Wind, MD, Uniformed Services University of the Health Sciences, Bethesda, Md.

a

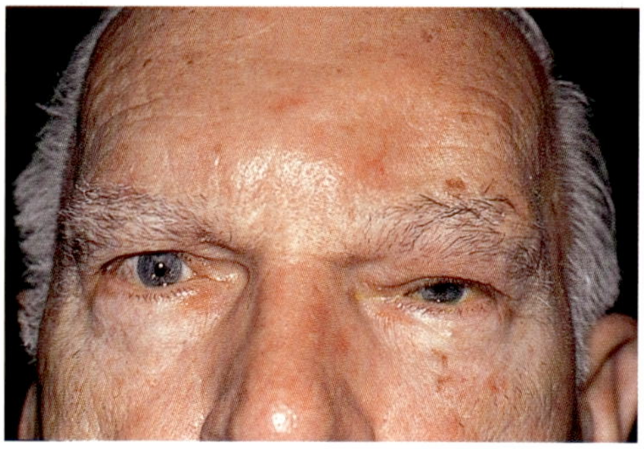

b

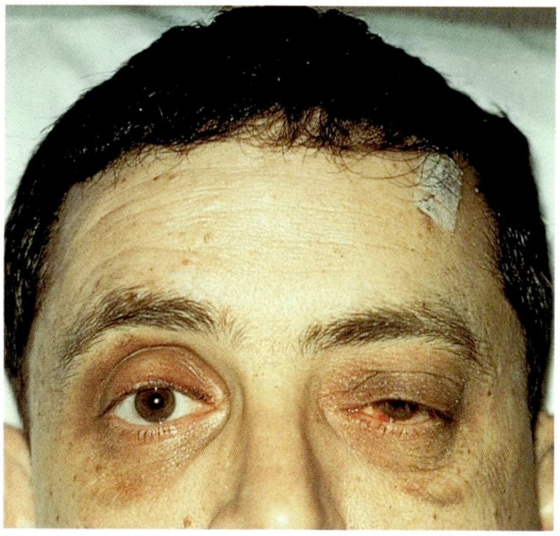

c

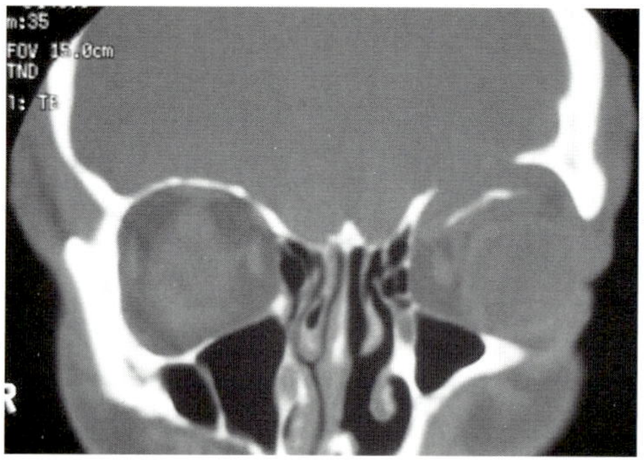

Fig. 20-27. Roof fractures with subperiosteal hemorrhage. Fractures of the orbital roof are rare in adults, and are indicative of high-energy injury. Surprisingly, not all patients are neurosurgically unstable, and many will present to the ophthalmologist for initial evaluation. (**a**) This 65-year-old man presented to the ophthalmology clinic complaining of diplopia after falling from a ladder. He was neurologically intact, despite the obvious depressed frontal fracture. The patient had restricted motility in up-gaze and dysesthesia over cranial nerve V_1. A computed tomography (CT) scan revealed a displaced roof and frontal sinus fracture. He was referred to a neurosurgeon for evaluation and treatment.

(**b**) This 45-year-old soldier struck his left brow and forehead in a motor vehicle accident. He never lost consciousness. On presentation, he complained of vertical diplopia, ptosis, and proptosis in the left eye. He was numb over left V_1 and had pulsatile proptosis. (**c**) A CT scan demonstrated an isolated fracture of the orbital roof with an associated subperiosteal hemorrhage. Such fractures are usually associated with significant intracranial or sinus injury and require neurosurgical and otorhinolaryngological evaluation.

scurvy; barotrauma from activities like strenuous Valsalva pressure (from weightlifting, childbirth, and vomiting), or rapid decompression (from underwater diving and explosive aeronautical decompression); and remote chest compression.[12–15] SPH is commonly associated with orbital fractures (Figure 20-27) and is best verified by CT and MRI. Classically, the mass assumes a lenticular shape, conforming to the bony orbital plate on one side and the displaced periosteum on the other. Its extension is limited by the periosteal attachments to the bony sutures. Orbital structures are displaced centrally. A clean fat stripe that separates the rectus muscles from the mass is often seen, distinguishing SPH from infectious subperiosteal abscess, in which the tissues adjacent to the muscles and mass are inflamed (see Figures 20-17 and 20-22). MRI characteristics will otherwise vary with the age of the hemorrhage and the strength of the magnet used. While some authors have recommended percutaneous needle aspiration of the hematoma, we caution against this practice—especially if the roof is involved—because of the inability to ensure against accidental perforation of the roof and subsequent neurological injury. Rather, we prefer orbitotomy and evacuation under direct visualization (after confirmation by CT).

Like other orbital hemorrhages, most subperiosteal hematomas will resolve on their own over time. However, like subdural hematomas of the central nervous system, they can become chronic processes, with episodic expansion from rebleeding. Chronic subperiosteal hematomas can transform into cholesterol granulomas (phantom tumors of the orbit), which are capable of large-scale bony destruction. Consequently, although acute hematomas can be managed conservatively, they must be (1) observed for expansion and (2) evacuated if (*a*) vision is threatened or (*b*) resolution does not occur within 3 to 6 weeks.[16]

ORBITAL FOREIGN BODIES

The diagnosis and treatment of IOFBs is covered in Chapter 14, Management of Penetrating Injuries with a Retained Intraocular Foreign Body. This section briefly covers the diagnosis and management of orbital FBs that do not involve the eye itself.

FBs are a frequent cause of orbital trauma. Small objects and missiles, which would be harmless were they to impact anywhere else on the body, are capable of creating devastating injury around the eye and orbit. Had the victims been wearing *any* kind of eye protection, the great majority of ocular and orbital FB injuries would have been prevented.[10,17,18] Slivers of glass, plastic, metal, or vegetable matter—whether by-products of motor vehicle or other accidents, on-the-job hazards, metal-on-metal impacts, or the result of intentional harm via combat or other assault—are all capable of inflicting serious orbital injury (see Figures 20-23, 20-24, and 20-25). Most orbital FBs themselves are inert—with the notable exception of vegetable FBs—and cause few long-term problems solely by their presence, but the damage they cause in the acute setting can be impressive and intimidating to the ophthalmologist who is charged with the initial evaluation and management of the injuries (Figure 20-28).

It is not difficult to maintain a high index of suspicion for an orbital FB when the history is highly suggestive. Well-recounted histories of metal-on-metal contact, the sensation that "something flew into my eye," "I got hit by a branch," "I stepped on a landmine," and so forth are not to be disbelieved, and they should quickly prompt the search for a retained orbital FB in addition to the treatment of any obvious injury (Figures 20-29 and 20-30). A much higher index of suspicion must be maintained when the history is vague or the casualty has combined traumas (eg, blunt trauma and multiple superficial lacerations from a motor vehicle accident,

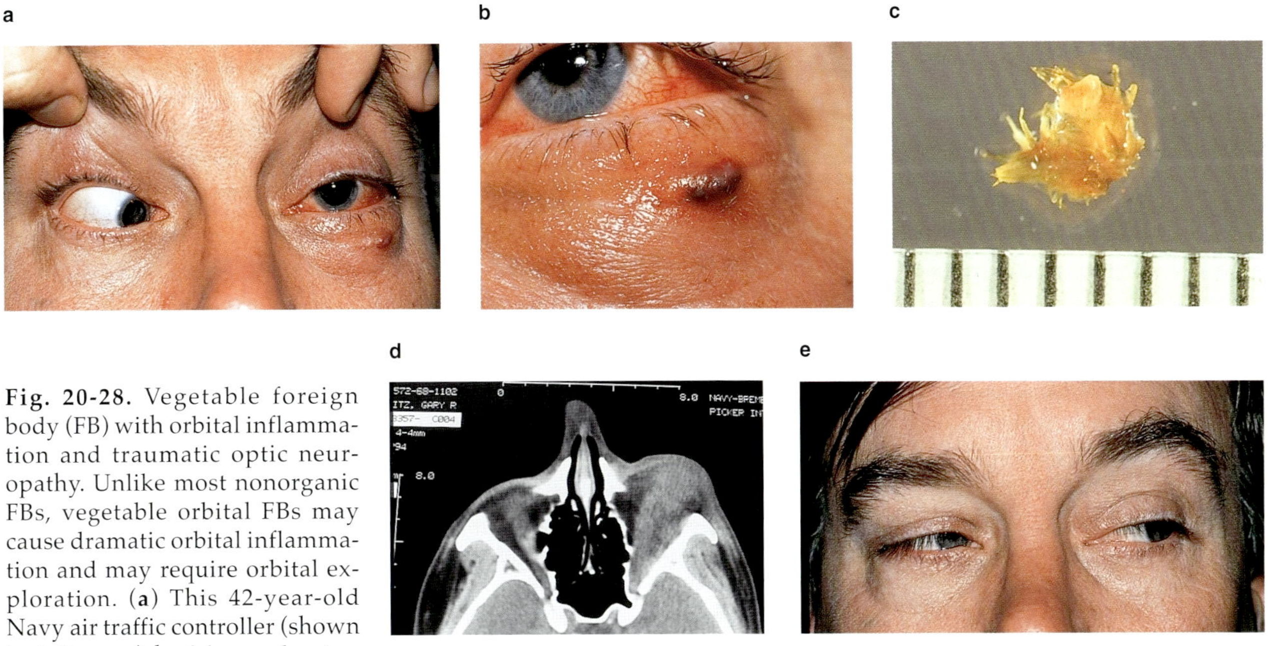

Fig. 20-28. Vegetable foreign body (FB) with orbital inflammation and traumatic optic neuropathy. Unlike most nonorganic FBs, vegetable orbital FBs may cause dramatic orbital inflammation and may require orbital exploration. (**a**) This 42-year-old Navy air traffic controller (shown in left gaze) had been clearing land when he removed his safety goggles to hand-cut a vine-maple tree branch. The branch recoiled, striking him in the left eye and orbit. He presented for care 1 week later with increasing orbital pain, decreased vision (20/50), a subtle afferent pupillary defect, a tense proptotic orbit, and decreased motility. (**b**) A suppurative pustule was explored, revealing (**c**) a small vegetable FB, which was later identified as moss. Serial computed tomography (CT) and magnetic resonance imaging (MRI) scans failed to demonstrate any other frank FBs. (**d**) This CT image shows dramatic inflammatory "dirty fat" and proptosis. The patient was treated with systemic megadose corticosteroids (see Figure 20-16) and antibiotics and underwent exploratory orbitotomy, which yielded more small moss fragments. After 1 year, motility and vision were essentially normal. (**e**) Although slight optic atrophy, mild color desaturation, and a subtle afferent pupillary defect persisted, he retained 20/25 vision.

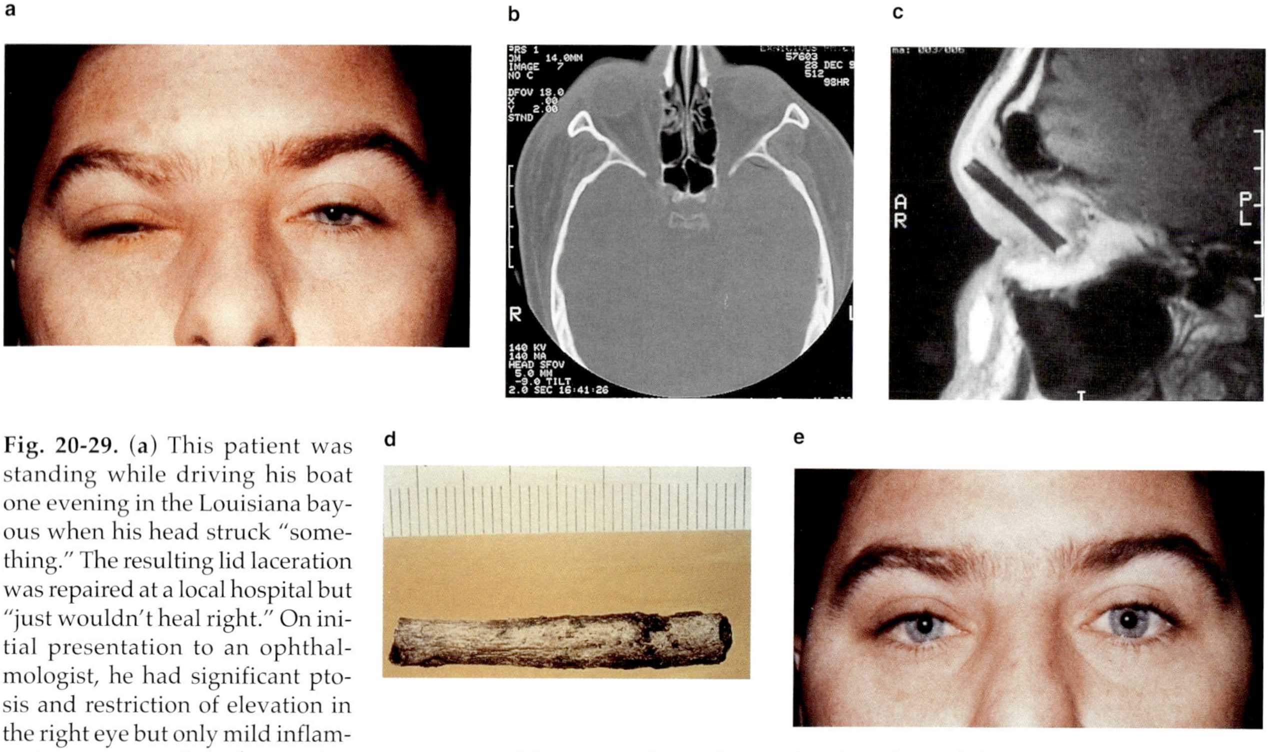

Fig. 20-29. (**a**) This patient was standing while driving his boat one evening in the Louisiana bayous when his head struck "something." The resulting lid laceration was repaired at a local hospital but "just wouldn't heal right." On initial presentation to an ophthalmologist, he had significant ptosis and restriction of elevation in the right eye but only mild inflammatory signs and erythema. An entrance wound is seen in the region of the right brow. (**b**) A noncontrast computed tomography (CT) scan shows a lucency along the medial wall just posterior to the nasolacrimal sac, with a zone of surrounding inflammation. (**c**) A magnetic resonance imaging (MRI) T1 image clearly demonstrates a large, retained, orbital foreign body (FB). (**d**) At orbitotomy, a large wooden FB was removed. Dry wood is often visible on T1 MRI scans, owing to the lack of hydrogen protons. (**e**) The same patient, 6 months postoperatively.

or massive blunt injury and hemorrhage/ecchymosis from unknown mechanism) (see Figures 20-4, 20-9). Even penetration by a known implement can create retained FBs, such as the broken-off tip of a knife (see Figure 20-11). A typically misleading history is that of "I was poked in the eye with this pencil (or stick, nail), but I pulled it right out, all in one piece. See? Here it is."

Because the orbit is so vascular, hemorrhage is always a sensitive indicator of deep orbital injury. Medial penetration is especially noted for brisk hemorrhage because of the location of the anterior and posterior ethmoidal arteries at the frontoethmoidal junction. Certainly, hemorrhagic chemosis should bring to mind not only the possibility of globe rupture but also of orbital hemorrhage secondary to one or more FBs. On the other hand, many small, sharp missiles (such as shards of metal, glass, and plastic) can penetrate deep into the orbit without notable outward signs. Many patients who are struck by FBs but have few outward signs acutely will forget the incident and may never seek medical care unless other symptoms arise later (see Figure 20-25). Vegetable FBs may incite inflammatory reactions long after the entrance wound has healed. In these cases, it is incumbent on the ophthalmologist to *always* suspect a retained FB.

Unfortunately, even if the suspicion for an FB is high, detecting it is still difficult. As sophisticated as imaging modalities are, many FBs still escape detection by even the most sensitive instruments. Detection is highly variable and depends on the density of the material, its CT number (Hounsfield units), the amount of air and water it contains, its ferromagnetic character, and its size. Some FBs with high CT numbers, such as some glass (eg, windshield glass), metal, and bone, may be readily visible on plain film radiographs, especially on hypocycloidal views. Other types of glass and most plastics—including that from which plastic landmines are made—may be invisible to plain film, CT, and MRI. Some FBs that would otherwise be visible can be camouflaged by accompanying hemorrhage and inflammation. In general, CT is the best first choice for imaging, with MRI a strong adjunct.

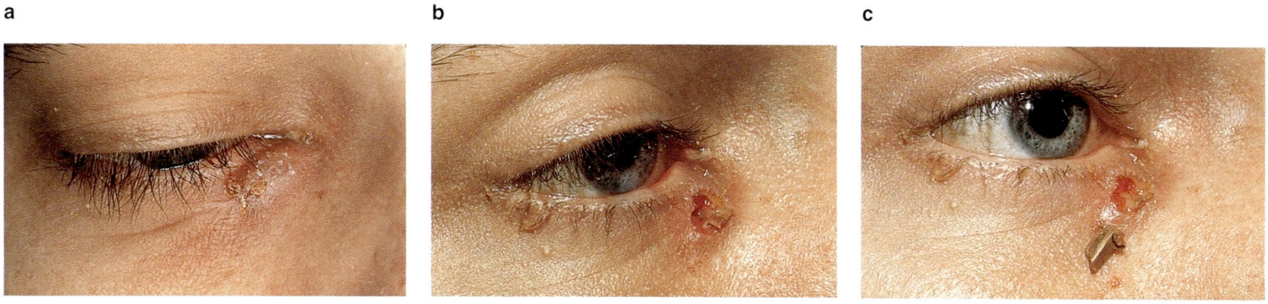

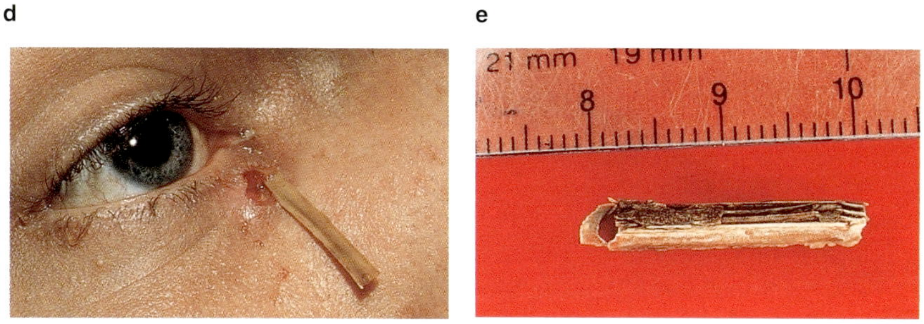

Fig. 20-30. Vegetable orbital foreign body (FB). Organic FBs can lead to significant orbital complications. (**a**) This 19-year-old Army Ranger student was on night patrol in Florida when he tripped and fell, feeling something strike him below the right eye. He experienced immediate pain and total loss of vision. On return to his home station after a week at a local hospital, vision was no light perception with an amaurotic pupil and total paralysis of motility. Although a healing laceration was noted in the nasojugal area, surprisingly few signs of orbital inflammation were found. Serial, fine-cut computed tomography (CT) scans searching for a retained FB were negative. (This injury predated the wide availability of magnetic resonance imaging.) (**b, c**) Three weeks later, the lid laceration dehisced and several small wooden splinters extruded spontaneously. (**d, e**) Further exploration of the wound produced the wooden FB seen in these photographs. The wound healed permanently, but the patient was left with a blind, immobile eye.

As stated earlier, MRI cannot be the first mode of imaging without first ruling out a metallic FB, and plain film studies are of little help for all but metallic FBs. Ultrasound is of proven value in the diagnosis of intraocular FBs but is of little benefit in orbital diagnosis, having limited penetration beyond the anterior third of the orbit.[7,8,10,18,19]

Imaging of FBs is subject to several important limitations. Plastic and vegetable FBs are notoriously difficult to detect either on CT or MRI. In particular, dry wood—because it lacks the water content of fresh or green wood—can initially manifest as an air density on CT. However, the density is not as dark as the free air seen in orbital emphysema (or compared with the sinus air); rather, it is typically a "partial air density"—a mid-density lucency between the densities of free air and water (see Figure 20-29). Wood and other vegetable matter is often surrounded by focal inflammation, and many scans have incorrectly been interpreted as "intraorbital air with surrounding inflammation," even though *air within the orbit* NEVER *causes "surrounding inflammation."* Another common indicator of vegetable matter is a finding of a linear intraorbital density on CT; however, *there are no linear structures in the orbit.* The ophthalmologist must personally review these films.

Modern digital CT displays that do not rely on conventional film processing allow active computer manipulation of the window / contrast levels at the desktop, but this must be done with caution. Such manipulation may allow the FB to be seen more clearly when the levels are changed, but when actively "playing with the contrast" it is possible to overcall or undercall any abnormality: nonexistent lesions can be "created," and existing lesions can be erased. Because the low water content of dry wood means few free protons for radioexcitation, on MRI, dry wood can often easily be identified as a dark mass against the bright fat of T1 images (see Figure 20-29).[9,10] Similar properties can help identify some plastics as well, but every material has its own, unique MRI characteristics. Fresh vegetable FBs, such as green wood, are much more difficult to detect, as the higher water content allows the material to blend in much more readily into the water densities of fat and orbital hemorrhage on CT images. Likewise, the high proton content of fresh wood will diminish the contrast on T1 MR images. With time, dry wood may hydrate, and the CT and MR characteristics will become more like wet wood. Such chronicity is usually accompanied by chronic orbital findings clinically, such as chronic redness or pain, or chronic drainage and fistula formation. Some chronic vegetable FBs will extrude spontaneously (see Figure 20-30).[8–10,18,19]

ORBITAL FRACTURES

Le Fort Midfacial Fractures

The well-known traditional classification scheme for midfacial fractures was developed by the 19th-century French surgeon and gynecologist Léon C. Le Fort, after he observed the patterns of injuries created by experimentally battering the heads of corpses. Since Le Fort's time, with the development of the motorcycle and other high-speed conveyances, and with the increased availability of handguns and semiautomatic, military-style weapons, the energies associated with facial traumas have increased dramatically. Because of the complexity of modern fractures and the recent progress in diagnostic and management techniques, Le Fort's traditional classification is neither very useful nor universally applicable in acute orbital trauma management. Frankly, most modern facial fractures do not fall neatly into one of Le Fort's three categories. Nevertheless, it is worthwhile for ophthalmologists to be familiar with the classification, as it conveys a common and easily understood description about the complexity and areas involved in a fracture, even if the fracture does not fit a "pure" Le Fort category. Currently, the classification scheme is more useful in the field of reconstructive craniofacial and maxillofacial surgery, as it accurately describes the various *planned* osteotomies performed in facial reconfiguration.

Common to all three Le Fort classes—and integral to the diagnosis of a true Le Fort fracture—is involvement of the pterygoid plates: all Le Fort fractures extend internally to involve the pterygoids. If the pterygoids are intact, then the fracture is *not* a true Le Fort fracture but can be considered an incomplete Le Fort. Extensive trauma can involve multiple Le Fort levels, usually asymmetrically.[2,4]

For additional information on the categories of Le Fort fractures, see Chapter 18, Injuries to the Face and Neck, in *Anesthesia and Perioperative Care of the Combat Casualty,* another volume in the Textbooks of Military Medicine series.[20]

Le Fort I: Low Transverse Maxillary Fractures

A horizontal fracture across the maxillary ridge and alveolus at the base of the nasal (pyriform) aperture is a classic Le Fort I fracture. This creates a free-floating maxilla. These fractures are the only ones that do not involve the orbit. Le Fort I fractures are created intentionally during orthognathic maxillary surgery (see Figure 20-16).

Le Fort II: Pyramidal Fractures

Fractures at the Le Fort II level (Figure 20-31) roughly parallel the pyriform aperture. Bilateral fractures extend across the bridge of the nose to involve the nasal bones. They also involve the medial orbital floor and rim. Consequently, the nasolacrimal duct is usually damaged, leading to traumatic dacryostenosis (see Figure 20-16).

Le Fort III: Craniofacial Dysjunction

Le Fort III fractures—total separation of the facial bones from the cranial base—are the result of significant trauma energies. Facial disarticulation occurs at the zygomatic arch, the lateral rim and wall, the posterior orbit and roof, the upper rim, and the root of the nose. Given the extent of orbital involvement, ocular symptoms are common. Because of the proximity of the fracture to the optic canal, the devastating complication of optic canal and nerve injury is not unusual. Nasolacrimal damage is also common. Such dysjunction is necessarily created intentionally during reconstructive craniofacial surgery for dysostotic syndromes, such as Apert's and Crouzon's syndromes (see Figures 20-16 and 20-31).

Orbital Floor

The isolated floor fracture (blowout) is the most common fracture that presents primarily to the ophthalmologist. It occurs after low- or moderate-energy impact, such as fist strikes, sports impacts, and injury with small missiles such as balls (Figure 20-32).[1,3,4] The most common location of the fracture is the posteromedial floor, because (*a*) the bone in this area is the thinnest of the floor and (*b*) it lacks the medial wall's corrugated reinforcement of the ethmoid air cells (see Figure 20-15). Various theories have been forwarded to explain the mechanics of

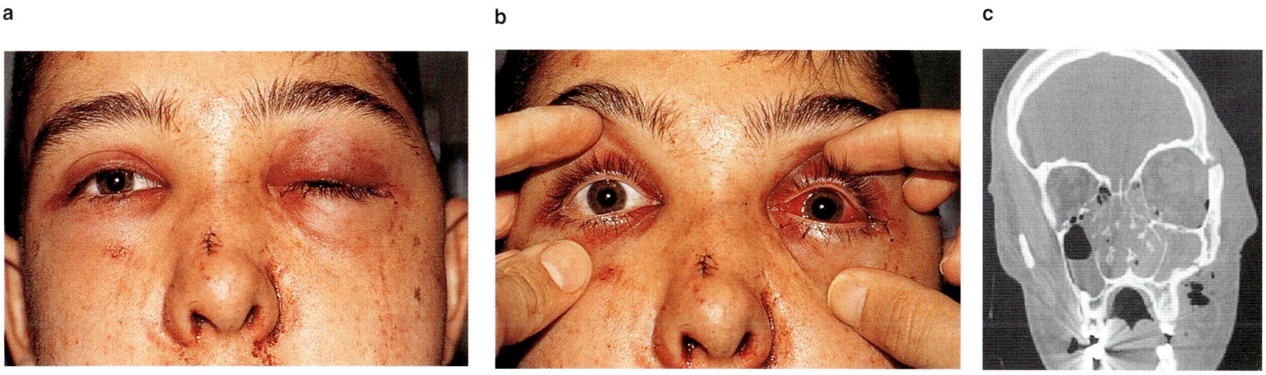

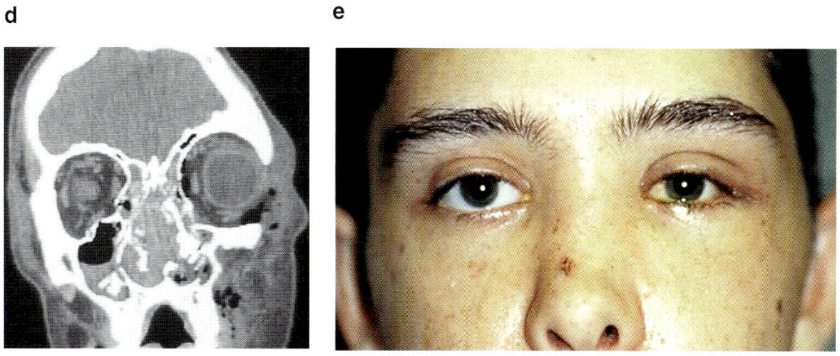

Fig. 20-31. Naso-orbital-ethmoid (NOE) fractures are the result of high-energy midfacial trauma. (**a**) This soldier was involved in a motor vehicle accident in which his face struck the steering wheel. Despite panfacial fractures, his eyes were minimally affected. Vision and motility were normal. (**b**) Although the patient suffered a marked nasal fracture with saddle deformity, he did not have traumatic telecanthus. (**c**) A computed tomography (CT) scan showed fractures of the left lateral wall, both floors, and the left zygomaticomaxillary complex, along with marked comminution of the midline buttresses (vomer, septum, ethmoid). (**d**) NOE fractures almost invariably affect the nasolacrimal system at the Le Fort II level. They are very likely to cause traumatic optic neuropathy. (**e**) The same patient 6 weeks after open reduction and internal fixation of the fractures.

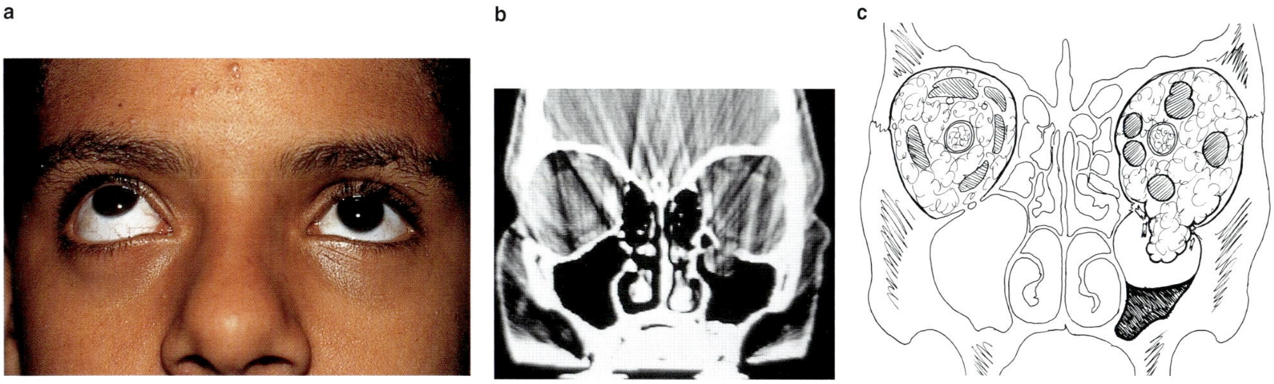

Fig. 20-32. This 13-year-old boy struck his left cheek and orbit in a snowboarding accident. He complained of vertical diplopia and numbness over the left cheek but denied dental dysesthesia; his vision was unaffected. (**a**) Examination revealed a restrictive deficit in up-gaze. (**b**) A coronal computed tomography (CT) scan demonstrates a small medial floor fracture with herniation of orbital fat. The left inferior rectus muscle is seen within the fracture. Notice the rounding of the muscle, indicating loss of the suspensory ligaments and rupture of the periorbita. (**c**) A schematic diagram illustrates the CT findings. Small fractures such as these are often the most symptomatic. Given the mechanism of injury, it is important to ensure that the patient did not suffer a concomitant zygomaticomaxillary complex fracture. This patient required open reduction and internal fixation to free the tethered tissues. Small fractures such as these can be repaired with absorbable implants (eg, Gelfilm and Vicryl mesh). Drawing prepared for this textbook by Gary Wind, MD, Uniformed Services University of the Health Sciences, Bethesda, Md.

blowout fractures. Most accepted are the theories of increased orbital hydrostatic pressure leading to primary bony failure, and compression of the rim with transmission of buckling forces across the floor with subsequent failure. Scientific testing has validated both of these theories.[3,21] Many objects—such as baseballs, tennis balls, and squash balls—can deform sufficiently so as to actually protrude into the orbit well beyond the orbital rim. Not only can the increased hydrostatic tissue pressure thus exerted fracture the bony walls, it also can obviously cause significant concussive ocular trauma (eg, angle recession, hyphema, retinal dialysis, commotio retinae, vitreous hemorrhage, etc). Therefore, a complete ophthalmological examination is essential.

Symptoms and Signs

Vertical Diplopia. Vertical diplopia, with limitation of up- or down-gaze, is the most common presenting complaint and stems primarily from entrapment of orbital tissues in the fracture plate (see Figures 20-15 and 20-32). Although the inferior rectus and oblique muscles may become frankly entrapped within the fracture, the more common cause of restriction is entrapment of the fibrovascular septa of the orbital tissues (the ligaments of Koornneef), while the muscles themselves remain free (Figures 20-33 through 20-37).

Paradoxically—but not surprisingly—the larger and more comminuted the fracture, the less likely entrapment and diplopia are to occur. Smaller fractures tend to create trapdoor defects (opening long enough to allow tissue prolapse and then closing shut, thereby entrapping the tissue and creating restrictive diplopia), but more-comminuted and larger fractures, such as extensive floor fractures or zygomaticomaxillary complex (ZMC) fractures, are less able to create the trapdoor effect. The small, comminuted, bony pieces have neither rigidity nor elasticity and cannot entrap anything. *In these situations ocular motility is often normal, without diplopia* (see Figure 20-20). Examiners must be aware of this

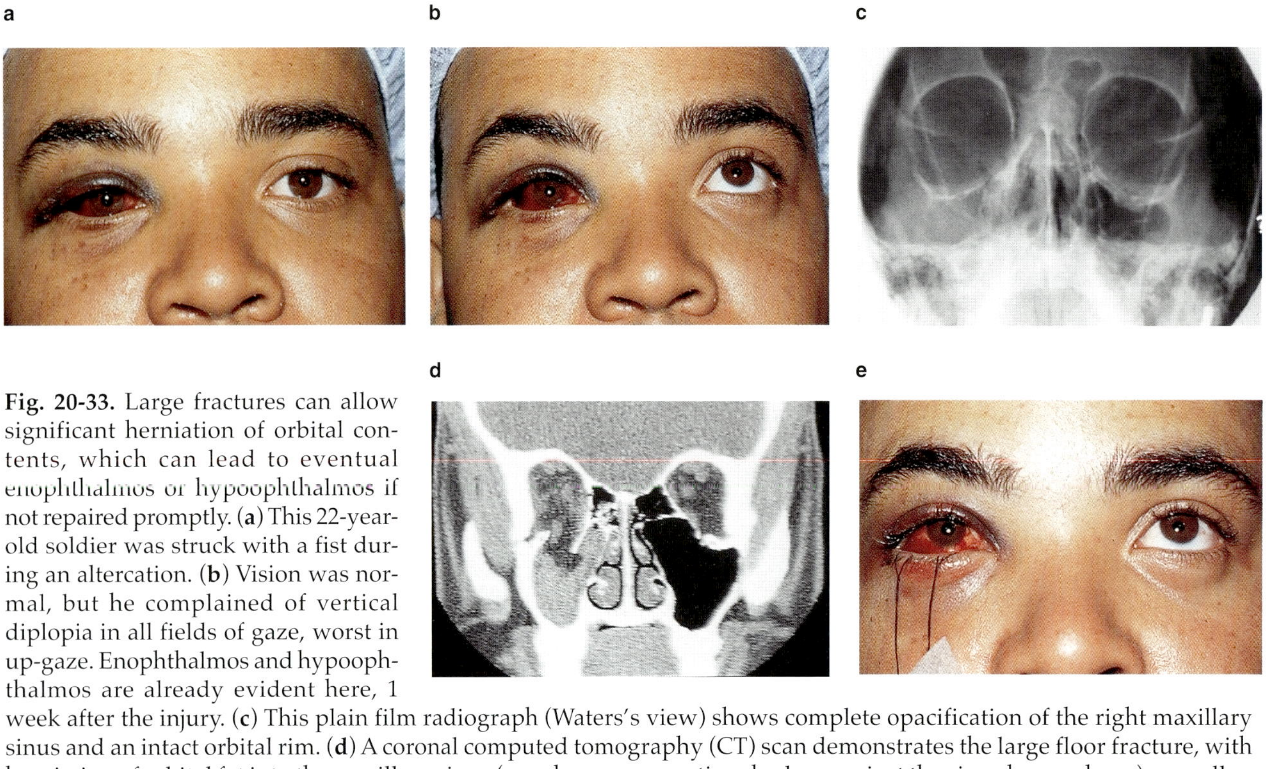

Fig. 20-33. Large fractures can allow significant herniation of orbital contents, which can lead to eventual enophthalmos or hypoophthalmos if not repaired promptly. (**a**) This 22-year-old soldier was struck with a fist during an altercation. (**b**) Vision was normal, but he complained of vertical diplopia in all fields of gaze, worst in up-gaze. Enophthalmos and hypoophthalmos are already evident here, 1 week after the injury. (**c**) This plain film radiograph (Waters's view) shows complete opacification of the right maxillary sinus and an intact orbital rim. (**d**) A coronal computed tomography (CT) scan demonstrates the large floor fracture, with herniation of orbital fat into the maxillary sinus (seen here as a negative shadow against the sinus hemorrhage), as well as frank herniation of the right inferior rectus muscle. The fracture was seen in 10 of the 12 coronal images in which the floor was identifiable. Unless repaired, such large fractures usually result in hypoglobus or enophthalmos. Because of orbital hemorrhage and proptosis, surgery was delayed for 1 week to allow swelling to subside. (**e**) The same patient, 1 day postoperatively after open reduction and internal fixation with placement of a rigid floor plate. Dramatic improvement of upward motility is evident. A Frost lid-traction suture was placed for 5 days.

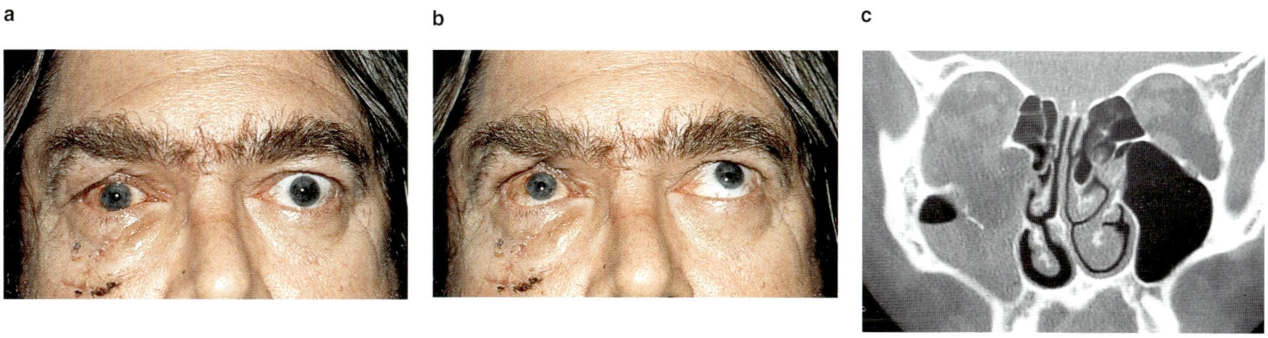

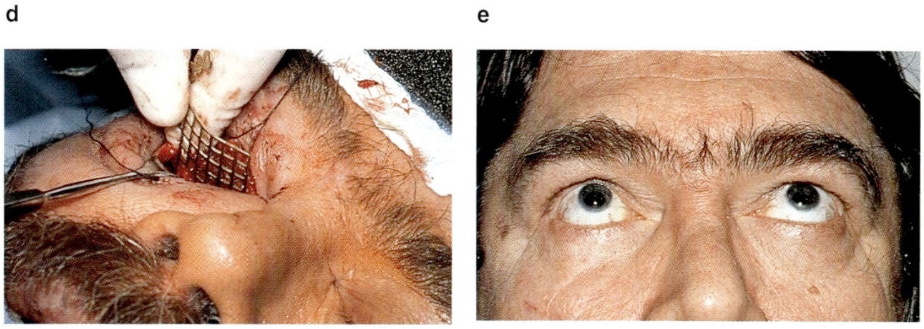

Fig. 20-34. This man tripped and fell in his house, striking his right cheek on a pot-bellied stove. His complaints included diplopia in all fields but worst in up-gaze, and numbness across cranial nerve V_2 and the upper bank of teeth. (**a**) Examination of the patient shows significant right enophthalmos and (**b**) limitation of motility. The orbital rim and the zygomaticomaxillary complex buttress were not tender. (**c**) This computed tomography (CT) scan shows a large fracture of the orbital floor, with herniation of both the orbital fat and the inferior rectus muscle into the maxillary sinus. Notice the rounding of the muscle shadow. The orbital volume is dramatically enlarged. The bony fracture plate has broken off at the orbital strut, the junction of the floor, and the ethmoid sinus. Reconstructing such a cavernous defect requires a rigid plate that can be cantilevered over the sinus and may require fixation to the orbital rim. Current choices for such plates include calvarial bone, porous polyethylene, silicone sheeting, and (**d**) titanium mesh of various designs. It is very difficult to reduce the most posterior aspect of these injuries because of possible surgical damage to the optic nerve. (**e**) This photograph shows the patient 1 year postoperatively, with resolution of all diplopia. He has mild, residual enophthalmos and sensory dysesthesia over V_2, both of which are inconsequential to the patient.

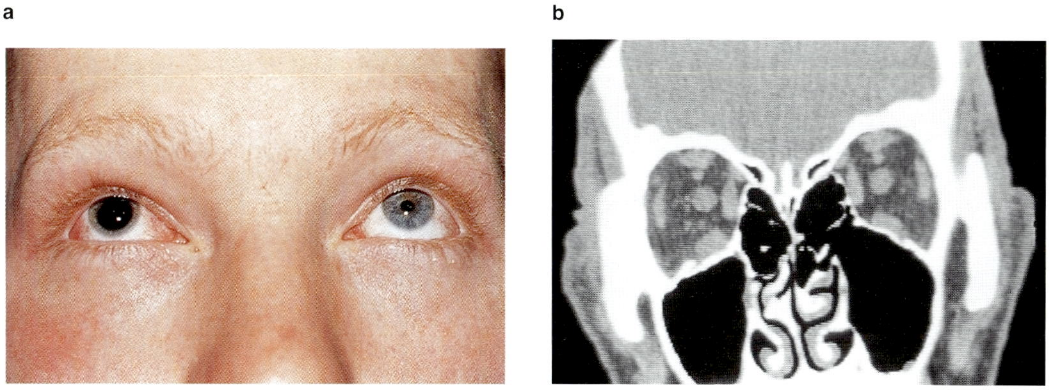

Fig. 20-35. Diplopia and dysmotility are not necessarily pathognomonic for orbital fracture. (**a**) This 21-year-old man suffered blunt trauma to the right orbit. He presented with diplopia, up-gaze limitation, and mildly decreased sensation over cranial nerve V_2. (**b**) Despite this cluster of symptoms, no frank fracture was identified on computed tomography (CT) scan. However, enlargement of the right inferior rectus muscle is seen, suggesting muscular contusion and intramuscular hemorrhage. Forced duction testing demonstrated free passive motility without restrictions. The patient was observed conservatively and all symptoms promptly resolved.

a

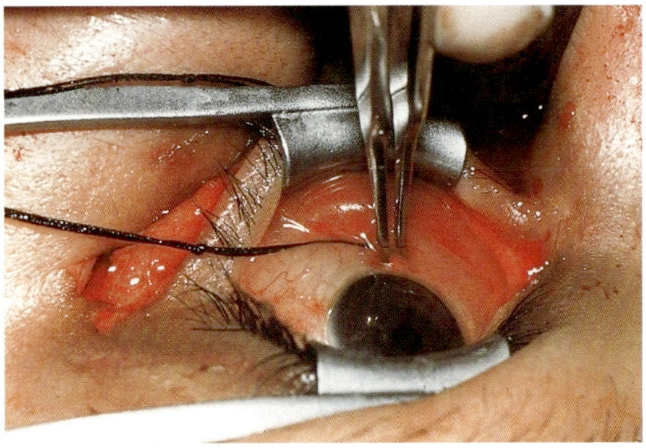

b

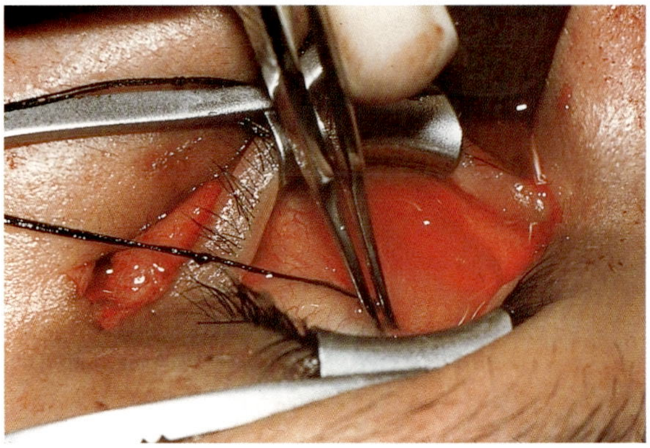

Fig. 20-36. Forced duction and force generation testing. Forced duction testing is extremely useful in determining whether dysmotility is restrictive or paralytic, and it can be used to test any muscle. Forced duction testing can be performed easily in the examination chair with topical anesthesia and should be the first step at surgery. The insertion of the muscle being tested is grasped firmly, and the eye is pushed into the desired field of gaze. These photographs illustrate (**a**) restricted duction of the inferior rectus before release of entrapped orbital tissues and (**b**) normal range of motion after release. In testing force generation, the muscle insertion is grasped and the patient is asked to look into the muscle's field of action. A paretic muscle will feel weak when compared with the fellow eye. Surgeons should avoid speaking in terms of "positive" and "negative" forced ductions and force generation, as these terms are imprecise and lead to confusion. Rather, the terms "restricted" and "unrestricted" should be used.

a

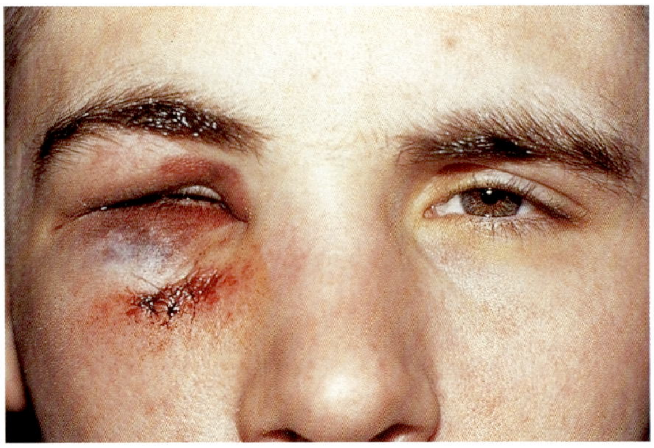

b

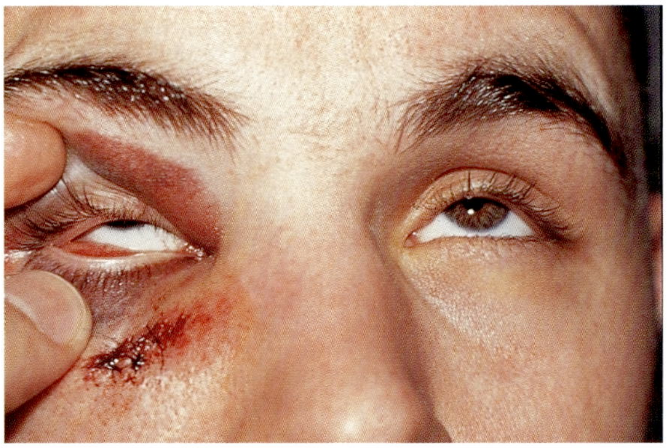

c

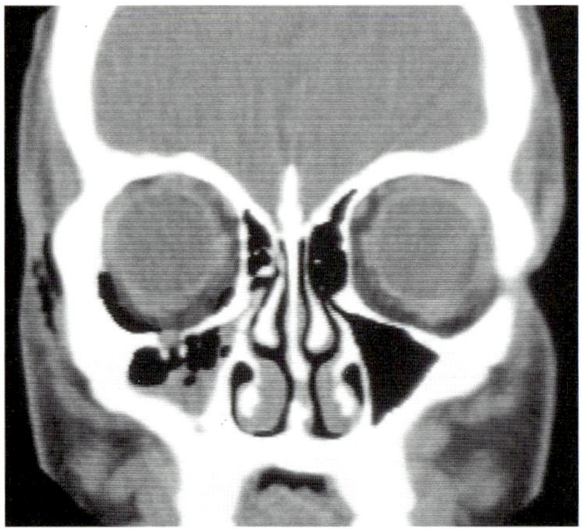

Fig. 20-37. (**a**) This man was elbowed on the right cheek while playing touch football. Other than a small laceration (sutured in the emergency department) and mild ecchymosis, the patient complained only of mild V_2 dysesthesia not involving the teeth. Close examination, however, revealed lid swelling out of proportion to the ecchymosis. Palpation confirmed subcutaneous emphysema. This finding is virtually pathognomonic for sinoorbital communication and orbital fracture. (**b**) Notice the overelevation of the right eye in up-gaze, although the patient denied diplopia (probably secondary to obstruction by the lid). (**c**) A computed tomography (CT) scan disclosed a small floor fracture without significant herniation or entrapment of tissues. Significant orbital emphysema sequestered to the floor caused the eye to assume a more hyperophthalmic position. Likewise, air sequestered to the roof can create the illusion of hypoglobus, leading the ophthalmologist to suspect a large fracture when none exists. This patient was followed conservatively and became asymptomatic without surgery as the emphysema resolved over the next few days.

a b c

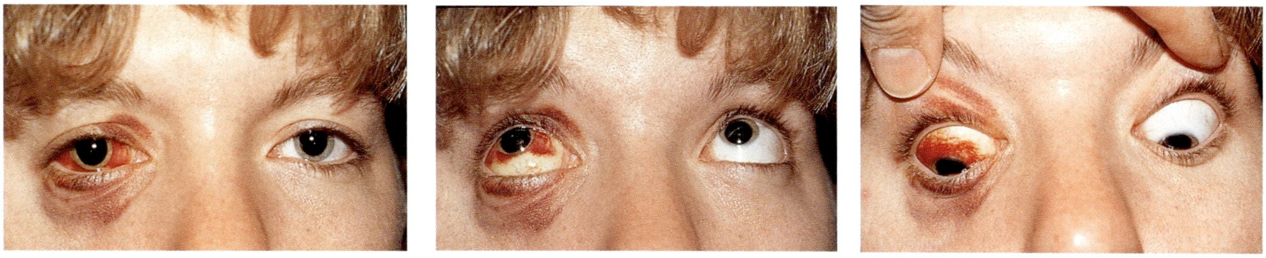

d e

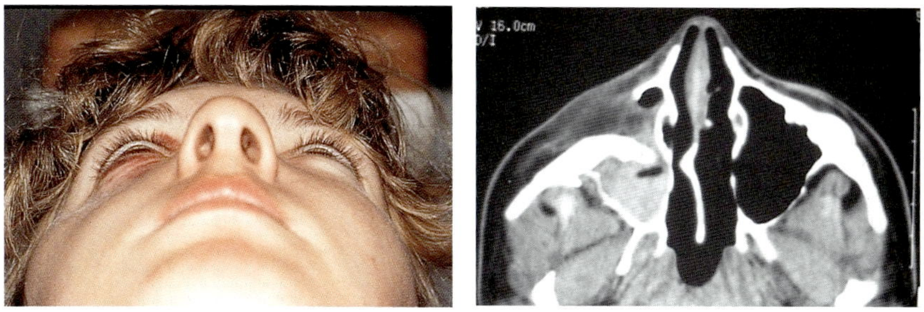

Fig. 20-38. Large fractures are often visually asymptomatic, and the ophthalmologist must have a high index of suspicion to pursue the evaluation. Associated symptoms and findings often herald a larger fracture. (**a**) This 24-year-old woman was accidentally struck on the right cheek with a softball bat. She denied diplopia, but persistent pain led her to seek care at the eye clinic. (**b, c**) She had full ocular motility but when questioned admitted dysesthesia of the cheek, nose, and teeth, as well as trismus (which was improving) and malocclusion. Palpation revealed point tenderness over the zygomaticofrontal suture and a large step-off deformity at the zygomaticomaxillary suture. (**d**) The patient had significant malar flattening but no appreciable canthal dystopia. (**e**) A computed tomography (CT) scan showed a large but noncomminuted zygomaticomaxillary complex fracture. Notice the flatness of the normal left zygomatic arch. This is the position to which a fractured arch must be reduced to maintain proper facial proportion.

possibility so as not to be fooled into thinking that there is no fracture (Figure 20-38). If doubt exists, a CT scan should be ordered.

Diplopia may also occur because of contusion of the inferior muscles. This temporary apraxia often clears over the span of 7 to 10 days (see Figure 20-35). Forced duction and force generation testing can usually distinguish paretic from restrictive diplopia (see Figure 20-36). Sometimes, a course of oral corticosteroids (40–60 mg prednisone daily for 5–7 d) can speed the resolution of swelling and make it easier to conclude whether diplopia is restrictive, mechanical, or paretic, but these medications should only be used selectively and not routinely.

Extraocular Muscle Rounding. CT can often reveal that the involved muscle has assumed a more rounded appearance than its typical flat or elliptical shape (see Figure 20-35). This rounding is probably due either to disruption of the normal fibrovascular septa holding the muscle in its elongated form, or to hemorrhage and fibrosis within the muscle sheath. In cases where the diagnosis of a fracture is equivocal, extraocular muscle rounding can help establish the presence of a fracture.

Hypesthesia of Infraorbital Cranial Nerve V_2. Hypesthesia of cranial nerve V_2 occurs from contusion or transection of the infraorbital neurovascular bundle, which traverses the orbital floor before it exits from the infraorbital foramen (see Figures 20-33 and 20-34). More posteriorly, involvement of the superior alveolar branch may cause numbness across the ipsilateral upper bank of teeth. Fractures of the inferior rim often extend along the anterior maxillary face to disrupt the nerve as it exits from the infraorbital foramen. The numbness across V_2 may become denser after surgery but generally resolves, although resolution may take months and may be incomplete.

Orbital Emphysema. Communication with the underlying maxillary sinus allows air and bacteria from the sinus to enter the orbit. Many patients will relate an accurate history of sneezing or nose blowing, followed immediately by the eyelids abruptly swelling. The emphysema is most readily diagnosed as dramatic, visible, swelling of the lids out of proportion to the limited ecchymosis present. Orbital emphysema can be felt with gentle palpation over the lids, but this is a subtle feeling at best. The sensation is not as dramatic as that felt along the chest and neck in the presence of pneumothorax but is rather likened to that of gently crushing crisped rice cereal through a glove. Emphysema may be significant enough to cause optic nerve compression and loss of vision. In such cases of acute pneumo-orbita, urgent orbital paracentesis can be sight-saving.

Occasionally, sufficient orbital emphysema will be sequestered to a wall so as to push the globe away, creating symptomatic hyper- or hypo-ophthalmia; the symptoms will resolve when the orbital air has resorbed (see Figure 20-37). Emphysema can also be so significant as to cause subcutaneous emphysema of the head and neck and has even been known to cause pneumomediastinum.[22] Patients should be told *not* to blow the nose. The role of prophylactic antibiotics in these cases is controversial but administering them is, nonetheless, common practice. If prescribed, a general, broad-spectrum antibiotic should be chosen (eg, amoxicillin/clavulanic acid or cephalexin) to prevent orbital cellulitis from common nasal pathogens, such as *Staphylococcus* species, *Streptococcus* species, and *Haemophilus influenza.*

Hypo-ophthalmos and Enophthalmos. Increased orbital volume associated with large fractures may result in axial retraction of the globe (enophthalmos) or downward vertical displacement (hypo-ophthalmos, hypoglobus). Loss of floor support lets the orbital contents and globe sink into the maxillary sinus (see Figures 20-16, 20-19, 20-33, and 20-34). The resulting deformity requires anatomical reconstitution of the floor, with restoration of the proper bony orbital volume and configuration.

Enophthalmos is primarily a consequence of increased orbital volume, *not*, as some believe, a result of orbital tissue atrophy. Tissue atrophy and resorption undoubtedly occur, but these are secondary factors.[23,24] Consequently, accurate restoration of the bony orbital volume is critical to the prevention of this complication. Two millimeters of enophthalmos is generally regarded as within normal variation and not cosmetically noticeable in most people. But, because of the tissue edema, hemorrhage, and swelling associated with acute orbital trauma, patients may not initially manifest either enophthalmos or hypoglobus. However, in the presence of a large fracture (> 50%), the risk of developing either hypo-ophthalmos or enophthalmos is high.

Late correction is difficult due to the development of significant fibrosis and Volkmann's contractures within the orbital tissues, which oppose mobilization of bony structures (see Figures 20-14, 20-19).[25] Although the primary abnormality, as stated above, is enlarged (ie, inadequately reduced) orbital volume, contracted orbital tissues make late attempts at reducing orbital volume difficult. If significant tissue swelling confounds the acute assessment of enophthalmos or hypo-ophthalmos, a short course of oral corticosteroids can speed resolution of the swelling and therefore help in making the diagnosis. As in the case of extraocular muscle paresis discussed above, steroids should only be used sparingly and should not be a routine first-line management tool.

Many patients will be asymptomatic to axial enophthalmos or purely vertical hypo-ophthalmos, because the visual axes are still essentially parallel (see Figures 20-14 and 20-16). If, however, a rotational component displaces the visual axis, then diplopia will most likely become intolerable (Figure 20-39).[23]

Oculocardiac Reflex and the White-Eyed Blowout. Attempting to move an eye that is entrapped by a blowout fracture may cause increased vagal tone, thereby stimulating the oculocardiac reflex, similar to that seen during strabismus surgery. This can manifest as nausea, vomiting, or severe bradycardia or heart block to the point of syncope on attempted ocular movement. Such symptoms must be specifically queried and noted; urgent surgical intervention is warranted in this potentially fatal condition. This may be more common in young patients (< 18 y), in whom the orbital bones are more flexible and consequently more likely to demonstrate greenstick fractures and trapdoor fractures of the floor. In these cases, the bony plate does not fracture completely but opens long enough to allow orbital tissues to herniate. The fracture plate then closes, entrapping the tissues. Very often, there is a corresponding paucity of external physical findings, with the exception of diplopia. In such cases (known as "white-eyed blowout"), clinical symptoms are often out of proportion to external findings. Unfortunately, long-term tissue ischemia can result from delayed release of the entrapped tissue, resulting in less-than-optimal surgical success, chronic diplopia, enophthalmos, and fibrosis—and disappointment for both patient and surgeon. Ophthalmologists should have a high index of suspicion for such injuries, especially if the mechanisms and energies involved in the injuries are sufficient to cause a fracture. Early surgery (within 24 h) is warranted for both conditions.[26–28]

Pupillary Abnormalities. Pupillary abnormalities result from damage to the pupillary fibers traveling with the inferior oblique muscle. The damage can occur as a consequence of either the primary injury or the corrective surgery.

Indications for Surgery

Surgery is indicated to correct or prevent functional visual loss or significant cosmetic deformity.

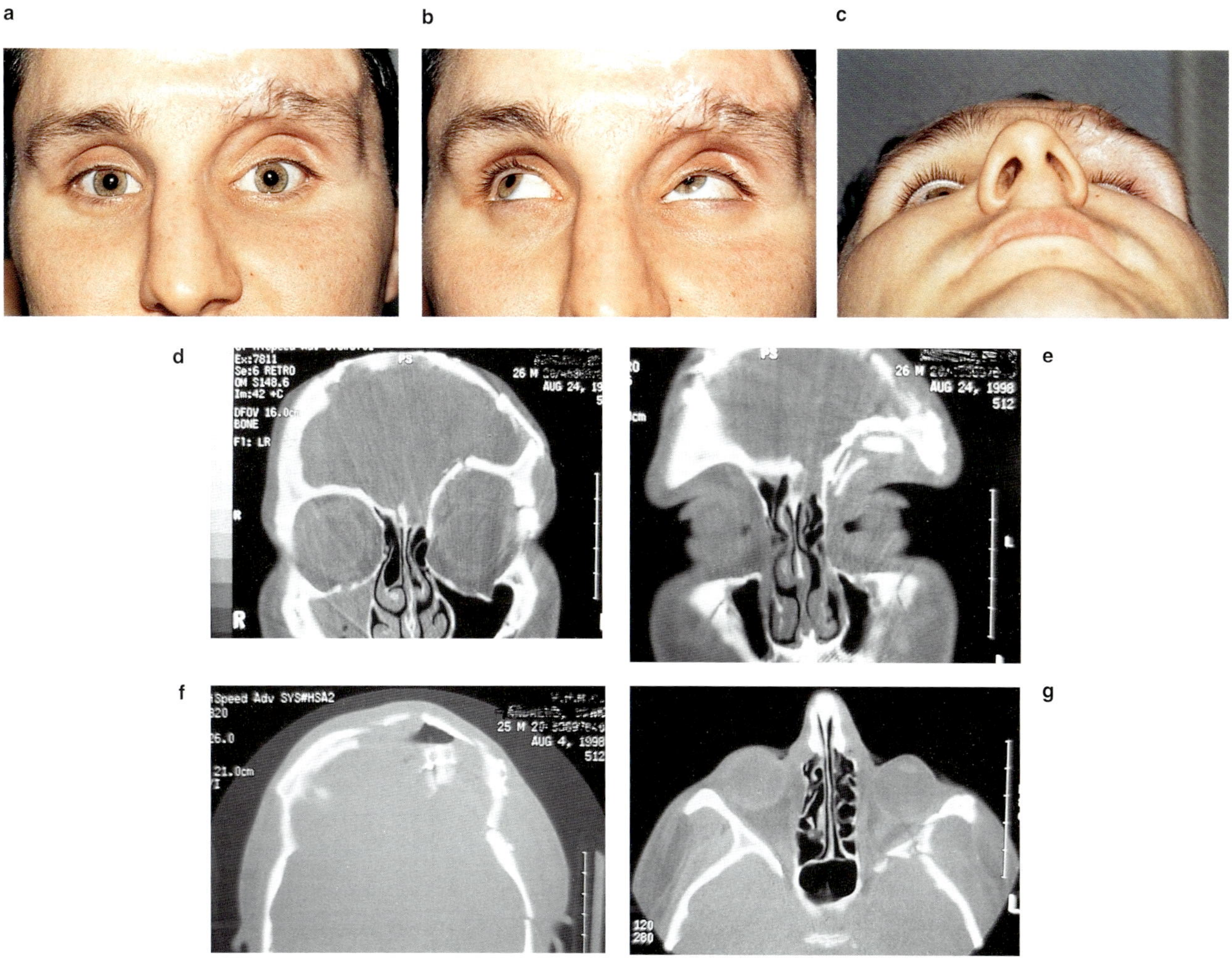

Fig. 20-39. Fractures involving the orbital roof are typically the result of significant head injury. This 24-year-old Coast Guard sailor was walking on his ship's outside deck when an inside boiler exploded. He was struck by a portion of a ship's door that was blown off by the force of the explosion. The patient suffered a massive craniofacial injury, which required emergent neurosurgery to save his life. The cranial defects were repaired concomitantly, using titanium mesh and plates to secure calvarial bone grafts that were used to reconstruct the orbit. (**a**) Two years later, the patient is left with marked orbital deformity and cicatricial contraction of the overlying skin. (**b**) He also has intractable diplopia in all fields of gaze, and (**c**) such significant enophthalmos that his left lids do not appose the globe. Fortunately, the patient's naturally deep-set eyes help disguise the enophthalmos. (**d**) A postreconstruction computed tomography (CT) scan shows the extent of the injury, with marked orbital enlargement, (**e**) intraorbital bone grafts, cranialization of the frontal sinus, and (**f**) intracranial titanium mesh. (**g**) This CT image shows the posterior extent of the fracture, involving the orbital apex and middle cranial fossa. Despite prior reconstruction, the posterior 50% of the orbital roof was absent. With such a defect, ophthalmologists would expect the orbit to be pulsatile. Although acute roof fractures typically cause *ex*ophthalmos, *en*ophthalmos can result from such extensive injuries.

Specific indications include the following:

- restrictive diplopia in a functional field of gaze (either primary gaze or within 30° of primary in either up-gaze or down-gaze);
- CT evidence of entrapped muscle or orbital tissue;
- enophthalmos greater than 2 mm (asymmetry < 2 mm is normal and is not cosmetically noticeable);
- oculocardiac reflex (nausea, vomiting, bradycardia, syncope with attempted gaze) should prompt immediate surgery if a young patient (< 18 y) has a white-eyed blowout;
- hypo-ophthalmos; and

- large floor fracture (> 50%), based on CT estimate of the fracture size.

Failure to repair large fractures can lead to significant hypo-ophthalmia and enophthalmos. Late repair of these cosmetic deformities is difficult, and it is as frustrating for surgeons as it is for patients and their families. Fracture size can be estimated by simply counting the number of coronal images in which the fracture is seen versus the number in which the floor is seen.

Medial Wall

Medial wall fractures are much less common than floor blowouts and are probably found more often as an extension of a floor fracture or a component of naso-orbital-ethmoid (NOE) fractures than as an isolated entity. They occur secondary to moderate-to-high-energy impacts (Figures 20-40 and 20-41).[2,4]

Symptoms and Signs

Horizontal Diplopia. In contrast to the vertical diplopia associated with floor fractures, horizontal diplopia is usually the primary complaint when medial orbital tissues are involved. However, a vertical or oblique component is often found (see Figure 20-41).

Orbital Emphysema. It was previously taught that orbital emphysema was almost always indicative of a medial wall fracture.[11] We know this not to be the case, however, because a fair number of floor fractures also create orbital emphysema. Nevertheless, the mechanism is the same in either case: fracture into the adjacent sinus allows sinus air (and bacteria) into the orbit. The consequences are also the same, as are the general precautions regarding nose blowing and prophylactic antibiotics.

Orbital Hemorrhage. As noted above, because of the rich vascular supply to the orbit, hemorrhage is a constant companion to orbital trauma. Certainly, disruption of the highly vascular maxillary sinus mucosa by a floor fracture can create significant orbital hemorrhage; however, much of this hemorrhage will drain inferiorly with gravity into the maxillary sinus. Orbital hemorrhage from a medial wall fracture, on the other hand, can be more dramatic because it may lack the natural drainage afforded by a floor fracture. Additionally, the proximity and caliber of the anterior and posterior ethmoidal arteries—located at the frontoethmoidal suture line above the ethmoid plate—makes them exquisitely susceptible to disruption or transection with medial wall trauma and can make the bleeding more considerable (see Figure 20-41).

a

b

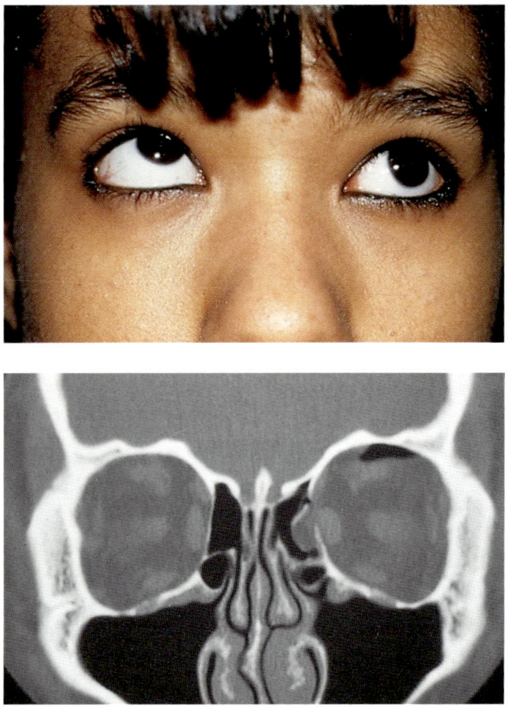

Fig. 20-40. Medial wall fracture. (**a**) Entrapment of the medial tissues results in horizontal diplopia, as demonstrated by this patient, who was kneed in the left orbit while playing soccer. (**b**) This computed tomography (CT) scan of a different patient demonstrates soft-tissue entrapment along the medial wall, as well as superior orbital emphysema. In such limited fractures, open reduction and internal fixation can be accomplished with thin absorbable or permanent implants, such as Gelfilm (absorbable) or porous polyethylene (permanent).

Enophthalmos. A sufficiently large medial wall fracture allows prolapse of enough orbital tissue to create significant loss of globe projection. This is the reason why the medial wall is intentionally removed in thyroid decompression.

Indications for Surgery

Indications for medial wall repair are similar to those for floor fracture:

- restrictive diplopia in a functional field of gaze;
- CT evidence of entrapped muscle or orbital tissue; and
- enophthalmos greater than 2 mm.

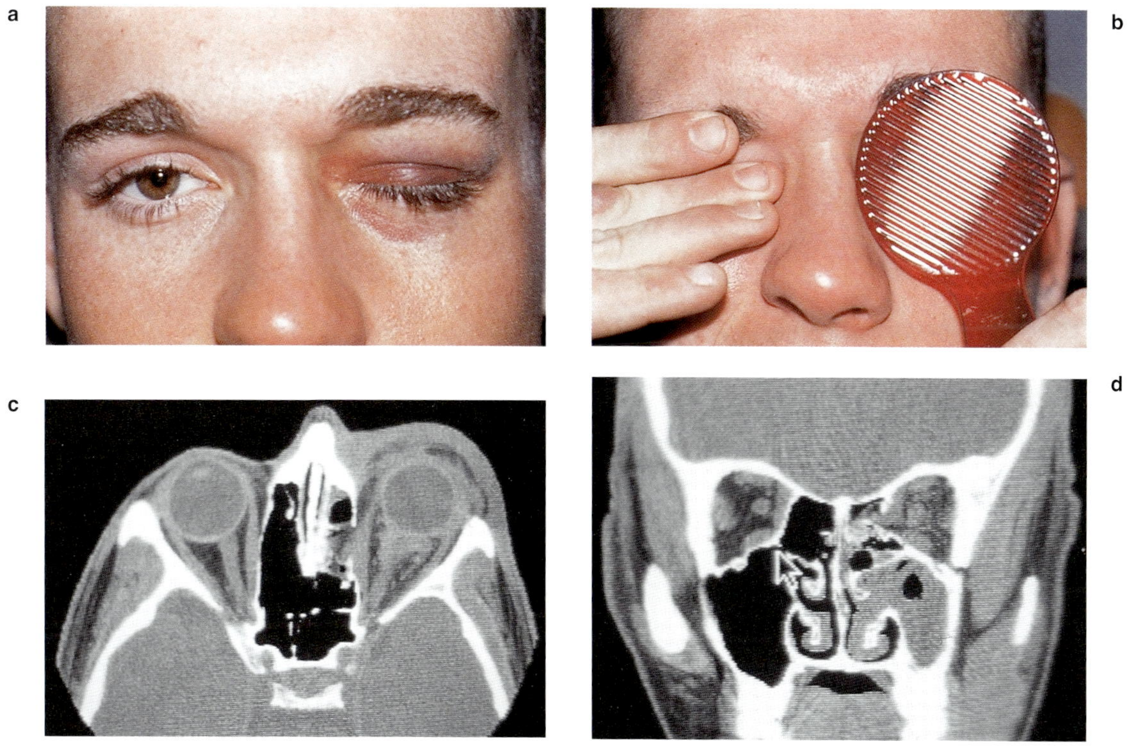

Fig. 20-41. Medial wall fracture. (**a**) This 19-year-old soldier was struck with a fist during a barracks fight. Marked lid and orbital hemorrhage prevented complete ocular examination for several days, although vision was always preserved. (**b**) When swelling abated, the patient complained of oblique and torsional diplopia in all fields, as demonstrated by the Maddox rod. (**c**) A computed tomography (CT) scan showed a large medial wall fracture with significant orbital hemorrhage. (**d**) Close inspection of the coronal CT scan shows the left orbital floor to be moderately thicker than the right (arrow). The patient later reported a history of a previous blow to the orbit with possible fracture but no surgery. This may explain why the medial wall, rather than the floor, buckled. The patient underwent open reduction and internal fixation via external ethmoidectomy incision, with placement of a thin (0.4-mm) porous polyethylene sheet implant. He was asymptomatic postoperatively.

Orbital Roof

Isolated roof fractures are distinctly uncommon, being almost always the result of moderate-to-high-energy injuries. As such, they are invariably associated with significant concomitant nonocular injury, such as frontal sinus fractures and intracranial injury.[2,4] Therefore, ophthalmologists are rarely the primary physicians managing these cases but are often called as consultants (see Figure 20-39).

Surprisingly, many patients are fully alert and oriented despite what is, in essence, a depressed skull fracture. Just as surprisingly, many patients will present initially to the ophthalmologist rather than the neurosurgeon, complaining of diplopia or ptosis after striking the head during, for example, a motor vehicle accident or a fall from a ladder (see Figure 20-27). Because other orbital fractures and ocular adnexal findings may be more impressive than the roof findings, primary physicians may, in addition, initially refer the patient to an ophthalmologist (Figure 20-42). On the other hand, there can be such a paucity of associated findings that physicians may discount the possibility that an isolated roof fracture can occur in such a setting and will simply never look for it, referring the patient to the ophthalmologist for evaluation of traumatic ptosis or management of the black eye. Therefore, the prudent ophthalmologist should always look for an associated roof fracture—even if the suspicion is low and he or she might end up not being the primary manager.

Symptoms and Signs

Restricted Up-Gaze and Ptosis. These findings develop secondary to (*a*) the inward displacement of the levator/superior rectus muscle complex by

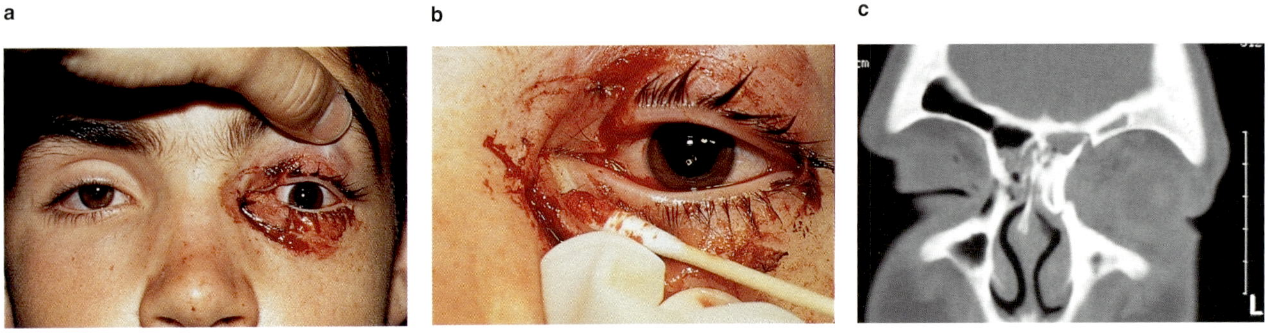

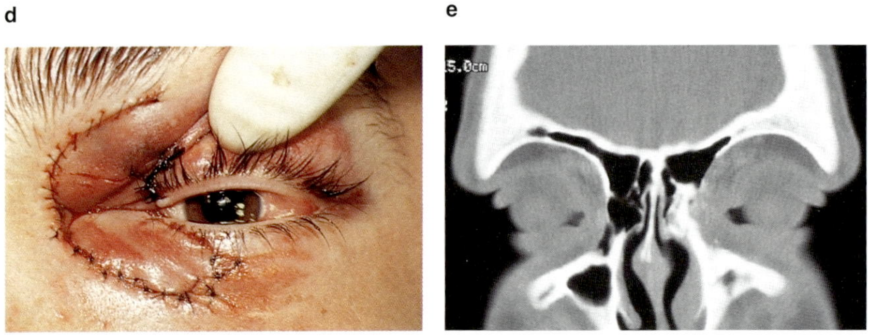

Fig. 20-42. Orbital roof fracture with combined injuries. External injuries should always prompt the search for significant associated injuries. (**a**) This 19-year-old man was struck with a polyvinylchloride pipe during a street fight. He was referred to the eye clinic for treatment of medial canthal and lower-lid lacerations. Lacerations in the medial canthal area should always prompt evaluation for associated canalicular damage. (**b**) The patient was fortunate to escape canalicular injury but sustained a full-thickness upper-lid laceration just lateral to the punctum. The location and extent of the lacerations prompted computed tomography (CT) evaluation. (**c**) The coronal CT scan shows a fracture of the floor of the frontal sinus, which also constitutes the partially pneumatized roof. Blood within the frontal sinus is easily seen. The injury was repaired via an external ethmoidectomy incision. (**d**) The lid laceration was repaired in conventional fashion. (**e**) Three months after open reduction and internal fixation, the orbit and frontal sinus are well reconstructed.

the bony fracture plate and (*b*) associated subperiosteal hematoma. Physical disruption of the nerve to the levator/superior rectus complex can occur, but it is uncommon. Even though traumatic ptosis occurs most commonly as aponeurotic damage unrelated to roof injury, ophthalmologists must, nevertheless, evaluate for roof injury when patients present to the medical treatment facility with ptosis after head trauma.

Epistaxis, Cerebrospinal Fluid Rhinorrhea, and Anosmia. Roof fractures often extend to the very thin bones of the ethmoid and cribriform plates, resulting in epistaxis. Additionally, if the dura is torn in these areas, cerebrospinal fluid (CSF) can drain from the anterior cranial fossa through the frontonasal recesses as clear fluid rhinorrhea. Anyone who has suffered a significant blow to the nose should also be queried regarding these symptoms. Fractures involving the cribriform plate can also damage the olfactory nerves, resulting in a decreased sense of smell. Because of the sensitivity of these nerves to trauma, smell sensations might never be fully recovered.

Occasionally, the frontal and ethmoid sinuses extensively pneumatize the orbital roof. In these cases, the roof has both an inner (calvarial) and an outer (orbital) table. In such a circumstance, a roof fracture represents the equivalent of an outer-table sinus fracture. Unless the inner table is also disrupted, however, CSF leakage will not occur.

Depression of the Supraorbital Rim. Roof fractures often involve the upper rim, which is also the anterior table and floor of the frontal sinus. The rim usually caves into the depth of the sinus, creating the hollow of a depressed skull fracture over the brow. The upper rim is also an important horizontal buttress.

Hypesthesia of Cranial Nerve V_1. Just as floor fractures extend through the infraorbital canal and foramen, disrupting infraorbital nerve (V_2) function, roof fractures often crack through the supraorbital notch or foramen, creating numbness across the forehead and scalp (cranial nerve V_1). Because multiple orbital fractures may coexist, and given the gravity of missing a roof fracture, ophthalmologists should routinely check V_1 sensation (on the forehead) in all orbital traumas.

Hypo-ophthalmos and Pulsatile Exophthalmos. Orbital floors tend to blow *out*, and roofs tend to blow *in*, because the orbit is more compressible than the brain, which is, after all, what is on the other side of the roof. Therefore, the bony fracture plate usually dislocates into the orbit, displacing the orbital contents anteriorly (exophthalmos) and inferiorly (hypo-ophthalmos). The open connection to the pulsatile intracranial pressure causes the globe to pulse, a phenomenon that is sometimes best seen when the patient is in the supine position. If the orbital periosteum is intact, a subperiosteal hematoma may be present. If the periorbita has been torn, blood and CSF can both dissect into the orbit proper. Care should be taken not to cavalierly perform a canthotomy and cantholysis for retrobulbar hemorrhage in these situations without neurosurgical approval, because CSF instead of blood can be liberated into the environment.

Indications for Surgery

Surgery is usually performed under the direction of neurosurgery, with extensive assistance from ENT. Craniotomy is often necessary for repair of dural tears and CSF leaks. Repair of the bony roof defect requires reestablishment of a rigid barrier between the anterior cranial fossa and the orbit. Various implant materials can be used, such as split-thickness calvarial bone; thin, porous polyethylene; or vascularized pericranial flaps. Whichever implant is selected, it should be well-secured to the surrounding bones, so as to prevent migration and transmission of intracranial pulsation (see Figure 20-39).

Indications for surgery of an orbital roof fracture include the following:

- depressed skull fracture (if the anterior cranial fossa is compromised, a craniotomy is often required);
- significant diplopia;
- significant exophthalmos; and
- frontal sinus fracture with compromise of the nasofrontal duct.

Even if the posterior sinus (calvarial) table is intact, the sinus must be explored and repaired so as to prevent the development of chronic sinusitis, mucocele, and mucopyocele. If the posterior table is intact, the sinus may be exenterated of its mucosa and the nasofrontal duct obliterated. If only the posterior table is fractured, the sinus may be opened widely and obliterated via craniotomy, thus "cranializing" the sinus.

Zygomaticomaxillary Complex

Fractures of the ZMC were formerly termed the "tripod" or "trimalar" fractures, because the zygoma was widely believed to have but three articulations: the zygomaticomaxillary (ZM) suture at the inferior rim, the zygomaticofrontal (ZF) suture along the lateral rim, and the zygomaticotemporal (ZT) suture along the zygomatic arch (ZA). The older terms are still commonly used, but since the introduction and common acceptance of the buttress concept, the zygoma is now believed to be a quadripod. Its articulations include the three of traditional teaching, plus a fourth—the ZMC buttress (see Figure 20-12). This last is probably the single most important component of the midfacial buttresses.

ZMC fractures occur as a result of moderate-to-high-energy injury. The greater the energy, the more comminution seen. Lower-energy injuries may be associated with variable degrees of displacement and dislocation, depending on the angle of impact. With higher energies, it is not unusual to find associated fractures of other midfacial buttresses and the mandible.[4,5]

After isolated orbital floor fractures, ZMC fractures are probably the second-most-common fracture presenting initially to the ophthalmologist. They are also among the most commonly missed. Patients suffering from facial trauma may initially present to, or be initially referred to, an ophthalmologist because of significant lid ecchymosis (a black eye), transient blurry vision, diplopia, or merely the history of "I got hit in the eye." Because the orbital and ocular symptoms associated with a ZMC fracture can be variable—including fully absent—it is incumbent on the ophthalmologist to always look for a ZMC fracture (see Figures 20-20 and 20-38). Just as large floor fractures can have minimal effect on ocular motility, ZMC fractures can have minimal effect on ocular function while still being significant enough to warrant surgical repair (Figures 20-43 and 20-44). Prompt recognition and diagnosis lead to timely surgical intervention and optimal results. Stated another way, delaying or missing the diagnosis of a ZMC fracture can lead to late intervention and suboptimal return of function, particularly cosmesis and dental occlusion (see Figure 20-14).

Symptoms and Signs

As stated above, symptoms and signs of ZMC fracture are highly variable, depending on the amount of energy causing the injury and the degree of bony displacement. Most patterns of ZMC

a b

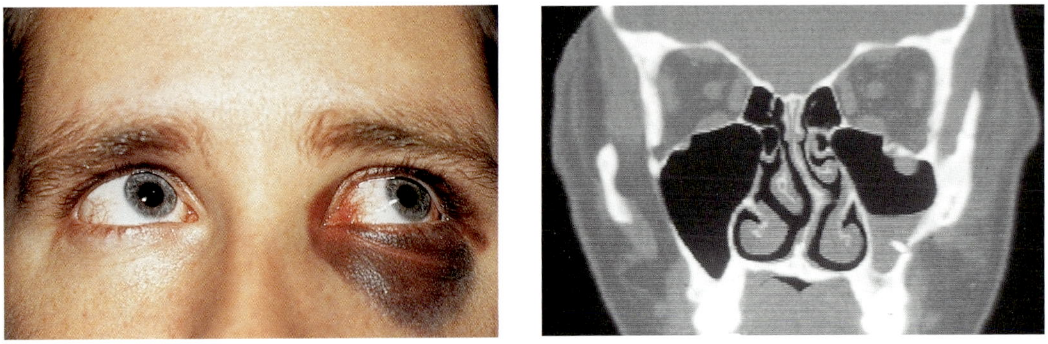

Fig. 20-43. Nondisplaced fracture of the zygomaticomaxillary complex (ZMC) with ocular symptoms. Small fractures can tether orbital contents due to a "trap-door" effect, producing symptomatic diplopia. (**a**) This 22-year-old man was the victim of an assault by his "best friend." The patient denied diplopia in primary gaze, dysesthesia of cranial nerve V_2, or trismus. On examination, however, he had significant diplopia in upper left gaze. (**b**) A computed tomography (CT) scan revealed a small, minimally displaced left ZMC fracture with probable herniation of orbital tissues. Inspection of the inferior rectus does not demonstrate significant rounding. The patient was followed conservatively for a week to allow contusion paresis to resolve. When the patient remained symptomatic at that point, he was taken to surgery for open reduction and internal fixation of the orbital floor. A small amount of orbital tissue was frankly entrapped. The floor was repaired with an absorbable gelatin plate (Gelfilm). Diplopia resolved completely by 1 day postoperatively.

a b

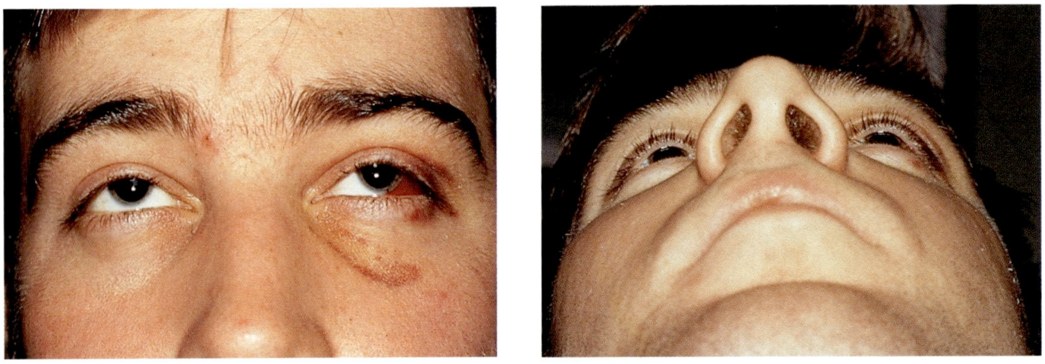

c

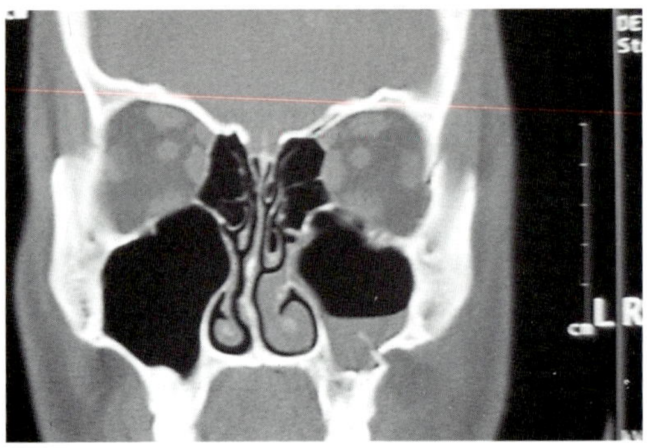

Fig. 20-44. Not all fractures cause ocular symptoms. (**a**) This patient fell on the ice, striking his left cheek. He was referred for evaluation of the "black eye." Examination revealed mild decreased sensation over cranial nerve V_2 and tenderness to palpation over the zygomaticomaxillary (ZM) and zygomaticofrontal (ZF) sutures as well as the ZMC buttress. He denied trismus, and had full ocular motility. (**b**) No enophthalmos or malar flattening were observed. (**c**) Because of the bony and intraoral tenderness, a computed tomography (CT) scan was obtained, which showed a minimally displaced zygomaticomaxillary complex (ZMC) fracture. The orbital floor was not significantly involved, but the inferior rectus muscle does show mild rounding. The patient went on to have open reduction and internal fixation for stabilization of the ZM and ZF sutures. At surgery, the orbital floor was explored, revealing a hairline fracture but no orbital incarceration. A gelatin implant was placed on the floor.

fractures exhibit some common findings, however.

Point Tenderness and Ecchymosis. Fractures of the ZMC affect all of its articulations to some degree. Frank dislocation of any of these articulations depends on the amount and direction of energy delivered. Palpation of the entire circumference of the bony rim usually discloses localized pain and tenderness at the ZF and ZM sutures. If pain is elicited, then the ZA and ZMC buttress should also be palpated. If the zygoma is dislocated, a tender rim step-off or separation can be felt, either inferiorly or laterally.

The ZMC buttress is best evaluated via intraoral examination. Ecchymosis at the gingival sulcus and upper vestibule are strong indicators of bony disruption (Figure 20-45). The buttress can be palpated by placing a finger into the upper gingival sulcus and following the anterior maxillary face laterally to just under the malar eminence. The bony pillar is easily felt as a prominent thickening of the bone. Point tenderness here indicates bony disruption, although not necessarily dislocation. While examining the ZMC buttress intraorally, the ophthalmologist can palpate the anterior maxillary face for comminution and examine the maxillary alveolus for Le Fort I stability. External palpation of the ZA can easily be performed.

Malar Flattening and Increased Facial Width. Because the zygoma is the major structure providing malar prominence, dislocation of the structure results in significant distortion of the cheek. Malar flattening typically occurs if at least one suture is frankly separated or dislocated. It can occur if the ZM suture is disrupted with rotation around an in-

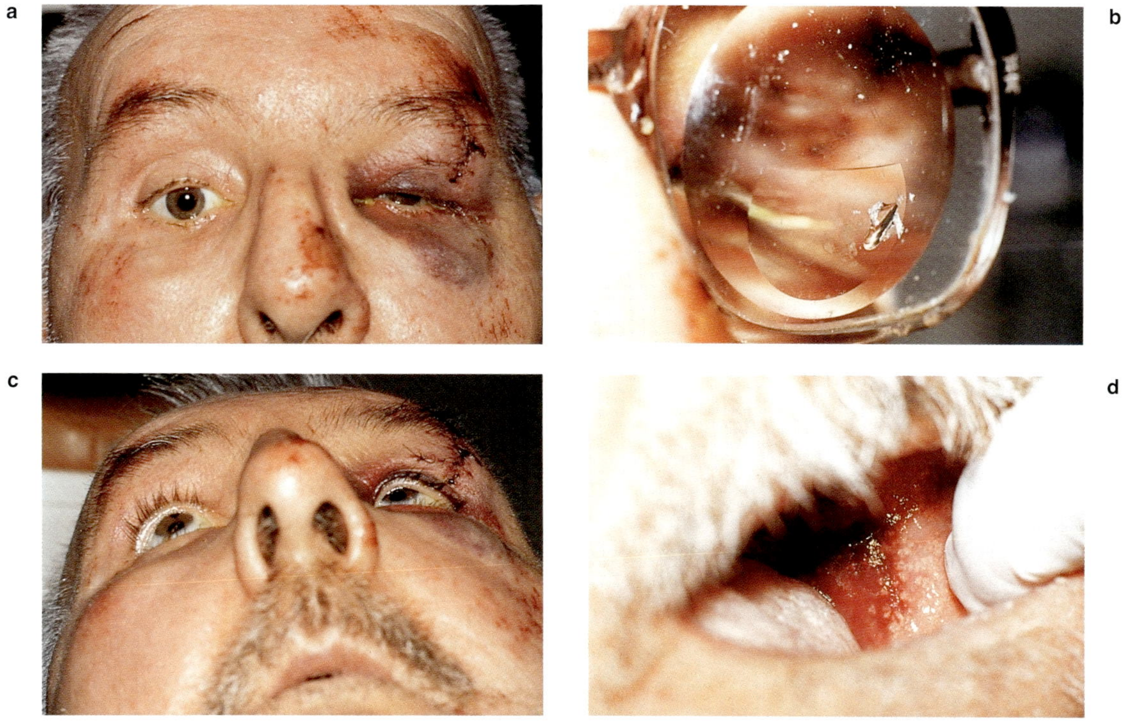

Fig. 20-45. Visually asymptomatic zygomaticomaxillary complex (ZMC) fracture. (**a**) This institutionalized patient passed out from unknown causes, falling onto a step, suffering an unprotected blow to his left cheek. (**b**) He was wearing his aphakic spectacles at the time, which exhibited significant damage. Fortunately, vision and the globe were unaffected. He complained of trismus and cranial nerve V_2 dysesthesia extending to the teeth. He denied diplopia and had full ocular range of motion. (**c**) Clinical examination showed point tenderness over the zygomaticofrontal suture and the zygomatic arch with a step-off deformity at the inferior orbital rim and malar flattening. (**d**) Oral examination showed buccal ecchymosis and significant tenderness at the ZMC buttress. Oral examination is an important part of the ophthalmologist's evaluation of a fracture, during which Le Fort I- and II-level fractures can also be identified. This patient refused treatment.

tact ZF suture, or vice versa, and it certainly occurs when more than one articulation is involved. If the ZA is affected, it generally dislocates laterally, increasing facial width (see Figures 20-14, 20-20, 20-38, 20-44, and 20-45).

Lateral Canthal Dystopia. If the lateral canthal tendon is still attached at the lateral orbital tubercle, downward canthal dystopia can be seen. The lid can also be dragged downward by the same mechanism.

Dysesthesia of Cranial Nerve V_2. The ZM suture runs very close to the infraorbital foramen along the anterior maxillary face. Therefore, fractures often compromise the neurovascular bundle, resulting in numbness of the cheek and, often, the ipsilateral teeth and gums.

Trismus and Malocclusion. The temporalis muscle originates along the temporalis fossa and passes medial to the ZA to insert on the coronoid process of the mandible. The masseter muscle arises from the inferomedial aspect of the ZA and the posterior-inferior aspect of the zygomatic body. It lies lateral to the temporalis and inserts along the ramus of the mandible. Together, the temporalis and masseter constitute the primary muscles of mastication.

Disruption of the zygoma, the ZA, or both dramatically affects the normal operation of these muscles. Significant bony dislocation of these structures—leading to direct impingement of the coronoid process as well as muscular swelling and hemorrhage—can lead to trismus (pain on opening the mouth) and limitation of movement. Likewise, tissue swelling and distortion can lead to frank misalignment of dental occlusion. Even though many patients have dental anesthesia, they can still perceive proper bite. Of course, malocclusion can also be a sequela of Le Fort I fracture or dental injury.[29]

Inferior or Lateral Rim Step-Off. Disruption or dislocation of the ZM or ZF sutures creates point tenderness and palpable separation.

Associated Floor Fracture Findings. Because the zygoma contributes to the lateral aspect of the floor, typical findings of floor fracture can be present. As stated above, this is why many ZMC fractures are sent initially to the eye clinic to rule out isolated blowout fracture. A good clinical examination can disclose the underlying larger fracture. However, as mentioned previously, a large fracture may not impede motility (see Figure 20-38).

Indications for Surgery

Minimally displaced or nondisplaced fractures can be followed conservatively. If orbital floor symptoms accompany a nondisplaced ZMC fracture (eg, restrictive diplopia), the floor should be explored independently. Occasionally, a minimally displaced ZMC fracture can be treated via closed, external reduction, but this is now uncommon practice. More typically, patients proceed to surgical reduction and fixation, via open reduction with internal fixation (ORIF). The goal of surgery is to restore stability of the four articulations. As previously mentioned, reestablishment of the buttresses—especially the ZMC buttress and arch—is the key to overall midfacial stability. Adequate ZMC fixation and stability require at least two points of rigid plate fixation. Wire fixation alone is insufficient to anchor the bone in three dimensions against the forces of normal jaw action, let alone the strong contractile forces of healing, fibrosis, and scarring.[24] Proper fixation is best accomplished with metal (titanium; see Figure 20-34) miniplates and microplates, but at times, interosseous wire techniques are still useful adjuncts.

Various surgical approaches are used, depending on the degrees of dislocation and comminution. The greater the injury, the wider the surgical exposure required. The ZMC buttress is typically approached via an intraoral gingival incision (eg, Caldwell-Luc procedure, Keen incision). The ZA can be exposed and reduced through a coronal flap or Gilles's approach. The ZM suture is typically repaired through any traditional approach to the orbital floor, although most oculoplastic surgeons would vastly prefer the transconjunctival or subciliary methods to a direct rim incision. Currently (2002), we believe the transconjunctival approach to be superior even to the subciliary, as the likelihood of postoperative cicatricial lid retraction and ectropion appears to be lower.

The ZF suture can be stabilized through an extended lid-crease incision, a direct lateral rim incision, or a coronal flap. Accurate reduction and alignment of the zygoma are critical to a good cosmetic result postoperatively, but relying solely on the external appearance of the reduction can be misleading. A more accurate perspective of proper reduction is gained by inspecting the internal (orbital) contour of the lateral wall and trying to attain a smooth internal contour at the zygomaticosphenoidal junction. Such reduction requires three-dimensional control of the zygomatic body. A handy instrument for achieving control in three dimensions is the Carroll-Girard screw, which temporarily secures into the body of the zygoma like a joystick. The bone can then be manipulated in multiple axes. Once the proper reduction is achieved, the zygoma is plated in place.[4] Another key concept in reconstruction is the reduction of the ZA, which, despite its name, is actually a rather flat, straight structure (see Figure 20-38). Taking pains to accurately reestablish the proper flat orientation of the ZA helps ensure proper reduction of increased facial width and the reestablishment of proper midfacial projection.[4]

If surgery is to be performed, then the orbit and floor should be explored to prevent orbital tissues from becoming inadvertently incarcerated during manipulation and reduction (see Figure 20-20). Additionally, as stated above, the internal aspect of the lateral wall is a very good indicator of correct alignment of the ZA.

Specific indications for surgical intervention include the following:

- significant malar flattening,
- lateral canthal dystopia or lower-lid malposition,
- trismus or malocclusion,
- significant orbital enlargement, with or without orbital floor symptoms, and
- significant displacement or comminution.

Naso-Orbital-Ethmoid

NOE fractures are the result of high-energy trauma that impacts on the central midface. By definition, these are complex, multilevel injuries, and they require management by several services. NOE fractures are almost always associated with significant craniofacial trauma, such as that resulting from high-speed motor vehicle accidents, and may be life-threatening because of vascular damage or airway compromise (particularly if the injuries are to the lower face). As the most complex of the facial fractures, more often than not they require more than one surgery for complete repair. Surgical stages may include initial ORIF with or without primary bone grafting, subsequent bone-graft harvests, several soft-tissue surgeries (such as scar revisions, telecanthus repair, and orbital volume augmentation), lacrimal repair, strabismus surgery, and oral surgery.[4,30]

The NOE region is typically injured in direct frontal impact, and the high energies involved crumple the bones of the nose and midface. The nasoethmoid labyrinth, however, often acts as a safety "crumple zone," absorbing much of the energy as it collapses internally (Figure 20-46). Although the crumpling creates tremendous midfacial and orbital disruption, it can sometimes prevent serious ocular injury (see Figures 20-1, 20-2, 20-16, and 20-31).

The NOE region includes the confluence of various facial buttresses. Not only do the nasomaxillary, upper-rim, and lower-rim buttresses all converge in the area of the nasal root bilaterally, but the vertical buttresses also meet here (see Figure 20-12). Consequently, NOE fractures are invariably bilateral. Comminution is the rule. Loss of the buttresses leads to three-dimensional collapse of the midface (see Figures 20-31 and 20-46). As the nasofrontal processes of the maxillary and frontal bones and the ethmoid telescope, the bridge of the nose is depressed, which causes loss of facial projection. Loss of the anterior medial wall (particularly the anterior and posterior lacrimal crests) leads to instability of the medial canthal tendons and telecanthus, as well as to injury of the nasolacrimal duct. Telecanthus requires accurate reduction and fixation of the posterior horn of the medial canthal tendons (the more posterior and superior, the better). This can be done by cantilevered plates suspended from the anterior nasofrontal process, or may require transnasal wire fixation. Lacrimal drainage injury may eventually require dacryocystorhinostomy.

Loss of the horizontal stabilizers—the upper and lower rims and the maxillary alveolus—leads to decreased midfacial width. Injury at the Le Fort I level is common. Loss of the vertical buttresses can lead to loss of facial height, especially if the mandible is affected as well. Malocclusion and chronic open bites can persist, even after attempted ORIF, if the lower buttresses are not accurately reconstructed.

NOE fractures usually cause some degree of damage at the Le Fort II and III levels as well. Multiple orbital walls, as well as the cribriform plate, can be fractured. Energy transmitted posteriorly along the medial wall can result in frank fracture of the optic canal or concussive damage to the optic nerve (traumatic optic neuropathy) (see Figure 20-16). Consequently, vision must be monitored meticulously, but because these patients often suffer significant brain injury and may be comatose, vision is not always assessable early in the course of treatment. Damage to the cribriform plate can also lead to CSF leaks and anosmia.

Soft-tissue reconstruction in this area can be challenging. Despite the excellent vascular supply to the tissues, fibrosis and tissue contraction can make any reconstructive attempt unsatisfying. Unlike other areas of the face and body that have relatively large, flat areas of homogenous skin, the midface is characterized by compound curves of tissue of varying

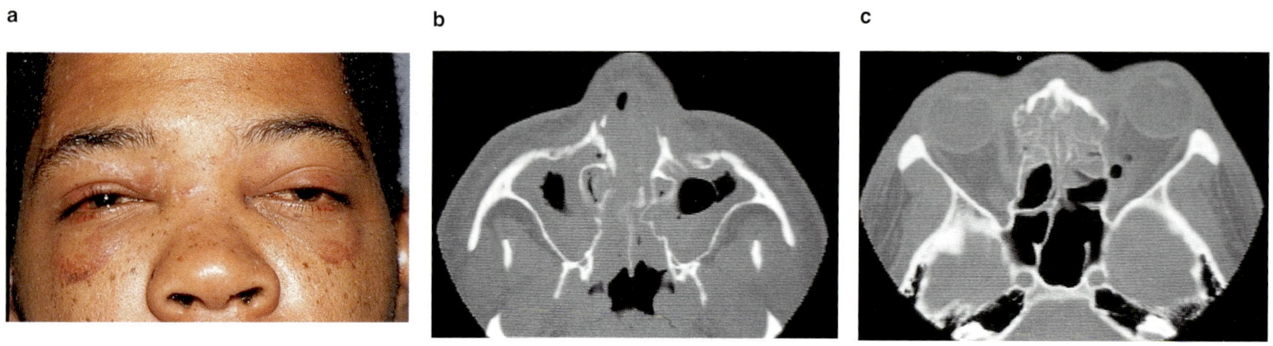

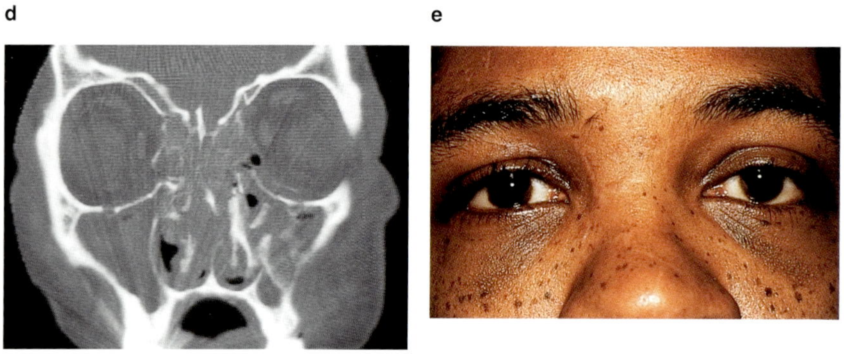

Fig. 20-46. (**a**) This man lost control of his car on ice and slid into a ditch, striking his face against the steering wheel. Vision and ocular examination were normal. The patient demonstrated the typical nasal fracture with saddle nose deformity and widening of the radix. Traumatic tele-canthus is common in naso-orbital-ethmoid (NOE) fractures, although this patient did not suffer it. Axial computed tomography (CT) scans show the massively telescoped collapse of (**b**) the midfacial skeleton, with marked comminution of the septum, bilateral medial maxillary walls, and (**c**) the ethmoid complex. The pterygoid plates are not fractured; therefore, these fractures are not true Le Fort fractures. (**d**) A coronal CT shows the degree of comminution of the vertical midfacial skeleton. Notice the marked hemorrhage, which fills all the sinus spaces. Notice also that the orbits are relatively spared, which is sometimes seen in NOE fractures. Fractures as extensive as these require early repair, and wide surgical exposure is required. (**e**) The same patient 3 weeks after open reduction and internal fixation, with a well-healed Lynch ethmoidectomy incision and normal intercanthal distance but with residual nasal depression. It is not unusual for NOE fractures to require further nasal, sinus, or lacrimal surgery.

thickness, pilosebaceous composition, and variable healing ability (see Figures 20-19 and 20-39).

Symptoms and Signs

The symptoms and signs of an NOE fracture are as follows:

- facial flattening,
- traumatic telecanthus,
- damage to the nasolacrimal system,
- epistaxis, CSF rhinorrhea, or anosmia,
- signs and symptoms of associated fractures, and
- traumatic optic neuropathy or optic canal fracture.

Indication for Surgery

The presence of an NOE fracture is the only indication necessary for surgery. Reconstruction of NOE fractures is difficult. Unlike other fractures described above, in which even comminuted bony fragments can often be salvaged for use in ORIF, NOE fractures often require bone grafts to replace the very small pieces of bone remaining (usually along the medial wall and nasomaxillary buttress). Wide exposure is mandatory, usually requiring bicoronal flap, bilateral gingival sulcus incisions, and orbital exposure. Total facial degloving in the subperiosteal plane allows mobilization of the facial soft tissues.

Early surgical intervention is crucial to successful facial restoration. Failure to operate in the acute setting can lead to irreversible contraction of the facial structures. In this setting of massive facial trauma, a delay of even a few days can lead to significant fibrosis. It is axiomatic that the soft tissues contract to conform to the underlying facial skeleton—wherever that framework should be. Contraction begins almost immediately after injury and, once set in motion, is very difficult to reverse.

Additionally, delaying surgery creates a separate traumatic insult. Soft tissues that suffered contusion damage during the initial injury are reinjured. Convalescing tissues are edematous and highly vascular. Operating soon after the initial insult takes advantage of the acute process and "disguises" the surgical insult within that of the original trauma. Soft tissues that were degloved traumatically or surgically can be redraped and reattached appropriately. In this way, contractile forces can be better controlled, and a better functional and cosmetic outcome results.

MANAGEMENT OF ORBITAL FRACTURES

The primary objective in managing orbital trauma is to *ensure the integrity of the globe*. Remember that any type of orbital trauma can cause loss of vision through either direct concomitant ocular trauma, or indirect optic nerve damage. Once the ocular injury has been evaluated, proceed with the orbital evaluation. A good clinical evaluation should look for all of the major fractures listed above. Remember that fractures can often be multiple: just because the patient has what looks to be (and probably is) an isolated floor fracture does not eliminate the possibility of an associated roof or ZMC fracture as well. The only way to be sure is to look for associated fractures. Ask about trismus and malocclusion. While checking for cranial nerve V_2 dysesthesia, check V_1 as well. Run a finger around the upper gingival sulcus and press on the ZMC buttress.

The thorough clinical examination can give a good idea of what to expect on imaging.[2] First, get good CT images through the orbit, and, if needed, the sinuses. As stated before, 3-mm axial and true coronal views usually suffice to evaluate the bone and most soft tissue. Consider thinner slices if looking for FBs, dealing with children, looking for optic canal trauma, or if true coronal views cannot be obtained. Depending on the type of FB or soft-tissue injury, an MRI may be needed as well, but only after metallic FBs have been ruled out.

Orbital fractures are considered "dirty" (ie, contaminated) whether the fracture is open or not, but thanks to the rich facial vascular supply, posttrauma infection is uncommon. Nevertheless, most surgeons feel that a course of prophylactic antibiotics is warranted. A broad-spectrum oral antibiotic will usually do, but, depending on the mechanism and extent of injury, intravenous dosing may be appropriate. To prevent orbital emphysema, tell the patient to refrain from nose blowing.

The orbit has several important neighboring structures that also may be involved. Even if the orbital injury is isolated, however, consider asking for help from other surgical services, such as ENT, OMFS, or plastic surgery. Trauma is always managed best when several minds work together. In addition, members of each service bring different perspectives and experiences to the case, enriching the learning experience for all.

Having put together a clinical picture of the extent of the trauma, the ophthalmic surgeon must now formulate a surgical plan. If the fractures are comminuted, will a plating set be needed? If so, where is the set kept? If multiple services are collaborating, whose plating set will be used? Is it a miniplate set, or a microplate set? Will one of each be needed? Is a microdrill available, and does it have a bit of the proper size for the particular plating set being used? Can all the needed specialties be present? Which instrument sets are needed? Who will do what first? (In complex trauma, OMFS or ENT will probably want to stabilize dental occlusion first, with intermaxillary fixation. If bone is missing, a calvarial graft may be harvested, in which case a bicoronal flap will be raised before the orbit is approached.) Will special cultures be needed?

Make sure that all needed equipment will be available at the time of surgery. Remember that each plating system has its own peculiarities: miniplate screws will not fit into microplate holes; one manufacturer's screws may not accept another's screwdrivers; mixing one type of screw with another type of plate throws off the profile, because each is milled for its own particular system.

When to operate depends on the nature and extent of the injury, but—unless vision is threatened—isolated orbital trauma rarely requires absolutely emergent intervention.[1–6,21,30] Most can be delayed at least overnight, when the regular eye surgical team is available, and many cases can be postponed for several days without jeopardizing the outcome. However, do not delay surgery needlessly, especially if the patient needs surgery anyway. For example, if the patient has a large floor blowout, or frank entrapment on CT with restriction on forced ductions and diplopia, or a frank surgical ZMC, or an injury in which surgery is clearly indicated, little or nothing will be gained by waiting 7 to 10 days; the decision that surgery is needed has been made. If there is significant edema, it is reasonable to wait for some of the edema to go down (corticosteroids may help speed the resolution), but in general, once the decision to operate has been made, the sooner the better. Waiting longer than 7 to 10 days allows significant fibrosis to set up. This may impair distraction of orbital tissues from sinuses and prevent accurate alignment of the buttresses, with resultant loss of facial proportion and projection.[2,4,5] To a large extent, the first operation sets the course for the eventual outcome, and in complex trauma, a delay of even 7 days can have a deleterious effect on results. As a general rule, the more complex the fracture, the sooner the operation.[2]

SURGICAL TECHNIQUES

The goal of treatment is to restore the orbital bony contour and volume. For the most part, this is accomplished through surgical ORIF. Currently, reduction and fixation are best accomplished by means of three-dimensional rigid plate fixation.[2,4,5,31]

Incision

Placement of the incision can be the single most important step in the surgical procedure. In orbital surgery—whether for trauma or tumor—exposure is the key. The desire to minimize a scar must not compromise surgical goals. Nevertheless, the surgeon should avoid making a huge incision if it is not necessary, and if the needed exposure can reasonably be achieved through an existing laceration or a hidden incision, then that is preferable to a new cutaneous incision. Experience has shown that almost every orbital structure can be reached via a variety of hidden incisions. These incisions include the bicoronal flap and transconjunctival, transcaruncular, and gingival sulcus incisions. In general, if a fracture fragment is at the furthest reaches of where an invisible incision would end, then the surgeon is better off not even attempting that incision.[5] Some bleeding invariably occurs once the area is exposed. Frank hemorrhage is rare, however; bleeding will most likely be a slow ooze. Resist the temptation to use monopolar electrocautery (eg, Bovie) in the orbit. Because of the prolapsed orbital tissue and its fibrovascular connections, not to mention the danger of inadvertently touching one of the metal orbital retractors and causing widespread damage, low-power bipolar cautery is preferred.

The pupil should be continually monitored throughout the case. If light is effectively obstructed from entering the fellow eye, pupillary size and reaction give a gross estimation of optic nerve function. To prevent iatrogenic direct optic nerve damage, posterior dissection beyond 30 mm should be undertaken only with extreme caution.[32]

Implants

Various implants are available for use in orbital reconstruction. If a bony wall is fractured with entrapment of tissues but the bony plates are relatively intact and not significantly displaced, then an absorbable implant can be used to span the defect and prevent reentrapment while the fracture heals. Examples of absorbable implants are fascia lata, gelatin film (Gel*film*, not Gel*foam*), polyglactin (Vicryl) mesh, and anterior maxillary wall (Figure 20-47).[33] The disadvantage of both Gelfilm and Vicryl mesh

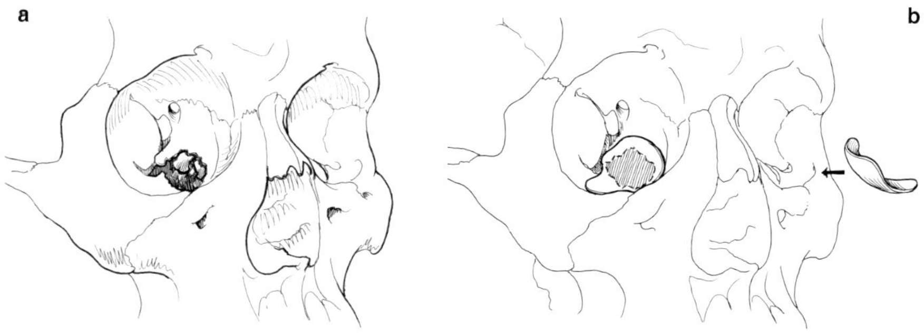

Fig. 20-47. The overriding premise of orbital fracture repair is twofold: to release all entrapped tissues and to prevent recurrence of herniation by placing a barrier over the fracture site while the fracture heals. If the fracture is small, an absorbable implant can suffice. (**a**) If the fracture is large or comminuted, the implant must (**b**) be large enough to span the defect and substantial enough to withstand the weight of the orbital tissues. A variety of materials is available for use. Axiomatic to the placement of any plate is that the plate must accurately reconstruct the normal intraorbital contour. Drawings prepared for this textbook by Gary Wind, MD, Uniformed Services University of the Health Sciences, Bethesda, Md.

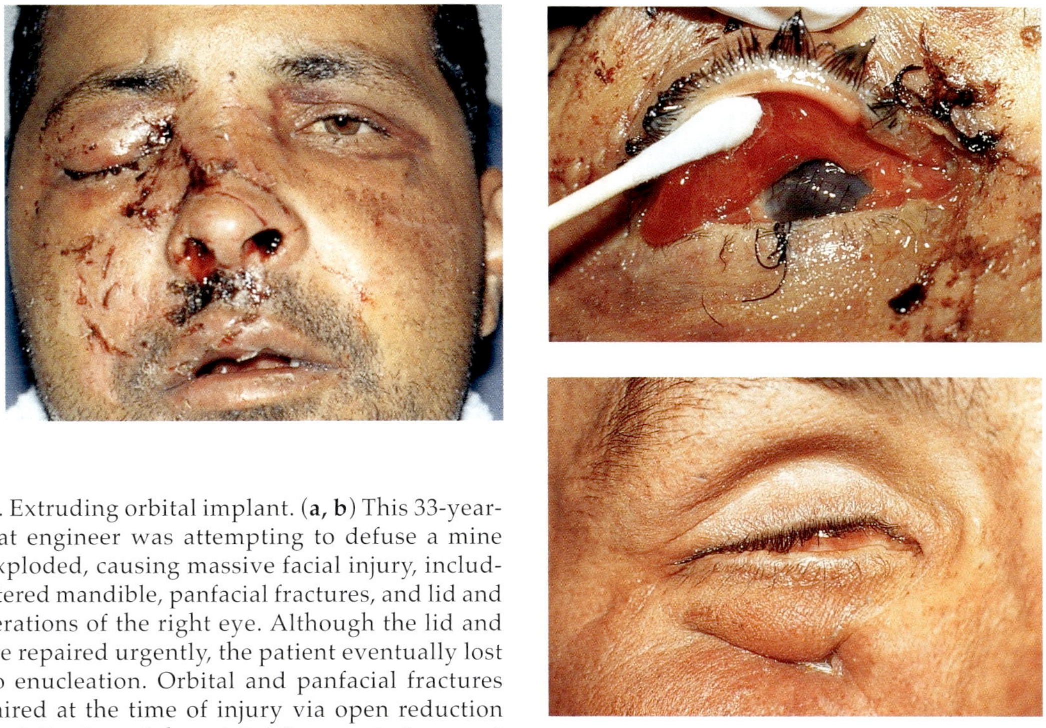

Fig. 20-48. Extruding orbital implant. (**a, b**) This 33-year-old combat engineer was attempting to defuse a mine when it exploded, causing massive facial injury, including a shattered mandible, panfacial fractures, and lid and globe lacerations of the right eye. Although the lid and globe were repaired urgently, the patient eventually lost the eye to enucleation. Orbital and panfacial fractures were repaired at the time of injury via open reduction and internal fixation of the orbital floor and placement of a silicone plate. One year later, the patient developed increasing swelling, erythema, and discomfort of the right eye. (**c**) The floor plate eventually extruded and was removed surgically.

is their lack of rigidity, especially when wet; therefore, they may not be suitable for spanning large, open fracture cavities. In patients with these types of large defects, a more rigid implant that can be cantilevered over the defect is needed.

Silicone plastic (Silastic) sheets are still widely used and are available in a variety of thicknesses (rigidities). A major drawback to these implants is that they occasionally migrate or extrude because of their smooth, nonporous surfaces (Figure 20-48). Various methods have been used to secure these plates in place more permanently, including bending a tab into the fracture, suturing or wiring the plate to the rim, or spot welding the plate to the floor with high-temperature thermal cautery. *We strongly advise against the latter method* because the cautery temperature is generally well above the flashpoints of these petroleum-based silicone plastic materials, and they may ignite if this maneuver is performed.

Alternatives include porous implants, which allow incorporation of fibrovascular tissue into the material, thereby preventing migration (at least in theory). Porous polyethylene (Medpor), titanium mesh orbital floor plates, and split-thickness calvarial bone are examples of porous implants. These implant materials have the added advantage of being moldable or sculptable, which allows specific configuration to restore proper orbital volume. A significant drawback to these materials is the difficulty in removing them, should that become necessary.

The most dramatic recent advance in surgical technique is the increasing use of titanium plates to reduce comminuted fractures. These plates have allowed the accurate reduction and reconstruction of the major buttresses, with restoration of structural integrity to a degree not previously seen with surgical wire (Figure 20-49). Both miniplates and the lower-profile microplates are easier to place than surgical steel wire. Current technology allows the manufacture of very strong 1.0-mm, 1.3-mm, and 1.5-mm plates. Unfortunately, the availability of titanium plates on the battlefield is dubious. So although the use of steel wire during peacetime may be limited, military ophthalmologists should be familiar with it. Titanium has the added advantage of being nonmagnetic, whereas steel is not. Patients—particularly battlefield casualties—in whom wire is used must be told of its presence in the event of future MRI.

Before placing any implant on the orbital floor, all orbital tissue that has prolapsed into the maxil-

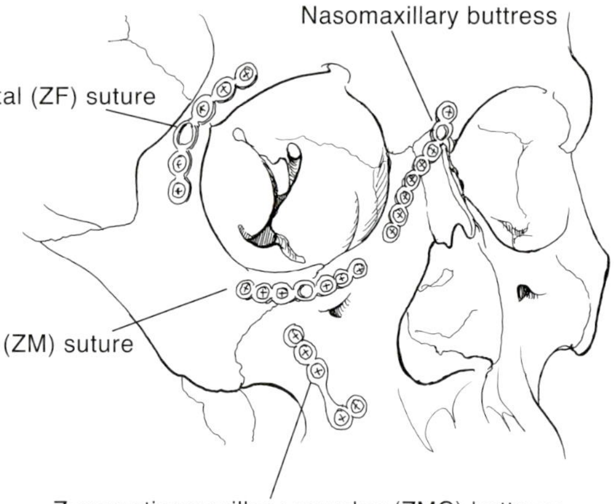

Fig. 20-49. Titanium microplates and miniplates allow more-accurate reconstruction of the facial skeleton in three dimensions than was previously possible with wire fixation. Plates are best used to reconstruct the facial buttresses. At least two screws should anchor the plates on each side of the fracture line. Drawing prepared for this textbook by Gary Wind, MD, Uniformed Services University of the Health Sciences, Bethesda, Md.

lary sinus must be extracted, using gentle hand-over-hand technique with a ribbon retractor and a blunt elevator as the primary tools. Occasionally, a bayonet forceps can help raise tissue that is tenaciously scarred in. Above all, remember that the neurovascular bundle of cranial nerve V_2 runs through the orbital floor and is supposed to be adherent to the floor. Unfortunately, many orbital tissues look alike after trauma, and it is not uncommon for even experienced surgeons to mistake the V_2 neurovascular bundle for incarcerated orbital tissue. During the heat of surgery, the surgeon must not tug overmuch on tissue and accidentally rip the nerve. *And under no circumstances should the surgeon cut it.*

Closure

In closing the incision, the surgeon should avoid suturing deep tissues. Incarceration of the septum into a microplate or deep closure often leads to lid retraction, particularly of the lower lid (Figure 20-50). The surgeon must also avoid the temptation to place an excessive number of deep sutures. The inflammatory response to trauma is active enough that adding another potential nidus of reaction only adds fuel to the fire. Most orbital incisions can be closed with simple cutaneous or vertical mattress sutures. Always consider placing a lid-traction suture at the end of the case to counteract early contraction.

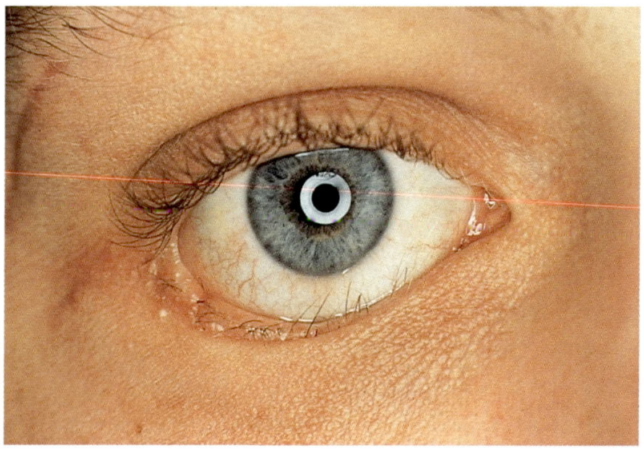

Fig. 20-50. Middle lamellar cicatricial retraction. Postoperative lower-lid retraction is typically secondary to contraction and scarring of the orbital septum and middle lamella. This patient underwent open reduction and internal fixation of an orbital fracture via a subciliary incision. In closing the periosteum, the orbital septum was inadvertently incarcerated, resulting in progressive lid retraction. Repair of this deformity required extensive lysis of scar bands; placement of a spacer graft; Frost traction suture; and corticosteroids administered topically, intralesionally, and systemically. Transconjunctival approaches to the orbital rim and floor may be less prone to this complication.

POSTOPERATIVE CARE

Many surgeons opt against pressure patching the eye after orbital surgery, fearing devastating loss of vision from increased orbital pressure in the face of an unexpected postoperative orbital hemorrhage. Such concerns are valid. Other surgeons argue that an orbital hemorrhage may drain through any fracture into the adjacent sinus, thereby decompressing the orbit. This reasoning, too, is valid. However, we have seen compressive optic neuropathy and loss of vision from orbital hemorrhage in the face of large orbital fractures, which nonetheless required canthotomy and cantholysis to decompress. There is no absolute right or wrong answer. We prefer to patch lightly overnight and then to remove the patch the next day. Overnight vision checks are recommended, and we routinely prescribe antinausea medications.

Surprisingly, postoperative pain is usually mild to moderate after orbital surgery and only rarely requires strong narcotic pain medication to control. Aggressive treatment with cold or ice packs helps in several ways. First, it helps decrease postoperative swelling and ecchymosis. Additionally, it helps decrease pain. After several days of cold packs, the patient can switch to warm-water compresses. Oral corticosteroids may also help resolve postoperative swelling.

As stated previously, the risk of postoperative orbital cellulitis is extremely low, despite the frank communication between the orbit and contaminated sinuses. Nevertheless, most surgeons will prescribe at least a short course of prophylactic oral antibiotics; a broad-spectrum antibiotic that covers *Staphylococcus* and *Streptococcus* species and *Haemophilus influenza* is most appropriate. To guard against both producing orbital emphysema and inoculating the orbit with sinus bacteria, patients should refrain from nose blowing and vigorous straining for at least 2 weeks.

Diplopia resolves in a variable length of time. If preoperative diplopia was mostly restrictive, then postoperatively, the patient should be markedly improved. Some limitation of motility may persist, however, because of contusion, apraxia, or ischemic contracture of the muscle. Active range-of-motion exercises can help expand the field of single binocular vision over time.

If a lid-traction suture was placed, it should be left in place for several days. If the lower lid begins to retract, gentle upward massage can sometimes reverse the process. Topical corticosteroids, especially the potent fluorinated steroids (eg, clobetasol), can be very effective. These topical medications are not formulated for the eye and must be used very judiciously, as they pose all the risks of ocular steroids in addition to having potential systemic effects. Intralesional steroid injections can also help.

Return to duty is obviously predicated on the extent of the trauma, the complexity of the repair, and the patient's occupation. Most patients with isolated floor or medial wall fractures can be discharged from the hospital the same day or after overnight observation. These patients can return to light duty quickly, usually within 2 weeks. (It is not unusual to find professional athletes returning to full contact within a few weeks of facial fracture repair.) They should be encouraged to use the eye as much as possible, with the previously stated warnings about nose blowing and straining. There is a paucity of information regarding the timing and safety of flight or of diving after orbital fracture, but we believe that such patients should not be exposed to these conditions for 2 to 3 weeks. If a patient must fly, he or she should be counseled to watch for signs of compressive pneumo-orbita (increasing proptosis, increased orbital pressure, decreased vision), and the cabin should be immediately repressurized. More extensive traumas, especially those that may require additional surgery, should be evacuated to the higher level of care as quickly as possible to minimize soft-tissue fibrosis.

SUMMARY

Orbital trauma requires extensive evaluation. The injured anatomical structures can range from one to many, and cooperation and participation of multiple surgical services—of which ophthalmology must be a part—are required to repair the damage. Because extended formal training in oculoplastics is probably not realistic, the general ophthalmologist must be comfortable with the evaluation and treatment of myriad orbital injuries, ranging from FBs to fractures. He or she must also be conversant with the basic nomenclature and techniques of consulting services and must be suspicious enough of any injury to seek consultation quickly. Above all, the ophthalmologist must serve as the guardian of vision, ever vigilant to the potential threat to the globe, regardless of how well disguised that threat may be.

REFERENCES

1. Wesley RE, Anderson SR, Weiss MR, Smith HP. Management of orbito-cranial trauma. In: Bosniak SL, Smith BC, eds. *Orbital Trauma.* Part 2. In: Bosniak SL, Smith BC, eds. *Advances in Ophthalmic Plastic and Reconstructive Surgery*. Vol 7. New York, NY: Pergamon Press; 1987: 3–26.

2. Guttenberg SA. Complicated orbital fractures. In: Bosniak SL, Smith BC, eds. *Orbital Trauma.* Part 2. In: Bosniak SL, Smith BC, eds. *Advances in Ophthalmic Plastic and Reconstructive Surgery.* Vol 7. New York, NY: Pergamon Press; 1987: 41–59.

3. Green RP, Peters DR, Shore JW, Fanton JW, Davis H. Force necessary to fracture the orbital floor. *Ophthal Plast Reconstr Surg.* 1990;6:211–217.

4. Manson PN. Dimensional analysis of the facial skeleton. In: Manson PN, ed. *Problems in Plastic and Reconstructive Surgery: Cranio-Maxillofacial Trauma.* Philadelphia, Pa: Lippincott; 1991: 213–237.

5. Phillips JH, Gruss JS. Choice of plates or screws for midfacial fixation. In: Manson PN, ed. *Problems in Plastic and Reconstructive Surgery: Cranio-Maxillofacial Trauma.* Philadelphia, Pa: Lippincott; 1991: 333–349.

6. Mayer MH, Manson PN. Plate and screw fixation in craniofacial skeletal fractures. In: Manson PN, ed. *Problems in Plastic and Reconstructive Surgery: Cranio-Maxillofacial Trauma.* Philadelphia, Pa: Lippincott; 1991: 290–310.

7. Mauriello JA, Lee HJ, Nguyen L. CT of soft tissue injury and orbital fractures. *Radiol Clin North Am.* 1999;37(1):241–252.

8. Lakits A, Steiner E, Scholda C, Kontrus M. Evaluation of intraocular foreign bodies by spiral computed tomography and multiplanar reconstruction. *Ophthalmology.* 1998;105:307–312.

9. Woolfson JM, Wesley RE. Magnetic resonance imaging and computed tomographic scanning of fresh (green) wood foreign bodies in dog orbits. *Ophthal Plast Reconstr Surg.* 1990;6:237–240.

10. Wilson WB, Driesbach JN, Lattin DE, Stears JE. Magnetic resonance imaging of nonmetallic orbital foreign bodies. *Am J Ophthalmol.* 1988;105:612–617.

11. Trokel SL. Radiologic evaluation of ophthalmologic trauma. In: Freeman HM, ed. *Ocular Trauma.* New York, NY: Appleton-Century-Crofts; 1979: 15–22.

12. Wolter JR. Subperiosteal hematoma of the orbit in young males: A serious complication of trauma or surgery in the eye regions. *Trans Am Ophthalmol Soc.* 1979;77:104–120.

13. Andenmatten R, Piguet B, Klainguti G. Orbital hemorrhage induced by barotrauma. *Am J Ophthalmol.* 1994;118:536.

14. Amrith S, Baratham G, Khoo CY, Low CH, Sinniah R. Spontaneous hematic cysts of the orbit presenting with acute proptosis: A report of three cases. *Ophthal Plast Reconstr Surg.* 1990;6:273–277.

15. Katz B, Carmody R. Subperiosteal orbital hematoma induced by the Valsalva maneuver. *Am J Ophthalmol.* 1985;100:617–618.

16. Dobben GD, Philip B, Mafee MF, Choi K, Belmont H, Dorodi S. Orbital subperiosteal hematoma, cholesterol granuloma, and infection: Evaluation with MR imaging and CT. *Radiol Clin North Am.* 1998;36(5):1185–1200.

17. Mader TH, Aragones JV, Chandler AC, et al. Ocular and ocular adnexal injuries treated by US military ophthalmologists during Operations Desert Shield and Desert Storm. *Ophthalmology.* 1993;100:1462–1467.

18. Nasr AM, Haik BG, Fleming JC, Al-Hussain HM, Karcioglu ZA. Penetrating orbital injury with organic foreign bodies. *Ophthalmology.* 1999;106:523–532.

19. Koornneef L, Zonneveld FW. Penetrating orbital injuries. In: Manson PN, ed. *Problems in Plastic and Reconstructive Surgery: Cranio-Maxillofacial Trauma.* Philadelphia, Pa: Lippincott; 1991: 395–407.

20. Matson MD. Injuries to the face and neck. In: Zajtchuk R, Grande CM, eds. *Anesthesia and Perioperative Care of the Combat Casualty.* In: Zajtchuk R, Bellamy RF, eds. *Textbook of Military Medicine.* Washington, DC: Department of the Army, Office of The Surgeon General, Borden Institute; 1995: 437–453.

21. Lisman RD, Barna N, Smith BC. Internal orbital fractures: Controversies in the surgical decision. In: Manson PN, ed. *Problems in Plastic and Reconstructive Surgery: Cranio-Maxillofacial Trauma*. Philadelphia, Pa: Lippincott; 1991: 365–394.

22. Almog Y, Mayron Y, Weiss J, Lazar M, Avrahami E. Pneumomediastinum following blowout fracture of the medial orbital wall: A case report. *Ophthal Plast Reconstr Surg.* 1993;9:289–291.

23. McCord CD, Shore JW, Moses JL. Orbital fractures and late reconstruction. In: McCord CD; Tanenbaum M, eds. *Oculoplastic Surgery*. Philadelphia, Pa: Lippincott-Raven; 1987: 155–168.

24. Watmull D, Rohrich RJ. Zygoma fracture fixation. In: Manson PN, ed. *Problems in Plastic and Reconstructive Surgery: Cranio-Maxillofacial Trauma*. Philadelphia, Pa: Lippincott; 1991: 350–364.

25. Lisman RD, Smith BC, Rogers R. Volkmann's ischemic contractures and blowout fractures. In: Bosniak SL, Smith BC, eds. *Orbital Trauma.* Part 2. In: Bosniak SL, Smith BC, eds. *Advances in Ophthalmic Plastic and Reconstructive Surgery*. Vol 7. New York, NY: Pergamon Press; 1987: 117–132.

26. Burnstine MA. Clinical recommendations for repair of isolated orbital floor fractures: An evidence-based analysis. *Ophthalmology*. 2002;109:1207–1213.

27. Sires BS, Stanley RB Jr, Levine LM. Oculocardiac reflex caused by orbital floor trapdoor fracture: An indication for urgent repair [letter]. *Arch Ophthalmol*. 1998;116:955–956.

28. Jordan DR, Allen LH, White J, et al. Intervention within days for some orbital floor fractures: The white-eyed blowout. *Ophthal Plast Reconstr Surg.* 1998;14:379–390.

29. Bedrossian EH, Della Rocca RC. Management of zygomaticomaxillary (tripod) fractures. In: Della Rocca RC, Nesi FA, Lisman RD, eds. *Smith's Ophthalmic Plastic and Reconstructive Surgery*. St Louis, Mo: CV Mosby; 1987: 506–522.

30. Petrelli RL. Naso-orbital fractures: Management and complications. In: Bosniak SL, Smith BC, eds. *Orbital Trauma.* Part 2. In: Bosniak SL, Smith BC, eds. *Advances in Ophthalmic Plastic and Reconstructive Surgery*. Vol 7. New York, NY: Pergamon Press; 1987: 27–32.

31. Patipa M, Slavin A. Axial dynamic compression plates in the management of complex orbital fractures via transconjunctival orbitotomy. *Ophthal Plast Reconstr Surg.* 1990;6:229–236.

32. Mauriello JA Jr. Complications of orbital trauma surgery. In: Bosniak SL, Smith BC, eds. *Orbital Trauma.* Part 2. In: Bosniak SL, Smith BC, eds. *Advances in Ophthalmic Plastic and Reconstructive Surgery*. Vol 7. New York, NY: Pergamon Press; 1987: 99–115.

33. Mauriello JA Jr, McShane R, Voglino J. Use of Vicryl (polyglactin-910) mesh implant for correcting enophthalmos and hypo-ophthalmos: A study of 16 patients. *Ophthal Plast Reconstr Surg.* 1990;6(4):247–251.

Chapter 21

EXTRAOCULAR MUSCLE TRAUMA

SCOTT K. McCLATCHEY, MD*

*Commander, Medical Corps, US Navy; Director, Motility Service, Department of Ophthalmology, Naval Medical Center San Diego, San Diego, California 92134; Clinical Assistant Professor, Department of Surgery, Uniformed Services University of Health Sciences, 4301 Jones Bridge Road, Bethesda, Maryland 20814-4799

INTRODUCTION

Diplopia (ie, double vision; a symptom) after extraocular muscle trauma following a head injury is not uncommon, and it can be disabling. In addition to the distress diplopia generates, the cosmetic appearance due to ocular misalignment is usually unacceptable. *Traumatic strabismus* (ie, lack of parallelism between the eyes' visual axes; a sign) has three main causes: direct injury to the muscles, orbital injury, and neurological injury. A careful workup, including a complete eye examination and measurements of alignment, is used to evaluate the cause and suggest a treatment. In addition, imaging studies and forced ductions are sometimes required.

Treatment of patients with traumatic strabismus is closely related to the cause, and it varies from waiting for spontaneous recovery to prisms to surgery. The surgical decision process can be quite complex and should be based on an accurate knowledge of the etiology of the misalignment and on the principles of strabismus surgery.

ETIOLOGY OF TRAUMATIC STRABISMUS

Direct Trauma to Extraocular Muscles

Direct injury to the extraocular muscles can cause immediate diplopia with obvious misalignment of the eyes. Although uncommon, it is dramatic when it occurs (Figure 21-1). A report of ocular injuries after the Oklahoma City bombing documented only one rectus muscle transection in 115 injuries.[1] In a series from South Africa of 25 patients with traumatic muscle loss, 81% of the injuries were due to stab wounds and none were associated with significant globe penetration or optic nerve damage.[2] Most injuries that cause strabismus are in the anterior, relatively exposed, segment of the extraocular muscles' tendons. A few patients, however, have a posterior laceration of the muscle or trauma to the trochlea of the superior oblique (Figure 21-2).

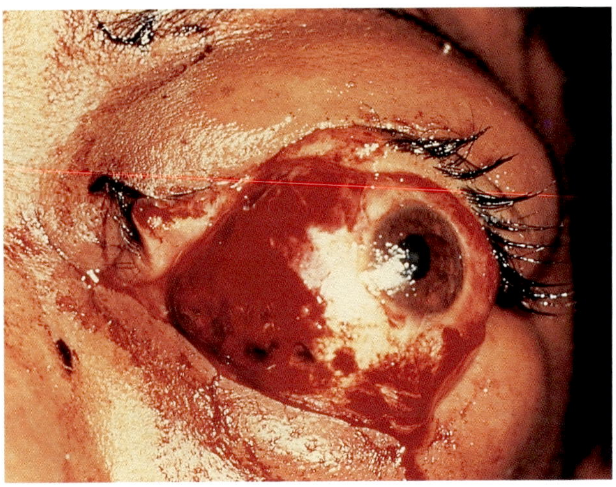

Fig. 21-1. Traumatic laceration of the inferior rectus muscle. This patient received a blow to the eye in a fight; a finger between the eye and the inferior orbital rim cut the inferior rectus. Photograph: Courtesy of Miguel Paciuc, MD, Mexico City, Mexico.

When eyes with an anterior injury are explored surgically, most are found to have a superficial scleral laceration, with the muscle some 5 to 6 mm from its original insertion. The inferior rectus is the most commonly affected muscle, followed by the medial rectus, the lateral rectus, the superior rectus, the inferior oblique, and the superior oblique.[2]

Orbital Fracture

An orbital fracture is one of the most common causes of traumatic diplopia. The classic blowout fracture of the floor of the orbit is the most common, followed by medial wall fractures. The roof of the orbit is uncommonly affected, and the lateral wall is protected by its strong bone structures. Approximately one third of patients with a blowout fracture have diplopia despite early repair of the fracture.[3]

Hypotropia from entrapment of the muscle or of orbital septae is the most common misalignment in cases of an orbital fracture. The muscle itself may be trapped by the sharp edge of the fracture or may be herniated into a sinus. Because the numerous connective tissue septae of the orbit are connected to the muscle sheaths, entrapment of the septae alone give a similar clinical result to muscle entrapment. Not infrequently, the orbital fracture repair itself causes entrapment of the muscle or incomplete release of an entrapped muscle. Forced duction testing generally shows a restriction of the entrapped muscle.

Hypertropia has also been described with posterior fractures.[3,4] The condition is thought to be caused by (*a*) one of the inferior rectus muscles being caught posteriorly on a sharp fracture step-off

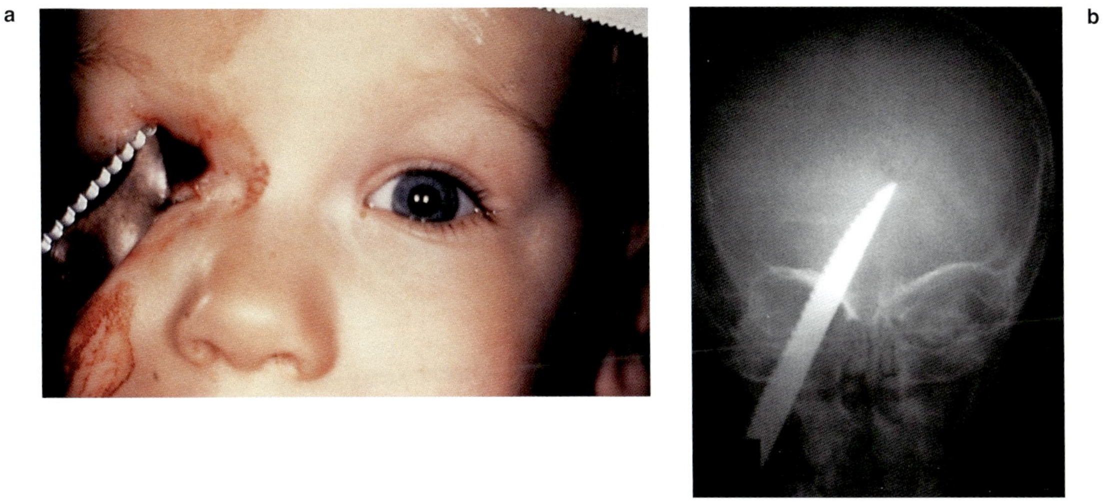

Fig. 21-2. Traumatic laceration of the superior oblique muscle. (**a**) This child picked up a knife from a counter and fell on it while running away from his grandmother. The only significant injury was to the superior oblique tendon, leaving him with a complete superior oblique paresis. (**b**) Plain film radiograph of the same patient. Photograph and radiograph: Courtesy of Julia Stevens, MD, University of Kentucky, Lexington, Ky.

or (*b*) a change in the angle of contact of the inferior rectus with the globe. Patients with traumatic hypertropia have negative forced ductions, and 80% of the conditions are corrected with surgical elevation of the orbital contents to the posterior extent of the fracture.[4]

It is important to realize that nerve and muscle contusion can cause a temporary muscle dysfunction and that orbital swelling can also restrict ocular motility.[5] Although a substantial number of patients with a blowout fracture experience spontaneous resolution of diplopia during the first 2 to 4 weeks after the injury,[3] large fractures should be operated on earlier before scarring makes repair more difficult.

Neurological Injury

Cranial nerve palsies can occur in severe or mild head trauma, but palsy of the third cranial nerve is usually seen only in the setting of severe head injury. However, cranial nerve IV, with its long path, is susceptible to lesser trauma and may be paretic even when the patient had head trauma without loss of consciousness. Palsies of cranial nerve VI are relatively common. In the initial period after an injury to the sixth nerve, the alignment shows an obvious incomitance. With time there is a spread of comitance, however, as the antagonist shortens to match its chronically deviated position.[6]

When dealing with a traumatic diplopia from neurological causes, military ophthalmologists should look carefully for other causes of the nerve damage. Otitis media can inflame the petroclinoid ligament and affect the sixth cranial nerve as it passes through Dorello's canal.[6] Diplopia after relatively mild head trauma also may occur with a previously asymptomatic brain tumor.

DIFFERENTIAL DIAGNOSIS

Underlying strabismus and diplopia from other causes should be excluded. Long-standing strabismus should be considered in any case in which the ocular misalignment does not match the injury, but strabismus can confuse the examiner in the setting of a concussion. In addition to those with a known history of strabismus, patients with an absence of previous symptoms may have mild, congenital, fourth nerve palsies, phorias, and Duane's syndrome. The stress of trauma or illness can cause some patients with phorias to break down into frank strabismus with diplopia, but these cases usually resolve in a few weeks. Careful measurements, old photographs, and occasionally forced ductions or examination under anesthesia may be necessary to differentiate congenital fourth nerve palsies and Duane's syndrome from traumatic nerve injury.

Nonstrabismic diplopia is not uncommon in the setting of trauma and should be differentiated from diplopia-induced ocular misalignment. Usually the diplopia is monocular because of cataract or regular or irregular astigmatism and is eliminated when the patient looks through a pinhole. In addition, a patient who has unilateral traumatic aphakia that is corrected by an anisometropic spectacle lens may see two images due to aniseikonia. This problem is usually easily corrected with a contact lens.

EVALUATION

History

Past ocular history should include specific questions about childhood strabismus, previous muscle operations, and any family history of strabismus. A head posture from an unsuspected congenital superior oblique palsy or Duane's syndrome may be obvious from old photographs such as one appearing on a driver's license.

Military ophthalmologists should inquire carefully about diplopia. A patient with childhood strabismus usually has little or no diplopia. A patient with a resolving muscle contusion or a recovering nerve injury, on the other hand, may describe improving diplopia or an increasing diplopia-free field of gaze.

Ocular Examination

Sensory Tests

When an asymmetrical visual acuity is uncorrectable by refraction and not caused by another obvious source, check for amblyopia with the crowding phenomenon. If the patient complains of diplopia but the eyes appear straight, occlude one eye to rule out monocular diplopia.

The double Maddox's rod test is useful when palsy of the fourth cranial nerve is suspected. Bilateral traumatic fourth nerve palsies are common and usually have more than 10° of excyclotorsion between the eyes on this test.

Stereopsis and the Worth four-dot test (or better, the circularly polarized four-dot test) help to define the binocular status of the patient and can be used to demonstrate improvement after surgery.

Pupils

A careful pupil examination can reveal dilation from a third nerve injury. If a dilated pupil is observed, the pupil should be carefully examined with a slitlamp to rule out traumatic rupture of the iris sphincter or a tonic pupil.

Alignment

Alignment should be measured with the best spectacle correction. Traumatic misalignment can be complex, so measurements should be made in primary position, near-, up-, down-, left-, and right-gaze. In cases with a component of hypertropia or suspected fourth nerve palsies, the alignment should also be measured on head tilt to the left and to the right. In addition to standard prism testing, one of the most useful tests of alignment is the Lancaster red–green test. The Lancaster test gives a standard graphic plot of misalignment and can dramatically demonstrate torsional misalignment.

In cases of incomitant misalignment, the prism should be placed over the apparently paretic or restricted eye and the *primary deviation* measured. If the prism is placed over the apparently normal eye, the resulting measurement is called the *secondary deviation* and is larger than the primary deviation. Because muscle surgery is usually done on the eye with abnormal motility, the primary deviation is the most useful measurement to determine the quantity of recession or resection.

Versions should be tested in all the cardinal positions of gaze. Testing of saccades can be useful to demonstrate a mild nerve paresis that is undetected on version testing: saccades tend to be slow in paresis.

A dilated fundus examination should be done to look for torsion. In straight eyes, the fovea will be observed to be in line with the lower third of the optic nerve head. Patients with fourth nerve palsy usually have observable excyclotorsion of 5° to 15°. Fundus photography can be used to document this torsion with a single photograph that includes both the fovea and the optic nerve.

Refraction

A cycloplegic refraction is important in cases of horizontal misalignment that could have an accommodative component. If an uncorrected hyperopia of greater than 1 diopter is discovered in the setting of concomitant esotropia, then putting this prescription in a trial frame (on another day, when the cycloplegia has worn off) may reduce or eliminate the misalignment.

Clinical Tests

Forced ductions are often useful in the setting of traumatic strabismus and help to confirm a suspected diagnosis of rectus muscle restriction. In the setting of acute orbital injury, soft-tissue swelling by itself can cause restriction, so the results are most reliable 1 week after the injury. Most adults tolerate the procedure well with topical anesthesia alone, but occasionally it must be first done as part of the surgical repair of the misalignment. Caution and gentle technique should be used in patients older than 60 years of age, because the relatively friable conjunctiva of older adults may tear easily. A five-tooth Lester forceps tends to be gentler on the conjunctiva than a three-tooth standard forceps.

The eye is grasped at the limbus nearest the suspected restricted muscle and rotated in the direction of maximum deviation. It is important to avoid depression of the globe while rotating the eye, as this relaxes the muscle being tested. If the muscle is restricted, there usually is an apparent limitation in ocular rotation. Limitation is usually obvious when the restricted eye alone is rotated, but comparisons of the forced ductions of both eyes are sometimes necessary.

Some clinicians use a cotton-tipped applicator to rotate the eye, but I have found this technique to be useful only when the restriction is severe. The applicator must be applied with significant downward pressure, depressing the globe and relaxing the rectus muscle.

The results of clinical forced ductions should be confirmed at the time of surgery. Small amounts of restriction that were not revealed by clinical testing may become apparent. In addition, forced duction testing of the oblique muscles should be done under anesthesia. To test the superior oblique muscle, grasp the limbal conjunctiva nearest the medial rectus muscle. Depress and excyclotort the globe. This exaggerated forced duction puts the tendon on stretch and the examiner should feel the eye roll over the tight tendon. This test is useful to differentiate congenital from acquired unilateral fourth nerve palsy. In congenital cases, the superior oblique tendon is usually quite lax owing to a congenitally anomalous tendon. This test is also useful in diagnosing traumatic Brown's syndrome. The inferior oblique can be tested in a similar fashion, incyclotorting the globe.

Force generation testing is especially useful to differentiate paretic from restrictive misalignment and must be done while the patient is awake. The eye is grasped using the same technique as described for forced ductions, and the patient is instructed to look in the direction of maximum deviation.

Ancillary Tests

Binocular visual fields to determine the field of binocular single vision are especially useful in patients with blowout fractures, for whom the surgical goal may be to shift this field to the most useful areas: primary position and reading position (down-gaze).

Computed tomography (CT) scans with direct axial and coronal views are most useful in the management of orbital-fracture-associated strabismus but can also be used in some cases to evaluate lacerations of the muscle belly (Figure 21-3).

Magnetic resonance imaging (MRI) provides high-resolution imaging of the muscles and is especially useful in evaluating cases of suspected laceration or loss of the muscle. In some cases, MRI

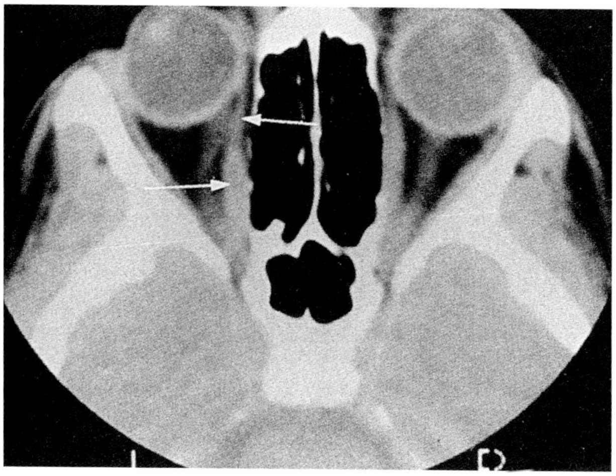

Fig. 21-3. Computed tomography scan. The bottom arrow (pointing right) denotes a slipped left medial rectus, and the top arrow (pointing left) denotes a muscle capsule still attached to the sclera. Reproduced with permission from Murray AD. Slipped and lost muscles and other tales of the unexpected. *J AAPOS*. 1998;2:135.

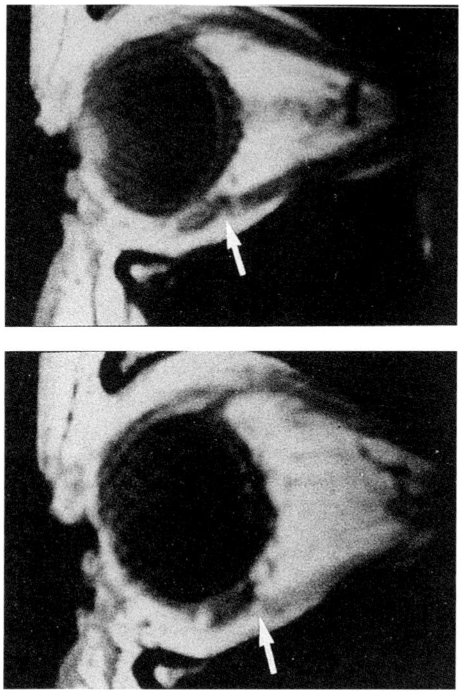

Fig. 21-4. Saggital magnetic resonance imaging scan. The patient is a 31-year-old man who fell onto a standpipe, striking his right lower eyelid and causing a 40-prism-diopter right hypertropia with severe limitation of infraduction due to disinsertion of the inferior rectus muscle. The arrows in both the upper and the lower views point to a defect in the contour of the inferior rectus muscle. A previous computed tomography scan had failed to show the disinsertion. Reproduced with permission from Ward TP, Thach AB, Madigan WP, Berland JE. Magnetic resonance imaging in posttraumatic strabismus. *J Pediatr Ophthalmol Strabismus*. 1997;34:132.

has shown the correct etiology of posttraumatic strabismus prior to surgical exploration and repair (Figure 21-4).[7] High resolution and a reduced signal-to-noise ratio can be obtained by using surface coils. The use of fat-suppression MRI helps reduce artifacts from the otherwise-bright orbital fat. Dynamic MRI (imaging the extraocular muscles during different gaze positions) can be used to differentiate a paretic muscle from a detached, functioning muscle.[8] Muscle bellies with normal contractility thicken when the patient attempts to gaze in the direction of action of that muscle.

MANAGEMENT

Preferred management options to treat the problems caused by extrocular muscle trauma include tincture of time, the use of spectacles and prisms, and occlusive filters in spectacles. In many cases, surgery should be considered only as a last resort.

Medical Options

Cranial nerve paresis often recovers spontaneously over a period of several months, and muscle contusions may recover in a few weeks. One long-term, prospective study[9] of traumatic sixth nerve palsy or paresis showed that spontaneous recovery is common. In this series, 76% of the cases were unilateral and 24% bilateral. Spontaneous recovery at 6 months occurred in 84% of the unilateral cases and in 38% of the bilateral. The prognosis was better if there was some sixth nerve function on the initial examination.

A few patients with concomitant esotropia and significant hyperopia benefit from spectacle correction. Before prescribing lenses, it is wise to evaluate the effect on alignment by putting the corrective lenses in a trial frame.

Prisms can help treat diplopia caused by small amounts of concomitant tropias. In some cases they are the only treatment needed. They are easier to use if the patient already wears spectacles, as small quantities of prism can be obtained simply by displacing the optical center of the lenses. Most patients who did not previously wear spectacles will find those with prisms intolerable. Fresnel prisms are useful as a therapeutic trial and on a short-term basis.

Occasionally a patient has a strabismus that cannot adequately be treated with surgery or prisms, or has incomitance such that the field of binocular single vision is nearly useless (eg, complete third nerve palsies). These patients should be offered the option of cosmetically acceptable occlusive filters. In a few cases, the diplopia is only in one direction (eg, down or laterally) and a partial occluder on the spectacle lens in the field of diplopia should be considered. In some cases of traumatic nerve paresis, occlusion is also useful while awaiting nerve recovery.

General Principles for Surgical Management

The choice of operation depends on the etiology of the misalignment, clinical measurements, forced duction and force generation findings, and, occasionally, imaging results. Tables of recommended surgical quantities for a given deviation are available in other textbooks, such as the *Color Atlas of Ophthalmic Surgery: Strabismus*.[10]

Military ophthalmic surgeons should bear in mind the following principles for surgical management of patients with extraocular muscle dysfunction:

1. The patient should have realistic expectations. Although muscle surgery is generally successful, some patients will never have useful binocular single vision and should clearly understand this caveat before proceeding to surgery. They should also understand that reoperation may be required.
2. If orbital surgery is planned, do that first. Orbital surgery can relieve strabismus if there is an entrapped muscle, or it can worsen the misalignment.
3. It is wise to delay surgery up to 6 months in cases of traumatic nerve paresis. Spontaneous recovery generally begins by about 3 months, and the alignment is usually stable by 6 months.
4. Optimize the field of binocular single vision. One of the primary goals of surgery in nonconcomitant cases is to increase the field of binocular single vision. This zone should be optimized for the individual patient; most need primary gaze and reading position. Consider the patient's occupation (eg, professional drivers may need single vision in left gaze to avoid diplopia when looking out the driver's-side window).
5. Use adjustable-suture surgery. Adjustment can be made up to 1 week after surgery if hyaluronic acid is placed between the muscle and the sclera.[11]
6. Reduce the risk of anterior segment ischemia. Blood supply to the anterior segment comes from three main sources: ciliary vessels running through the rectus muscles, the limbal conjunctiva, and the long posterior ciliary vessels at 3 o'clock and 9 o'clock. Anterior segment ischemia is rare but can be devastating in severe cases, resulting in chronic iritis, cataract, or even phthisis. To prevent this, avoid performing surgery on all four rectus muscles on one eye, even if the operations are separated in time by years. To preserve the limbal blood supply, use fornix conjunctival incisions in patients younger than age 60. If the patient is known to have compromised blood supply or requires surgery on three muscles, consider the use of vessel-sparing procedures.[12]
7. Recess muscles that are tight on forced duction testing.
8. Operate on the muscle active in the field of greatest deviation. For example, in cases of long-standing fourth nerve paresis, the antagonist inferior oblique muscle is usually shortened, resulting in excyclotorsion and a deviation that is greatest in the action of the inferior oblique muscle. In these cases, the procedure of choice is to weaken the inferior oblique. This dictum must be tempered by the results of intraoperative forced ductions, however. For example, a tight superior rectus muscle will cause the greatest deviation to be in the field of action of the ipsilateral inferior rectus, but the procedure of choice is to weaken the tight superior rectus.
9. Cripple the yoke muscle in nonconcomitant strabismus using either recession of this muscle or a Faden procedure (posterior fixation suture). This intervention increases the field of binocular single vision. For example, a patient with a sixth nerve palsy will have a nonconcomitant esotropia, with greatest deviation in the field of gaze of the flaccid lateral rectus muscle. In this case, a transposition of the ipsilateral vertical recti to the lateral rectus combined with botulinum toxin injected into the ipsilateral medial rectus muscle will help straighten the eye, but a recession of the contralateral medial rectus will increase the field of binocular single vision.
10. Partial nerve palsies are often adequately treated with recession of the antagonist and resection of the weak (but functional) muscle. In some cases, crippling the yoke muscle and injecting botulinum toxin into

the antagonist gives the best results. If the muscle is completely palsied, however, it is not worth resecting, as little effect will be obtained.

11. Transpositions of recti combined with injection of botulinum toxin into the antagonist are generally the best approach to complete isolated rectus muscle palsy (eg, sixth nerve palsy).

Management of Lacerated Muscles

The management of most lacerated muscles is similar to that of slipped or lost muscles. If repaired early, a muscle that has been lacerated at its insertion is usually found 5 to 6 mm away from the original insertion. In one series[2] of such cases, 53% were repaired with reattachment of the muscle to its original insertion, whereas 29% of the muscle insertions could not be found and had to be treated with transpositions (eg, transposing the superior and inferior rectus muscle insertions to the site of a lacerated lateral rectus insertion). With time, the lacerated muscle and its antagonist shorten, making retrieval more difficult and requiring recession or botulinum toxin injection of the antagonist muscle.

When looking for the lacerated muscle, good illumination and exposure using malleable retractors are critical. Loupes and a strong overhead surgical light are usually sufficient, but a headlight or operating microscope may also be useful in some cases. The muscle is often found at its penetration through Tenon's capsule. If the patient has not received systemic atropine or a similar medication as part of anesthesia, then tugging on the muscle may help differentiate it from the surrounding tissue by inducing the oculocardiac reflex.[13] If the muscle cannot be found after diligent efforts, it is not useful to open Tenon's capsule in a usually futile search for the stump: this procedure risks causing a fat adherence syndrome. Instead, the muscle should be declared lost and a transposition procedure performed to align the eyes.

SUMMARY

When a trauma patient complains of double vision, a careful clinical history and examination can in most cases clearly define the etiology, differentiating among direct trauma to the extraocular muscles, fracture of the orbit, and neurological causes. In some cases, imaging of the orbits or the head is necessary to make the final diagnosis. Infrequently, a surgical exploration of the muscles is required.

The examination should include a complete standard eye examination including refraction, confrontation visual fields, pupils, anterior segment, and fundus examination. The motility examination should include, at a minimum, a careful measurement of alignment in relevant positions of gaze, versions, and a fundus examination looking for torsion. In addition, parts of the examination should be carefully tailored to the individual patient, such as alignment in head-tilt positions for patients with vertical deviations, double Maddox's rod testing to measure subjective torsion, and the Lancaster red–green test in cases of complex misalignment. In many cases, forced duction and force generation testing are also required to look for restrictive and paretic causes of misalignment. Many patients with traumatic strabismus need imaging studies to define the course of the muscles, orbital fractures, and central nervous system injury.

The preferred management is determined in part by the motility examination and orbital scan (in the case of orbital fractures). Many cases of diplopia caused by nerve or muscle contusion recover spontaneously in weeks to months; some can be treated with spectacles or prisms. Patients who eventually require surgery to relieve diplopia should be carefully counseled to have realistic expectations, and surgery should be guided by the several principles outlined above.

REFERENCES

1. Mines M, Thach A, Mallonee S, Hildebrand L, Shariat S. Ocular injuries sustained by survivors of the Oklahoma City bombing. *Ophthalmology*. 2000;107:837–843.

2. Murray AD. Slipped and lost muscles and other tales of the unexpected. *J AAPOS* 1998;2:133–143.

3. Good WV, Hoyt CS, eds. *Strabismus Management*. Boston, Mass: Butterworth-Heinemann; 1996: Chap 20.

4. Seiff SR, Good WV. Hypertropia and the posterior blowout fracture: Mechanism and management. *Ophthalmology*. 1996;103:152–156.

5. von Noorden GK. Diagnosis of trauma-related strabismus. In: Freeman HM, ed. *Ocular Trauma*. New York, NY: Appleton-Century-Crofts; 1979: Chap 33.

6. Rubin SE. How to diagnose and manage paralytic strabismus. *Rev Ophthalmol*. 1999;6(10):103–116.

7. Ward TP, Thach AB, Madigan WP, Berland JE. Magnetic resonance imaging in posttraumatic strabismus. *J Pediatr Ophthalmol Strabismus*. 1997;34:131–134.

8. Shin GS, Demer JL, Rosenbaum AL. High resolution, dynamic, magnetic resonance imaging in complicated strabismus. *J Pediatr Ophthalmol Strabismus*. 1996;33:282–290.

9. Holmes JM, Droste PJ, Beck RW. The natural history of acute traumatic sixth nerve palsy or paresis. *J AAPOS*. 1998;2:265–268.

10. Wright KW, ed. *Color Atlas of Ophthalmic Surgery: Strabismus*. Philadelphia, Pa: JB Lippincott Company; 1991: 241–243.

11. Granet DB, Hertle RW, Ziylan S. The use of hyaluronic acid during adjustable suture surgery. *J Pediatr Ophthalmol Strabismus*. 1994;31:287–289.

12. McKeown CA, Lambert HM, Shore JW. Preservation of the anterior ciliary vessels during extraocular muscle surgery. *Ophthalmology*. 1989;96:498–507.

13. Reineke RD. Treatment of ocular motility problems following trauma. In: Freeman HM, ed. *Ocular Trauma*. New York, NY: Appleton-Century-Crofts; 1979: Chap 34.

Chapter 22

TRAUMATIC OPTIC NEUROPATHY

KIMBERLY PEELE COCKERHAM, MD*

*Director, Ophthalmic Plastics, Orbital Disease and Neuro-Ophthalmology, Allegheny General Hospital, 420 East North Avenue, Pittsburgh, Pennsylvania 15212; Assistant Professor, Department of Ophthalmology, Drexel University College of Medicine, Philadelphia, Pennsylvania 19102; formerly, Major, Medical Corps, US Army; Director, Neuro-Ophthalmology, Orbital Disease, and Plastic Reconstruction, Department of Ophthalmology, Walter Reed Army Medical Center, Washington, DC

INTRODUCTION

Approximately 1.5% to 5% of patients with closed head injuries have damage to the visual pathways (4–6 / 100,000 general population / y). These injuries can be divided into anterior and posterior lesions. Anterior lesions show ophthalmoscopic abnormalities (eg, central retinal artery occlusion) and are usually associated with a variety of easily recognized injuries to the globe. Anterior lesions may include optic nerve avulsion, traumatic anterior ischemic optic neuropathy, anterior optic nerve sheath hematoma, and optic nerve compression from an anterior orbital hematoma. Posterior lesions, on the other hand, are often free of ophthalmoscopic findings, but disc edema (acutely) and optic nerve pallor (eventually) do occur. Posterior traumatic optic neuropathy is characterized by visual loss that occurs in the presence of an afferent pupillary defect (APD) but without evidence of injury to the eye or optic nerve.[1–3] This chapter focuses primarily on the diagnosis and management of posterior traumatic optic neuropathy.

Etiology

Blunt trauma, penetrating injuries, and self-mutilations are the most common causes of optic nerve injury. Blunt trauma classically occurs following rapid deceleration injuries to the anterofrontal regions of the head. Trauma to the outer third of the superior orbital rim is transmitted directly to the optic canal, where the optic nerve is tethered at both ends by dura. Conversely, the optic nerve is redundant in the orbit and protected by orbital fat and resistant to injury at this site.[1,4]

The severity of the trauma does not always correlate with the degree of visual loss. Incidents such as minor falls after tripping, or hitting the side of the head against a solid object resulting in a frontal blow are adequate to produce a posterior traumatic optic neuropathy. The most common mechanism of injury is bicycle accidents, followed by motor vehicle accidents. Most bicycle accidents (90%) are solo spills; the protective impact of bicycle helmets has not been studied with respect to incidence of optic neuropathy.[1]

Also, the presence or severity of orbital fractures neither directly predicts the severity of visual loss nor determines prognosis. Fractures of the medial orbital wall, optic canal, zygoma, or floor may be present.[1] One patient with an optic canal fracture may regain normal vision without intervention, but another with no fractures may present with no light perception (NLP) vision that persists despite all interventions.

Traumatic optic neuropathy is most often seen in boys in their first or second decade of life, but case series have included a wide age range and both genders. In one series,[5] patients older than 40 years of age were found to have a worse visual outcome independent of mechanism of injury, severity of visual loss, or intervention utilized.

Pathology

The optic nerve axons lie in two compartments: the intradural and the intrafascicular. Closed-space edema, contusion necrosis, nerve fiber tears, and infarction due to thrombosis or spasm have all been implicated as potential mechanisms of optic nerve injury. Shearing, stretching, compression, and contusion at the level of the intracanalicular optic nerve are probably all important in creating the dysfunction. Surgery can only open the dura and cannot relieve intrafascicular pressure elevations. Interruption of venous flow may also play an important role. Myelin is more sensitive to edema and acidosis than axonal structures. Typical findings found at autopsy include hemorrhage, demyelination, focal necrosis, and axonal changes.[4,6]

NEUROOPHTHALMIC EVALUATION

The complete ophthalmic examination has been detailed in this textbook in Chapter 3, Ocular Trauma: History and Examination. Identification of optic nerve injury can be challenging, especially in uncooperative, inebriated, or unresponsive patients. Best-corrected visual acuity is usually quantitated at the bedside with a near card. Patients who are 45 years old or older should be offered plus correction if vision is less than 20/20 on initial testing. Formal color testing is not essential, but comparing red saturation is very helpful and can easily be performed at the bedside. Even a patient who has been mistakenly or traumatically dilated can see a red-topped eyedrop container. Red desaturation, a characteristic of optic nerve dysfunction, causes the cherry-red color to appear orange or brown. The gold standard for identifying a unilateral or asymmetrical optic neuropathy is, of course, the swinging flashlight test. This test is performed using a penlight, muscle light, or indirect ophthalmoscope. The light is moved from the left to the right pupil and back again. The amount and timing of constriction and redilation are then computed.

Asymmetry of constriction (1+ to 3+) or redilation (trace) is consistent with an APD. Even if the pupil on the side of interest is unreactive, the status of the optic nerve pathways can be evaluated by looking for a reverse APD. The optic nerve head is usually normal in appearance even when vision is NLP. Other associated abnormalities (eg, peripapillary choroidal rupture, hemorrhage, edema) should be sought as well. If sectoral swelling of the optic nerve head is present, especially in the presence of a small cup-to-disc ratio and altitudinal field defect, then posttraumatic anterior ischemic optic neuropathy should be suspected.

Clinical Features

Posterior traumatic optic neuropathy is often difficult to recognize in patients with multiple injuries, especially in unconscious patients. Care must be taken to examine the patient as early as possible in the evaluation process, as APD may be the only sign of injury. Typically, the optic nerve head is initially normal. Visual deficits range from normal vision with subtle visual field defects (inferior altitudinal is most common) to complete loss of light perception. In most cases, the visual loss is severe and instantaneous.[1,6–8]

Even seemingly trivial trauma may result in dramatic optic nerve impairment. The severity of visual loss does not necessarily correlate with the degree of overall trauma, but total loss of vision has been associated with the presence of fractures. Nau and colleagues[4] found that 90% of patients with total visual loss had evidence of bony fracture by computed tomography (CT); 33% presented with Le Fort III fractures, 33% had orbital fractures, and 33% had frontobasal fractures. This same study also revealed that all the patients had a laceration in the region of the eyebrow on the affected side.[4] On the other hand, Lessel,[1] reporting 33 cases in which the most common cause of injury was a bicycle accident, found no correlation between fractures and degree of visual loss. Visual evoked potentials (flash) have limited utility and may give false-negative results prior to the onset of optic atrophy.

Imaging

Although most patients with posterior traumatic optic neuropathy have normal imaging studies, CT without contrast should be performed in all cases. Spiral CT allows rapid data acquisition in uncooperative adults and children. Imaging will allow identification of associated fractures (Figure 22-1), optic nerve avulsion, optic nerve sheath hematoma (Figure 22-2), and optic nerve compression due to an orbital hematoma (Figure 22-3). The optic nerve injury may not be isolated (Figure 22-4); associated

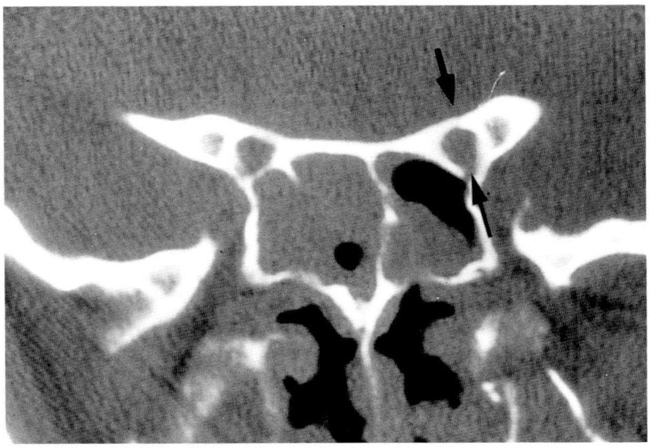

Fig. 22-1. A computed tomography (CT) scan demonstrating a fracture of the optic canal (arrows). CT scan: Courtesy of Department of Ophthalmology, Allegheny General Hospital, Pittsburgh, Pa.

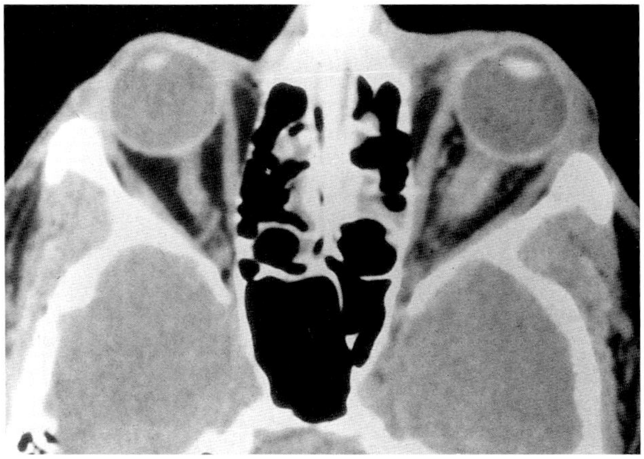

Fig. 22-2. A computed tomography (CT) scan demonstrating a left optic nerve sheath hematoma. Preseptal swelling is also present. CT scan: Courtesy of Department of Ophthalmology, Allegheny General Hospital, Pittsburgh, Pa.

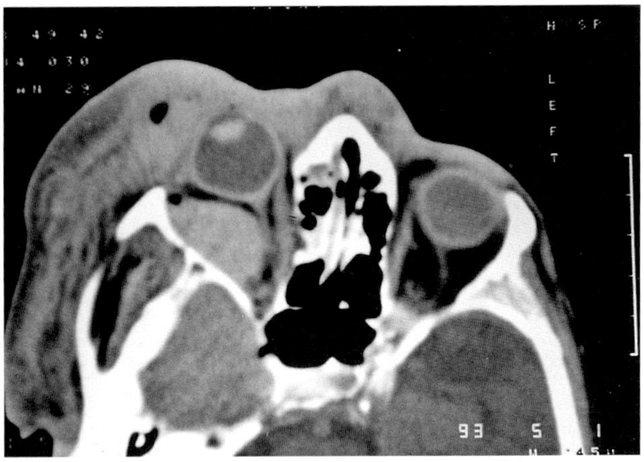

Fig. 22-3. Massive blunt trauma has resulted in preseptal swelling and a lateral orbital hematoma (arrow) that is compressing the right optic nerve, as seen in this axial computed tomography (CT) scan. CT scan: Courtesy of Department of Ophthalmology, Allegheny General Hospital, Pittsburgh, Pa.

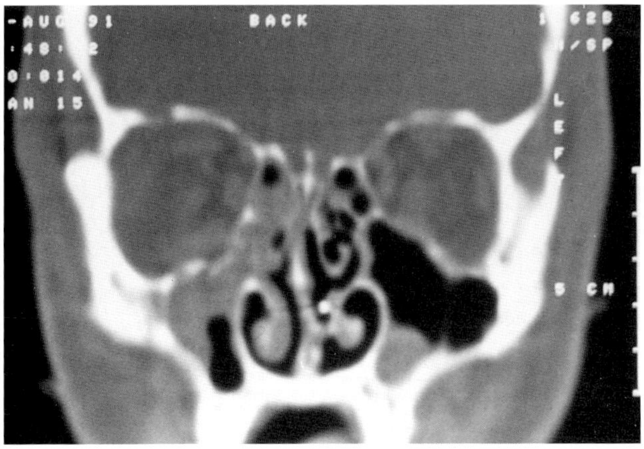

Fig. 22-4. Medial wall and blowout fractures are present in a patient with optic nerve dysfunction due to indirect blunt trauma (posterior posttraumatic optic neuropathy). As seen in this computed tomography (CT) scan, optic nerve avulsion is not present and the optic canal is intact. CT scan: Courtesy of Department of Ophthalmology, Allegheny General Hospital, Pittsburgh, Pa.

fractures and injuries can be identified when the scope of evaluation is expanded to include otolaryngology, oral, maxillofacial, and neurosurgery colleagues. Magnetic resonance imaging is only indicated if intracranial injuries are present that are inadequately detailed with CT imaging.[1,6,9]

NATURAL HISTORY

TABLE 22-1

NATURAL HISTORY OF TRAUMATIC OPTIC NEUROPATHY

Author (Year of Study)	Number of Patients	Spontaneous Improvement (%)
Tang (1986)[1]	13	38
Millesi (1988)[2]	7	57
Lessell (1989)[3]	25	20
Seiff (1990)[4]	15	33
Levin (1999)[5]	9	57

Data sources: (1) Tang R, Li H, Regner V, Bridges MB, Prager TC. Traumatic optic neuropathy: Analysis of 37 cases. *Invest Ophthalmol Vis Sci.* 1986;27(suppl):102. (2) Millesi W, Hollmann K, Funder J. Traumatic lesions of the optic nerve. *Acta Neurochir.* 1988;93:50–54. (3) Lessell S. Indirect optic nerve trauma. *Arch Opthalmol.* 1989;107:382–386. (4) Seiff SR. High dose corticosteroids for treatment of vision loss due to indirect injury to the optic nerve. *Ophthalmic Surg.* 1990;21:389–395. (5) Levin LA, Beck RW, Joseph MP, Seiff S, Kraker R. The treatment of traumatic optic neuropathy: The International Optic Nerve Trauma Study. *Ophthalmology.* 1999;106:1268–1277.

The natural history of traumatic optic neuropathy is difficult to characterize because each patient is different. Attempts to study patient outcomes have also been hindered by the assumption that corticosteroids are helpful and that not offering them would be unethical. Visual prognosis and likelihood of spontaneous improvement are independent of the initial visual acuity.[10,11]

The natural history of indirect optic nerve injuries has been described in several clinical series. The rate of spontaneous visual improvement ranges from 20% to 57% (Table 22-1). Even patients who had a return of normal central visual acuity did not regain an entirely normal afferent examination. Persistence of visual field and color defects, and APD are typical. Optic nerve pallor or nerve fiber layer changes also develop over the months following the injury. Patients with NLP on presentation can sometimes recover-useful vision without intervention.[1,11]

The prognosis tends to be better for patients who have a lucid interval or an enlarged nerve sheath[12] but poorer for patients older than 40 years.[5] The following factors do not appear to correlate with visual outcome[5]:

- gender,
- level of consciousness,
- mechanism of injury,
- initial visual acuity (including NLP),
- presence of fractures (including optic canal fracture), and
- time from injury to intervention (within the first 7 d).

TREATMENT

During the mid 1970s, observation was replaced by steroid therapy and surgery as a variety of case series promoted the success rates of these interventions, and since then, significant improvement without treatment has been well documented (see Table 22-1). Despite the rate of spontaneous improvement, however, the standard of care has been to offer high-dose corticosteroids. The role of surgical intervention is still debated. The International Optic Nerve Trauma Study[13] (published in 1999) demonstrated no clear benefit from either corticosteroid therapy or optic canal decompression surgery. Observation has again become an acceptable option when there is no evidence of intrasheath hematoma, orbital hematoma, or optic canal fracture fragments (Figure 22-5).

Corticosteroid Therapy

Widely used for several decades, corticosteroids are thought to stabilize lipid membranes, reduce spasm, increase blood supply, and reduce neural

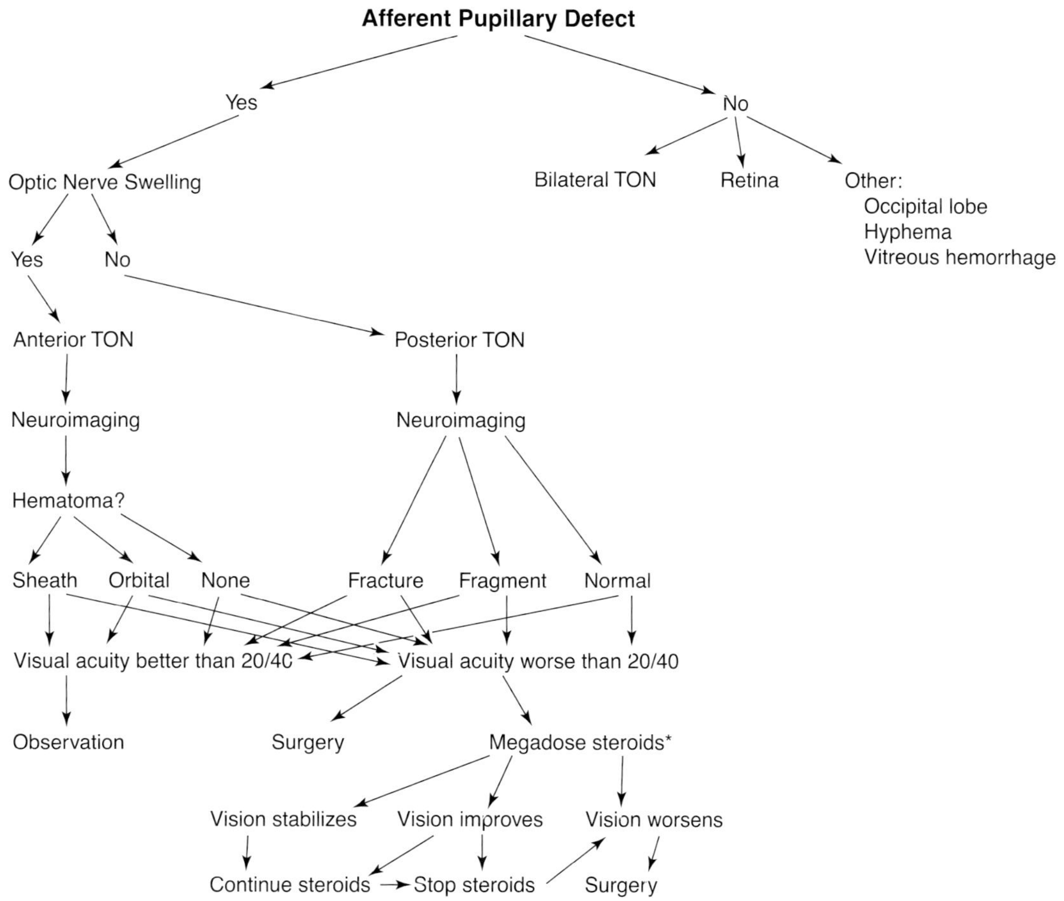

*Loading dose: 30 mg/kg followed by 15 mg/kg 2 h later. The maintenance dose could then be 15 mg/kg at 6-h intervals or 5.4 mg/kg/h for at least 48 h before deciding whether response has occurred.
TON: traumatic optic neuropathy

Fig. 22-5. Algorithm for medical and surgical management of traumatic optic neuropathy tissue edema and necrosis. Megadose steroids were first studied in animal models with brain edema and then in humans with spinal cord injuries.[14] Spoor and colleagues[15] were the first to use spinal cord doses for patients with traumatic optic neuropathy. They divided their patients into two groups, and treated

- one group (13 patients) with methylprednisolone (30 mg/kg initially, then 15 mg/kg given 2 h later, and then in divided doses every 6 h), and
- the second group (8 patients) with high-dose dexamethasone (20 mg every 6 h).

Both therapies were continued for 48 hours, then followed by a rapid taper. Of the treated eyes (one per patient), 17 of 21 (81%) improved in visual function during these protocols. The relative dose of steroid was much higher for the methylprednisolone group, but the overall outcome was no different. The methylprednisolone group appeared to make a more-rapid recovery, however. A delay in treatment did not appear to alter outcome in this study. The mean onset of therapy was 4.2 days. The authors of the study believed that neither the initial severity nor the type of nerve injury allowed the response to steroid therapy to be predicted, as five of eight eyes in this study initially had NLP but regained significant function.

Another series by Bendel and colleagues[16] described 17 patients treated with 2 g methylprednisolone initially, then 1 g, divided, every 6 hours for 48 hours. Vision improved in all patients, with an average pretreatment vision of 20/100 and average posttreatment vision of 20/25. Best vision occurred between 1 and 6 days after treatment (mean = 2.9 d). Three patients demonstrated deteriorating visual function during steroid taper and were treated with extracranial optic nerve decompression; all three had eventual improvement.

Mauriello and colleagues[12] reported a series in which 9 of 16 patients (56%) treated with a more-conventional steroid dose had significant improvement (1 g loading dose, then 250 mg in divided doses every 6 h for 48 h). Almost all patients who did not improve had NLP vision initially. They also noted that all 5 of their patients with a lucid interval following injury had eventual improvement.

In summary, a short course of high-dose steroid may be considered unless there is clear evidence of optic nerve transection or avulsion by clinical or radiographic criteria. A delay in onset of therapy and the degree of visual loss have not been clearly shown to alter prognosis (Table 22-2).[6–8,12,15,17,18]

Surgical Intervention

Optic canal decompression was first described in 1916, wherein a transcranial unroofing was performed in patients with afferent dysfunction who required craniotomies for other reasons.[19] Extracranial techniques were later described to minimize the possible complications associated with craniotomy. A transethmoidal approach was investigated as early as 1926 but not popularized until the 1960s.[6] External, transantral, Caldwell-Luc, and transnasal approaches have all been tried.[20] Comparison of different clinical series is difficult because of differences in techniques, selection criteria, and quantification of visual improvement. Many patients also

TABLE 22-2

REPORTED OUTCOMES USING CORTICOSTEROIDS

Author (Year of Study)	Number of Patients and (Treatment Received)*	Visual Improvement (%)
Tang (1986)[1]	5 (C)	20
	11 (M)	36
Millesi (1988)[2]	2 (U)	50
Lessel (1990)[3]	4 (U)	25
Seiff (1990)[4]	21 (M)	62
Spoor (1990)[5]	22 (M)	86
Bendel (1993)[6]	17 (M)	100
Levin (1999)[7]	85 (M)	52

*C: conventional steroid dose (1 g methylprednisolone loading dose followed by 250 mg methylprednisolone qid)
M: megadose steroid doses (30mg/kg methylprednisolone loading dose followed by 15 mg/kg every 6 h or 5.4 mg/h for 24–48 h)
U: unspecified dose

Data sources: (1) Tang R, Li H, Regner V, Bridges MB, Prager TC. Traumatic optic neuropathy: Analysis of 37 cases. *Invest Ophthalmol Vis Sci.* 1986;27(suppl):102. (2) Millesi W, Hollmann K, Funder J. Traumatic lesions of the optic nerve. *Acta Neurochir.* 1988;93:50–54. (3) Lessell S. Indirect optic nerve trauma. *Arch Opthalmol.* 1989;107:382–386. (4) Seiff SR. High dose corticosteroids for treatment of vision loss due to indirect injury to the optic nerve. *Ophthalmic Surg.* 1990;21:389–395. (5) Spoor TC, Hartel WC, Lensink DB, Wilkinson MJ. Treatment of traumatic optic neuropathy with corticosteroids. *Am J Ophthalmol.* 1990;110: 665–669. (6) Bendel RE, McHenry JG, Ramocki JM, Spoor TC. Traumatic optic neuropathy and intravenous megadose corticosteroids. *Invest Ophthalmol Vis Sci.* 1993;34(suppl):1215. (7) Levin LA, Beck RW, Joseph MP, Seiff S, Kraker R. The treatment of traumatic optic neuropathy. The International Optic Nerve Trauma Study. *Ophthalmology.* 1999;106:1268–1277.

receive at least conventional doses of corticosteroids in the perioperative period, further confusing the ability to attribute improvement to the surgical intervention. The frequency of reported visual improvement ranges from 12% to 79%.[5,6,13,17–19,21–26] In many medical centers, the decision to operate is governed by the criteria established in 1966 by Walsh (Exhibit 22-1).

Mauriello and colleagues[12] treated 23 patient with steroids and operated on 7 nonresponders based on CT evidence of surgical pathology (optic nerve sheath enlargement or narrowing of the optic canal by bone spicules). Of the 3 patients treated with optic nerve sheath fenestration alone, only 1 had significant improvement. The remaining 4 patients were treated with both fenestration and optic canal decompression. Only 1 patient had significant improvement (NLP to 20/200).

Joseph and colleagues[26] reported visual improvement in 11 of 14 patients treated with steroids and transethmoidal decompression of the optic canal. This report was a retrospective review and not compared to any large, steroid-only treatment group, but the results are similar to those in the study of Spoor and colleagues,[15] who used megadose corticosteroids (described above).

Levin and colleagues[13] reported the outcome of the International Optic Nerve Trauma study in 1999. The goal of this endeavor was to compare the visual outcome of traumatic optic neuropathy treated with corticosteroids, treated with optic canal decompression surgery, or observed without treatment. Patients who were randomized to the surgical group did not receive steroids in the perioperative period. Intervention occurred within the first 7 days following injury. The main outcome measure was defined as visual acuity improvement of three or more lines of Snellen acuity. The Inter-

EXHIBIT 22-1

CRITERIA GOVERNING SURGICAL INTERVENTION IN PATIENTS WITH TRAUMATIC OPTIC NEUROPATHY

Absolute Surgical Contraindication:

- Optic nerve avulsion is present on CT imaging

Relative Surgical Contraindications:

- Patient is unconscious
- Total loss of vision and pupillary response

Relative Surgical Indications:

- If visual loss develops despite steroid treatment
- If visual decline occurs during the steroid taper
- If an optic canal fracture is accompanied by potentially compressive bone fragment
- If an optic nerve sheath hematoma is present
- If the visual evoked potential (VEP) response deteriorates over time

Sources: (1) Levin LA, Joseph MP, Rizzo JF. Optic canal decompression in indirect optic nerve trauma. *Ophthalmology.* 1994:101:566–569. (2) Levin LA, Beck RW, Joseph MP, Seiff S, Kraker R. The treatment of traumatic optic neuropathy. The International Optic Nerve Trauma Study. *Ophthalmology.* 1999;106:1268–1277. (3) Mine S, Yamakami I, Yamaura A, et al. Outcome of traumatic optic neuropathy: Comparison between surgical and nonsurgical treatment. *Acta Neurochir.* 1999;141:27–30. (4) Pomeranz HD, Rizzo JF, Lessell S. Treatment of traumatic optic neuropathy. *Int Ophthalmol Clin.* 1999;39(1):185–194. (5) Li KK, Teknos TN, Lai A, Laurentano AM, Joseph MP. Traumatic optic neuropathy: Result in 45 consecutive surgically treated patients. *Otolaryngol Head Neck Surg.* 1999;120:5–11. (6) Li KK, Teknos TN, Lauretano A, Joseph MP. Traumatic optic neuropathy complicating facial fracture repair. *J Craniofacial Surg.* 1997;8:352–355. (7) Kuppersmith RB, Alford EK, Patrinely JR, Lee AG, Parke RB, Holds JB. Combined transconjunctival/intranasal endoscopic approach to the optic canal in traumatic optic neuropathy. *Laryngoscope.* 1997;107:311–315. (8) Cook MW, Levin LA, Joseph MP, Pinczower EF. Traumatic optic neuropathy: A meta-analysis. *Arch Otolaryngol Head Neck Surg.* 1996;122:389–392. (9) Girard BC, Bouzas EA, Lamas G, Soudant J. Visual improvement after transethmoid-sphenoid decompression in optic nerve injuries. *J Clin Neuro Ophthalmol.* 1992;12:142–148. (10) Joseph MP, Lessell S, Rizzo J, Momose KJ. Extracranial optic nerve decompression for traumatic optic neuropathy. *Arch Ophthalmol.* 1990;108:1091–1093.

national Optic Nerve Trauma study found that only 32% in the surgery group (n = 33) improved significantly. This was in contrast to the visual improvement observed in the untreated group (57%, n = 9) and steroid group (52%, n = 85). The study concluded that there was no clear benefit for intervention. In addition, they confirmed the findings of others that the timing of corticosteroids or surgery within the 7-day window did not affect outcome.

SUMMARY

Traumatic optic neuropathy is a rare but significant cause of posttraumatic visual loss. The responsible blunt trauma to the frontal region may be minor or severe and accompanied by multiple adjacent fractures. Careful documentation of visual acuity, pupillary function, and red desaturation is essential to guide management. CT imaging should be performed to document such structural abnormalities as optic nerve avulsion, optic nerve sheath hematoma, orbital hematoma, or optic canal fracture with fragments.

Based on the data from the International Optic Nerve Trauma Study, observation without intervention is a viable option. Patients and their families should be made aware of the information regarding megadose corticosteroid therapy and participate in an informed decision. In particular, if visual acuity begins to deteriorate, then corticosteroid therapy should be considered. If a structural abnormality is present that may be contributing to optic nerve dysfunction (hematoma or fragment) or if the patient's visual acuity deteriorates on corticosteroids, optic canal decompression should be offered. Management of this disorder remains very controversial; involvement of other appropriate subspecialists and careful discussions with the patient and family are essential to maximize visual outcome.

REFERENCES

1. Lessell S. Indirect optic nerve trauma. *Arch Ophthalmol.* 1989;107:382–386.

2. Brodsky MC, Wald KJ, Chen S, Weiter JJ. Protracted posttraumatic optic disc swelling. *Ophthalmology.* 1995;102:1628–1631.

3. Wyllie AM, McLeod D, Cullen JF. Traumatic ischemic optic neuropathy. *Br J Ophthalmol.* 1972;56:851–853.

4. Nau HE, Gerhard L, Foerster M, Nahser HC, Reinhardt V, Joka T. Optic nerve trauma: Clinical, electrophysiological and histological remarks. *Acta Neurochir (Wien).* 1987;89:16–27.

5. Levin LA, Joseph MP, Rizzo JF. Optic canal decompression in indirect optic nerve trauma. *Ophthalmology.* 1994:101:566–569.

6. Berestka JS, Rizzo JF. Controversy in the management of traumatic optic neuropathy. *Int Ophthalmol Clin.* 1994;34(3):87–96.

7. Millesi W, Hollmann K, Funder J. Traumatic lesions of the optic nerve. *Acta Neurochir (Wien).* 1988;93:50–54.

8. Tang R, Li H, Regner V, Bridges MB, Prager TC. Traumatic optic neuropathy: Analysis of 37 cases. *Invest Ophthalmol Vis Sci.* 1986;27(suppl):102.

9. Al-Qurainy A, Stassen LFA, Dutton GN, Moos KF, El-Attar A. The characteristics of midfacial fractures and the association with ocular injury: A prospective study. *Br J Oral and Maxillofac Surg.* 1991;29:291–301.

10. Feist RM, Kline LB, Morris RE, Witherspoon CD, Michelson MA. Recovery of vision after presumed direct optic nerve injury. *Ophthalmology.* 1987;94:1567–1569.

11. Wolin MJ, Lavin PJM. Spontaneous visual recovery from traumatic optic neuropathy after blunt head injury. *Am J Ophthalmol.* 1990;109:430–435.

12. Mauriello JA, DeLuca J, Krieger A, Schulder M, Frohman L. Management of traumatic optic neuropathy: A study of 23 patients. *Br J Ophthalmol*. 1992;76:349–352.

13. Levin LA, Beck RW, Joseph MP, Seiff S, Kraker R. The treatment of traumatic optic neuropathy: The International Optic Nerve Trauma Study. *Ophthalmology*. 1999;106:1268–1277.

14. Bracken MB, Collins WF, Freeman DF, et al. Efficacy of methylprednisolone in acute spinal cord injury. *JAMA*. 1984;251(1):45–52.

15. Spoor TC, Hartel WC, Lensink DB, Wilkinson MJ. Treatment of traumatic optic neuropathy with corticosteroids. *Am J Ophthalmol*. 1990;110: 665–669.

16. Bendel RE, McHenry JG, Ramocki JM, Spoor TC. Traumatic optic neuropathy and intravenous megadose corticosteroids. *Invest Ophthalmol Vis Sci*. 1993;34(suppl):1215.

17. Mine S, Yamakami I, Yamaura A, et al. Outcome of traumatic optic neuropathy: Comparison between surgical and nonsurgical treatment. *Acta Neurochir (Wien)*. 1999;141:27–30.

18. Pomeranz HD, Rizzo JF, Lessell S. Treatment of traumatic optic neuropathy. *Int Ophthalmol Clin*. 1999;39(1):185–194.

19. Pringle J. Monocular blindness following diffused violence to the skull: Its causation and treatment. *Br J Surg*. 1916;4:373–385.

20. Kennerdell JS, Amsbaugh GL, Myers EN. Transantral-ethmoidal decompression of optic canal fracture. *Arch Ophthalmol*. 1976;94:1040–1043.

21. Li KK, Teknos TN, Lai A, Laurentano AM, Joseph MP. Traumatic optic neuropathy: Result in 45 consecutive surgically treated patients. *Otolaryngol Head Neck Surg*. 1999;120:5–11.

22. Li KK, Teknos TN, Lauretano A, Joseph MP. Traumatic optic neuropathy complicating facial fracture repair. *J Craniofacial Surg*. 1997;8:352–355.

23. Kuppersmith RB, Alford EK, Patrinely JR, Lee AG, Parke RB, Holds JB. Combined transconjunctival/intranasal endoscopic approach to the optic canal in traumatic optic neuropathy. *Laryngoscope*. 1997;107:311–315.

24. Cook MW, Levin LA, Joseph MP, Pinczower EF. Traumatic optic neuropathy: A meta-analysis. *Arch Otolaryngol Head Neck Surg*. 1996;122: 389–392.

25. Girard BC, Bouzas EA, Lamas G, Soudant J. Visual improvement after transethmoid-sphenoid decompression in optic nerve injuries. *J Clin Neuro Ophthalmol*. 1992;12:142–148.

26. Joseph MP, Lessell S, Rizzo J, Momose KJ. Extracranial optic nerve decompression for traumatic optic neuropathy. *Arch Ophthalmol*. 1990;108:1091–1093.

Chapter 23

ENUCLEATION AND EVISCERATION

ASA D. MORTON, MD*

*Commander, Medical Corps, US Navy; Chief, Oculoplastics Section, Naval Medical Center San Diego, San Diego, California 92134

INTRODUCTION

Although historically the eyes have suffered an inordinately high rate of injury relative to the total body surface area in harm's way,[1] the loss of an eye in combat is an exceedingly costly, largely preventable catastrophe (Figure 23-1). During the Vietnam War, at least 1,200 eyes were removed secondary to a combat-related injury, and the US Library of Congress estimates that the long- and short-term costs associated with serious eye injuries in that war exceeded $4 billion.[2] The incidence of eye injuries has increased with each conflict in the 20th century. For example, World War I data document an incidence of eye injuries of 2.0% to 2.5%, but the rate of such injuries during the Persian Gulf War was 13%[3]; fragments from explosive munitions accounted for 78% of the serious eye injuries and 94% of the enucleations reported during the latter war.[4] Most of these injuries could have been prevented with readily available ballistic eye armor. Military ophthalmologists must be versed in enucleation and evisceration, but greater efforts should be directed toward force education and injury prevention (Figure 23-2).

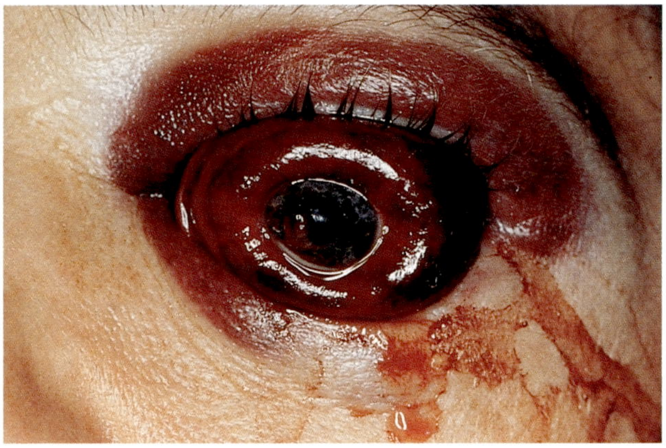

Fig. 23-1. Massive retrobulbar hemorrhage associated with a low-velocity metal fragment. Surgical attempts to repair this double, perforating globe injury (entrance and exit wounds) were unsuccessful, and the eye was enucleated. This injury could have been prevented with appropriate eye protection.

HISTORY OF EYE REMOVAL AND PROSTHESES

References to ocular surgical procedures predate 2000 BCE (before the common era). Sumerian law limited what a practitioner could charge for successful eye operations; for those procedures deemed unsuccessful, the penalty was amputation of the surgeon's hands.[5] In the mid 16th century, extirpa-

a

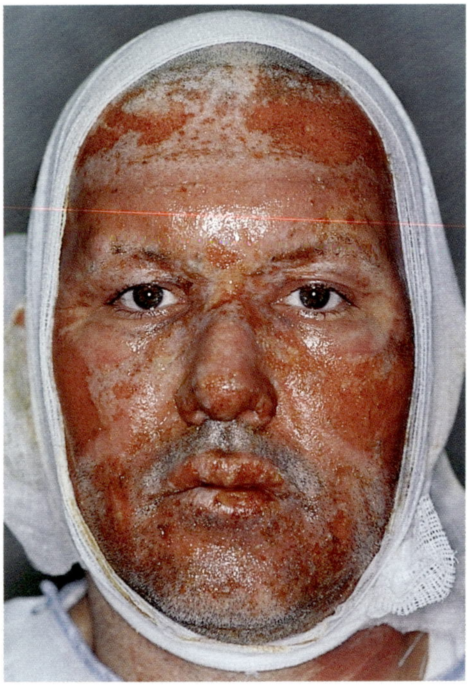

b

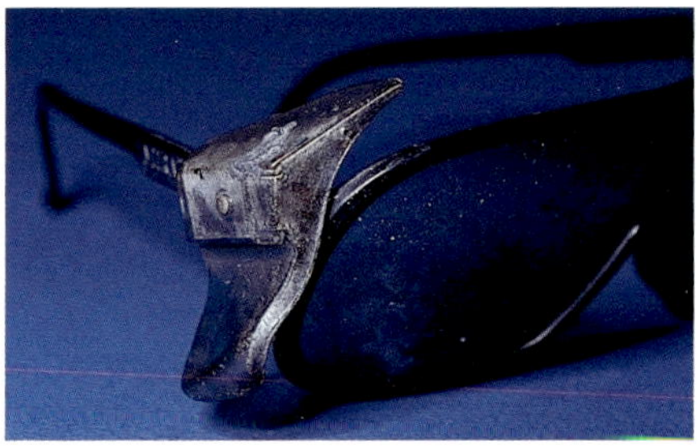

Fig. 23-2. (**a**) A short-range thermal blast induced significant damage to the face of this individual. The periocular area was spared by the patient's protective eyewear. (**b**) The polycarbonate lenses have been significantly pitted by the heat and flying debris. The blast was of sufficient intensity that its heat melted the side shields.

tion of the eye was described.[6] The disfiguring procedure was more akin to a subtotal exenteration, including removal of portions of the conjunctiva, extraocular muscles, and orbital fascia. The patient could not be fitted with an ocular prosthesis. In the mid 1800s, O'Ferral and Bonnet[7] developed a more accepted technique, which involved transecting the extraocular muscles at their scleral insertions and preserving Tenon's capsule. Their description is most consistent with enucleation as we know it today.[8]

The first description of an evisceration is credited to Beer in 1817.[9] While he was performing a glaucoma procedure, the eye experienced an expulsive hemorrhage and Beer removed the ocular contents. In 1874, Noyes[10] published his experience in removing the contents of severely infected eyes, and it is he who is credited with first using evisceration as a routine procedure.

In 1884, Mules[11] placed a glass sphere into an eviscerated scleral shell, initiating the search for the perfect implant. The early implants were hollow glass spheres and had unacceptably high extrusion rates. Throughout the early part of the 20th century, numerous implant materials were investigated, including gold, silver, vitallium (a cobalt–chromium alloy), platinum, aluminum, cartilage, bone, fat, fascia lata, sponge, wool, rubber, silk, catgut, peat, agar, asbestos, cork, ivory, paraffin, and cellulose. Concerns about the simple spheres' tendency to migrate, incomplete translation of socket motility to the prosthesis, and inadequate volume replacement led to the development of several unique implants. Shape and texture modifications sought to isolate the extraocular muscles to their respective quadrants to limit implant migration. Anterior implant projections, some with exposed coupling pegs, were engineered to create a direct linkage with the prosthesis and maximize motility. Several implants met the goal of improved prosthesis motility but at the expense of unacceptably high exposure and extrusion rates. Others developed donor sclera–covering techniques for the acrylic and silicone spheres, historically the best tolerated of any implant design, allowing the muscles to be sutured to the implant. The latter technique remains an acceptable adjunct to enucleation surgery today, with the same acrylic and silicone spheres acceptable as evisceration implants.

Since the early to mid 1990s, porous implants (hydroxyapatite and porous polyethylene) have become the choice for many surgeons. The interconnecting porous channels allow fibrovascular ingrowth throughout the implant. This ingrowth stabilizes the implant position and limits migration. After the implant has completely fibrovascularized, it may be drilled and an anterior projecting coupling peg placed. Although early results of the pegging process have been promising, recent reports of complications are emerging.[12] The long-term prognosis for drilling of implants and placing of pegs is not yet known.

PREOPERATIVE PLANNING

Decision to Remove the Eye

The psychological effect of losing an eye may present greater difficulties for the patient than the physical disability.[13] The preoperative time spent addressing eye removal, as well as discussing life after losing an eye, will reap benefits in postoperative recovery and acceptance. Photographs of other anophthalmic patients are useful as the prospective patient tries to understand the process. It may be helpful to facilitate a meeting between the patient facing eye removal and one who has completed the process. Psychiatric referral is appropriate for patients who manifest increased difficulty coping with the loss.

Preoperative Counseling

It is vitally important that the patient be prepared for surgery and the rehabilitation to follow. Pain is variable in the immediate postoperative period, and patients should be assured that appropriate medication will be provided. The patient must be prepared to wear a conformer for 5 to 7 weeks until the socket is ready to be fitted with a prosthesis. In addition, the patient must understand that the fitting process may require several appointments over as many weeks.

Goals of Rehabilitating the Anophthalmic Socket

Communication between the ophthalmologist and the ocularist is integral to a good outcome. The ophthalmologist must select an implant of appropriate volume to allow for optimal prosthetic size. Too small an implant necessitates an inappropriately large prosthesis to fill the orbital volume, and this may limit motility and transmit excess weight to the lower eyelid. Over time, the excess weight will result in laxity of the lower eyelid with a resultant asymmetric appearance. On the other hand, too large an implant limits the ocularist's ability to fashion a prosthesis with simulated anterior chamber depth without imparting a proptotic appearance to the orbit.

The ocularist can modify the prosthesis to adjust lid position, correct for a shortened conjunctival cul-de-sac, and improve motility. The posterior surface of the prosthesis can be vaulted in cases of conjunctival irritation or breakdown. Patients who elect to undergo implant pegging to maximize prosthetic motility (discussed later) rely on the ophthalmologist and the ocularist to coordinate their care. The ocularist can provide a prosthetic template to assist the ophthalmologist in peg placement and centration. Following the peg placement, the ocularist will modify the implant to allow implant–prosthetic coupling.

Eye removal and socket rehabilitation are not procedures to relegate to minimally supervised junior residents. This is the primary procedure that will determine long-term success and promote rapid patient rehabilitation. Less-than-optimal surgical technique can lead to subsequent procedures to address implant exposure, implant extrusion, implant migration, socket contraction, chronic pain, and lid malposition. The same impeccable attention that the ophthalmologist commits to microsurgical ocular procedures is essential for surgery of the anophthalmic socket. Preservation of conjunctiva, implant placement and sizing, anatomical reinsertion of extraocular muscles, and tension-free wound closure are integral to a successful outcome.

Decision to Enucleate or Eviscerate

The patient needs to understand the available options and to participate in the choice between *enucleation* (removal of the globe and a segment of the anterior optic nerve) and *evisceration* (removal of the ocular contents with preservation of the sclera and, in some cases, the cornea). The ophthalmologist must guide the patient to the most appropriate procedure if absolute indications or contraindications exist. Some patients may take comfort in evisceration and equate the retention of the scleral shell to keeping the eye. Conversely, the appropriately selected evisceration candidate may find the minimal risk of sympathetic ophthalmia to be unacceptable and elect for enucleation. (Although a consensus does not exist, most authors agree that penetrating trauma increases the risk of sympathetic ophthalmia and is a contraindication to evisceration. For war-related ocular trauma that leads to loss of useful vision, enucleation removes the uveal tissue implicated in inciting inflammation in the sympathizing eye. For further information, see Chapter 16, Sympathetic Ophthalmia.)

Otherwise-untreatable intraocular malignancies and cases that require histopathological review for assessment of the tumor margins dictate enucleation. In addition, a small, phthisical eye may preclude adequate volume replacement following evisceration. On the other hand, in cases of endophthalmitis, evisceration offers a relative barrier to posterior spread of the infection, assuming that no posterior scleral incisions are necessary to accommodate the appropriately sized implant. Evisceration may impart less disruption to the orbital tissues, does not require disinsertion of the rectus muscles, and may enhance cosmesis. In cases appropriate for either procedure, the surgeon should pursue the technique that allows for the most consistent results in his or her hands.[14]

ENUCLEATION

Enucleation involves removing both the globe and a segment of the anterior optic nerve, with care taken to preserve the conjunctiva, Tenon's capsule, and the extraocular muscles. The goals of enucleation and evisceration surgery are found in Exhibit 23-1. The indications for enucleation include severe trauma, intraocular tumors, and cases at risk for sympathetic ophthalmia. In the setting of eye injury secondary to war wounds, enucleation is more commonly the procedure of choice. It is these severe wounds with uveal prolapse that are at greater risk for sympathetic ophthalmia, and early removal of the inciting eye minimizes this risk. The presence of a known or suspected ocular tumor that is untreatable by other means dictates enucleation over evisceration. In a blind, painful eye with opaque media, enucleation is the better choice and precludes the possibility of eviscerating an occult tumor.

Enucleation surgery is best performed under general anesthesia but, with a cooperative patient, can successfully be undertaken with a retrobulbar anesthetic block alone. An epinephrine-containing retrobulbar block is a recommended adjunct to general anesthesia. Lidocaine with epinephrine is injected into the perilimbal bulbar conjunctiva to promote hemostasis, and the fluid wave assists in dissecting the conjunctiva and Tenon's capsule from the limbal sclera.

EXHIBIT 23-1

SURGICAL GOALS OF ENUCLEATION AND EVISCERATION

- To achieve a centrally placed inert implant with adequate anterior coverage.
- To achieve appropriate volume replacement in the orbit.
- To maintain deep fornices and eyelid support for the placement of a prosthesis.
- To provide symmetry with the contralateral orbit.
- To allow for maximum socket motility, with translation of forces to the prosthesis.

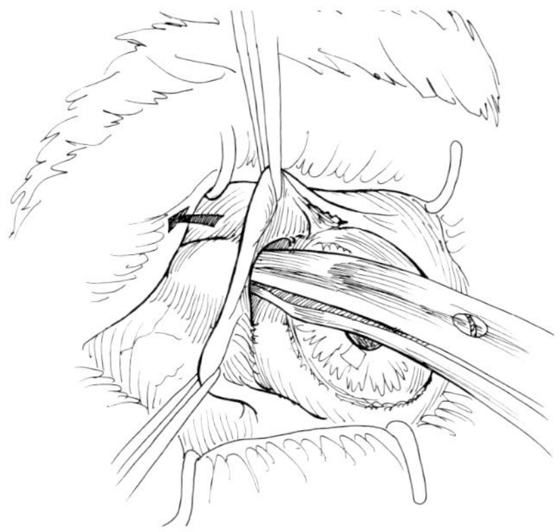

Fig. 23-4. Curved Stevens scissors are placed into the oblique quadrants (avoiding the rectus muscles), and the tips are slid posteriorly along the sclera. The natural curve of the scissors is used to follow the globe surface posteriorly. Drawing prepared for this textbook by Gary Wind, MD, Uniformed Services University of the Health Sciences, Bethesda, Md.

Curved tenotomy or Westcott scissors are used to perform a 360° limbal peritomy. In an effort to preserve the greatest amount of conjunctiva for closure, the tips of the scissors are used to elevate Tenon's capsule and the conjunctiva toward the corneal limbus before cutting (Figure 23-3). Curved Stevens scissors are then placed into the oblique quadrants and slid posteriorly along the sclera (Figure 23-4). The tips are spread and withdrawn to separate Tenon's capsule from the sclera (Figure 23-5).

The check ligaments are then identified by pulling the conjunctiva and Tenon's capsule away from the rectus muscles, and the anterior fibers are cut to better expose the insertion (Figure 23-6). Muscle hooks are passed in a serial fashion under the muscle to isolate and elevate it. As the toe of the hook emerges from under the muscle, it will be covered by a thin film of Tenon's capsule; a small snip in this tissue is necessary to complete the pass (Figure 23-7). A second muscle hook is passed through this track, and the muscle insertion is presented for

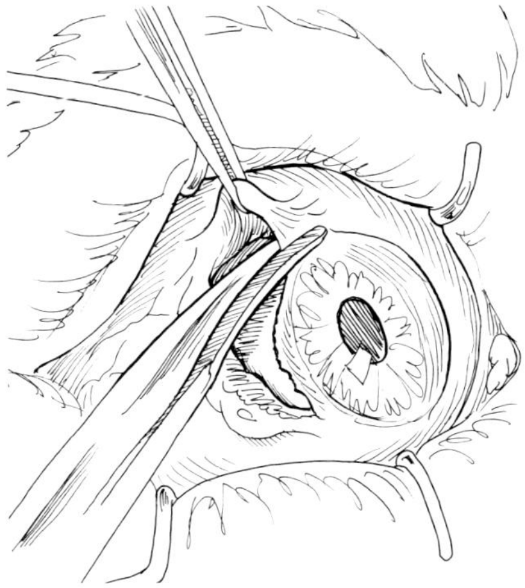

Fig. 23-3. A 360° limbal peritomy is performed. The scissors blade, deep to Tenon's capsule and conjunctiva, is slid firmly against the limbus before cutting. This step maximizes the amount of conjunctiva and Tenon's capsule preserved for closure over the implant. Drawing prepared for this textbook by Gary Wind, MD, Uniformed Services University of the Health Sciences, Bethesda, Md.

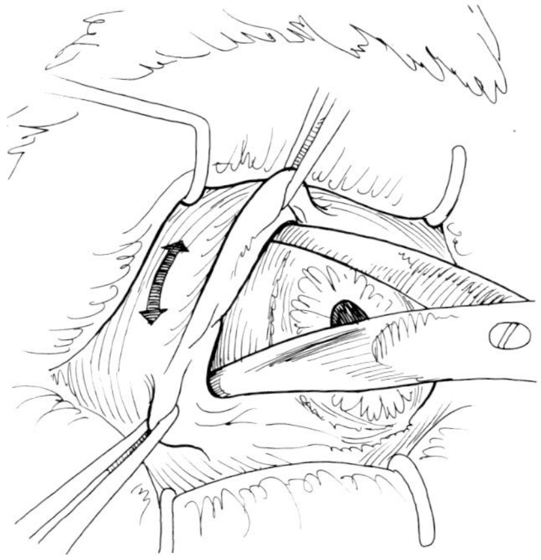

Fig. 23-5. The scissors tips are spread and withdrawn slowly (with the blades open). This action, repeated in each of the four oblique quadrants, separates Tenon's capsule from the outer surface of the globe. Drawing prepared for this textbook by Gary Wind, MD, Uniformed Services University of the Health Sciences, Bethesda, Md.

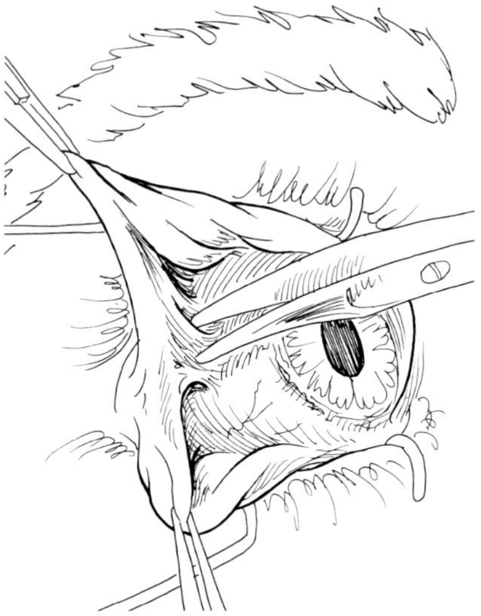

Fig. 23-6. The Tenon's capsule and conjunctival flap are elevated away from the globe to identify the check ligaments of the rectus muscles. Lysing these anterior tissue bridges improves visualization of the rectus muscle insertion. Drawing prepared for this textbook by Gary Wind, MD, Uniformed Services University of the Health Sciences, Bethesda, Md.

traction suture placement.

A double-armed 6-0 Vicryl (polyglactin) suture with spatulated needles is passed through the muscle parallel to and 3 to 5 mm from the muscle insertion. A locking bite is secured at each pole of the muscle (Figure 23-8). The muscle is disinserted from its attachment to the sclera using Westcott or tenotomy scissors. This procedure is repeated for each of the four rectus muscles (Figure 23-9).

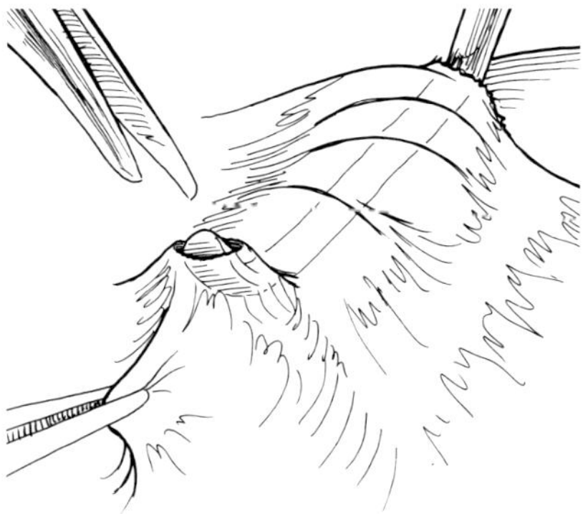

Fig. 23-7. Muscle hooks are used to isolate the insertions of the rectus muscles. As the toe of the hook emerges from under the muscle, it is covered by a thin layer of Tenon's capsule. A small snip in this tissue is necessary to complete the pass. Drawing prepared for this textbook by Gary Wind, MD, Uniformed Services University of the Health Sciences, Bethesda, Md.

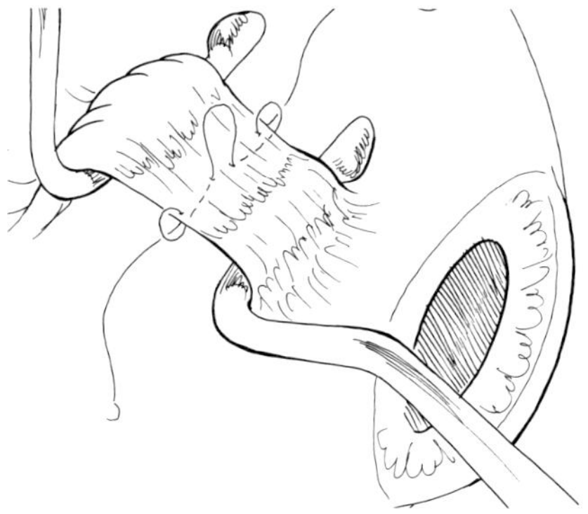

Fig. 23-8. Once the insertion has been isolated, a second hook is used to present the muscle for suture placement. A double-armed 6-0 Vicryl suture with spatulated needles is passed through the muscle parallel to and 3 to 5 mm from its insertion. A locking bite is secured at each margin of the muscle. Drawing prepared for this textbook by Gary Wind, MD, Uniformed Services University of the Health Sciences, Bethesda, Md.

When transecting the medial and lateral rectus, it is advisable to leave a small segment of tendon on the globe so that a traction suture can be attached to the eye. A 4-0 silk suture is whip-stitched through both tendon stumps to make manipulation of the eye easier.[15] This step facilitates oblique muscle identification and allows for controlled anterior

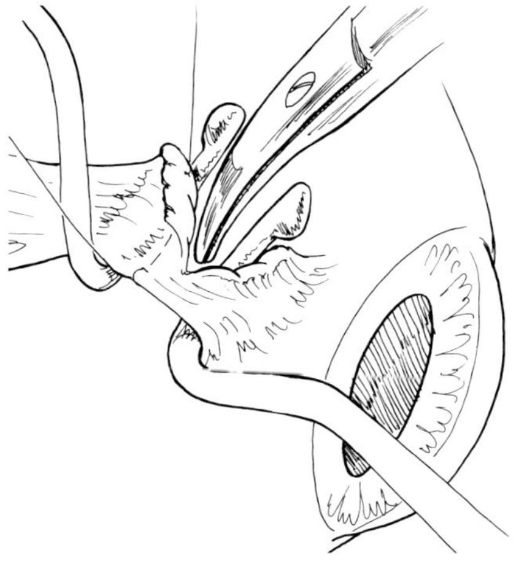

Fig. 23-9. The Vicryl-tagged rectus muscles are disinserted from their scleral attachments. The superior and inferior rectus muscles are cut flush with the sclera. When transecting the medial and lateral rectus muscles, a 3-mm stump of tendon is left on the globe to facilitate manipulation of the globe. Drawing prepared for this textbook by Gary Wind, MD, Uniformed Services University of the Health Sciences, Bethesda, Md.

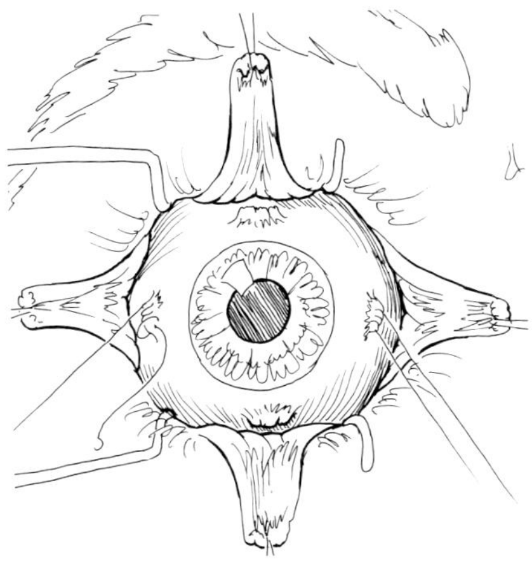

Fig. 23-10. A locking 4-0 silk traction suture is placed through both the medial and lateral rectus muscle stumps. This measure provides a handle to manipulate the globe during oblique muscle identification and also allows controlled anterior traction as the optic nerve is later transected. Drawing prepared for this textbook by Gary Wind, MD, Uniformed Services University of the Health Sciences, Bethesda, Md.

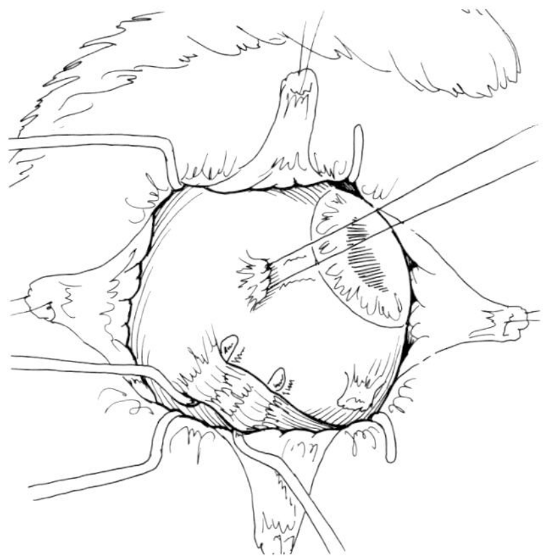

Fig. 23-12. Rotating the eye superiorly and medially presents the inferior oblique muscle, which is transected from its scleral insertion near the macula. Drawing prepared for this textbook by Gary Wind, MD, Uniformed Services University of the Health Sciences, Bethesda, Md.

traction as the optic nerve is later transected (Figure 23-10).

Rotating the eye inferiorly and medially allows for identification of the superior oblique tendon in the superolateral quadrant. The tendon is isolated with a muscle hook and transected at its scleral attachment (Figure 23-11). Next, the eye is rotated superiorly and medially to identify the inferior oblique muscle, which is transected free from its insertion near the macula (Figure 23-12).

Using silk traction sutures, the eye can be rotated about its primary axis to assess freedom of movement. Limitations to rotation suggest an incomplete rectus or oblique muscle disinsertion. Next, the eye is torted laterally, and curved enucleation scissors are inserted into the medial orbital space. The tips

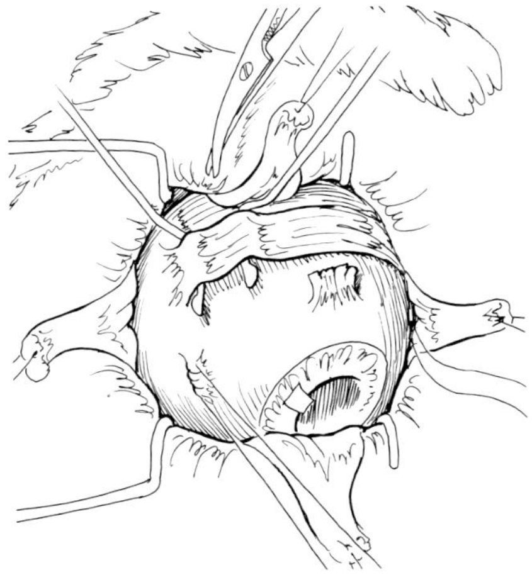

Fig. 23-11. The eye is rotated inferiorly and medially to expose the superolateral quadrant. The superior oblique tendon is isolated with a muscle hook and transected. Drawing prepared for this textbook by Gary Wind, MD, Uniformed Services University of the Health Sciences, Bethesda, Md.

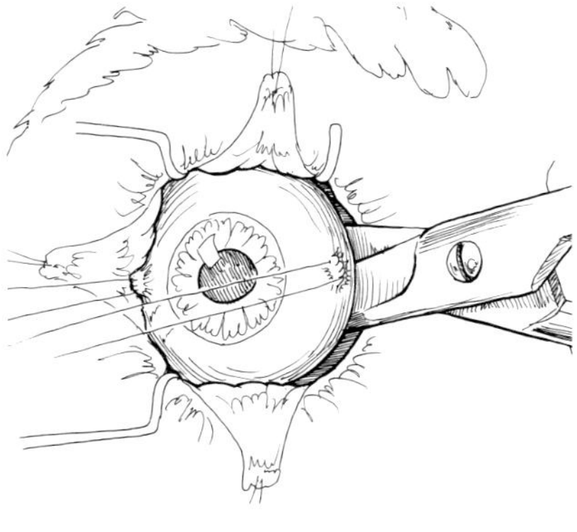

Fig. 23-13. The silk traction suture is used to rotate the globe and ensure that it is free from all muscular attachments. The eye is placed into lateral gaze, and enucleation scissors are slid into the medial space. With the tips of the scissors together, the optic nerve is strummed. Drawing prepared for this textbook by Gary Wind, MD, Uniformed Services University of the Health Sciences, Bethesda, Md.

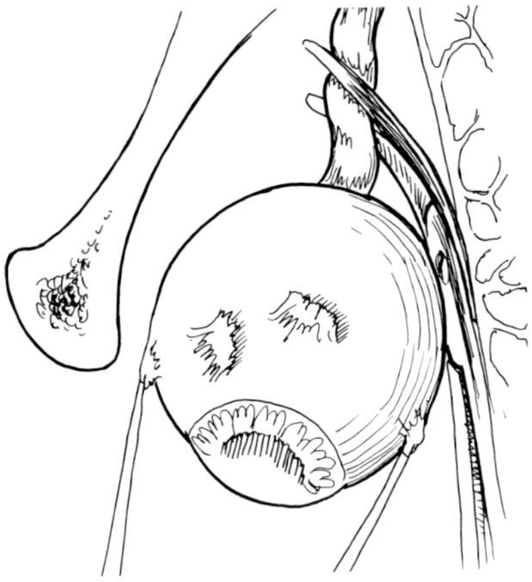

Fig. 23-14. The tips of the scissors are spread around the optic nerve. The silk traction sutures are used to distract the globe anteriorly as the enucleation scissors are slid posteriorly along the nerve. The optic nerve is transected. Drawing prepared for this textbook by Gary Wind, MD, Uniformed Services University of the Health Sciences, Bethesda, Md.

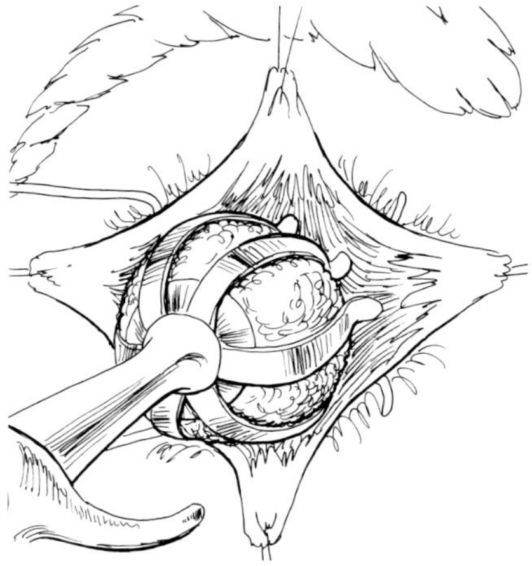

Fig. 23-16. The selected implant is placed into an inserter. The prongs of the device are placed deep into Tenon's capsule, and the plunger is depressed to eject the implant. Drawing prepared for this textbook by Gary Wind, MD, Uniformed Services University of the Health Sciences, Bethesda, Md.

of the scissors are used to locate the optic nerve by strumming it from above and below. The blades of the scissors are then spread to span the nerve (Figures 23-13 and 23-14). While applying anterior traction to the globe, the scissors are slid posteriorly and the optic nerve is transected. An attempt is made to take at least a 4-mm segment of nerve with the globe. The eye is removed from the socket, and any residual soft-tissue attachments are transected. Packing material is then placed into the socket for several minutes to control bleeding (Figure 23-15).

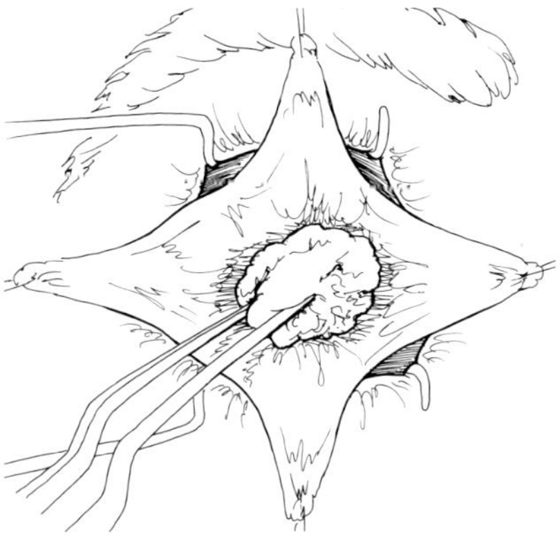

Fig. 23-15. Hemostasis is achieved by packing the socket with gauze soaked in cool normal saline solution. Drawing prepared for this textbook by Gary Wind, MD, Uniformed Services University of the Health Sciences, Bethesda, Md.

Sizing spheres may be used to determine an appropriate implant size. The implant should provide adequate volume replacement and when properly positioned should allow for a tension-free anterior closure of Tenon's capsule and conjunctiva. My own preference is the porous polyethylene sphere (Medpor, mfg by Porex Surgical Group, Newnan, Georgia) for three reasons: (1) a scleral wrap is not

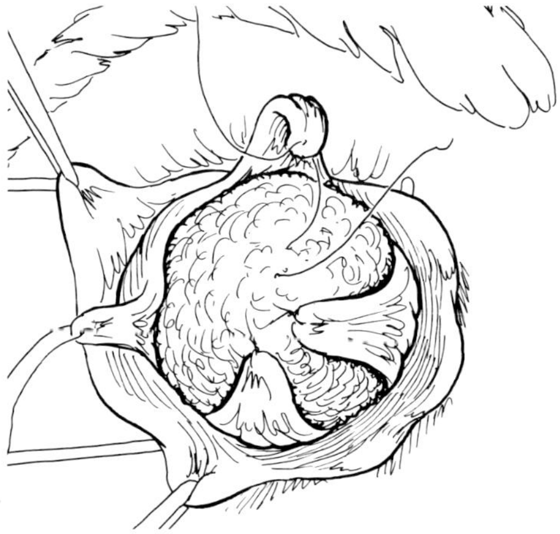

Fig. 23-17. The extraocular muscles are attached to the implant. Each needle of the double-armed suture, preplaced in the rectus muscles, is passed through the porous polyethylene implant. Anterior placement provides an additional layer of protection against implant exposure. Drawing prepared for this textbook by Gary Wind, MD, Uniformed Services University of the Health Sciences, Bethesda, Md.

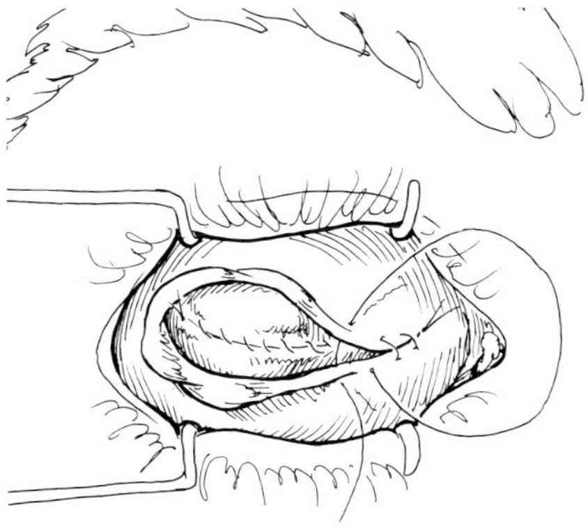

Fig. 23-18. A layered closure of Tenon's capsule and conjunctiva provides protection against implant exposure. 6-0 Vicryl is used to close Tenon's layer, and 7-0 Vicryl is used to close the conjunctiva. The tissue edges must approximate easily over the implant because wound traction increases the risk of breakdown and exposure. Drawing prepared for this textbook by Gary Wind, MD, Uniformed Services University of the Health Sciences, Bethesda, Md.

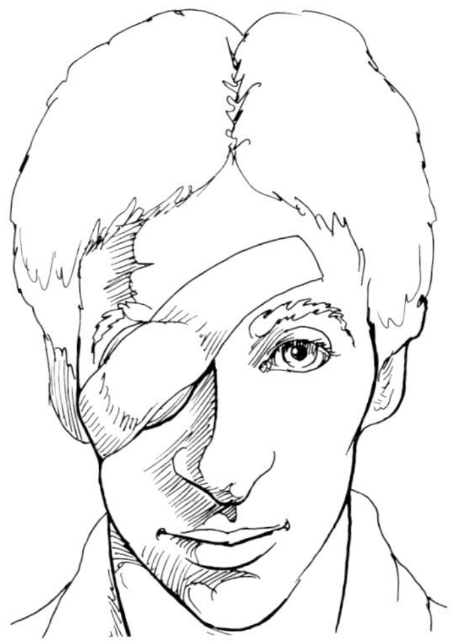

Fig. 23-19. A pressure patch is applied for 48 hours to maximize orbital hemostasis and to maintain the conformer in position. Drawing prepared for this textbook by Gary Wind, MD, Uniformed Services University of the Health Sciences, Bethesda, Md.

required, (2) the muscles may be sewn directly to the implant, and (3) future coupling-peg placement will be possible. The most frequently used implant is 20 mm in diameter. The implant is placed into the socket using a sphere introducer (Figure 23-16). If an introducer is not available, forceps are used in a hand-over-hand fashion to pull Tenon's capsule up and over the implant.

Next, the extraocular muscles are attached to the implant. Each needle of the double-armed suture, preplaced in the rectus muscles, is passed through the porous polyethylene implant (Figure 23-17). The needle tip is placed into a surface pore, and a shallow pass is made through the surface material of the implant. As these sutures are pulled tight and secured, the muscle becomes firmly attached to the implant in a position slightly anterior to the original anatomical placement. This positioning helps cover the anterior aspect of the implant and protects against its exposure. Each of the four rectus muscles is reattached in this fashion.

Tenon's capsule is draped anteriorly to ensure that it will cover the implant without tension across the wound. This layer is crucial, and several layers of interrupted 6-0 Vicryl sutures are used to close it. Care is taken to avoid trapping the conjunctiva, which will predispose to the development of inclusion cysts. Finally, a running 7-0 Vicryl suture closes the conjunctiva (Figure 23-18). The suture only approximates the conjunctival edges and does not add strength to the closure. Sterile antibiotic ointment and a plastic conformer are then placed behind the eyelids into the interpalpebral forniceal space. The largest conformer that allows for closure of the eyelids should be used. A pressure patch is applied over the closed eyelids for 48 hours (Figure 23-19).

EVISCERATION

The evisceration process removes the ocular contents but preserves the sclera and, in some cases, the cornea. The goals of evisceration and enucleation are the same (see Exhibit 23-1). Although no firm consensus exists on the indications for evisceration, most experts agree that a patient with a blind, painful eye without risk of intraocular malignancy is a good candidate. Additionally, eyes lost to endophthalmitis may be best treated with evisceration.

Evisceration is best performed under general anesthesia supplemented with a retrobulbar block but may also be performed with local retrobulbar anesthesia alone. The conjunctiva is injected with an epinephrine-containing local anesthetic mixture before the procedure. As described above for enucleation, a limbal peritomy is performed. The conjunctiva and Tenon's capsule are elevated off the sclera back to the insertions of the rectus muscle. A partial-thickness incision is made around the cor-

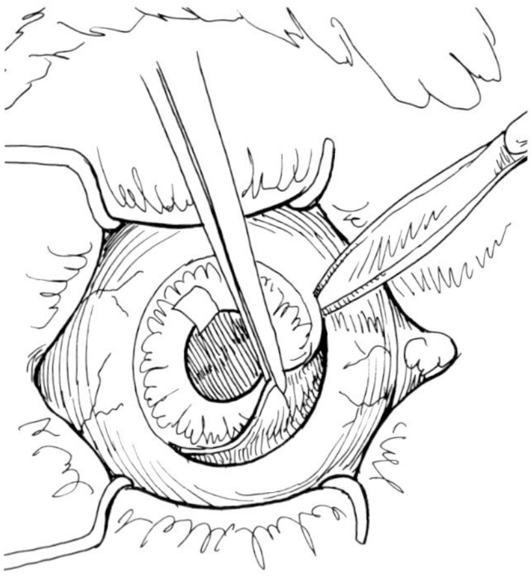

Fig. 23-20. The surgical limbus is incised with a surgical blade, and then corneal scleral scissors are used to remove the corneal button. Drawing prepared for this textbook by Gary Wind, MD, Uniformed Services University of the Health Sciences, Bethesda, Md.

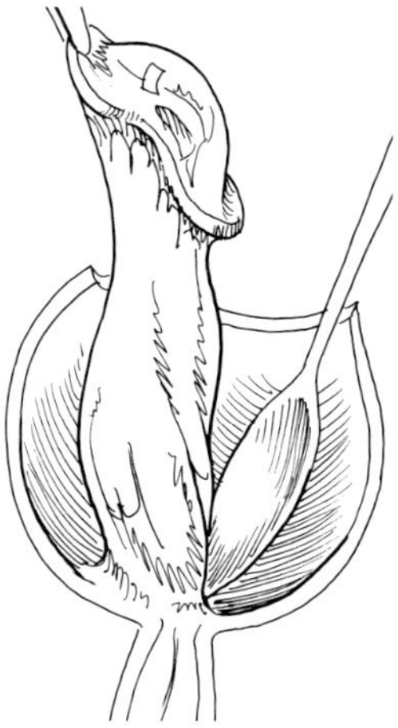

Fig. 23-22. The ciliary body is disinserted, and a plane deep to the choroid is dissected. Drawing prepared for this textbook by Gary Wind, MD, Uniformed Services University of the Health Sciences, Bethesda, Md.

neal limbus, and scissors are used to excise the corneal button (Figure 23-20). A cornea-sparing technique has also been described[16] but is not recommended by this author. An evisceration spoon is placed into the eye to scoop out the intraocular contents (Figure 23-21). The dissection plane is just internal to the sclera, and the entire uveal tract, vitreous, lens, and anterior ocular structures are removed (Figure 23-22).

Sterile, cotton-tipped applicators soaked with absolute alcohol solution are used to treat the internal aspect of the sclera, minimizing the potential for viable uveal tissue remnants (Figure 23-23). Small, radial incisions are made in the oblique quadrants of the sclera so that sizing spheres can be placed into the scleral shell. Care is taken to select an implant that will minimize any anterior traction on the scleral closure. An insertion device can be used to place the implant into the scleral shell, and forceps can be used to further position the implant and ensure that it is adequately seated. If the sclera does not easily close over the implant, then poste-

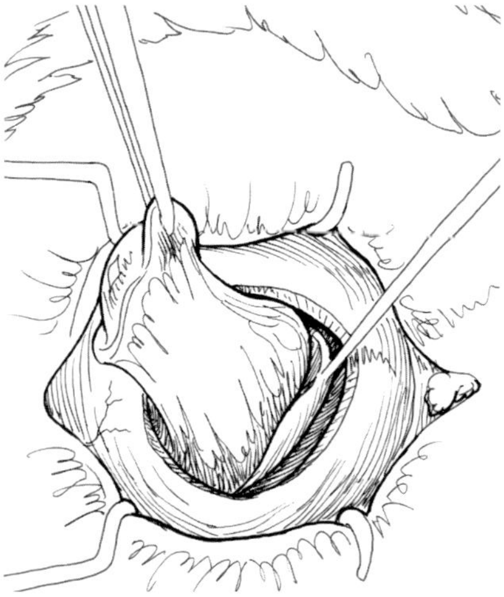

Fig. 23-21. An evisceration spoon is used to remove the ocular contents. Drawing prepared for this textbook by Gary Wind, MD, Uniformed Services University of the Health Sciences, Bethesda, Md.

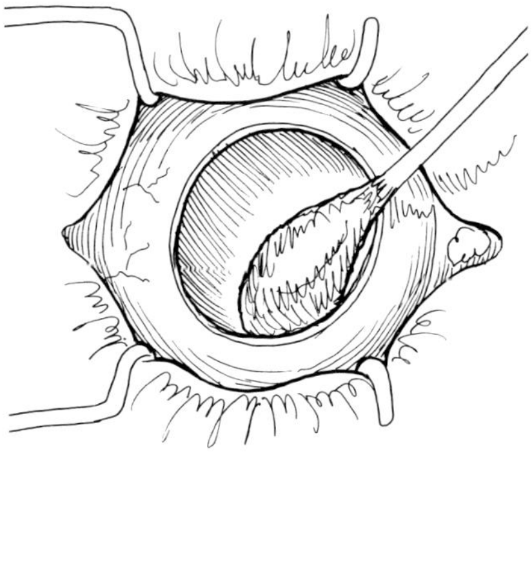

Fig. 23-23. A cotton-tipped swab soaked in absolute alcohol is used to clean the inside of the scleral shell. This step minimizes the survivability of uveal tissue and may reduce the risk of sympathetic ophthalmia. Drawing prepared for this textbook by Gary Wind, MD, Uniformed Services University of the Health Sciences, Bethesda, Md.

Fig. 23-24. A permanent suture (eg, Mersilene) is used to close the sclera over the implant. A tension-free, layered closure of Tenon's capsule minimizes the risk of implant exposure or extrusion. Drawing prepared for this textbook by Gary Wind, MD, Uniformed Services University of the Health Sciences, Bethesda, Md.

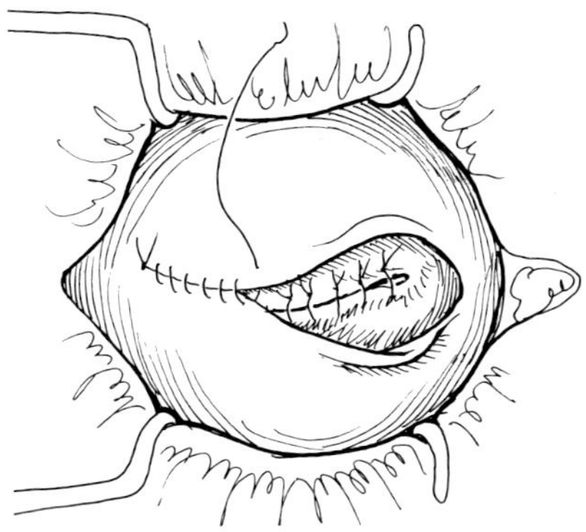

rior radial incisions may be made in the scleral shell to allow the implant to be placed deeper. A 4-0 nonabsorbable suture (eg, Mersilene) is then used to close the sclera over the implant. Tenon's capsule and the conjunctiva are now closed in separate overlying layers (Figure 23-24). A conformer is placed behind the eyelids, and a pressure patch is applied for 48 hours.

IMPLANTS

The history of implant development is fascinating but beyond the scope of this chapter. However, excellent reviews are available elsewhere (eg, in the Enucleation chapter in *Ophthalmic Plastic and Reconstructive Surgery*[17]). The most suitable options at present include (*a*) solid spheres, (*b*) autogenous dermis fat grafts, and (*c*) porous implants.

The solid spherical implants, either acrylic (polymethylmethacrylate) or silicone, are well tolerated, have low extrusion rates, and are inexpensive. Their disadvantages include a tendency to migrate within the orbit and decreased motility.[18] However, by wrapping the implant in donor sclera and reattaching the extraocular muscles, it may be possible to minimize both of these complications.

The autogenous dermis fat graft is readily available in all settings, and the implanted tissue can augment the lining of a contracted socket.[19] Disadvantages include decreased motility, unpredictable resorption, and increased operative time. Although it may not be the primary implant of choice, harvesting and implanting the dermis fat graft are procedures that battlefield ophthalmologists should be prepared to perform.

The graft is harvested from an area midway between the anterior superior iliac spine and the ipsilateral buttock. The area is injected with local anesthetic. A 20-mm circle is drawn and incised to a depth of approximately 20 mm or just above the underlying muscular fascia. Before removing this cylindrical core of tissue, the epidermis is sharply excised or abraded from the dermis and discarded. The dermis-covered fat plug is then separated from its deep attachments and transferred to the recipient orbit. The donor site is converted into an ellipse and closed primarily.

The dermis fat graft is inserted into the orbit. The tagged extraocular muscles are drawn up and sutured in correct anatomical position to the edge of the dermis cap. Tenon's capsule and the conjunctiva can now be positioned over the edge of the dermis graft and sutured into position. By minimizing the overlap at this junction, maximal socket surface area is maintained. The bare dermis will epithelialize under the conformer.

The porous implants are the ones most commonly used today. Both hydroxyapatite and porous polyethylene have interconnecting pores that provide a passive latticework for fibrovascular ingrowth. This ingrowth helps stabilize the implant position within the muscle cone and provides the implant with access to the patient's immune system. After fibrovascular ingrowth is complete, an optional pegging procedure may be considered, in which the prosthesis is directly coupled to the implant, allowing complete translation of socket motility (Figure 23-25). Many patients, however, are satisfied with the motility of the uncoupled prosthesis and decline to risk the potential complications associated with the pegging procedure. These complications include chronic discharge, peg extrusion, and implant exposure.[20]

Hydroxyapatite implants must be wrapped prior to placement. Donor sclera, readily available from eye banks, is commonly used for this purpose. The wrap covers the abrasive surface of the implant, decreasing the risk of conjunctival breakdown and providing a scaffold to which the extraocular muscles are reattached. Four small windows are cut

a b c

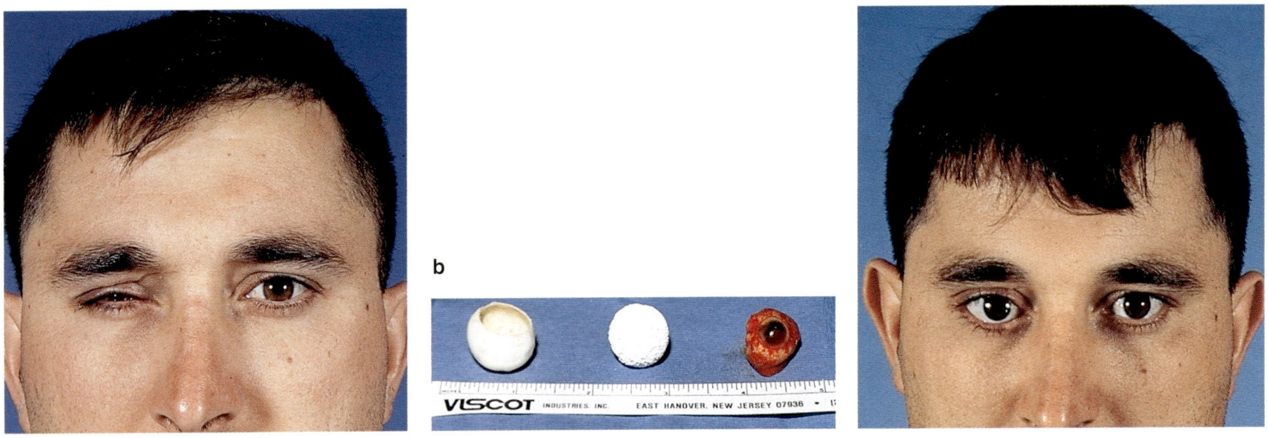

d(l) d(r)

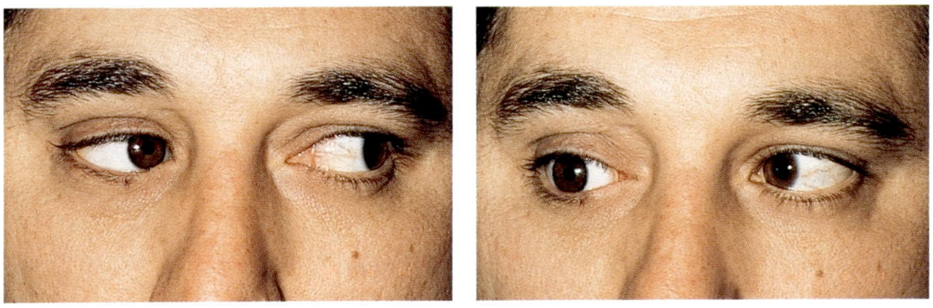

Fig. 23-25. (**a**) A US Marine with a phthisical right globe secondary to an injury by a low-velocity metal fragment during the Persian Gulf War. (**b**) The enucleated phthisical eye is presented alongside the hydroxyapatite implant and donor scleral shell prior to placement in the orbit. (**c**) Postoperatively, the patient was pleased by his orbital symmetry but elected implant pegging to increase the motility of the prosthesis. (**d**) Following a successful pegging procedure, the patient enjoyed excellent left and right lateral gaze. Photographs: Courtesy of William Bigham, Captain, Medical Corps, US Navy; Naval Medical Center San Diego, San Diego, Calif.

in the sclera to accept each of the four rectus muscles. The windows are positioned to approximate the anatomical insertion of the extraocular muscles. Each of the double-armed Vicryl suture needles is passed through the anterior edge of the scleral window. Securing these sutures pulls the muscle into the window and into contact with the hydroxyapatite implant. This provides the anterior implant with a source for fibrovascularization. Several windows may be cut in the posterior aspect of the implant wrap to accelerate the ingrowth there.

Porous polyethylene implants have a smooth surface and may be placed without a wrap. The material is also softer, and the suture needles used to attach the extraocular muscles can be passed through the surface of the implant. The curved needle engages the implant in a surface pore at a shallow angle. With steady force, the needle is passed forward and the natural curve of the needle returns it to the implant surface.

POSTOPERATIVE CARE

The use of systemic antibiotics should be dictated by the potential for infection. If endophthalmitis is present preoperatively, then an antibiotic that is appropriate for the cultured pathogen should be used. In cases of trauma specifically involving organic matter (ie, tree-branch perforation of the eye), a broad-spectrum antibiotic is appropriate. Routine enucleation or evisceration with minimal risk of infection need not be covered with antibiotics.

The pressure patch is applied following surgery to preclude orbital hematoma formation. It also serves to maintain the conformer in position under the eyelids, ensuring the preservation of deep superior and inferior fornices. The patch is removed 48 hours after surgery unless discharge or patient complaints of increasing orbital pain warrant earlier removal to allow inspection of the socket. Following removal of the pressure patch, the patient is instructed to instill an ophthalmic antibacterial ointment into the interpalpebral fissure twice daily for 7 days.

The conformer is first removed 1 week following surgery, and a careful inspection of the socket is performed. The conjunctival suture line is surveyed for breakdown and areas of implant exposure. Any indication of infection warrants aggressive management, including culture and appropriate antibiotics.

The patient is next seen 5 to 6 weeks following surgery. At that time, the conjunctiva should be pink and free of edema. The superior and inferior forniceal spaces should be deep and there should be no evidence of implant exposure. The patient is now ready for referral to the ocularist for socket evaluation and prosthesis fitting.

Most patients who receive porous implants are satisfied with the translation of socket movement to the prosthesis without pursuing direct coupling. The ocularist should be consulted before the option of implant pegging is entertained. Changes to the posterior prosthesis—in addition to overall size modifications—may provide satisfactory improvement in motility. If the patient still desires increased motility and a disparity between socket and prosthesis movement can be seen, then pegging can be considered 6 to 12 months after implant placement. The time delay is necessary to ensure adequate implant vascularization. Magnetic resonance imaging with gadolinium contrast medium may be useful in assessing vascularity of the implant.[21]

Pegging systems exist for both the hydroxyapatite and the porous polyethylene implants. Each system involves the placement of a post (ie, a peg) into the central implant along a line paralleling what would be the visual axis. A template prepared by the ocularist can assist the surgeon in achieving proper centration. A small portion of the post protrudes above the conjunctival tissues and engages a corresponding indentation on the posterior surface of the prosthesis. In addition to the potential for improved motility, such coupling may serve to distribute a portion of the weight of the prosthetic to the implant, effectively unweighting the lower eyelid. This may, over time, minimize lower-eyelid sag.

Although impressive results are possible following prosthesis–implant coupling (see Figure 23-25), the patient must be prepared to accept the potential complications of the procedure. Long-term effects of pegging are not known, but early problems include exposure, extrusion, and socket discharge.[12]

COMPLICATIONS

Blepharoptosis

Either true or pseudoblepharoptosis may follow eye removal. True blepharoptosis can be a result of aponeurotic dehiscence, levator palpebrae muscle injury, or damage to the innervation of the levator palpebrae. These complications may result from the initial trauma or the surgical procedure used to remove the eye. Careful preoperative assessment is necessary to document a preexisting problem. Enucleation surgery, by virtue of visitation to the retrobulbar space, has higher potential for damage to the levator palpebrae muscle or the orbital branches of the third cranial nerve.

Pseudoblepharoptosis can be associated with inadequate volume replacement or the shape of the prosthetic. An ideal implant replaces most of the globe volume, leaving only enough room for an adequately sized prosthesis. Too small an implant can create enophthalmos, and the lack of anterior projection changes the geometry of the levator palpebrae complex. The ocularist can increase the vertical height of the prosthesis or build up its superior margin—within the limits of acceptable weight and volume—to help correct eyelid position. Too large a prosthesis, though, can decrease motility and create lower-eyelid malposition.

Lower-Eyelid Malposition and Laxity

Both minimizing prosthetic size and coupling the implant to the prosthesis decrease the amount of weight that the lower eyelid must support. Over time, though, it is not uncommon for the lower eyelid to yield to gravitational forces, and a lower-eyelid-tightening procedure might be necessary. If recurrences of lower-eyelid malposition secondary to a large prosthetic occur, it may be necessary to replace the orbital implant with one of greater volume. The increased volume of the implant allows the ocularist to fit a smaller prosthesis.

Enophthalmos

As noted above, enophthalmos is usually related to inadequate volume replacement at the time of enucleation or evisceration. In cases of trauma, with concurrent damage to the bony orbital walls, spherical implants alone may be insufficient for volume

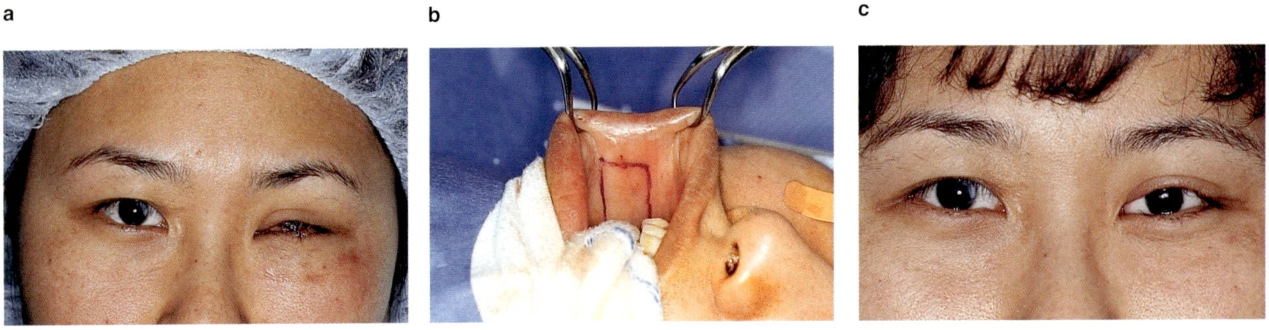

Fig. 23-26. (a) A severely contracted socket precluded the patient from wearing an ocular prosthesis. (b) Buccal mucosa grafts were harvested and used to expand the surface area of the socket. (c) Postoperatively, the prosthesis is maintained in the expanded socket.

replacement. Orbital fracture repair may be necessary to achieve satisfactory results.

Socket Contracture

One of the more difficult complications to manage is contracture of the socket and the associated foreshortening of the fornices. Depending on the degree of contracture, the patient may be unable to wear a prosthesis, and surgical expansion often requires tissue grafting to the mucosa-lined socket (Figure 23-26). In removing the eye, every effort should be made to preserve Tenon's capsule and the conjunctiva. Preserving these structures can be challenging in serious ocular injuries and may necessitate primary dermis fat grafting if insufficient tissue is available.

Following either enucleation or evisceration, a conformer of the largest possible size should be placed into the palpebral fornices as a socket maintainer. Patients should be instructed on how to replace the conformer should it dislodge and the potential consequences of not wearing one for prolonged periods.

Implant Exposure

Tension on the closure of Tenon's capsule and conjunctiva may predispose to wound breakdown and exposure of the implant (Figure 23-27). A rough implant surface (eg, uncovered hydroxyapatite spheres) has also been associated with anterior implant exposure and extrusion.

Small, stable defects of the conjunctiva may be observed. Progressive areas of exposure or those

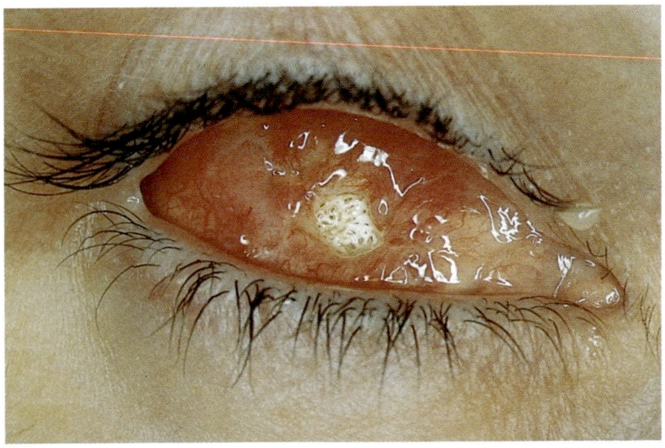

Fig. 23-27. Central area of breakdown exposes the surface of the porous implant.

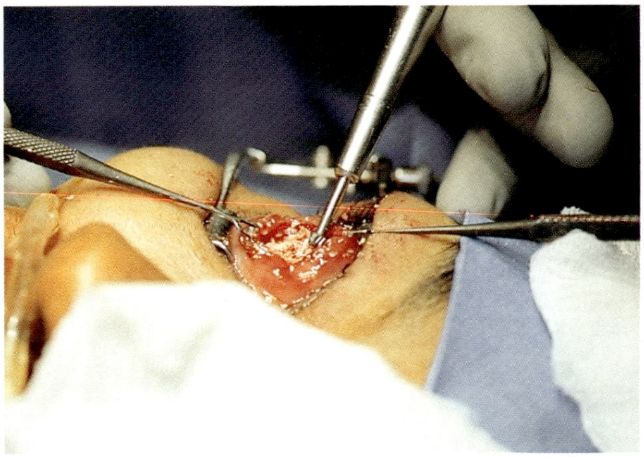

Fig. 23-28. An electric burr is used to reduce the anterior projection of the implant that underlies the area of exposure. This volume reduction may facilitate primary closure of the defect and provide a more vascular bed to support the overlying tissue.

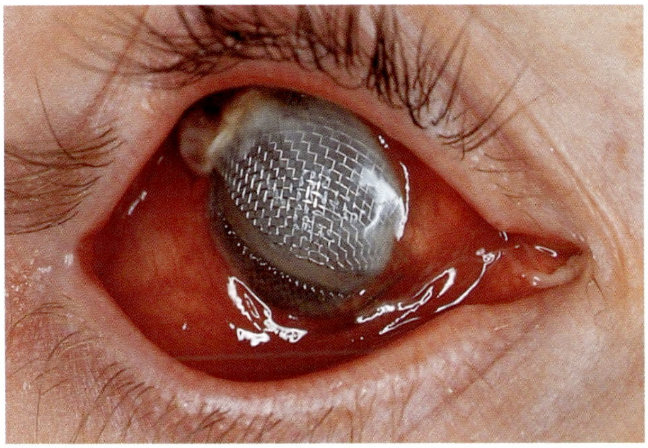

Fig. 23-29. An older, metallic-mesh implant is exposed to its equator and complete extrusion is impending. The implant was exchanged with a porous sphere, and the patient did well.

associated with infection require intervention. In some cases, the anterior projection of the porous implant may be reduced, allowing for a tension-free closure of Tenon's capsule and conjunctiva. An electric burr is used to remove portions of the anterior implant both to reduce its projection and to expose deeper vascularized areas (Figure 23-28). If the wound is sufficiently large to preclude primary closure, a small dermis fat graft can be used to span the defect. It may be necessary to replace the implant with a smaller one in cases of profound infection or impending extrusion (Figure 23-29).[22]

SUMMARY

Proportionally, the eyes receive more battlefield injuries than any other area of the body. Early care must be definitive, with every possible attempt made to preserve vision. In the event that this is not possible, the military ophthalmologist must be prepared to remove the traumatized eye.

Given the tools of modern warfare, ocular injuries with significant uveal exposure and increased risk of sympathetic ophthalmia can reasonably be expected. It is, therefore, most likely that enucleation will be the procedure of choice for those eyes deemed unsalvageable. In planning, the battle-ready ophthalmic surgeon must identify those essential supplies necessary to provide optimum care. Space and weight allowances will limit gear selection.

A single implant that is suitable for both enucleation and evisceration is ideal. Additionally, an implant that allows direct attachment of the extraocular muscles will save on the necessity to stock a wrapping material such as donor sclera. A selection of 18-mm, 20-mm, and 22-mm implants should be adequate. The advantages of stabilization and access to the immune system warrant consideration of porous implants (I prefer porous polyethylene implants). The military ophthalmologist should also ensure that an adequate supply of socket conformers is available, as the freshly operated socket will contract without one.

Eye removal surgery runs contrary to ophthalmologists' investment in preservation of vision. When circumstances necessitate, the military ophthalmic surgeon must be prepared to intervene and provide the best result possible. It is the initial surgery that defines a successful outcome or, conversely, commits the patient to future surgical management of complications arising from an inadequate repair. Finally, ophthalmologists must be prepared to recognize the psychosocial issues associated with eye removal and to treat or refer for treatment when necessary.

REFERENCES

1. Bowen TE, Bellamy RF, eds. *Emergency War Surgery NATO Handbook*. 2nd rev US ed. Washington, DC: Department of Defense, Government Printing Office; 1988: 310.

2. Hornblass A. Eye injuries in the military. *Int Ophthalmol Clin*. 1981;21:121–138.

3. Wong TY, Seet MB, Ang CL. Eye injuries in twentieth century warfare: A historical perspective. *Surv Ophthalmol.* 1997;41(6):433–459.

4. Mader TH, Aragones JV, Chandler AC, et al. Ocular and ocular adnexal injuries treated by United States military ophthalmologists during Operations Desert Shield and Desert Storm. *Ophthalmology.* 1993;100:1462–1567.

5. Prince. Cited by: Luce CM. A short history of enucleation. *Int Ophthalmol Clin.* 1970;10:681–687.

6. Shastid. Cited by: Luce CM. A short history of enucleation. *Int Ophthalmol Clin.* 1970;10:681–687.

7. Hirschberg. Cited by: Schaefer DP, della Rocca RC. Enucleation. In: Nesi FA, Lisman RD, Levine MR, eds. *Smith's Ophthalmic Plastic and Reconstructive Surgery.* 2nd ed. St Louis, Mo: Mosby–Year Book; 1998: Chap 55.

8. Luce CM. A short history of enucleation. *Int Ophthalmol Clin.* 1970;10:681–687.

9. Beer. Cited by: Luce CM. A short history of enucleation. *Int Ophthalmol Clin.* 1970;10:681–687.

10. Noyes. Cited by: Luce CM. A short history of enucleation. *Int Ophthalmol Clin.* 1970;10:681–687.

11. Mules. Cited by: Luce CM. A short history of enucleation. *Int Ophthalmol Clin.* 1970;10:681–687.

12. Jordan DR, Chan S, Mawn L, et al. Complications associated with pegging hydroxyapatite orbital implants. *Ophthalmology.* 1999;106:505–512.

13. Linberg JV, Tillman WT, Allara RD. Recovery after loss of an eye. *Ophthal Plast Reconstr Surg.* 1988;4(3):135–138.

14. Dortzbach RK, Woog JJ. Choice of procedure: Enucleation, evisceration, or prosthetic fitting over globes. *Ophthalmology.* 1985;92:1249–1255.

15. Moses K, La Piana F. Controlled enucleation. *Ophthalmic Surg.* 1987;18:379–382.

16. Ruedemann A. Evisceration with retention of the cornea. *Am J Ophthalmol.* 1958;45:433–434.

17. Schaefer DP, della Rocca RC. Enucleation. In: Nesi FA; Lisman RD; Levine MR, eds. *Smith's Ophthalmic Plastic and Reconstructive Surgery.* 2nd ed. St Louis, Mo: Mosby–Year Book; 1998: Chap 55.

18. Allen L. The argument against imbricating the rectus muscles over spherical orbital implants after enucleation. *Ophthalmology.* 1983;90:1116–1120.

19. Nunery WR, Hetzler KJ. Dermal-fat graft as a primary enucleation technique. *Ophthalmology.* 1985;92:1256–1261.

20. Edelstein C, Shields C, De Potter P, Shields J. Complications of motility peg placement for the hydroxyapatite orbital implant. *Ophthalmology.* 1997;104:1616–1621.

21. De Potter P, Shields CL, Shields JA, Flanders AE, Rao VM. Role of magnetic resonance imaging in the evaluation of the hydroxyapatite implant. *Ophthalmology.* 1992;99:824–830.

22. Christmas NJ, Gordon CD, Murray TG, et al. Intraorbital implants after enucleation and their complications. *Arch Ophthalmol.* 1998;116:1199–1203.

Chapter 24

EYE INJURIES ASSOCIATED WITH TERRORIST BOMBINGS

ALLEN B. THACH, MD[*]

[*]*Colonel, Medical Corps, US Army Reserve; Retinal Consultants of Arizona, Phoenix, Arizona 85214; formerly, Chief, Vitreoretinal Service, Ophthalmology Service, Walter Reed Army Medical Center, Washington, DC*

INTRODUCTION

On 23 October 1983, terrorists drove a truck into the US Marine Corps headquarters in Beirut, Lebanon, that exploded with the force of 12,000 pounds of TNT (trinitrotoluene), killing 241 and injuring 105.[1,2] On 26 February 1993, in the first terrorist bombing of the World Trade Center in New York, New York, terrorists detonated a bomb in the parking garage beneath the Twin Towers, killing 6 and injuring 548.[3] One of the most devastating terrorist attacks was the bombing of the Murrah Building in Oklahoma City, Oklahoma, on 19 April 1995, which killed 167 and resulted in 692 injuries.[4] The Olympic Games in Atlanta, Georgia, were marred by a bombing in Centennial Olympic Park on 27 July 1996, which caused 2 deaths and 111 injuries.[5] The bombing of the US Air Force barracks, Khobar Towers, in Saudi Arabia on 25 June 1996 caused 500 injuries and 19 fatalities (Figure 24-1).[6] On 7 August 1998, terrorists attacked the US embassies in Nairobi, Kenya, and Dar es Salaam, Tanzania, on the same day and at approximately the same time (Figure 24-2). The explosion in Kenya killed more than 240 individuals and injured more than 5,000.[7] And on 11 September 2001, two jet aircraft crashed into the World Trade Center in New York, New York. More than 3,000 individuals died as a result of this terrorist attack. Of the 790 survivors and rescue workers with injuries who reported to nearby hospitals, 204 (26%) had ocular injuries, most of which were attributed to smoke, dust, debris, or fumes.[8]

Statistics compiled by the Federal Bureau of Investigation from 1990 to 1995 show that there have

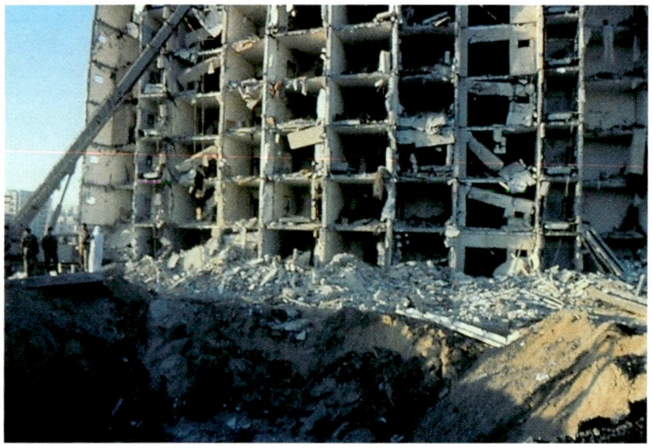

Fig. 24-1. Remains of Khobar Towers in Dhahran, Saudi Arabia. On 25 June 1996, terrorists bombed this complex, which was used as a barracks for US Air Force personnel. Note the large crater in front of the building and the loss of the building closest to where the truck bomb was parked. This bombing caused 19 deaths and 500 injuries.

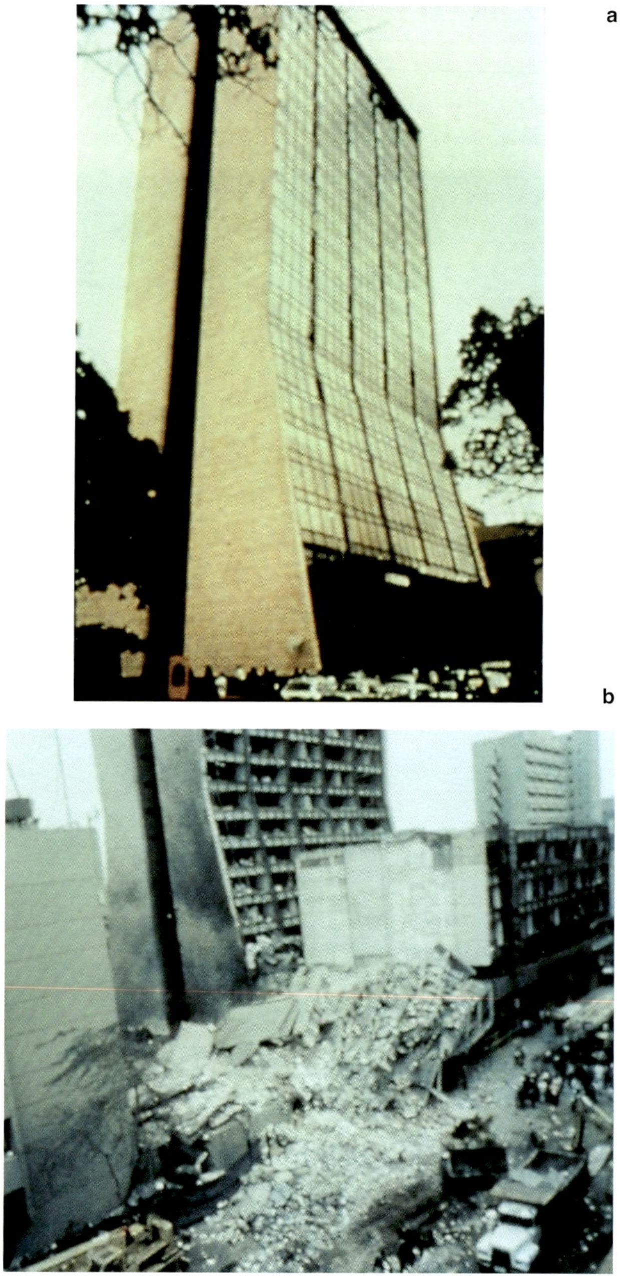

Fig. 24-2. (a) The bank building pictured was adjacent to the US embassy in Kenya before the terrorist bombing on August 7, 1998. (b) After the explosion, the same bank building (rear) has lost of most of the windows on the side closest to the explosion.

been 15,790 criminal bombing incidents in the United States that have killed 355 individuals, injured 3,176, and caused more than $650 million worth of damage.[9] These data do not, of course, include the horrendous loss of life and massive loss of property caused by the destruction of the World Trade Center on 11 September 2001, nor do they include the terrorist ramming of the USS *Cole* and its subsequent explosions, deaths, and injuries off the coast of Aden, Yemen, on 12 October 2000. Whether the targets were civilian or military, however, the bombings caused injuries that are usually associated with military conflicts. Eye injuries make up an important percentage of these injuries.

BLASTS

Detonation of an explosive device causes a high-speed chemical decomposition of a solid or liquid into a gas.[10–12] The explosion creates a wave of very high pressure that moves rapidly away from the point of explosion (10,000–30,000 m/s). The leading edge of the blast wave is a shock front that causes an instantaneous rise in the air pressure (Figure 24-3). The magnitude and duration of the pressure are principally governed by

- the size of the explosive charge, with larger explosions producing a shock wave of faster velocity and longer duration;
- the surrounding medium, with denser media (eg, water compared to air) allowing the shock wave to move faster and making the duration of the positive pressure longer; and
- the distance from the explosion, with greater distance from the explosion resulting in a slower shock-wave velocity and longer duration.

The blast wave front decreases exponentially in pressure and velocity as the distance from the explosion increases. The level of peak pressure and the duration of the shock wave determine the type and extent of the injury. At the end of the decay of the pressure front is an underpressure, which can last about 10 times longer than the overpressure phase. The negative pressure sucks debris into the explosion area, even pulling windows out of buildings.

Even small changes in atmospheric pressure can lead to high-velocity winds. For example, a peak pressure of as little as 0.25 psi can generate winds as high as 125 mph (Table 24-1). Loose objects,

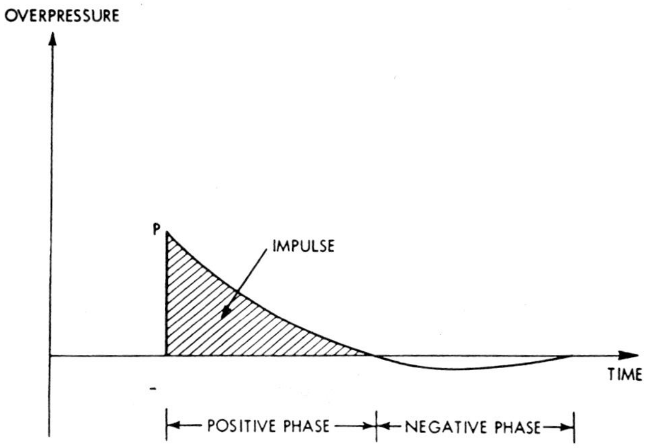

Fig. 24-3. The idealized graph shows the immediate pressure rise (overpressure; P represents peak overpressure) after an explosion with subsequent decrease in pressure after the explosion (underpressure). In an actual blast, the negative phase can last as much as 10 times longer than the positive. Reproduced from Stuhmiller JH, Phillips YY, Richmond DR. The physics and mechanisms of primary blast injury. In: Bellamy RF, Zajtchuk R, eds. *Conventional Warfare: Ballistic, Blast, and Burn Injuries.* In: Zajtchuk R, Bellamy RF, eds. *Textbook of Military Medicine.* Washington, DC: Department of the Army, Office of The Surgeon General, Borden Institute; 1990: 244.

TABLE 24-1

RELATIONSHIP BETWEEN PEAK PRESSURE AND WIND VELOCITY

Maximum Overpressure (psi, at Sea Level)	Wind Velocity (mph)
0.02	40
0.10	70
0.25	125
0.60	160
2.00	290
8.00	470
16.00	670
40.00	940
125.00	1,500

Adapted from Stuhmiller JH, Phillips YY, Richmond DR. The physics and mechanisms of primary blast injury. In: Bellamy RF; Zajtchuk R, eds. *Conventional Warfare: Ballistic, Blast, and Burn Injuries.* In: Zajtchuk R, Bellamy RF, eds. *Textbook of Military Medicine.* Washington, DC: Department of the Army, Office of The Surgeon General, Borden Institute; 1990: 252.

which may be moved by the initial shock wave, achieve their ultimate velocity depending on the blast wind. Blast winds are generated when large volumes of air are displaced by the expanding gases of the explosion (overpressure) or the subsequent underpressure. The victim of a blast may be struck by small objects that may penetrate the body, or the blast may accelerate the victim, hurling him or her with great velocity. The human body might be able to tolerate the instantaneous acceleration but would most likely be injured if it were to hit a hard, stationary object.

Explosive devices also create a short-lived pulse of thermal energy. The intense heat may cause burns of the skin or lead to combustion of surrounding materials. If an explosive device contains flammable fuel, the thermal injuries can be more severe and occur at greater distances from the source.

TABLE 24-2

RELATIONSHIP OF PRESSURE TO PRIMARY BLAST EFFECT

Critical Organ or Event	Related Maximum Overpressure (psi)
Eardrum Rupture	5
Lung Damage	15
Lethality:	
Threshold	30–42
50%	42–57
95%–100%	58–80

Adapted from White CS. *Biologic Blast Effects*. Albuquerque, NM: Lovelace Foundation for Medical Education and Research; 1959. USAEC Report TID-5564.

Types of Blast Injuries

Primary blast injuries are caused by the sudden change in environmental pressure associated with explosive blasts, and they tend to occur in tissues in which variations in tissue density are greatest.[10–16] The air-containing organs (eg, lungs, ears, bowel) are the most susceptible tissues to primary blast injury, although organs that contain both liquid and air (eg, the gastrointestinal tract) are also vulnerable. Damage to the lungs is the cause of the greatest morbidity and mortality. The blast can lead to massive hemorrhage, rupture of the alveoli, and air emboli. An air embolism can occlude the vascular system in the central nervous system and the coronary arterial system, leading to severe disability or death. Pulmonary contusion can cause pulmonary edema and make oxygenation difficult.

The ear is the most susceptible organ to primary blast injury. The eardrums may rupture after a shock wave with no evidence of injury elsewhere. The rupture can occur with an overpressure of as little as 5 psi, compared with the 15 psi needed to cause damage to the lungs (Table 24-2). In addition to eardrum rupture, the ossicles may also fracture or dislocate.

The bowel is also prone to primary blast injury. The large bowel is more susceptible than the small because of the greater volume of air within the colon. Most primary blast injuries of the bowel are associated with underwater explosions and are not as likely to occur with a detonation in air. Injuries range from small, serosal hemorrhages to rupture of the bowel.

Although unusual, rupture of the liver or spleen can occur without accompanying blunt abdominal trauma.

Secondary blast injuries are the result of missiles accelerated by the blast wave.[11–15] The missiles may be a part of the explosive device (primary fragment) or may be secondary missiles, such as glass, masonry, and trees. Depending on the mass and velocity of the projectile, the injuries can include contusions, lacerations, penetration, and fractures.

Tertiary blast injuries result from movement of the human body by the blast wind.[11–15] The acceleration injuries occur if the body is unprotected or only partly protected from the blast. Exposed body parts may suffer traumatic amputation. When the entire body is set in motion, it may be carried a considerable distance from the blast. The type and severity of injury depends mostly on the type of surface against which the body strikes and the body's velocity on impact. Most tertiary blast injuries are blunt in nature and result in fractures and damage to the solid organs of the body.

Thermal (quaternary) injuries result when very high temperatures are generated for a short time after the explosion.[11,12,15] The heat produced by the explosion can produce significant burns of the skin. Flash burns tend to be superficial because of the short exposure time, but the intense heat may ignite the victim's clothing, leading to more extensive and deeper burns. Although most burns are external, they can take the form of inhalational injury, due either to the thermal effects of the explosion or the release of gases.

Other blast-associated injuries, although not classified as one of the types above, include those caused by the collapse of walls and ceilings of build-

TABLE 24-3

TERRORIST INCIDENTS: MORBIDITY, MORTALITY, AND EYE INJURY RATES

Incident	Date	Deaths	Injuries	Eye Injuries (% of All Injuries)
Belfast, Northern Ireland[1]	1969–1972	117	1,532	12 (0.8)
Old Bailey, London[2]	1973	0	160	Not reported
Birmingham, England[3]	1974	2	80	5 (6.3)
Tower of London[4]	1974	0	37	4 (10.8)
Jerusalem[5]	1975–1979	26	340	Not reported
Bologna, Italy[6]	1980	73	218	7 (3.2)
Northern Ireland[7]	1972–1980	5+	339	16 (4.7)
Beirut (Marine Headquarters)[8,9]	1983	241	105	5 (4.8)
Paris, France[10]	1985–1986	20	248	12 (4.8)
Jerusalem[11]	1988	6	52	5 (9.6)
Victoria Station, London[12]	1991	1	50	1 (2.0)
World Trade Center[13]	1993	6	548	0 (0)
Oklahoma City, Oklahoma[14,15]	1995	167	684	55 (8.0)
Centennial Park, Atlanta, Georgia[16]	1996	2	111	Not reported
Manchester, England[17]	1996	0	208	6 (2.9)
Khobar Towers, Dhahran, Saudi Arabia[18]	1996	19	500	3 (0.6)
US Embassy in Kenya[19]	1998	247	> 5,000	> 70 (~ 1.4)
World Trade Center, New York, New York[20]	2001	> 3,000	790	204 (26)

Data sources: (1) Hadden WA, Rutherford WH, Merrett JD. The injuries of terrorist bombing: A study of 1532 consecutive patients. *Br J Surg.* 1978;65:525–531. (2) Caro D, Irving M. The Old Bailey bomb explosion. *Lancet.* 1973;1:1433–1435. (3) Waterworth TA, Carr MJT. Report on injuries sustained by patients treated at the Birmingham General Hospital following the recent bomb explosions. *Br Med J.* 1975;2:25–27. (4) Tucker K, Lettin A. The Tower of London bomb explosion. *Br Med J.* 1975;3:287–290. (5) Adler J, Golan E, Golan J, Yitzhaki M, Ben-Hur N. Terrorist bombing experience during 1975–1979. Casualties admitted to the Shaare Zedek Medical Center. *Isr J Med Sci.* 1983;19:189–193. (6) Brismar B, Bergenwald L. The terrorist bomb explosion in Bologna, Italy, 1980: An analysis of the effects and injuries sustained. *J Trauma.* 1982;22:216–220. (7) Pyper PC, Graham WJH. Analysis of terrorist injuries treated at Craigavon Area Hospital, Northern Ireland, 1972–1980. *Injury.* 1983;14:332–338. (8) Frykberg ER, Tepas JJ III. Terrorist bombings: Lessons learned from Belfast to Beirut. *Ann Surg.* 1988;208:569–576. (9) Frykberg ER, Tepas JJ III, Alexander RH. The 1983 Beirut airport terrorist bombing: Injury patterns and implications for disaster management. *Am Surg.* 1989;55:134–141. (10) Rignault DP, Deligny MC. The 1986 terrorist bombing experience in Paris. *Ann Surg.* 1989;209:368–373. (11) Katz E, Ofek B, Adler J, Abramowitz HB, Krausz MM. Primary blast injury after a bomb explosion in a civilian bus. *Ann Surg.* 1989;209:484–488. (12) Johnstone DJ, Evans SC, Field RE, Booth SJ. The Victoria bomb: A report from the Westminster Hospital. *Injury.* 1993;24:5–9. (13) Quenonmoen LE, Davis YM, Malilay J, Sinks T, Noji EK, Klitzman S. The World Trade Center bombing: Injury prevention strategies for high-rise building fires. *Disasters.* 1996;20:125–132. (14) Mallonee S, Shariat S, Stennies G, Waxweiler R, Hogan D, Jordan F. Physical injuries and fatalities resulting from the Oklahoma City bombing. *JAMA.* 1996;276:382–387. (15) Mines M, Thach A, Mallonee S, Hildebrand L, Shariat S. Ocular injuries sustained by survivors of the Oklahoma City bombing. *Ophthalmology.* 2000;107:837–843. (16) Anderson GV Jr, Feliciano DV. The Centennial Olympic Park bombing: Grady's response. *J Med Assoc Ga.* 1997;86:42–46. (17) Carley SD, Mackway-Jones K. The casualty profile from the Manchester bombing 1996: A proposal for the construction and dissemination of casualty profiles from major incidents. *J Accid Emerg Med.* 1997;14:76–80. (18) Thach AB, Ward TP, Hollifield RD, Cockerham K, Birdsong R, Kramer KK. Eye injuries in a terrorist bombing: Dhahran, Saudi Arabia, June 25, 1996. *Ophthalmology.* 2000; 107:844–847. (19) News Journal Online. Kenya struggles to cope with dozens blinded from embassy bomb. 2 Sep 1998. Available at: http://www.n-jcenter.com/1998Sep/2/WOR4.htm. Accessed 8 April 2000. (20) Centers for Disease Control and Prevention. Rapid assessment of injuries among survivors of the terrorist attack on the World Trade Center—New York City, September 2001. *MMWR.* 2001;51(1):1–5.

a

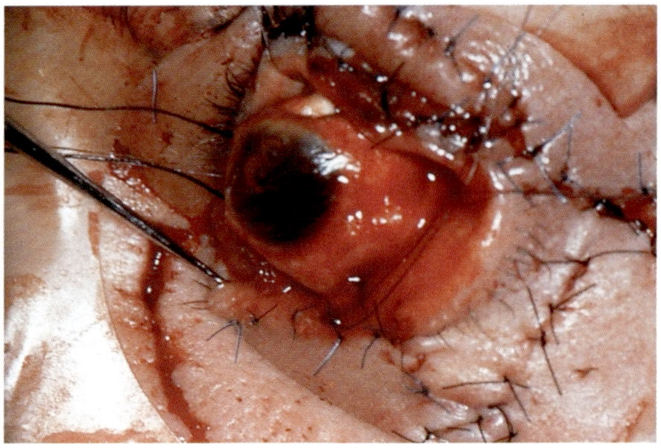

b

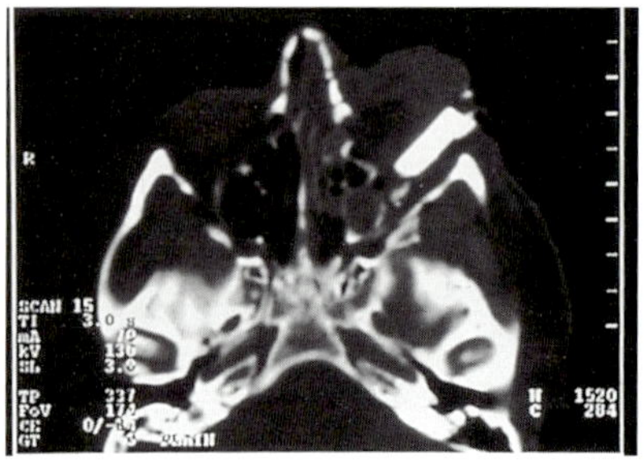

c

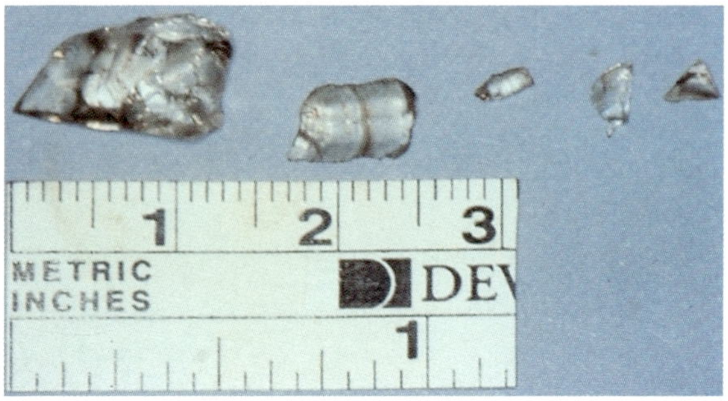

Fig. 24-4. (**a**) A victim from the blast of Khobar Towers, in Dhahran, Saudi Arabia, on 25 June 1996, had numerous facial lacerations in addition to an open globe injury. (**b**) A computed tomography image of the same patient showed numerous orbital foreign bodies. One of the foreign bodies caused a transection of the optic nerve. The glass foreign bodies imaged well because of the high lead content of this glass. (**c**) These glass foreign bodies were removed from the orbit of this patient. The longest piece of glass was thought to have caused the optic nerve transection. Reproduced with permission from Thach AB, Ward TP, Hollifield RD, Cockerham K, Birdsong R, Kramer KK. Eye injuries in a terrorist bombing: Dhahran, Saudi Arabia, June 25, 1996. *Ophthalmology.* 2000;107:846.

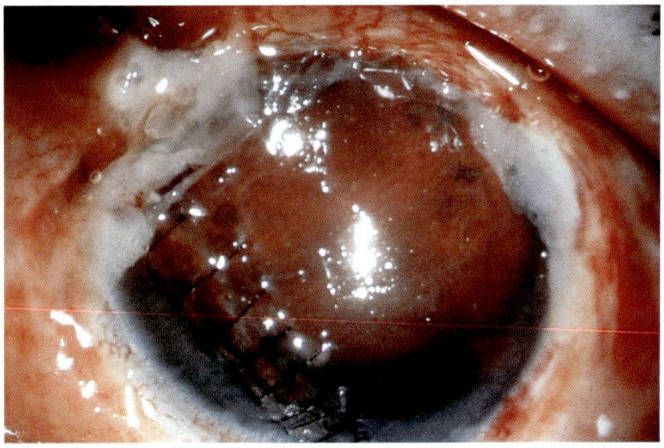

Fig. 24-5. A victim of the terrorist bombing of the Khobar Towers, in Dhahran, Saudi Arabia, on 25 June 1996. This individual suffered a bilateral corneoscleral laceration with loss of his lens at the time of injury. Associated injuries included a hyphema, vitreous hemorrhage, retinal detachment, and choroidal hemorrhage. Reproduced with permission from Thach AB, Ward TP, Hollifield RD, Cockerham K, Birdsong R, Kramer KK. Eye injuries in a terrorist bombing: Dhahran, Saudi Arabia, June 25, 1996. *Ophthalmology.* 2000;107:846.

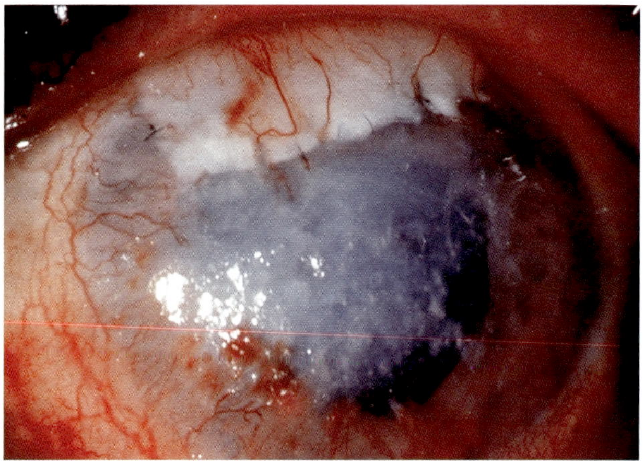

Fig. 24-6. This patient's cornea was "peppered" with small glass fragments as a result of the terrorist explosion at the US embassy in Nairobi, Kenya, on 7 August 1998. Additionally, the patient had a bilateral corneoscleral laceration, hyphema, vitreous hemorrhage, intraocular foreign bodies, and a retinal detachment. Photograph: Courtesy of Edward W. Trudo, MD, and K. Scot Bower, MD, Department of Ophthalmology, Walter Reed Army Medical Center, Washington, DC.

EXHIBIT 24-1

TYPES OF OCULAR INJURIES ASSOCIATED WITH TERRORIST EXPLOSIONS

- Eyelid, Orbit, and Adnexa
  - Eyelid and/or eyebrow laceration
  - Orbital fracture
  - Orbital foreign body
  - Lacrimal system injury
- Anterior Segment
  - Corneal abrasion
  - Corneal laceration
  - Corneoscleral laceration
  - Conjunctivitis and/or conjunctival irritation
  - Hyphema
  - Corneal burn
  - Traumatic cataract
  - Subconjunctival hemorrhage
- Posterior Segment
  - Scleral laceration
  - Retinal detachment
  - Intraocular foreign body
  - Vitreous hemorrhage
- Miscellaneous
  - Ocular contusion
  - Cranial and/or optic nerve injury
  - Rectus muscle transection

ings within the blast zone. These are a significant cause of death and injury. Victims in a building that collapses may suffer blunt and crush injuries without other injuries associated with a blast.

Ocular Injuries Associated With Explosive Blasts

Although the eye is subject to all the types of injuries described above, the most common and devastating ocular injuries result from the missiles created by a blast (ie, secondary blast injuries). Just as with wartime ocular injuries, those associated with terrorist blasts are most commonly due to fragments that damage the eye. Table 24-3 describes some of the terrorist bombings that have occurred over the last several years.[1–8,17–28] Most blasts cause at least some ocular injuries. A notable exception is the 1993 World Trade Center bombing, in which explosives were detonated underground and most injuries were therefore due to smoke inhalation, not fragmentation missiles. The other reported bombings occurred in crowded public places or in the open, causing injuries due to the blast itself, collapse of a building, or secondary missiles from the blast effect. Although most deaths are probably due to the initial blast or collapse of a building, most eye injuries are related to fragments (eg, glass, bomb casing, masonry, other unsecured items) and debris.

Ocular injuries due to missile fragments during wartime are very similar to ocular injuries that occur from a terrorist bombing. In recent conflicts, most eye injuries stemmed from fragmentation projectiles rather than bullets.[29,30] Unlike the metallic fragments that injure the eye in the military environment, most severe eye injuries from terrorist bombings occur from fragments of glass (Figures 24-4 through 24-6).[6,27,31,32] Glass, particularly monolithic glass, was a major contributing factor for eye injuries in the Oklahoma City bombing.[27,33] Such injuries might be prevented by the use of shatter-resistant glass, laminated glass, Mylar curtains, filmed glass, and catch bars over the windows.

Although the eye makes up much less than 1% of the frontal body surface area, it is very susceptible to injury. Small fragments that may not penetrate clothing or that barely penetrate the skin are able to cause blinding damage to the eye. Ocular injuries that occur in a terrorist blast can be as minor as a superficial foreign body from debris, a subconjunctival hemorrhage, or a corneal abrasion, and as severe as an open globe injury, orbital fracture, or damage to the optic nerve (Exhibit 24-1). Modern microsurgical techniques, the operating room microscope, and the use of vitrectomy enable the ophthalmologist to restore vision in eyes with injuries that in the past may have led to blindness and enucleation.

SUMMARY

Terrorist bombings—overseas and in the United States—affect military personnel and civilians alike. The detonation of an explosive device leads to a rapid increase in atmospheric pressure (blast wave) followed by a decrease in the atmospheric pressure, both of which lead to displacement of air creating a blast wind.

The blast wave can lead to primary blast injury,

which usually affects air-containing organs (lungs, ears, gastrointestinal tract). These injuries can cause air emboli, pulmonary contusion, ruptured eardrums, and ruptured bowel. Secondary blast injuries are due to missiles and fragments that are propelled by the explosion. Tertiary blast injuries are due to movement of parts of or the entire human body and can result in traumatic amputations and blunt injuries. Thermal injuries, including burns of the skin and inhalational injury, can also be produced by an explosion.

Although the eye constitutes only a small portion of the frontal body surface area, it is very susceptible to fragmentation missiles. Fragments that may cause minimal damage to other parts of the body can cause severe injuries to the globe. Most fragments tend to be glass, bomb casing, and masonry, but any unsecured item may act like a missile and cause damage to the eye. Injuries created by a terrorist explosion have included corneoscleral lacerations, orbital fractures, hyphemas, eyelid lacerations, traumatic cataracts, and optic nerve injuries, to name a few. Techniques developed over the years to treat ocular injuries have led to an improved prognosis for these once-devastating injuries.

REFERENCES

1. Frykberg ER, Tepas JJ III. Terrorist bombings: Lessons learned from Belfast to Beirut. *Ann Surg.* 1988;208:569–576.

2. Frykberg ER, Tepas JJ III, Alexander RH. The 1983 Beirut airport terrorist bombing: Injury patterns and implications for disaster management. *Am Surg.* 1989;55:134–141.

3. Quenonmoen LE, Davis YM, Malilay J, Sinks T, Noji EK, Klitzman S. The World Trade Center bombing: Injury prevention strategies for high-rise building fires. *Disasters.* 1996;20:125–132.

4. Mallonee S, Shariat S, Stennies G, Waxweiler R, Hogan D, Jordan F. Physical injuries and fatalities resulting from the Oklahoma City bombing. *JAMA.* 1996;276:382–387.

5. Anderson GV Jr, Feliciano DV. The Centennial Olympic Park bombing: Grady's response. *J Med Assoc Ga.* 1997;86:42–46.

6. Thach AB, Ward TP, Hollifield RD, Cockerham K, Birdsong R, Kramer KK. Eye injuries in a terrorist bombing: Dhahran, Saudi Arabia, June 25, 1996. *Ophthalmology.* 2000;107:844–847.

7. News Journal Online. Kenya struggles to cope with dozens blinded from embassy bomb. 2 Sep 1998. Available at http://www.n-jcenter.com/1998Sep/2/WOR4.htm. Accessed April 8, 2000.

8. Centers for Disease Control and Prevention. Rapid assessment of injuries among survivors of the terrorist attack on the World Trade Center—New York City, September 2001. *MMWR.* 2001;51(1):1–5.

9. Federal Bureau of Investigation. *1995 Bomb Summary.* Quantico, Va: US Department of Justice; 1995.

10. Stapczynski JS. Blast injuries. *Ann Emerg Med.* 1982;11:687–694.

11. Mellor SG. The pathogenesis of blast injury and its management. *Br J Hosp Med.* 1988;39:536–539.

12. Hull JB. Blast: Injury patterns and their recording. *J Audiovisual Med.* 1992;15:121–127.

13. de Candole CA. Blast injury. *Can Med Assoc J.* 1967;96:207–214.

14. Rawlings JSP. Physical and pathophysiological effects of blast. *Injury.* 1977;9:313–320.

15. Cooper GJ, Maynard RL, Cross NL, Hill JF. Casualties from terrorist bombings. *J Trauma.* 1983;23:955–967.

16. Phillps YY. Primary blast injuries. *Ann Emerg Med.* 1986;15:1446–1450.

17. Hadden WA, Rutherford WH, Merrett JD. The injuries of terrorist bombing: A study of 1532 consecutive patients. *Br J Surg.* 1978;65:525–531.

18. Caro D, Irving M. The Old Bailey bomb explosion. *Lancet.* 1973;1:1433–1435.

19. Waterworth TA, Carr MJT. Report on injuries sustained by patients treated at the Birmingham General Hospital following the recent bomb explosions. *Br Med J.* 1975;2:25–27.

20. Tucker K, Lettin A. The Tower of London bomb explosion. *Br Med J.* 1975;3:287–290.

21. Adler J, Golan E, Golan J, Yitzhaki M, Ben-Hur N. Terrorist bombing experience during 1975-1979: Casualties admitted to the Shaare Zedek Medical Center. *Isr J Med Sci.* 1983;19:189–193.

22. Brismar B, Bergenwald L. The terrorist bomb explosion in Bologna, Italy, 1980: An analysis of the effects and injuries sustained. *J Trauma.* 1982;22:216–220.

23. Pyper PC, Graham WJH. Analysis of terrorist injuries treated at Craigavon Area Hospital, Northern Ireland, 1972–1980. *Injury.* 1983;14:332–338.

24. Rignault DP, Deligny MC. The 1986 terrorist bombing experience in Paris. *Ann Surg.* 1989;209:368–373.

25. Katz E, Ofek B, Adler J, Abramowitz HB, Krausz MM. Primary blast injury after a bomb explosion in a civilian bus. *Ann Surg.* 1989;209:484–488.

26. Johnstone DJ, Evans SC, Field RE, Booth SJ. The Victoria bomb: A report from the Westminster Hospital. *Injury.* 1993;24:5–9.

27. Mines M, Thach A, Mallonee S, Hildebrand L, Shariat S. Ocular injuries sustained by survivors of the Oklahoma City bombing. *Ophthalmology.* 2000;107:837–843.

28. Carley SD, Mackway-Jones K. The casualty profile from the Manchester bombing 1996: A proposal for the construction and dissemination of casualty profiles from major incidents. *J Accid Emerg Med.* 1997;14:76–80.

29. Heier JS, Enzenauer RW, Wintermeyer SF, Delaney M, La Piana FG. Ocular injuries and diseases at a combat support hospital in support of Operations Desert Shield and Desert Storm. *Arch Ophthalmol.* 1993;111:795–798.

30. Mader TH, Aragones JV, Chandler AC, et al. Ocular and ocular adnexal injuries treated by United States military ophthalmologists during Operations Desert Shield and Desert Storm. *Ophthalmology.* 1993;100:1462–1467.

31. Boffard KD, MacFarlane C. Urban bomb blast injuries: Patterns of injury and treatment. *Surg Annu.* 1993;25:29–47.

32. Karmy-Jones R, Kissinger D, Golocovsky M, Jordan M, Champion HR. Bomb-related injuries. *Mil Med.* 1994;159:536–539.

33. Norville HS, Harvill N, Conrath EJ, Shariat S, Mallonee S. Glass-related injuries in Oklahoma City bombing. *Journal of Performance of Constructed Facilities.* 1999;13:50–55.

Chapter 25

OCULAR LASER INJURIES

RODNEY D. HOLLIFIELD, MD*

*Vitreoretinal Surgeon, Retina Consultants of Nevada, Las Vegas, Nevada 89144; formerly, Lieutenant Colonel, Medical Corps, US Army; Chief, Vitreoretinal Service, Walter Reed Army Medical Center, Washington, DC

INTRODUCTION

Laser use continues to proliferate on the modern battlefield. They are used routinely for target designators, rangefinders, and radar warning.[1] More ominously, the use of lasers as antipersonnel devices by enemy forces is a real and increasing threat. Given these facts, it is likely that healthcare providers will encounter individuals with possible ocular laser injuries. The ability of medical personnel to identify and properly manage suspected laser casualties is crucial to sustaining the fighting force.

In a combat situation, laser emissions by both hostile and friendly forces can lead to potential ocular injury. An unclassified list of known US Army lasers is provided in Table 25-1.[2]

With advances in solid-state electronics, frequency-doubled neodymium:yttrium-aluminum-garnet (Nd:YAG) lasers operating at a wavelength of 532 nm are commonplace and should also be expected in a battlefield environment. These lasers emit in the green color band. Potential threat lasers include, at a minimum, the lasers listed in Table 25-1, as well as the frequency-doubled Nd:YAG laser. Additionally, lasers that operate at multiple wavelengths are now available. These lasers offer the operator the ability to instantaneously choose and switch the operating wavelength, thus making the prevention of laser injuries more difficult.

Laser pointers, now commonplace in society, are also found in the combat environment. With their momentary exposure, most commercially available laser pointers have insufficient power to cause permanent retinal injury.[3,4] Nevertheless, the visible emission of the laser pointer can cause glare and dazzle (ie, flash blindness). Many individuals who are exposed to a laser pointer emission seek medical attention and will require reassurance. Proper diagnosis and management of these patients can prevent unnecessary loss of personnel and possible panic among otherwise healthy individuals.

Ocular injuries in military personnel have been reported[5] from friendly laser sources. Most of these incidents have involved exposure to target designators and rangefinders operating in a Q-switched (ie, rapidly pulsed) mode at 1,064 nm (infrared). Although the technology is available to produce antipersonnel lasers, no use of such a laser has been documented to date. Nevertheless, with increasing use of lasers, healthcare providers in future conflicts should be prepared to evaluate and treat ocular laser injuries.

LASER PHYSICS

The word "laser" is an acronym for *l*ight *a*mplification by *s*timulated *e*mission of *r*adiation. The unique properties of lasers allow for the production of an intense, single wavelength of electromagnetic energy with minimal divergence. These properties allow the lasers to concentrate sufficient energy to destroy a target. Laser emissions are visible or invisible, depending on the wavelength of the particular laser.

The damaging effects of a laser on a target depend largely on the amount of energy delivered. At a constant distance, the total energy delivered by a laser is a function of three variables: power, exposure time, and spot size (diameter of the laser beam). For a constant exposure time and spot size, increasing the power increases the total energy delivered

TABLE 25-1

WAVELENGTHS OF COMMON US ARMY LASERS

Type	Device	Wavelength (nm)	Band
Helium-Neon	Tank, gunnery trainer	642.8	Visible (red)
Ruby	Rangefinder	694.3	Visible (red)
Gallium-Arsenide	MILES	905.0	Near-infrared
Nd:YAG	Rangefinder, target designator	1,064.0	Near-infrared
Carbon Dioxide	Rangefinder	10,600.0	Far-infrared

MILES: multiple integrated laser engagement system
Nd:YAG: neodymium:yttrium-aluminum-garnet
Adapted from Headquarters, Department of the Army. *Prevention and Medical Management of Laser Injuries.* Washington, DC: DA; 8 Aug 1990: 19. Field Manual 8-50.

to a target. For a constant power and spot size, decreasing the exposure time increases the energy delivered to a target. In this scenario, a rapidly pulsed (Q-switched) laser delivers more energy than a laser operating in a continuous wave mode. For a given power setting and exposure time, decreasing the spot size of the laser increases the total amount of energy delivered.

Mechanisms of Bioeffects

A laser interaction with tissue causes damage by one or more of the following mechanisms: (*a*) photochemical reaction, (*b*) thermal effects, (*c*) vaporization, or (*d*) optical breakdown.[6]

After laser exposure—usually with ultraviolet or visible light—chemical bonds are destroyed or formed because of photochemical reactions. Opacities or haziness of the cornea or lens, or both, may result from ultraviolet or visible light laser emissions.

Absorption of the laser energy results in a 10°C to 20°C rise in temperature of the affected tissue.[6] As a result, the absorbing tissue denatures. This thermal effect is most commonly encountered with visible or infrared laser exposure to pigmented areas of the eye, such as the layer of cells under the retina known as the retinal pigment epithelium (RPE). Clinically, the patient may present with an area of whitening of the RPE. Within days to weeks, many of these same areas may become heavily pigmented.

When the temperature of water within tissue rises above its boiling point, a microexplosion occurs and the tissue vaporizes. This type of injury might follow a particularly intense visible-wavelength laser exposure in the RPE, or an exposure to a carbon dioxide laser.

In optical breakdown, an extremely high-power laser exposure strips electrons from an atom, which results in the formation of plasma. The shock wave created by the plasma formation physically disrupts tissue, causing injury. Optical breakdown is independent of ocular pigment and can occur anywhere in the eye. Because of the eye's focusing power, though, these types of injuries are more likely to be encountered in the retina. Optical breakdown is most commonly seen with lasers operating with a pulse duration of 10^{-6} seconds or less.

Ocular Bioeffects

The human eye absorbs electromagnetic wavelengths between 400 and 1,400 nm. The greatest absorption occurs in the visible and near-infrared spectrum, 500 through 950 nm (Figure 25-1).[2]

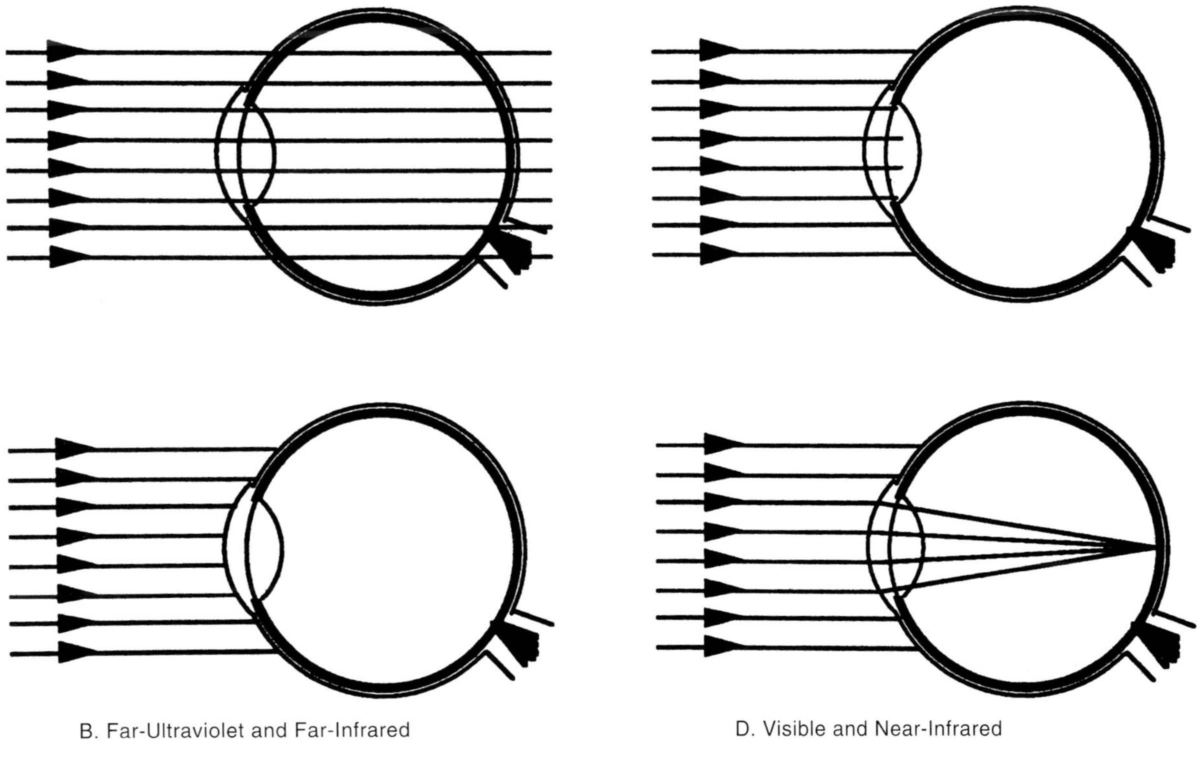

Fig. 25-1. Schematic diagram of the absorption of electromagnetic radiation in the eye. Adapted from Headquarters, Department of the Army. *Prevention and Medical Management of Laser Injuries.* Washington, DC: DA; 8 Aug 1990: 4. Field Manual 8-50.

TABLE 25-2

LASER ABSORPTION BY FUNDUS PIGMENTS

	XAN	HEM	MEL
Argon blue-green (488 nm)	+ + +	+ + +	+ +
Argon green (514 nm)	–	+ + +	+ + + +
Nd:YAG green (532 nm)	–	+ + + +	+ + + +
Dye yellow (577 nm)	–	+ + + +	+ + + +
Dye red (630 nm)	–	+	+ + +
Krypton red (647 nm)	–	+	+ + +
Diode (810 nm)	–	–	+ +

XAN: xanthophyll
HEM: hemoglobin
MEL: melanin
Adapted with permission from Bloom S, Brucker A. *Laser Surgery of the Posterior Segment.* Philadelphia, Pa: Lippincott-Raven; 1997: 7.

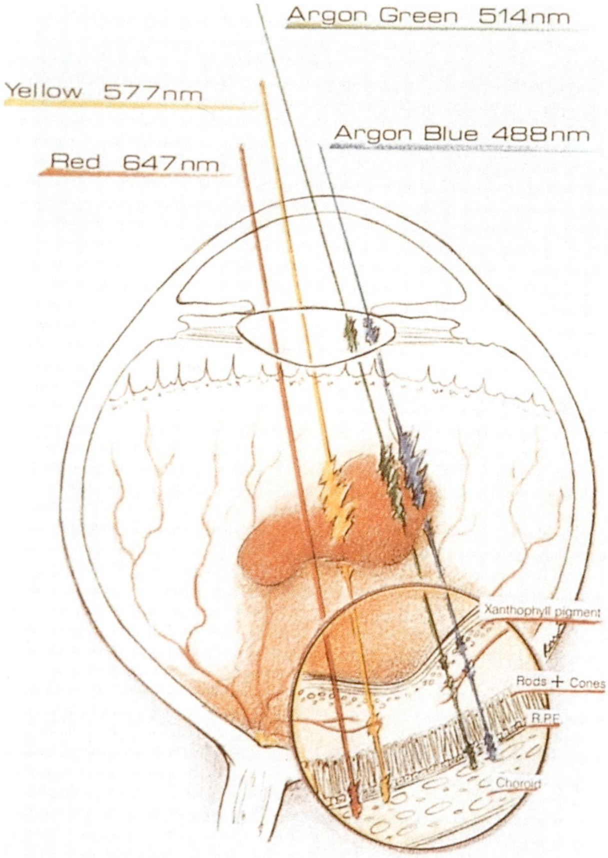

Fig. 25-2. Absorption characteristics of the major ocular pigments. Adapted with permission from Bloom S, Brucker A. *Laser Surgery of the Posterior Segment.* Philadelphia, Pa: Lippincott-Raven; 1997: Figure 1-4.

Because of the focusing power of the lens and cornea of the eye, energy transmitted to the retina can intensify by a factor of 10,000.[2] The use of optical sighting devices, such as binoculars or rangefinders, further increases the amount of laser energy delivered to the retina. Absorption of laser energy inside the eye depends on pigmentation. Pigments within the retina near the fovea (xanthophyll) and within blood vessels throughout the retina (hemoglobin) readily absorb laser energy (Table 25-2 and Figure 25-2). However, most absorption of laser energy occurs in the RPE. This layer of cells contains melanin, which readily absorbs laser energy. Laser energy absorbed in the RPE usually causes injury to the adjacent retina and choroid.

Depending on the laser intensity and wavelength, exposure to laser light may have temporary or permanent effects. With subthreshold laser emissions in the visible spectrum, most individuals experience glare and dazzle resulting from the saturation of the photoreceptors with light. This effect is similar to looking into the flash of a camera. Vision usually returns to baseline within several minutes. Nevertheless, during this refractory time, an exposed individual is visually handicapped. Tasks like firing a weapon, flying an aircraft, or driving a vehicle are severely hampered. Even minor tasks like map reading are affected. Laser emissions intense enough to cause ocular injury are known as threshold emissions. Threshold emissions in the visible spectrum usually cause glare and dazzle along with ocular injury.

SYMPTOMS

Individuals with ocular laser injuries experience a variety of symptoms depending on the type of laser and the location of the injury within the eye. Most individuals exposed to laser emissions in the visible spectrum present with complaints of glare or dazzle. Individuals with laser burns involving the cornea may complain of decreased visual acuity, pain, and tearing. Individuals with laser injuries involving the retina may complain of decreased visual acuity, blind spots (scotomas), or both in the visual field. Loss of contrast sensitivity and color vision may be presenting complaints. Lesions near or directly involving the fovea may result in metamorphopsia (distortion of straight lines) along with decreased visual acuity. Individuals who experience hemorrhage in the eye from a laser lesion may complain of floaters or a red discoloration to their vision. It is important to note that an individual presenting with laser burns to the peripheral retina may be asymptomatic.

DIAGNOSTIC MODALITIES

History

All suspected laser injury evaluations begin with a thorough history. In addition to aiding subsequent evaluation and treatment, the questions posed by the examiner are helpful for determining the possible threat laser wavelengths. These data are helpful when selecting appropriate laser protection to prevent subsequent injury. The following list of questions, developed by the US Army Medical Research Detachment of the Walter Reed Army Institute of Research, should be included in the history of an individual with a suspected laser injury:

- What were you doing at the time of the incident?
- How long did the incident last?
- Can you describe the color of the light?
- Was the light continuous or interrupted?
- Was there an after-image?
- Did the incident impact the mission?
- Has there been any pain associated with the light?
- Did you rub your eyes?

Physical Examination

The physical examination begins with assessment of the patient's visual acuity. If available, Amsler grid testing is done to check for metamorphopsia and scotomas (Figure 25-3). The Amsler grid test is administered one eye at a time at the patient's normal reading distance. If reading spectacles are worn by the patient, they should be worn during the test.

Testing for color vision and contrast sensitivity should be documented. Most permanent laser injuries involving the retina have a decrement in one or both of these parameters. Color vision testing is done with each eye separately, at the patient's nor-

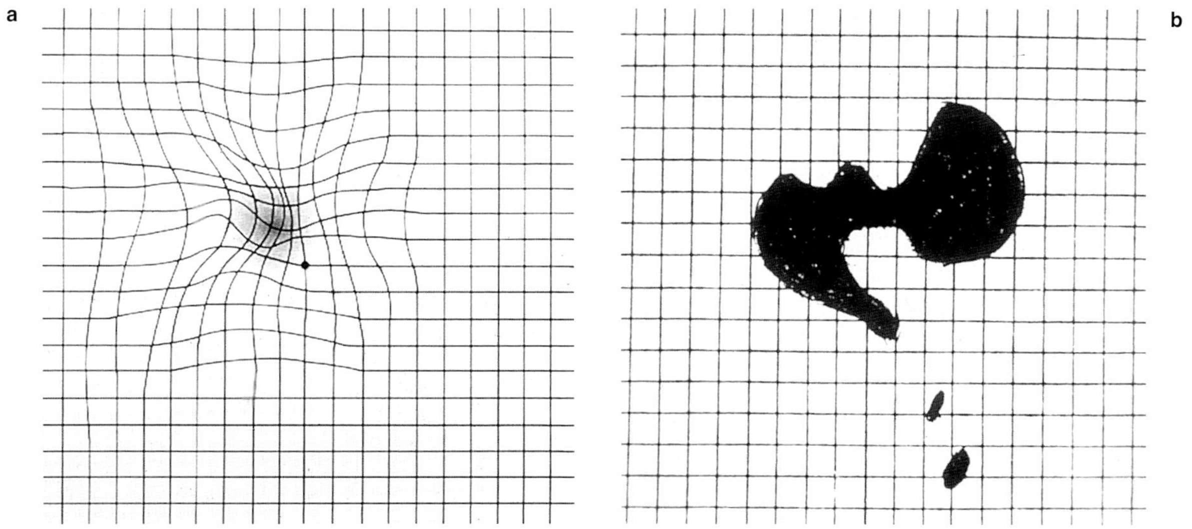

Fig. 25-3. (**a**) Metamorphopsia and relative scotoma on Amsler grid after laser injury to the retina. Test one eye at a time with the Amsler grid held 14 in. away. If the patient routinely wears spectacles, they should be worn for this test. (**b**) Absolute scotoma on the Amsler grid following a laser injury to the retina. Such a finding is suggestive of severe laser injury to the macula. The patient should be referred to an ophthalmologist for further evaluation. Photograph (a): Reproduced from Retina Research Fund. *For My Patient: Macular Degeneration*. San Francisco, Calif: Retina Research Fund; 1997; 18. Photograph (b): Courtesy of Bruce Stuck, US Army Medical Research Detachment, Walter Reed Army Institute of Research, Washington, DC.

mal reading distance and with spectacle correction, if needed. Pseudoisochromatic color plate (PIP) testing may be used to screen for color deficits. Detailed color tests such as the Farnsworth panel D-15 and the Farnsworth-Munsell 100 hue test are more sensitive for detecting color deficits but are not likely to be available in a combat environment. Contrast sensitivity testing requires the patient to look at a series of gratings at a fixed distance. The lowest amount of contrast to see the grating is known as the contrast threshold, and it is recorded for the various-sized gratings for each eye. Unfortunately, this test requires special equipment that may not be available in tactical environments.

The external adnexa and periorbital skin should be inspected. Swelling and erythema are findings consistent with possible carbon dioxide (10,600 nm) laser exposure. Attention is then directed inside the eye. Clouding and opacities of the cornea and lens are consistent with possible ultraviolet or far-infrared laser injury (Figure 25-4). Perforation of the cornea may be noted in high-energy exposures.

Injuries involving the posterior segment usually result from visible and near-infrared wavelengths. Laser injury to the retina can cause vitreous hemorrhage. In a combat environment, however, more common causes of vitreous hemorrhage (eg, blunt

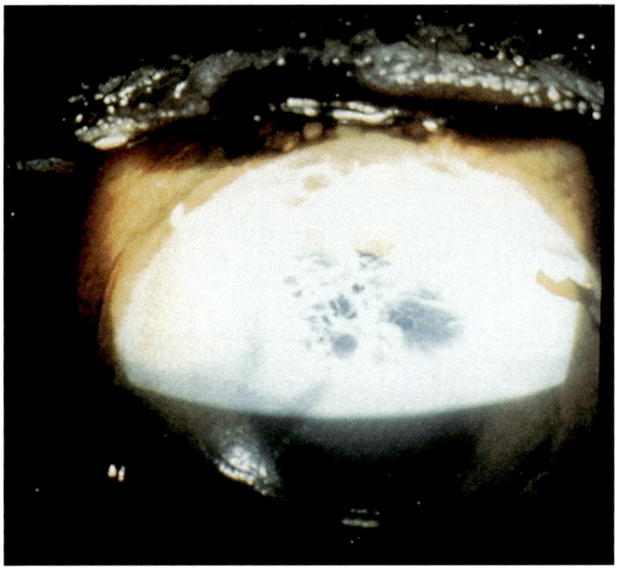

Fig. 25-4. Corneal opacification after an ocular injury with a high-energy infrared laser (laser operating parameters unknown). Acute corneal injuries without perforation should be treated with topical antibiotics. A pressure patch may be used to help make the patient more comfortable. Reproduced from Headquarters, Department of the Army. *Prevention and Medical Management of Laser Injuries.* Washington, DC: DA; 8 Aug 1990: Figure 6. Field Manual 8-50.

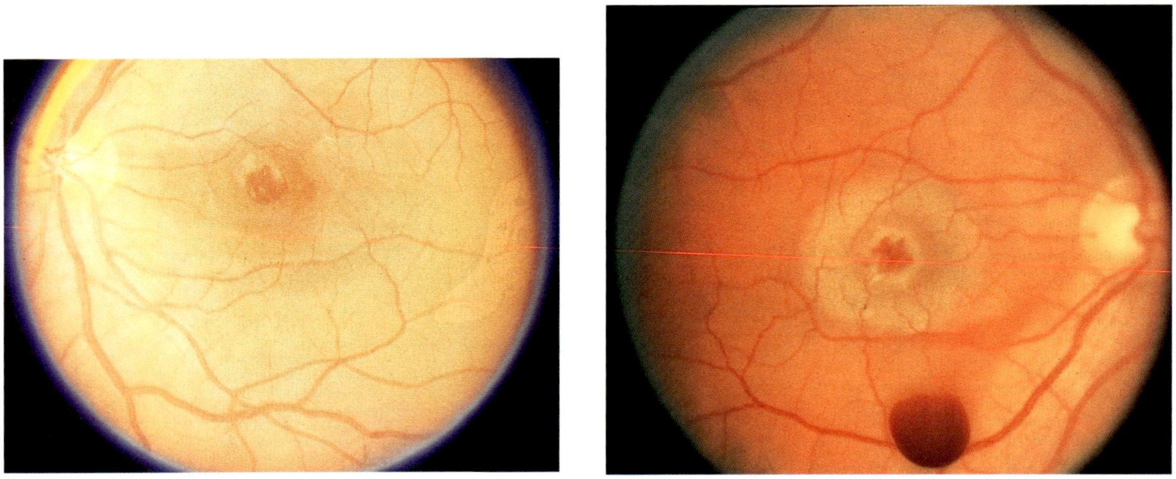

Fig. 25-5. (**a**) A full-thickness retinal hole after exposure to a neodymium:yttrium-aluminum-garnet (Nd:YAG) laser (1,064 nm) with pulse energy 150 mJ, frequency 10 Hz, and duration 10 nanoseconds. Some macular holes may be surgically closed with improvement of vision. (**b**) The retinal photograph shows preretinal hemorrhage, intraretinal hemorrhage, and retinal edema after exposure to an Nd:YAG laser. Photographs: Courtesy of Allen Thach, MD, Phoenix, Ariz.

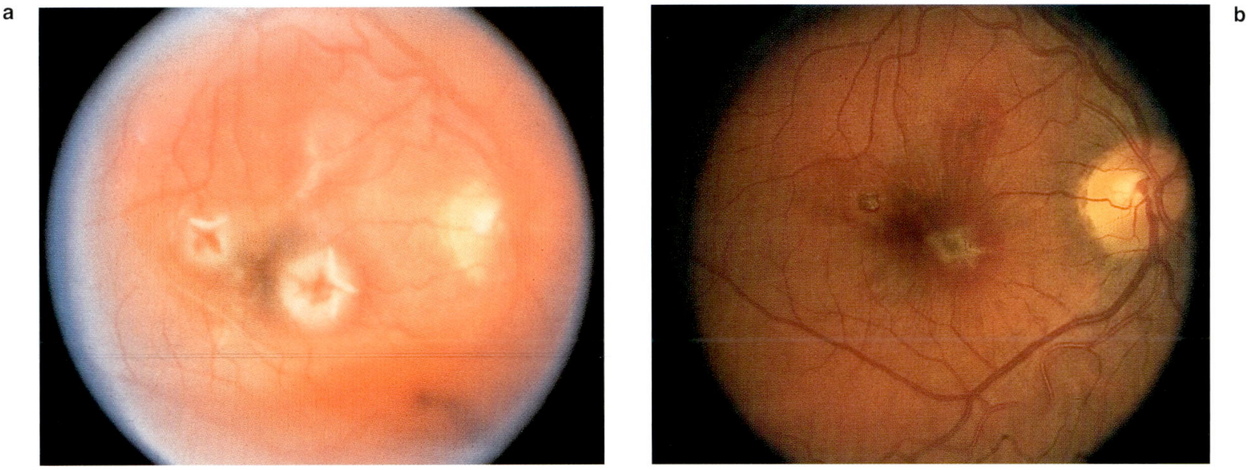

Fig. 25-6. (**a**) A retinal photograph made after the patient received multiple acute retinal burns from a Q-switched neodymium:yttrium-aluminum-garnet (Nd:YAG) laser (1,064 nm) rangefinder. (**b**) Several weeks after the laser injury, the same individual's retina was photographed again. Retinal striae and subretinal hemorrhage are present. Visual acuity is 20/200 with eccentric fixation. Photographs: Courtesy of Bruce Stuck, US Army Medical Research Detachment, Walter Reed Army Institute of Research, Washington, DC.

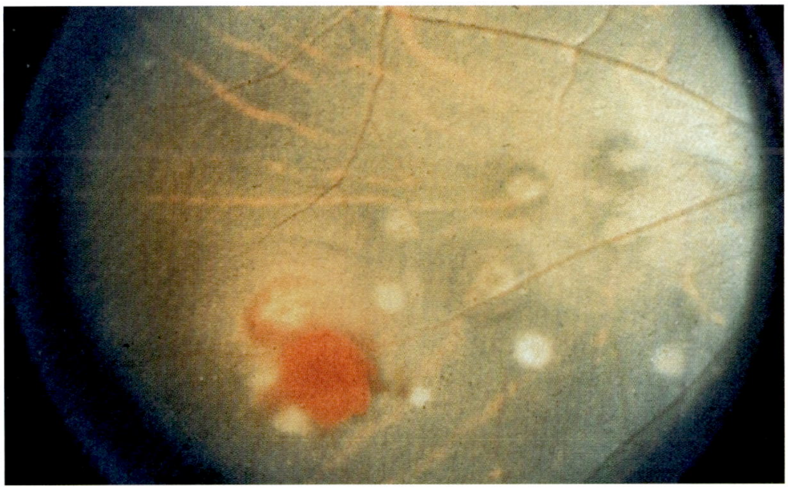

Fig. 25-7. Creamy colored retinal pigment epithelium changes after acute retina injury. Note the presence of preretinal hemorrhage. Reproduced from Headquarters, Department of the Army. *Prevention and Medical Management of Laser Injuries.* Washington, DC: DA; 8 Aug 1990: Figure 7. Field Manual 8-50.

trauma, penetrating trauma, retained intraocular foreign body) should be ruled out. If the visual axis is clear, the retina is inspected. The spectrum of retinal findings from a threshold laser exposure includes edema, necrosis, full-thickness holes, and retinal detachment (Figures 25-5 and 25-6). Hemorrhage may accompany retinal injuries and localize in front of the retina (preretinal), in the retina (intraretinal), under the retina (subretinal), or within the vitreous cavity. Preretinal fibrosis and retinal striae may present weeks to months after severe laser retinal injuries.[7]

The RPE in acute retinal injuries appears cream colored or white (Figure 25-7). Within a few weeks, these areas manifest varying degrees of pigment hyperplasia and atrophy.

TREATMENT

Laser injuries involving the external adnexa should be treated similarly to thermal burns from other sources. Topical antibiotics should be applied to the exposed area. Ophthalmic antibiotic ointment preparations are used to prevent toxic damage to the eye that may result from the use of nonophthalmic preparations.

Anterior Segment

Nonpenetrating injuries involving the cornea are treated similarly to corneal abrasions. Topical ophthalmic antibiotic preparations should be applied directly to the globe. If the individual has severe discomfort from corneal injury, a pressure patch can be placed over the affected eye to prevent eyelid movement. This patch is similar to that applied for a corneal abrasion. Patching is contraindicated in wearers of soft contact lenses. If both eyes are affected, the more severely affected eye should be patched. Corneal injuries should be seen daily until the epithelium has healed. Perforating laser injuries involving the cornea are treated similarly to perforating injuries from other sources. A Fox shield is placed over the eye, and systemic antibiotics are instituted to cover Gram-negative and Gram-positive organisms. Analgesics and antiemetics are used as needed. *No drops or ointment of any kind are placed on an eye with a suspected perforating injury.*

Posterior Segment

Treatments for laser injuries to the posterior segment of the eye are limited. In the absence of a retinal detachment, vitreous hemorrhages are initially treated with bed rest and at least 30° elevation of the head. Dense vitreous hemorrhages may require ultrasound evaluation to rule out a retinal detachment. The fundus should be examined frequently as the hemorrhage clears, to rule out underlying retinal holes or retinal detachment. If these are found, the patient should be immediately referred to an ophthalmologist for further treatment. Bilateral vitreous hemorrhages that obscure the visual axis require evaluation by an ophthalmologist for consideration of pars plana vitrectomy.

Retinal tears and retinal detachments resulting from laser injuries require urgent evacuation to an ophthalmologist for further care. Patients with retinal detachments should refrain from reading and remain sedentary to prevent extension of the retinal detachment. Individuals with macular holes from laser exposure should be referred to an ophthalmologist for evaluation. Some of these patients may benefit from pars plana vitrectomy with air–fluid exchange to close the edges of the macular hole and possibly improve vision.[8]

Individuals with subretinal hemorrhage under the fovea should be evaluated by an ophthalmologist as soon as possible. Early evacuation of subretinal hemorrhage with pars plana vitrectomy may limit subsequent damage to retinal photoreceptors and, in some cases, may improve visual prognosis.[9] Research is ongoing in this area.

To date, there are no proven medical interventions for the treatment of laser injuries involving the retina. The use of intravenous steroids in the acute setting to limit subsequent epiretinal and subretinal fibrosis is controversial and unproven to date. Intravitreal injection of tissue thromboplastin activator (TPA) has been successful in removing subfoveal blood.[10]

PREVENTION

Because treatment options are limited for individuals with laser injuries, prevention is extremely important. In an environment where laser use is suspected, individuals should be instructed to refrain from looking directly at bright lights. The use of optical sighting devices such as binoculars and rangefinders should be limited, as these devices increase any laser energy delivered to the eye. If available, all personnel should wear laser eye protection at all times (Figure 25-8). The laser eye protection must correspond to the threat wavelength to be effective. In many cases, simple measures such as taking cover or setting up a smoke screen can prevent harmful laser exposure.[2] The use of indirect viewing methods for target acquisition and surveillance can prevent laser injuries, as well.

It is also important to avoid laser injury from friendly laser sources. Rangefinders and target designators should not be pointed directly at personnel, and individuals using these lasers should avoid looking at the output end.

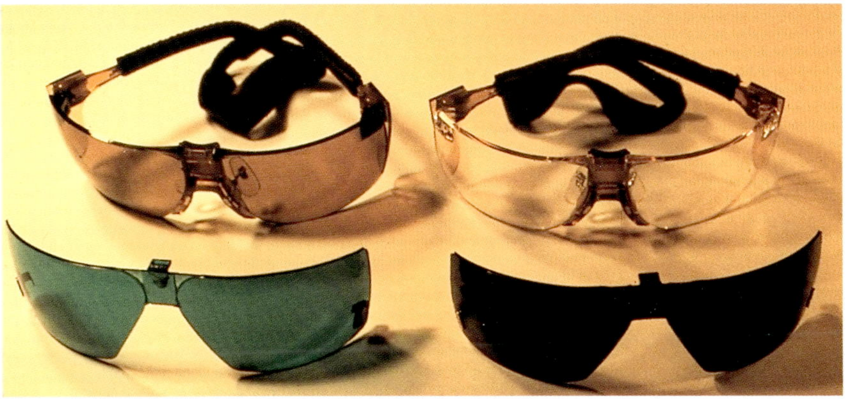

Fig. 25-8. Examples of ballistic laser eye protection currently in US Army inventory.

SUMMARY

Increasing military applications of lasers will lead to a concomitant increase in ocular laser exposure and ocular laser injuries. Laser exposure of the unprotected eye may result in injury to the eyelids, cornea, lens, retina, and choroid. Hemorrhage into the vitreous cavity may also be encountered if adjacent ocular structures bleed. Patients with prolonged visual loss or intraocular hemorrhage after possible laser exposure should be referred to an ophthalmologist for further care. Conversely, personnel exposed to laser emissions with mild or no ocular injury should be returned to duty as soon as possible to minimize secondary gain and limit the potential psychological impact on fellow personnel. Proper identification and treatment of laser injuries by medical personnel will allow friendly forces to sustain the fighting strength.

REFERENCES

1. Hudson S. Eye injuries from laser exposure: A review. *Aviat Space Environ Med.* 1998;69:519–524.

2. Headquarters, Department of the Army. *Prevention and Medical Management of Laser Injuries.* Washington, DC: DA; 8 Aug 1990. Field Manual 8-50.

3. Mainster M. Pointers on laser pointers. *Ophthalmology.* 1997;104:1213–1214.

4. Zamir E, Kaiserman I, Chowers I. Laser pointer maculopathy. *Am J Ophthalmol.* 1999;127:728–729.

5. Stuck B, Zwick H, Molchany J, Lund D, Gagliano D. Accidental human laser retinal injuries from military laser systems. *SPIE: The International Society of Optical Engineering.* 1996;2674:7–20.

6. Bloom S, Brucker A. *Laser Surgery of the Posterior Segment.* Philadelphia, Pa: Lippincott-Raven; 1997: 3–36.

7. Kearney J, Cohen H, Stuck B, Rudd P, Beresky D, Wertz F. Laser injury to multiple retinal foci. *Lasers Surg Med.* 1987;7:499–502.

8. Custis P, Gagliano D, Zwick H, Schuschereba S, Regillo C. Macular hole surgery following accidental laser injury with a range finder. *SPIE: The International Society of Optical Engineering.* 1996;2674:166–174.

9. Toth C, Morse L, Hjelmeland L, Landers M. Fibrin directs early retinal damage after experimental subretinal hemorrhage. *Arch Ophthalmol.* 1991;109:723–729.

10. Coll G, Sparrow J, Marinovic A, Chang S. Effect of intravitreal tissue plasminogen activator on experimental subretinal hemorrhage. *Retina.* 1995;15:319–326.

Chapter 26

THE DEVELOPMENT OF EYE ARMOR FOR THE AMERICAN INFANTRYMAN

FRANCIS G. LA PIANA, MD, FACS*; AND THOMAS P. WARD, MD†

This chapter is a modified reprint of La Piana FG, Ward TP. The development of eye armor for the American infantryman. *Ophthalmology Clinics of North America*. 1999;12(3):421–434. Reproduced with permission from Harcourt Health Sciences.

*Colonel, US Army (Ret); Ophthalmology Residency Program Director, Department of Ophthalmology, The Washington Hospital Center, Washington, DC 20010, and Professor of Surgery, Uniformed Services University of the Health Sciences, 4301 Jones Bridge Road, Bethesda, Maryland, 20814-4799; formerly, Consultant in Ophthalmology to The Surgeon General, US Army, and Ophthalmology Residency Program Director, Ophthalmology Service, Walter Reed Army Medical Center, Washington, DC

†Colonel, Medical Corps, US Army; Ophthalmology Residency Program Director, Ophthalmology Service, Walter Reed Army Medical Center, Washington, DC 20307-5001; Associate Professor of Surgery, Uniformed Services University of the Health Sciences, 4301 Jones Bridge Road, Bethesda, Maryland 20814-4799

"If protection of the eyes of combat soldiers were a simple affair, that protection would have been provided long ago."

—J. Fair, 1952[1]

INTRODUCTION

Attempts to protect the soldier's body in war have been made at least since the fifth millennium BC.[2] Although many energetic and creative individuals have attempted to develop eye armor, the great majority of emmetropic American infantrymen, the soldiers most at risk, continue to enter combat with their eyes as exposed to the hazards of war as were the eyes of the first bellicose hominid. The following is an account of the development of eye protection for the American infantry, a twenty-year effort which culminated in the production and distribution of such eye armor for the emmetrope and ametrope, protective against the small missile and blunt-force threat, and against some of the eye-threatening laser wavelengths. This article will be concerned primarily with the protection of the eyes of infantrymen, the soldiers who suffer by far the preponderance of injuries in war and who are "the most valued component of the military force."[3]

It is necessary to define *eye armor* as the term is used in this report because the eye is vulnerable to many threats, but protection against only some of them is necessary and possible. The major threat to the eye of the infantryman in combat is the small missile, as has been true since World War I.[4] *Eye armor* is defined primarily, though not exclusively, as that component of personal body armor that can protect the eyes of the infantryman from such a threat.

EYE INJURIES IN WAR

Injuries to the eye and its adnexal structures are of increasing significance in war. The incidence of eye injuries sustained by our forces has increased 18-fold since the US Civil War, reaching 9% in the Vietnam War (see Table 26-1). Conflicts since Vietnam have continued to demonstrate the increasing

TABLE 26-1

OCULAR WAR INJURIES AS A PERCENTAGE OF TOTAL WAR INJURIES

War	Year(s)	Percentage	Soldiers Involved
Crimean War	1854–1856	0.65	British
		1.75	French
US Civil War	1861–1865	0.5	American
Franco–Prussian War	1870–1871	0.86	Prussian
		0.81	French
Russo–Japanese War	1904–1905	2	Russian
		2.22	Japanese
World War I	1914–1918	2	American
World War II	1939–1945	2	American
Korean War	1950–1953	2.8	American
6-Day War	1967	5.6	Israeli
Yom Kippur War	1973	6.7	Israeli
Vietnam War	1962–1974	9	American
Lebanon War	1982	6.8	Israeli
Desert Storm	1991	13	American

Data from Belkin M, Treister G, Dotan S. Eye injuries and ocular protection in the Lebanon War, 1982. *Isr J Med Sci* 1984;20:333-338. Heier JS, Enzenauer RW, Wintermeyer SF, Delaney M, La Piana FG. Ocular injuries and diseases at a combat support hospital in support of Operations Desert Storm and Desert Shield. *Arch Ophthalmol* 1993;111:795-798. Wong TY, Seet MB, Ang CL. Eye Injuries in twentieth century warfare: A historical perspective. *Surv Ophthalmol* 1997;41:433-459.

frequency of ocular injuries on the battlefield. Data derived from experience in highly mobile armored combat (Yom Kipper War, 1973) show that 6.7% of all combat injuries were isolated ocular injuries. This compares to figures of 2.0% in WW II and 2.8% in Korea. In the Yom Kipper War 70% of the eye casualties were among tank crews and armored infantry, whereas only 44% of the total war casualties served in the armored corps.[5] Ocular injuries accounted for 13% of the patient volume at a major combat support hospital during the ground phase of the recent Gulf War.[6] Making these figures even more ominous is the finding that 20% to 50% of ocular injuries are penetrating or perforation globe injuries and up to 28% are bilateral (see Fig. 26-1).[7,8] Eye injuries are a common occurrence on the modern battlefield.

Not only are ocular injuries common in combat they are also devastating. A soldier who sustained a penetrating wound of the globe in combat in Vietnam had a 50% of losing the eye no matter how prompt and expert the care.[6] This figure should be compared with the dramatic decrease in the percentage of wounded dying from their wounds (from 14.1% in the US Civil War to 4.5% in World War II, 2.5% in the Korean War and 2.6% in the Vietnam War).[3,9] Only 25% of the Vietnam eye casualties could return to active duty, while 83% of all surviving wounded could do so.[10,11] The Wound Data and Munitions Effectiveness in Vietnam (WDMEV) team determined that 7.4% of interviewed casualties reported "eye disability" after wounding.[12] Of these eye casualties, 79% were partially disabled and 21% completely disabled (at least temporarily).

The cost to our society of eye injuries (both combat-related and during peacetime) is significant, both monetarily and medically. For example, a 20-year-old E-4 (corporal) who loses one eye in the line of duty will receive at least $189,000 over his expected lifetime, and an O-5 (lieutenant colonel) with 18 years of service will receive at least $477,000.[13] Fortunately the great majority of these accidents can be prevented.[14] This fact has resulted in the general requirement of the American National Standards Institute (ANSI) Z-87.1-1979 standard that "...eye protection shall be required in hazardous environments where there is a reasonable probability that injuries can be prevented by the use of such protection."[15] It would seem appropriate that the same concern about eye injuries in the civilian workplace should exist for the soldier in combat.

Despite the obvious concern for ocular injuries on the battlefield, it must not be forgotten that soldiers are at risk for eye trauma even during peacetime. Tarabishy in 1983 reported that 40% (75 of 157) of injuries sustained by soldiers from four types of automatic weapons over a six-year period in peacetime were to the eye.[16] McMarlin and Connelly reported that 5% of injuries seen in a Army field hospital during a military training exercise were to the eyes.[17]

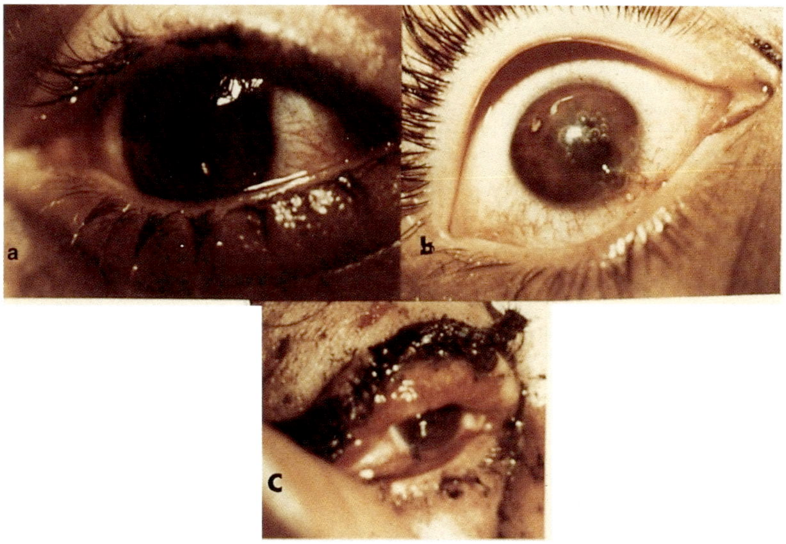

Fig. 26-1. Vietnam eye injuries. (**a**) Fragment (probably aluminum) on anterior lens capsule. (**b**) Fragment of rock on iris, air bubbles in anterior chamber, and iris prolapse through wound of entry. (**c**) Penetrating wound of globe from "mud blast" injury. Photograph: Courtesy of Richard M. Leavitt, MD.

ELEMENTS IN EYE ARMOR DEVELOPMENT

The development of eye armor was begun during World War I but did not reach fruition until just prior to the Gulf War, in large part because of the complexity of the task. Five elements must be considered: 1) the tasks of the infantryman; 2) the ocular threats; 3) the mind-sets of those to be protected and of those in positions of leadership; 4) the materials available to provide protection; and 5) available funds to support the costs of development, testing, modification, provision, maintenance, and replacement of eye armor.

The missions of an infantryman in combat can be reduced to firing his weapon or weapons, moving, identifying friend or foe, estimating range, communicating, and surviving. His eyes are his primary fire control mechanism and are important in maneuvering (as he is often the hunted as well as the hunter), and in communicating (a significant amount of which is done primarily with the eyes). The sine qua non for eye armor for the infantryman is that it must not only protect his eyes against several threats but must neither interfere with his ability to accomplish his missions nor with his chances of surviving them unharmed. Because the infantryman trains and fights under the most rugged conditions, equipment provided him must be simple and very rugged. It must also be compatible with his equipment (eg, helmet and weapon). Eye protection suitable for a pilot who fights seated and protected by his aircraft canopy may not serve for the infantryman who often must run, jump, and hit the ground hard and often. The detection of movement in the periphery of his visual field is of such great importance to the infantryman, correlating directly with his chances of survival, that he will reject any eye armor that interferes with his peripheral vision. This fact has been appreciated for at least 70 years – "...the fighting man must keep his whole visual acuteness, or at least have it but slightly modified by the protecting apparatus placed before the cornea; the visual field must not be manifestly narrowed."[4]

In the 20th century, body armor (except for the helmet) has been worn mostly by those on the defensive.[18] If eyes are unprotected, soldiers on the defensive suffer more eye injuries than do those on the offensive.[19] Since the head and neck region of the soldier are the "locus of the major sensory equipment in the human ... continuous appraisal of his situation vis-a-vis the enemy forces the foot-soldier to expose his head more often than any other part of his body."[3] Even taking this into account, an infantryman's eyes are injured at a frequency at least ten times higher than might be expected based on target size alone.[20] Eye injuries, furthermore, are always important; a small corneal abrasion can completely incapacitate a soldier in combat and penetrating injuries of the globe require medical evacuation.

In wartime, the major ocular threat is from fragments generated by detonating munitions (see Table 26-2), and we must expect that laser weapons will also be employed against our soldiers' eyes in any future conflicts. Eye-hazardous laser range finders and target designators are widely deployed now. The problem of protecting the eye against even a few wavelengths in such a way as not to impair the soldier's performance is a monumental task. The advent of the frequency-agile laser on the battlefield will only increase the problem.[21] Other significant immediate or potential threats to the eye are fragments from improved conventional munitions, flechettes (dart-like missiles released from artillery projectiles), ultraviolet light, flash from nuclear weapon detonation, sunlight, wind, dust, microwaves, particle beams, blast, heat, and poison gases. There is no way to protect against all of the threats all of the time, but it is now possible to protect against the small missile, the ultraviolet light, and blunt-force threats very well, and also against some of the eye-hazardous laser wavelengths. An analysis of ocular injuries to American servicemen in Vietnam estimated that the wearing of 2-mm poly-

TABLE 26-2

CAUSES OF NONFATAL WOUNDS

Agent	World War II (%)	Korean War (%)	Vietnam War (%)
Bullets	19.7	27	30
Fragments*	66.1	65.5	68
Other	14.2	7.5	2

*Fragments generated from explosive projectile shells, rockets and bombs, grenades, booby traps, land mines, and other munitions

Data from Reister FA. *Battle Casualties and Medical Statistics: US Army Experience in the Korean War.* Washington, The Surgeon General, Department of the Army, 1973, pp 48, 51. *Evaluation of Wound Data and Munitions Effectiveness in Vietnam.* US Departments of the Army, Navy and Air Force, Washington, 1970 (Vol 1), p D-51.

carbonate eye protection would have prevented fully 39% of all ocular injuries.[13]

The element in eye armor development that has been least appreciated is the mind-sets of both those who need protection and those who lead the Army. The complexity of the objective has frequently been ignored and the infantryman has often been regarded as just another industrial worker needing eye protection. In fact, the infantryman is usually young, emmetropic, unsophisticated, skeptical, denial-practicing, and body-image-conscious, with a variety of highly dangerous tasks to perform (most of which require unimpeded vision) and burdened already with much personnel equipment. He tends to regard ametropia for what it is, an eye abnormality. He is likely to reject eye protection that resembles ordinary spectacles, both because of the implications of wearing it and the interference with his field of vision produced by the spectacle frame. Only three of the 92 American soldiers treated for ocular complaints at one combat support hospital in the Gulf War were wearing their eye protection at the time.[6] It is important, therefore, not only to provide the infantryman with eye protection that provides a nearly unimpeded field of vision, but also to term it "eye armor" rather than "goggles" or "spectacles."

The mind-sets of those in senior positions are also of critical importance. Senior officers have often regarded eye injuries as being of little overall consequence and not preventable. The threat of injury to the infantryman's eyes has been in part consciously and in part unconsciously denied because to recognize it would saddle the Army with a major additional task that in the past could not be accomplished. Certain groups of combatants have, however, been judged to need eye protection (eg, aviators, tankers), reflecting the elitist division between cavalry and infantry known since antiquity. Sometimes it is the developers of eye armor who have failed to involve the user of the armor in its planning and development.[22]

Materials available for the production of soldier-acceptable eye armor have been readily available for only a relatively short period of time. Eye armor development was retarded by the belief that the generation of secondary missiles by shattered glass lenses made their use for the protection of emmetropes unwise. The plastic lens, CR-39, was easily scratched, and neither glass nor plastic could be formed in a configuration that would protect the temporal potion of the glove without obstructing peripheral vision. The development of injection-moldable optical-grade polycarbonate and scratch-resistant coatings has obviated all of these problems.

Fortunately for the US soldier, Army leadership has made available the monies required for the development, testing, and initial procurement of eye armor. Polycarbonate is intrinsically inexpensive and the cost to the US taxpayer for the infantryman's eye protection will be far less than the cost of his boots. The elements that have been of greatest importance in the successful development of eye armor are the availability of injection-moldable polycarbonate, the decision of the Infantry School to make eye armor a requirement for the infantryman, and the fear of laser weapons.

THE HISTORY OF EYE ARMOR DEVELOPMENT IN AMERICA

Pre-Colombian Period to World War I

The Incan and Aztec warriors of pre-Colombian America wore quilted cotton jackets and padded helmets that did not incorporate eye protection.[23] The Colonial period saw the gradual abandonment of the metal body armor that the earliest settlers had brought with them from Europe because it was "...too burdensome for the long treks and rapid movements of woodland warfare"[24] despite its effectiveness against Indian arrows.[23] "Soft" armor of buckram (a stiff armor of cotton or linen and silk covered with leather), fustian (a type of cotton or linen fabric), or canvas was also used by the colonists but was discarded because it was hot and uncomfortable.[25] Though eye protection for the helmet wearer was attempted in the 15th century by means of "metal-rimmed protective lenses of glass ... hinged to drop over the eyes,"[26] such eye protection was not present on helmets worn in the New World. Some of the Spanish infantrymen who accompanied DeSoto wore a type of helmet called a salade or sallet, some of which bore a hinged visor, and others themselves covered the face, in which case vision was provided for by means of a slot (ocularium).[24] These partial eye protective devices were abandoned in part because the limitation of visual field they produced prevented the effective handling of pistols. Dupuy and Dupuy comment that "by 1650, European armor, although effective against Indian projectiles, had been largely abandoned ... and was replaced by lighter and less cumbersome protective garb of cloth and leather."[27]

In the American Revolutionary War and the War of 1812, the cavalry continued to wear leather helmets and a few combat engineers wore steel breastplates.[18,23] Breastplates were also worn in the American Civil War by combatants of both sides, although they were never formally authorized.[28] The Indian and Spanish-American Wars were fought apparently without body armor of any kind, though "push-shields" were considered for use in the latter.[18] The American Indians, however, "...used buffalo-hide shields and breastplates of bone tubes strung together, both of which were a good defense against arrows and lances, and were even able to stop a half-spent bullet."[23] By the onset of World War I, the use of body armor was regarded as "dead as Queen Anne."[25]

World War I and the Interwar Period (1914–1940)

Although all belligerent nations embarked on World War I providing little if any body armor for their infantrymen, almost all (including the United States) made efforts during that war to develop and distribute armor, including eye armor. The head was protected first, largely through the efforts of General Adrian of the French army, but ophthalmologists soon attempted to stimulate and assist in efforts "...to try and realize for the eye sockets what has been obtained for the skull."[4,18] Unfortunately, no acceptable eye armor could be developed and development of eye armor for the infantryman practically stopped at war's end.

The major impetus for the interest in the development of body armor early in World War I was the employment by all armies of munitions generating a myriad of small fragments upon detonation, the extensive use of the machine gun, and the rapid replacement of a war of maneuver with a war of position ("trench warfare"), which made many combatants especially vulnerable to small fragment injuries. The trench war became a war of artillery and over half the casualties were caused by shellfire.[29] The static war of the trenches led to a peak of 8% of injuries being eye injuries, and 10% of all patients seen in base hospitals required eye examinations and treatment.[9,30,31] Three-quarters of the casualties were due to missiles of low velocity, less than a thousand feet per second.[25] A British 1917 attempt at eye armor (see Fig. 26-2) was based upon a French automobile driver's goggle. Because of the inherent visual field limitations of these "lunettes," however, they would not have to be worn by soldiers, except when the wearer was "...under bombardment or menaced by bullets."[32]

Senior American Army ophthalmologists, such as Wilmer and Greenwood,[33] were familiar with the various types of eye armor developed by our allies and with their deficiencies. Wilmer, at the request of the Ordnance Department, had developed an eye shield of Hadfield (manganese) steel with a single horizontal stenopeic slit and a circular opening below to permit a view of the ground (see Fig. 26-2). The idea for the shield came to Wilmer from the "single slotted eye shield which is used against snow blindness by the Indians of our northwest."[18] Greenwood devised an "eye shield" with two stenopeic slits, one vertical and one horizontal, but concluded that Wilmer's shield, designed to be compatible with the standard British helmet, was superior.[30] The US Army ordered 30,000 of Wilmer's shield but they were rejected by the headquarters of the American Expeditionary Force because they were "not readily kept in position."[18] This unfortunate result mirrored the fate of all body armor (except the helmet).

Although visors of different types were tested on experimental helmets of many different designs, all visors were rejected and the helmets that became standard at the outset of World War II made no provision for eye protection. In fact, many line officers in positions of authority during this period of time

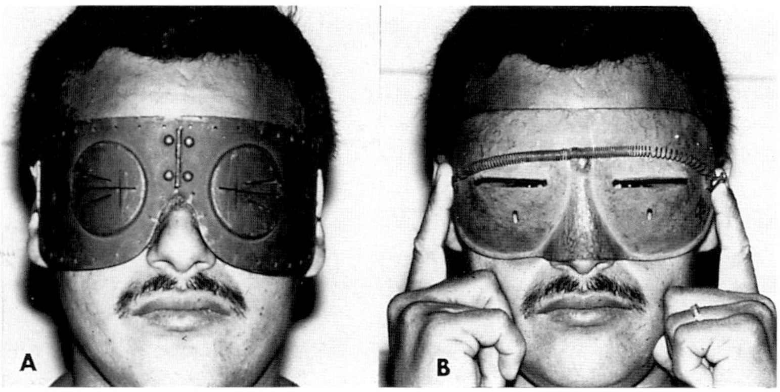

Fig. 26-2. World War I eye armor. (**a**) British, 1917. (**b**) US Wilmer-type, 1918.

believed that eye protection would "spoil the image of the soldier" who was apparently expected to be farsighted in every sense of the word (personal communication, Lowrey, 1979). Efforts did continue to improve flying goggles for the Army and Navy aviators, for "it had long been realized that the task of flying was more dependent on vision than on any other of man's senses."[34] It is interesting, though not surprising, that many of the issues dealt with by developers of better eye protection for military aviators in the 1920s and 1930s (field of vision, peripheral protection) are the same issues dealt with in the 1970s and 1980s for the infantryman.

Methacrylate (plastic) lenses (Lucite, Plexiglas) were introduced in the United States in 1937, but their softness and discoloration led to their rejection and they were not manufactured in this country after 1939.[26,35]

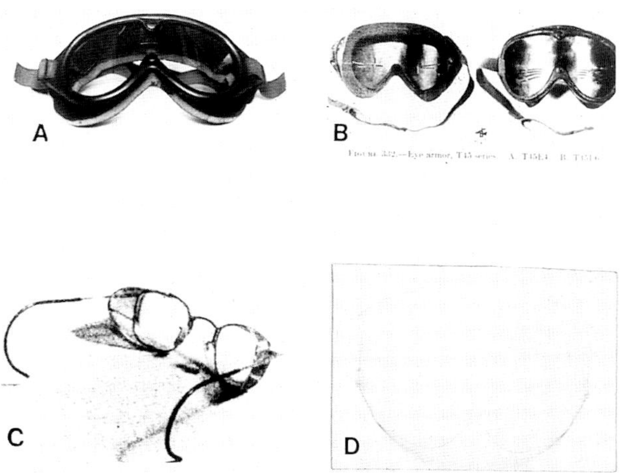

Fig. 26-3. US military eye protective devices. (**a**) World War II sun-wind-dust goggle, M1944. (**b**) World War II mine-clearance goggle, T45. (**c**) Korean War, Fair-type eye armor. (**d**) Vietnam War, polycarbonate eye shield (component of Army aviator's helmet).

World War II and the Interwar Period (1941–1949)

In contrast to the many efforts made in World War I, relatively few such efforts were made towards eye protection in World War II. Those in senior positions considered the incidence of eye injuries to be too low to necessitate eye armor development. Military planning in the pre-World War II period posited a war of movement, of maneuver, to obviate a recurrence of the static trench warfare of World War I. Body armor (except for the helmet) was believed to hinder the infantryman so much as to be ill advised.[22] In short, it was decided not to "sacrifice freedom of body movement for protection."[36] Hence, although the prevention of industrial eye injuries was well advanced, the United States entered World War II with no eye armor for its infantrymen.[37,38]

Eye injuries were again very significant.[20] As had been true in World War I, the devastating effects of miniscule fragments upon soldiers' eyes prompted attempts at eye armor development. Town[39] described a "metal eye protector," then in use by Soviet Union forces, which weighed 5 ounces and provided for vision through crossed stenopeic slits. Stieren[40] described a "metal safety and glare goggle" of aluminum (reminiscent of the British World War I eye armor in Fig. 26-2). An eyeshield of cellulose acetate was provided for members of the Chemical Corps for wear when they were in the vicinity of toxic gasses, and some soldiers employed this eyeshield as a dust protector. A sun-wind-dust goggle, M1944, bearing 1-mm cellulose acetate lenses (see Fig. 26-3) was provided to tankers and certain vehicle operators, but its size and shape made it unsuitable for use by foot soldiers. Towards the end of the war a metal eye shield, T45, was developed for engineers engaged in mine clearance (see Fig. 26-3).[22,41] It was composed of a plate of manganese steel bearing vision slits (similar to those of the World War I British eye armor in Fig. 26-2) mounted in a rubber sun-wind-dust goggle frame, and weighed 7 ounces.

United States Army Air Force aviators wore several types of eye protection and different types of sunglasses, but the restriction of visual field was a major problem.[34,42] The US Navy considered a visor for the standard M1 helmet to protect the face, but it was not fielded. Ironically, but not surprisingly, "industrial type" eye protection was provided to some soldiers performing equipment maintenance, and successful efforts were made by the US Armed Forces to protect the eyes of those working in defense industries.[43,44] The glass spectacles worn by ametropic soldiers were not case-hardened and secondary missile injuries occurred with enough frequency to stimulate a recommendation that increased protection be provided the ametrope: "Ordinary spectacles should be made of armor plate or shatter-proof glass."[20] Body armor, especially in the form of thoraco-abdominal protection, was investigated for infantry. "Flak suits" were developed for and extensively and effectively used by US Army Air Force flying personnel. Eye protection for these airmen was nonetheless suboptimal and many eye injuries occurred.[22]

The British did make efforts to develop eye protection for the infantry. Cruise,[45] who had developed a form of helmet-mounted eye armor termed the "chain mail veil" in World War I, had continued to work on such a protective device in the inter-war period. In 1940 he advocated a helmet-attached perforated visor of 22-gauge duraluminum that could, if necessary, be adjusted over spectacles. The visor "acted as a multiple stenopeic disk, and in that way vision would be improved for the people with refractive errors without their glasses."[46] The visors used by knights in the Middle Ages were also believed to correct refractive errors in a similar fashion. By 1941, three types of eye armor had been evaluated by the British military: 1) a perforated metal visor of the Cruise type; 2) slotted and round holed metal visors; and 3) methyl methacrylate and cellulose acetate plastic visors and goggles.[47] Cellulose acetate, 2 or 3 mm thick, was found superior to methyl methacrylate on impact resistance evaluation. The latter's proclivity to spall was to cost some airmen their sight during the war. The scratchability of the plastic was identified as a serious problem. Despite the efforts made to develop and field eye armor, British soldiers were provided no protection to the eye beyond cellophane anti-gas shields similar to the cellulose acetate shield provided US ground forces.

The Korean War and the Interwar Period (1950–1962)

The Korean War evolved from a war of maneuver to a war of position, and the resulting eye injuries again stimulated US Army ophthalmologists to attempt to enhance eye protection. King,[48] a US Army ophthalmologist, called for the provision of case-hardened lenses to ametropic combat arms soldiers and considered an eye shield that could be attached to the helmet. He recommended the testing of plastic lenses in front-line companies and stressed the importance of gauging the soldier's acceptance or rejection of eye armor.[49]

Freed, the inventor of the metal device described by Town,[39] attempted to interest the US Army in it without success. Fair[50] made the major eye armor development effort by advocating a "spectacle-type goggle with tempered glass lenses and side shields" (see Fig. 26-3). He noted that, "the only real problems foreseen are making the goggles acceptable to the soldier who has never before worn spectacles and providing lenses for the soldier with a significant refractive error."[50] Unfortunately for thousands of US soldiers, accomplishment of these objectives required 30 additional years. According to Stokes, "...although the eye armor that [Fair] was working on might be beneficial in decreasing eye injuries, it so impaired a soldier's peripheral vision and his ability to defend himself otherwise, that it was not practical in battle" (personal communication, Stokes, 1986). Despite the proposal to test various types of commercial safety glasses, no trials were conducted in Korea.[51]

The next significant attempt was made in 1962 by McNair, who advocated the development of a polycarbonate eye protective device for the infantryman based on the polycarbonate lenses provided to aviators (see Fig. 26-3).[52] This attempt was rejected by US Army commanders, who stated that "the line officers had enough trouble getting the foot soldier even to wear his helmet let alone to have him wear protective glasses or a shield" (personal communication, McNair, 1987). Nonetheless, in 1962, a joint effort by the Quartermaster and the Army Medical Department to develop eye armor was begun. It was to be an optically clear device suitably curved to provide maximum protection with minimum interference with soldiers' activities and include provision for optical correction. A major shortcoming of this effort was the absence of a formally approved Army statement of need for eye armor, and in fact such a "requirement document" was not generated until 1984.

Scientific studies of great relevance were conducted during this period by Stewart and Rose[53,54] and Williams[55] who, disturbingly, demonstrated that non-heat-treated glass lenses were more protective than heat-treated ones against small missiles and that, under some circumstances, eyes were probably safer uncovered than "protected" by glass lenses. Bryant[56] substantiated the greater impact resistance of plastic (allyl resin) lenses compared to tempered glass lenses. Fackler et al[57] studied wound ballistics and Davis[58] made valuable observations regarding the optical factors of plano lenses. The major development of the period, however, was the production of optical-grade polycarbonate by General Electric.[59] The marked advantage of polycarbonate over other lens materials was promptly appreciated and it has become the eye and face protective materials of choice.[60,61] Polycarbonate could withstand the impact not only of molten metal but also of a quarter-inch diameter steel ball moving at velocities of up to 500 feet/second (ft/s).[62] Such lenses of 2.47 mm thickness resisted the impact of 545 mg lead spheres and slugs with pointed heads traveling at 595 ft/s.[63]

The Vietnam War Era (1962–1969)

The overwhelming majority of emmetropic infantrymen entered combat in Vietnam without eye protection of any kind. Some drivers of large vehicles and helicopter loaders were provided the US M1944 sun-wind-dust goggle which, as had been true in World War II, provided only minimal protection from the small fragment threat because its lenses were made of 1 mm thick cellulose acetate. When struck with a fragment, this material readily disintegrated into small sharp-edged fragments (spall) which could themselves damage the eye.[64] The US Army aviator's visor was attached to the standard M1 helmet by Navy researchers in an attempt to protect the eyes of sailors serving on patrol boats in the Delta region of South Vietnam.[65] The visor was judged to be sailor-acceptable, protective, and capable of satisfactorily withstanding the deleterious effects of salt air and intense sun. Although US Army personnel were also equipped with the M1 helmet, no effort was made to evaluate the effectiveness of the helmet-mounted visor for them.

Once again the ocular threat came predominantly from small, low-velocity missiles (see Fig. 26-4). Bryant,[66] studying the lens retention of safety frames, concluded, "Polycarbonate plastic lenses exhibited a highly significant increased fracture resistance compared to industrial or dress thicknesses of tempered glass and CR-39 plastic lenses." Later reviews of wound data and foreign bodies from Vietnam led to the conclusion that the majority of foreign bodies which resulted in eye injury would have been stopped by 2-mm thick eye armor.[67–70] Thus, polycarbonate plastic lenses appeared to have a great potential for truly effective eye protection against flying missiles. Solution of the lens retention and scratch-resistance problems, among others, had to be achieved to permit a complete realization of this potential.

Modern Eye Armor Development—1969 to Present

The modern development of eye armor began by the testing of the Postoperative Eye Guard (Younger Manufacturing Company, Los Angeles, CA) by La Piana (see Fig. 26-5). Intended to protect an eye that had recently undergone cataract extraction, the protective qualities of these devices was demonstrated in demolition tests. Further testing conducted on soldiers during combat training exercises in Vietnam revealed a general dissatisfaction with the plastic ring on the back surface of the Guard (the ring was designed to hold the aphakic correction) because of its interference with their peripheral vision. Other frequently expressed complaints were of distortion in the far peripheral field (due to the cylindrical lens power in the lateral portion of the shield) and lack of firm stabilization of the shield on the face when sweating occurred (unpublished data, 1970).

An effort was made in 1971 to interest first the Army and then private industry in the development of eye armor, without success. Part of the problem was political: the failure to interest civilian industry may have been influenced by the widespread anti-military sentiment at the time. In fact, eye armor in the form now being manufactured (in-

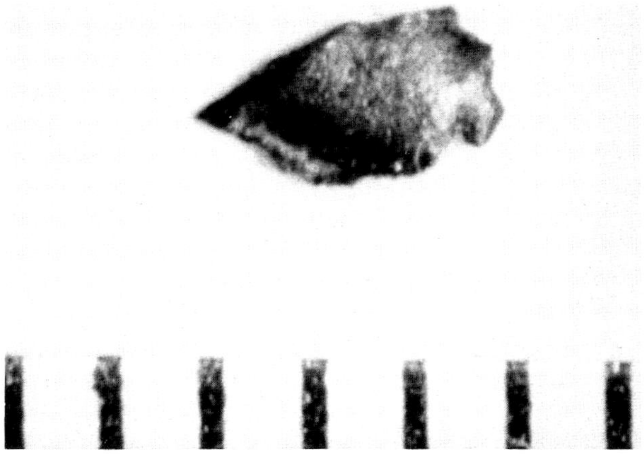

Fig. 26-4. Typical intraorbital foreign body removed in Vietnam weighing 12 mg (millimeter scale).

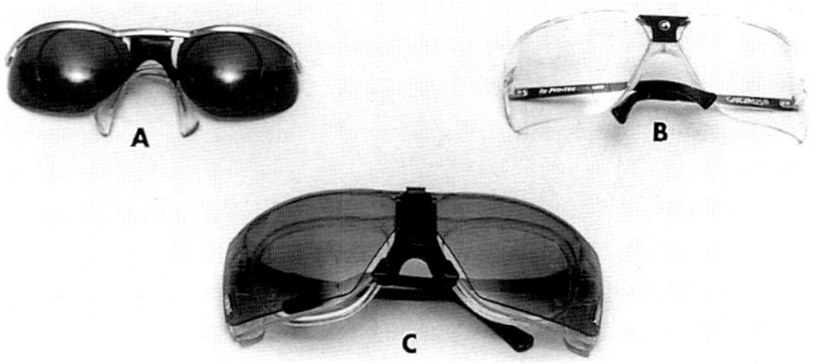

Fig. 26-5. Contemporary forms of eye armor. (**a**) Prototype eye armor-1 (PEA-1). (**b**) Prototype eye armor-2 (PEA-2). (**c**) Definitive eye armor (ballistic and laser protective spectacle [BLPS]) complete and assembled.

jection-molded polycarbonate in a toric-wrap configuration) could have been manufactured in 1971 (personal communication, LaMarre, 1987). Eye armor development was therefore in a sense another casualty of the Vietnam War, reminding us of Hirschberg's observation that "the history of medicine is part of the history of the entire civilization."[71]

Much effort has been devoted to convincing US Department of Defense (DOD) workers involved in eye armor development that the threat to the eye of the soldier in peace and in war is overwhelmingly from small missiles of 100 mg or less and that eye armor should be developed to protect against this threat (see Figs. 26-4 and 26-6). Many DOD workers were unrealistically calling for eye armor that could also protect against larger missiles, including bullets. In Desert Storm, not a single bullet injury was noted in a series of 160 American eye casualties.[72] Such unrealistic demands on the performance of eye armor only delayed the deployment of protection from the much more likely small-missile threat.

In the 1970s, studies had demonstrated the superior impact-resistance of polycarbonate but also demonstrated degradation in its strength when a scratch-resistant coating was applied.[73] This was a matter of great importance since polycarbonate must be so coated because it is easily scratched. Further studies demonstrated that polycarbonate lenses could protect the wearer from the small missile threat.[67–70] Among the findings, it was demonstrated that at 30 meters from a munitions burst, a polycarbonate eye shield could protect a soldier's eye from most (about 80%) of the fragments.

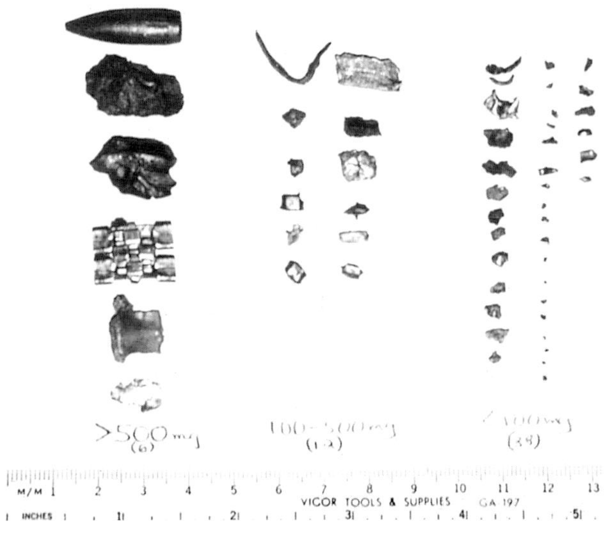

Fig. 26-6. Some of the intraocular and orbital foreign bodes removed by two military ophthalmologists in Vietnam from 1968 to 1969. Photograph: Courtesy of H. Dale Sponaugle, MD, and Robert T. McKinley, MD.

Prescription polycarbonate lenses became available in 1977 and their advantages over lenses made of glass or CR-39 were noted, including greater impact resistance, higher refractive index (making possible stronger lenses with either less curvature, thinner edges, or both), and low specific gravity (making polycarbonate prescription-bearing lenses approximately one-half the weight of an equivalent strength glass lens).[74] The increased lateral chromatic aberration of polycarbonate was a relative disadvantage, however, because patients wearing lenses greater than 2D may appreciate colored fringes along black-edged borders.[75]

A major conference on Combat Ocular Problems was held in 1980, and much attention was paid to the protection of the soldier's eye from all identified threats.[76] Partially as a result of this conference, the three following important decisions were made: 1) to link laser eye protection to missile and blunt force protection, 2) to make polycarbonate the material upon which all development efforts would center, and 3) to provide protection against the missile and blunt-force threat as soon as such became available, and not delay its provision until laser protection became available, as it was judged that the latter required much more time and effort than the former.

The need to protect the soldier's eye from laser wavelengths has concerned the US Army since the advent of this powerful and versatile directed energy source.[77] Many medium-power laser systems are being used in tactical military ground and airborne applications, which include range finding, target designation, ordnance guidance and, during periods of darkness, night vision illuminators. Viewing the collimated laser beam or the specularly reflected beam through a telescope or binoculars can increase the retinal irradiance considerably. Thus at locations where a laser might be considered safe to view by the unaided eye, it may not be safe when viewed through optical devices. Damage to the eye on the battlefield or the training ground can occur at distances of 400–4000 meters depending on the wavelength and power employed, whereas the M-16 rifle (the standard infantry weapon) is effective to only 400 meters (personal communication, Stuck, 1986). The inherent ability of polycarbonate to block ultraviolet and far infrared light (such as emitted by the CO_2 laser) added to its attractiveness. The spectral attenuation of a polycarbonate lens in the visible and near-infrared is insignificant, however, and of no value for laser protection in the retinal hazard region (400–1400 nm).[78]

A major stimulus to eye armor development was provided by the appearance on the commercial market of Gargoyles (Pro-tec, Inc., Kent, WA; see Fig. 26-5). Gargoyles are fabricated of optical-grade polycarbonate, the thickness of which varies from 2.5 mm in the optical center to 1.8 mm in the periphery, and weighs only one ounce. They are impact resistant, efficient UV absorbers, and cosmetically acceptable—a very important characteristic because "protective head gear and eyewear will be worn only if the design appeals to the intended wearer."[79,80] Gargoyles, or some variation of them, seemed to be an ideal foundation for the development of troop-acceptable eye armor. Some continued to propose the sun-wind-dust goggle fit with 4 mm thick polycarbonate, this despite the fact that the restriction of visual field caused it to be rejected by even many tank crewmen and a similar goggle was rejected by Israeli infantrymen engaged in combat.[64]

Testing of Gargoyles on US Army soldiers and Marines began in 1983. Initial results were encouraging, with high troop-acceptance. Several modifications were deemed necessary, however. The nose bridge required strengthening. The distance between the brow and lens had to be increased to minimize fogging. The integrated front had to be extended at least 8 mm posteriorly to provide full protection to the eyes of soldiers with large heads and widely spaced eyes. A polycarbonate lens cleaner was needed because soap and water often are not available in the field.

Because eye armor must protect the ametrope as well as the emmetrope, it was necessary to know the incidence and range of ametropia within the US Army. It had been stated that approximately half of the Army wore glasses,[81] but the incidence and degrees of ametropia in different types of units had not been studied adequately. Studies were initiated to determine the incidence and range of ametropia in three Army infantry divisions, the results of which are summarized in Table 26-3. The studies substantiated the impression that the incidence of ametropia is lowest in combat arms units, those units whose members are at greatest risk of eye injury in war. This information provided an additional stimulus to work for the development of troop-acceptable eye armor, for is clear that those most at risk (emmetropic combat arms unit members) had the least, and in most cases no, protection.

TABLE 26-3

INCIDENCE OF AMETROPIA IN THREE ARMY DIVISIONS

Investigator	Unit Type	Percentage
Rimm (25th Infantry Division)	Combat Arms	15–20
	Combat Support	25–30
	Combat Service Support	45–50
Bussa (82nd Airborne Division)	Combat Arms	27
	Combat Support	24
	Combat Service Support	35
Tressler (4th Infantry Division)	Combat Arms	25
	Combat Support	49
	Combat Service Support	33

The emergence of low energy lasers as a significant ocular hazard on the modern battlefield gave additional impetus towards the development of eye armor. Whereas up until recently the major threats to the infantryman's eye were ballistic in nature, now electromagnetic energy, in the form of lasers, was a significant and increasing threat. There have been a number of well documented laser injuries, usually as a result of incorrect usage of laser range finders, target designators, or other common laser devices utilized by modern armies.[82,83] Added to these accidental exposures are a number of suspected intentional laser exposures over the past two decades, usually directed towards pilots and other aircrew members.[82] There were two documented laser eye injuries during the recent Gulf War (personal communication, Brown, 2000). A number of countries are known or suspected to have developed laser devices with the direct purpose of causing either temporary or permanent eye injury; these countries include the United States, United Kingdom, and the former Soviet Union.[82] Thus modern eye armor needs to protect against both the ballistic and laser threats.

Contracts were let with the American Optical (Southbridge, MA) and Gentex Corporations (Carbondale, PA) in early 1985, and the American Optical product selected for final development and testing of eye armor (see Figs. 26-5 and 26-7). The American Optical eye armor, termed the ballistic and laser protective spectacle (BLPS), is composed of an integrated front (see Fig. 26-7) of medium molecular weight polycarbonate containing ultraviolet wavelength inhibitors and coated with an

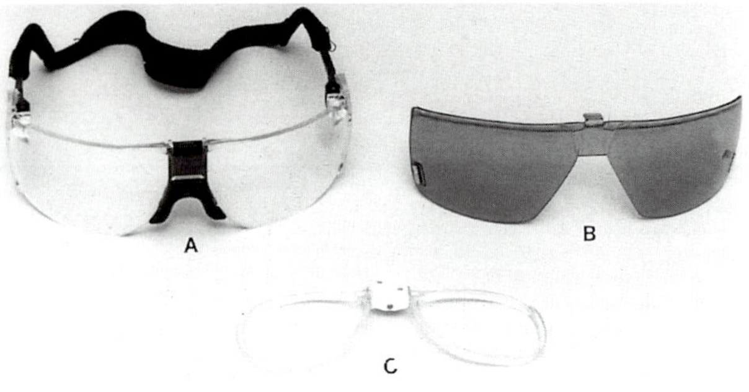

Fig. 26-7. Definitive eye armor (BLPS) components. (**a**) Polycarbonate eye armor. (**b**) Laser protective attachment. (**c**) Corrective lens carrier.

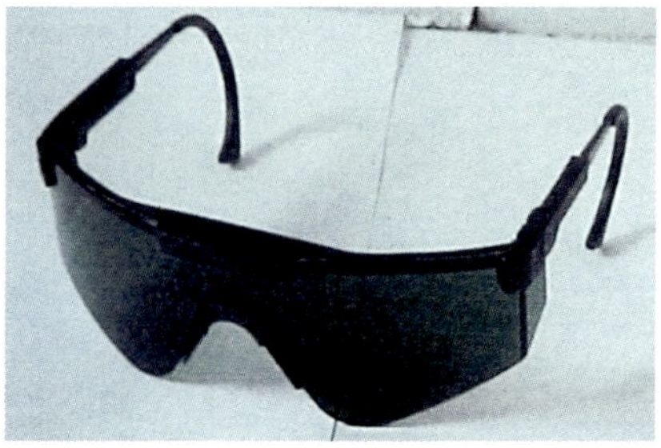

Fig. 26-8. SPECS. UVEX, Fürth, Germany.

organo-silane for abrasion and chemical resistance. Additional components include a laser-protective device of low molecular weight polycarbonate into which are incorporated specific laser wavelength absorbers, a lens carrier, and a retaining strap of neoprene and fabric (see Fig 26-7). Further testing determined that emmetropes preferred a new device manufactured by UVEX (Fürth, Germany), termed SPECS (see Fig. 26-8). Unfortunately, SPECS could not be modified to accept a spectacle correction and is unsuitable for use by ametropes. Thus the US Army is currently fielding two different forms of eye armor: BLPS for ametropes and SPECS for emmetropes.

CONCLUSION

The development of soldier-acceptable eye armor for the American infantryman, seemingly a straightforward, simple task has in fact required 70 years for successful realization. A thorough understanding of the elements of personal body armor development (missions of the infantryman, threats on the battlefield, materials available for eye protection, mind-sets of both the infantryman and his leaders, and monies for the development, provision and replacement of eye armor) and the sustained, dedicated efforts of many within and outside the Department of Defense have been required for the development of such eye armor.

In the *Iliad,* Homer sang, "Men grow tired of sleep, love, singing and dancing sooner than war." As threats to the eye of the soldier (and quite possibly the civilian) evolve, eye armor must also evolve. The development of eye protection for the American infantryman will continue to be a work in progress.

Acknowledgment

This work is dedicated to the memory of John Harry King, MD, FACS (COL, MC, USA, Retired), ophthalmologist, soldier, mentor, and friend who serves as an example for all military ophthalmologists. Melvin Alper, MD, William Glew, MD, and Robert Welch, MD, provided much encouragement and many suggestions. Mr Bernard Corona of the Human Engineering Lab made numerous critically important contributions to eye armor development. Paul Vinger, MD, provided much valuable encouragement and the example of his efforts to protect the athlete's eye. Mr Melvin Jee of the Natick Research Development and Engineering Center made numerous important contributions to eye armor development and provided the senior author with valuable information concerning prior attempts to protect the soldier's eye. Paul Whitmore, MD (COL, MC, USA, Retired), provided the statistical analysis of refractive error data. William Rimm, MD, JD (COL, MC, USA) and Kenyon Kramer, MD (COL, MC, USA, Retired) have provided valuable support during all stages of the eye armor development program. Gene Channing, OD (COL, MSC, USA, Retired) made significant contributions toward obtaining funding for the development of eye armor. Robert Joy, MD (COL, MC, USA, Retired), assisted the authors in the study of military medical history. Mrs. Maria Tama-Maggio reviewed the papers of Dr Wilmer for information concerning his efforts to develop eye armor. To all of them, and to all others who have assisted in this effort, the authors express their deep appreciation.

REFERENCES

1. Fair J. Protective goggles for the combat soldier. Read before the Meeting of Consultants Ocular Research Unit, Walter Reed Army Medical Center, Washington, DC, December 12, 1952.

2. Tarassuk L, Blair C (eds). *The Complete Encyclopedia of Arms and Weapons*. New York, Simon and Schuster, 1982, p 22.

3. Beebe GW, DeBakey ME. *Battle Casualties*. Springfield, Illinois, Charles Thomas Publisher, 1952, pp 42, 77, 167, 244.

4. Morax V, Moreau F. Etiologie des blessures oculaires par projectiles de querre. *Annales D'Oculistique (Paris)* 1916; 153:321-32.

5. Belkin M, Treister G, Dotan S. Eye injuries and ocular protection in the Lebanon War, 1982. *Isr J Med Sci* 1984; 20:333-8.

6. Heier JS, Enzenauer RW, Wintermeyer SF, Delaney M, La Piana FG. Ocular injuries and diseases at a combat support hospital in support of Operations Desert Storm and Desert Shield. *Arch Ophthalmol* 1993; 111:795-8.

7. La Piana F and Hornblass A: Army Ophthalmology in the Vietnam War. The Surgeon General, Department of the Army. *Doc Ophthalmol* 1997; 93:29-48.

8. Wong TY, Seet MB, Ang CL. Eye Injuries in twentieth century warfare: A historical perspective. *Surv Ophthalmol* 1997; 41:433-59.

9. Neel S. *Vietnam Studies: Medical Support of the US Army in Vietnam 1965-70.* Washington, Department of the Army, 1973, pp 50-51, 55.

10. Aker F, Schroeder DC, Baycar RS. Cause and prevention of maxillofacial war wounds: a historical review. *Milit Med* 1983; 148:921-7.

11. Tredici TJ. Management of ophthalmic casualties in Southeast Asia. *Milit Med* 1968; 133:355-62.

12. *Evaluation of Wound Data and Munitions Effectiveness in Vietnam.* US Departments of the Army, Navy and Air Force, Washington, 1970 (Vol 1), p D-51.

13. Cotter F, La Piana FG. Eye casualty reduction by eye armor. *Milit Med* 1991; 156:126-8.

14. Keeney AH. *Lens Materials in the Prevention of Eye Injuries.* Springfield, Illinois, Charles C. Thomas Publishers, 1957, p 62.

15. *American National Standard Practice for Occupational and Educational Eye and Face Protection,* ANSI Z87.1-1979. New York, American National Standards Institute, 1979.

16. Tarabishy R. Peacetime automatic weapon-related eye injuries: case reports. *Milit Med* 1983; 148:874-7.

17. McMarlin S, Connelly L. Reforger patient data: information collected in a CSH emergency room during a military training exercise. *Milit Med* 1985; 150:368-71.

18. Dean B. *General Surgery. In The Medical Department of the United States Army in the World War* (Volume XI: *Surgery*). Washington, Government Printing Office, 1927, pp 2, 3.

19. Reister FA. *Battle Casualties and Medical Statistics: US Army Experience in the Korean War.* Washington, The Surgeon General, Department of the Army, 1973, pp 48, 51.

20. Coates JB, Randolph ME, Canfield N (eds). *Medical Department, United States Army Surgery in World War II: Ophthalmology and Otolaryngology.* Washington, Office of the Surgeon General, Department of the Army, Government Printing Office, 1957, pp 32, 70, 85.

21. Sliney DH. *Standard-Item and Commercially Available Laser Eye Protection,* United States Army Environmental Hygiene Agency Nonionizing Radiation Protection Study No. 25-42-0337-86. Aberdeen Proving Ground, MD, 1986.

22. Coates JB, Beyer JC (eds). *Wound Ballistics.* Washington, Government Printing Office, 1962, pp XVIII, 592-3, 642, 662, 673, 679, 681, 684, 728.

23. Nickel H. *Warriors and Worthies: Armies and Armor Through the Ages*. New York, Atheneum, 1969, pp 66-67, 88, 105, 109.

24. Peterson HL. *Arms and Armor in Colonial America 1526-1783*. New York, Bramhall House, 1956, pp 5, 106, 111.

25. Dean B. *Helmets and Body Armor in Modern Warfare Including World War II Supplement.* Tuckahoe, NY, Carl J Pugliese Publisher, 1977, pp 1, 65-66, 145, 186, 234, 236, 237, 287; World War II Supplement, pp 3, 33.

26. Keeney AH. Lens materials and the prevention of eye injuries. *Trans Am Ophthalmol Soc* 1956; 54:521-65.

27. Dupuy RE, Dupuy TN. *The Encyclopedia of Military History.* New York, Harper and Row Publishers Inc, 1986, p 602.

28. Held R (ed). *Arms and Armor Annual.* Northfield, Illinois, Digest Books Inc, 1973, Vol 1, p 306.

29. Dyer G. *War*. New York, Crown Publishers Inc, 1985, p 82.

30. Greenwood A, DeSchweinitz GE, Parker WR. *Military Ophthalmic Surgery.* Philadelphia and New York, Lea and Febiger, 1918, pp 7, 46, 47.

31. Vail D. Military ophthalmology. *Trans Am Acad Ophthalmol Otolaryngol* 1950-1951; 55:709-15.

32. Terrien F, Cousin G. Prophylaxie des blessures du globe oculaire. *Archives D'Ophtalmologie (Paris)* 1914-1915; 34:811-7.

33. Whitham LB. Military ophthalmology. *Trans Am Ophthalmol Soc* 1919; 17:593-716.

34. Link MM, Coleman HA. *Medical Support of the Army Air Forces in World War II.* Washington, Government Printing Office, 1955, pp 305, 309, 334.

35. Nugent MW, Graham R. A hard plastic spectacle lens. *Am J Ophthalmol* 1950; 33:1763-8.

36. Thomson HC, Mayo L. *US Army in World War II The Technical Services The Ordnance Department: Procurement and Supply.* Washington, Office of the Chief of Military History, Department of the Army, Government Printing Office, 1960, p 186.

37. Kuhn HS. *Industrial Ophthalmology*. St Louis, CV Mosby, 1944.

38. Mayer LL. Eyesight in industry. *Arch Ophthalmol* 1942; 27:375-99.

39. Town AE. Metal eye protector. *Arch Ophthalmol* 1943; 29:633.

40. Stieren E. A metal safety and glare goggle. *JAMA* 1942; 120:26.

41. Wurdemann HV. Injuries of the head and eyes in warfare. *Milit Surg* 1921; 49:443-55.

42. Sweeting CG. *Combat Flying Clothing: Army Air Forces Clothing During World War II.* Washington, Smithsonian Institution Press, 1984.

43. Byrnes VA. Recent advances in military ophthalmology. *US Armed Forces Med J* 1951; 2:371-81.

44. Sylvia SW, O'Donnell MJ. *Uniforms, Weapons and Equipment of the World War II GI.* Orange, Virginia, Moss Publications, 1982.

45. Cruise R. Protection of the eyes in warfare. *Br J Ophthalmol* 1917; 1:489-92.

46. Cruise R. Preventable blindness in war. *Trans Ophthalmol Soc UK* 1944; 64:165-78.

47. Parsons J. Protection of the eyes from war injuries. *Trans Ophthalmol Soc UK* 1941; 61:157-78.

48. King JH. Research in the Army as it pertains to ophthalmology. *Trans Am Acad Ophthalmol Otolaryngol* 1951; 55:880-5.

49. Symposium on Operative Eye Surgery and Advances in Ophthalmology May 18-22, 1953. Army Medical Service Graduate School, Walter Reed Army Medical Center, Washington, DC.

50. Fair JR. Eye armor. *Am J Ophthalmol* 1957; 43:258-64.

51. King JH. Ophthalmology in the military services. *Trans Pa Acad Ophthalmol Otolaryngol* 1955; 8:5-10.

52. Lastnik AL, Cleavly BT, Brown JR. *Development and Fabrication of a Polycarbonate Eyeshield for the US Army Flyer's Helmet,* United States Army Natick Laboratories Technical Report 71-3-CE. Natick, Massachusetts, United States Amy Natick Laboratories, 1970.

53. Rose HW, Stewart GM. Eye protection against small high-speed missiles. *Trans Am Acad Ophthalmol Otolaryngol* 1957; 61:404-10.

54. Stewart GM. Eye protection against small high-speed missiles. *Am J Ophthalmol* 1961; 51:80-7.

55. Williams RL, Stewart GM. Ballistic studies in eye protection. *Am J Ophthalmol* 1964; 53:453-64.

56. Bryant RJ. Ballistic testing of spectacle lenses. *Am J Optom Arch Am Acad Optom* 1969; 46:84-95.

57. Fackler ML, Bellamy RF, Malinowski JA. Wounding mechanism of projectiles striking at more than 1.5 km/sec. *J Trauma* 1986; 26:250-4.

58. Davis JK. The optics of plano lenses. *Am J Optom Arch Am Acad Optom* 1957; 34:540-56.

59. *Modern Plastics Encyclopedia 1986-1987*. New York, McGraw-Hill Pub Co, 1986, vol 63, pp 39-40.

60. Newton AW. Industrial eye protection - an appraisal of some current safety lens materials. *J Inst Eng Australia* 1967; 39:163-70.

61. Quam GN, Shea J. An investigation of high impact shields for eyes and face. *Environmental Control and Safety Management* 1971:24-5.

62. Duke-Elder S, MacFaul PA: *System of Ophthalmology*. St Louis, CV Mosby, 1972, vol 14, pp 46-7.

63. Goldsmith W. Projectile impact on glass and polymeric ophthalmic lenses and circular plates. *Am J Optom Physiol Opt* 1974; 51:807-29.

64. Brand J, Reches M, Carroll MM. Eye protection for armor crewmen. *Armor* 1985; 94:25-7.

65. Hassett RJ, Hanlein SL, Goeller JE. *Protective Eye Shield Against Small Fragments,* United States Naval Ordnance Laboratory NOLTR 70-202. White Oak, MD, United States Naval Ordnance Laboratory, 1970.

66. Bryant RJ. Lens retention performance of safety frames. *Am J Optom Arch Am Acad Optom* 1969; 46:265-9.

67. Reches M. *Improved Ballistic Eye Protection.* Aberdeen Proving Ground, MD, US Army Materiel Systems Analysis Activity, 1976.

68. Carey ME, Sacco W, Merkler J. An analysis of fatal and non-fatal head wounds incurred during combat in Vietnam by US forces. *Acta Chir Scand [Suppl]* 1982; 508:351-6.

69. Robertson DM. Safety glasses as protection against shotgun pellets. *Am J Ophthalmol* 1976; 81:671-7.

70. Simmons ST, Krohel GB, Hay PB. Prevention of ocular gunshot injuries using polycarbonate lenses. *Ophthalmology* 1984; 91:977-83.

71. Hirschberg J. *The History of Ophthalmology,* Blodi FC (trans). Bonn, Wayenborgh, 1982, vol 1, p XIII.

72. Mader TH, Aragones JV, Chandler AC, et al. Ocular and ocular adnexal injuries treated by Unites States military ophthalmologists during Operations Desert Shield and Desert Storm. *Ophthalmology* 1993; 100:1462-7.

73. LaMarre DA. *Development of Criteria and Test Methods for Eye and Face Protective Devices,* DHEW (NIOSH) Publication No 78-110. Cincinnati, Ohio, National Institute for Occupational Safety and Health, 1977.

74. Donato JJ, Rengstorff RH. Polycarbonate ophthalmic lenses for eye protection. *Rev Opt* 1979; 116:87-8.

75. Davis JK. A polycarbonate ophthalmic-prescription lens series. *Am J Optom Physiol Opt* 1978; 55:543-52.

76. Proceedings of Combat Ocular Problems Conference, October 20-21, 1980. San Francisco, Letterman Army Institute of Research, 1980, p 94.

77. Sliney DH, Yacovissi R. Control of health hazards from airborne lasers. *Aviat Space Environ Med* 1975; 46:691-6.

78. Sliney DH. *Evaluation of Laser Protective Properties of Ballistic Plastics,* United States Army Environmental Hygiene Agency Nonionizing Radiation Protection Study No. 25-42-0343-84. Aberdeen Proving Ground, MD, 1984.

79. Vinger PF. The eye and sports medicine. *In* Duane TD (ed). *Clinical Ophthalmology.* Philadelphia, Harper and Row Publishers Inc, 1985, vol 5, chap 45, pp 1-39.

80. Vinger PF. Sports eye injuries: A preventable disease. *Ophthalmology* 1981; 88:108-13.

81. Rengstorff RH. Problems with optical inserts in military protective masks. *Milit Med* 1980; 145:334-7.

82. Anderberg B, Wolbarsht ML. *Laser Weapons: The Dawn of a New Military Age.* New York, Plenum Press, 1992, pp 5-6, 76, 93-94, 140-145, 150-166, 176-190.

83. Kearney JJ, Cohen HB, Stuck BE, Rudd FP, Beresky DE, Wertz FD. Laser injury to multiple retinal foci. *Lasers Surg Med* 1987; 7:499-502.

Chapter 27

GEOGRAPHICAL OPHTHALMOLOGY

RICHARD D. STUTZMAN, MD*

*Major, Medical Corps, US Army; Staff Ophthalmologist, Department of Ophthalmology, Walter Reed Army Medical Center, Washington, DC 20307-5001

INTRODUCTION

Geographical ophthalmology is an area within our specialty that is undergoing rapid changes. In addition to understanding the ophthalmological manifestations of disease, military ophthalmologists in developing nations need to consider disease processes from a public health standpoint. How does this disease process affect the country? The disease process and, more likely, its complications may result in large numbers of individuals being unable to contribute to the socioeconomic development of their country. Are there any identifiable factors that can prevent the disease or its complications? For example, the incidence of trachoma and its blinding complications have been significantly reduced by educating the populace regarding the importance of good hygiene, particularly facial cleanliness among children.

Although the disease processes that are seen in the West also affect developing countries, ophthalmology in the Third World is hindered by several factors, including poverty, inadequate community health education programs, and insufficient numbers of healthcare personnel and services. Underdeveloped nations also have a number of disease processes with significant ocular and systemic morbidity that have been eradicated to a large extent in developed nations. These diseases may manifest significant ocular morbidity, with the most significant sequela being blindness.

Data on the prevalence of blindness are difficult to ascertain. Worldwide there are variations in the definitions as well as the causes of blindness. The World Health Organization (WHO) has been instrumental not only in attempting to determine the prevalence of blindness but also, more importantly, in developing programs aimed at preventing and reducing the incidence of blindness. Worldwide, estimates are that at least 40 to 45 million people are blind, with an additional 160 to 180 million visually disabled.[1] The leading causes of blindness in Third World countries include cataract, glaucoma, trachoma, xerophthalmia, and onchocerciasis. Less common etiologies include Hansen's disease (leprosy), age-related macular degeneration, and diabetic retinopathy. WHO's goal is ultimately to have a blindness prevalence less than 0.5% globally or less than 1% in any country.[1]

Military ophthalmologists need an understanding of ocular diseases that affect countries in the developing world. We may be deployed to any of the underserved regions that are affected by these diseases. We need to be familiar with the disease, its manifestations, and its management. Management includes the treatment of acute and chronic manifestations of the disease and its complications. It also includes the ability to recognize factors that may be useful in the prevention of disease, ranging from the simple—implementing a community health education program—to the complex—providing instruction about surgical techniques to ancillary health personnel.

MEDICAL CARE IN THE THIRD WORLD

In developing countries, medical care is delivered in a tiered system. The first level provides the most basic healthcare to the greatest number of persons, with an emphasis on prevention. Because most of the population of developing nations usually lives in rural areas, these areas are the focus of the first level of care. The personnel providing medical services at this level have limited ophthalmological experience and few resources. They have been trained to evaluate large populations, make simple diagnoses, and provide basic treatments.

Many believe that early diagnosis of a particular disease process leads to a more favorable prognosis. For example, we know that the blinding complications of trachoma occur as a result of reinfection, and not of the acute infection. Therefore, the earlier the diagnosis can be made, the earlier the healthcare system can intervene (from both treatment and prevention standpoints) and potentially reduce the chance of visually significant sequelae. The personnel working at this level are trained to identify and manage the early and acute manifestations of many of the blinding conditions that will be reviewed in this chapter. As mentioned previously, a large part of geographical ophthalmology involves public health. At this echelon, healthcare providers play an important role in educating the population in the remote areas they serve. They promote proper sanitation, both personal and environmental.

The second level of care is more advanced; it has more numerous trained personnel, and hospitals are available. The resources are greater at this level compared with the first, yet more limited than at the third. The primary provider at this level is an ophthalmic assistant, with the occasional support of an ophthalmologist. Ophthalmic assistants are an invaluable asset. They receive extensive training and provide a broad range of care. They are responsible for examination, diagnosis, and management of most disease processes. Their management also includes the surgical treatment of various diseases. For example, many ophthalmic assistants are capable of providing eyelid repairs in patients with trachoma. The providers at this level give appropriate referrals to the third level of care, thereby improving the efficiency of an already overburdened system.

The most sophisticated level of care occurs at the third level, which usually consists of a central national hospital, typically located within an urban area. Medical subspecialists can be found at this level. Training of healthcare personnel, regardless of level of care, occurs at this level.

CATARACT

Worldwide, cataracts are the leading cause of blindness; the latest estimates reveal that approximately 16 million people are blind secondary to cataract.[2] In the Third World, the prevalence of cataracts is great because of limited material and financial resources, as well as the lack of adequately trained healthcare providers.

The risk factors for cataracts are similar for developed and underdeveloped countries. The most significant risk factor is probably age, and the most common type of cataract is the senile cataract. Other risk factors include gamma radiation, ultraviolet and ionizing radiation, nutritional factors, underlying metabolic disorders (eg, diabetes mellitus), medications (eg, steroids), alcohol, smoking, and geographical location. At present, there is no specific preventive measure to reduce the incidence of cataracts. The management of cataract remains one of surgical intervention. But in the Third World, management can be difficult because of patient fears, lack of access to healthcare, and the severe limitation of resources.

Screening and Assessment

The structure of a healthcare system must be integral to its delivery. In the Third World, the process begins with the promotion of ocular health. There is a strong public health mission imbedded in medical care provided in Third World countries. When a patient presents at the first level of care, he or she needs to be screened for the presence of cataract as well as other ocular diseases. This screening primarily occurs at the first and second levels of care. When a patient is suspected of having a cataract, he or she should be referred to the next level of care so that the ophthalmic assistant can confirm the presence of a cataract and determine whether the cataract warrants surgical intervention.

Cataract assessment is taken for granted in developed regions of the world, and diagnosis of cataract is relatively straightforward. In developing countries, however, examination is more difficult. There, assessment is frequently made with a handheld light and loupes rather than by slitlamp examination. Once a cataract has been determined to require surgical intervention, the patient must decide whether to undergo surgery. In Third World countries, many patients are apprehensive about undergoing surgical correction of cataracts. In India, "cataract camps" have been developed, which provide surgical services to large numbers of individuals. These camps have allowed reluctant patients to feel more comfortable because so many have received treatment and publicly applauded the surgical experience.

Management

In Western nations, the surgical procedure of choice is, without question, small-incision phacoemulsification with insertion of a foldable intraocular lens. In the Third World, the choice of procedure is not so simple. Most developing countries have provided their patients with intracapsular cataract extraction (ICCE), leaving the patients aphakic. Should these countries proceed to extracapsular cataract extraction (ECCE) with posterior chamber intraocular lenses (IOLs)? Most surgeons in developing countries are quite comfortable performing ICCE, and this procedure can be performed with the limited resources that are available. The ICCE technique is relatively straightforward and, once the initial learning period is over, can be performed with low rates of complications.

ECCE is a good procedure but is technically more difficult than ICCE and requires more sophisticated resources. In some of the less-developed countries, mass production of IOLs has reduced the financial burden associated with ECCE, but problems with IOLs need to be recognized. For example, the ability to determine the correct power IOL for a given patient is less precise in the Third World than it is in developed countries. There is greater variability among the IOL *A*-constants. Additionally, the powers and formulas used in Western nations depend on knowing corneal curvatures and the axial length of the eye. Sophisticated equipment is, therefore, required to determine the "correct" IOL power.

In addition, ECCE frequently is done with a microscope, which adds to the resource burden. ECCE also requires additional training. To reduce the number of patients with visual loss secondary to cataract, we must have an effective means of delivering eye care to large numbers of persons with limited access to care. Various camps have been established in an attempt to decrease the visual impairment associated with cataract. Such facilities include static eye facilities, mass cataract camps, and mobile eye units.[2] Once the surgery has been completed, however, the patient begins a rehabilitation period. It is important to keep the eye protected and free of contamination; therefore, it is important (1) to maintain a good level of personal hygiene and (2) to try to maintain environmental cleanliness, as well. Postoperative medications are frequently used in the West, but such drugs are limited in Third World countries (eg, they frequently have only a single steroid and one or two antibiotics).

The issue of visual rehabilitation must be addressed, as well. An aphakic individual may be provided with an array of aphakic spectacles and advised to try on multiple pairs and determine which pair provides the best subjective visual acuity. If an IOL is inserted, how do you refract the patient? And once a refraction has been determined, how do you provide the individual with a spectacle if neither a facility for making spectacles nor money to pay for them is available?

TRACHOMA

Following cataract and glaucoma, trachoma is the third leading cause of blindness, worldwide. It has been estimated that 150 million people are affected by trachoma and that 6 million are blind as a result of trachoma.[3] Trachoma is a chronic, infectious keratoconjunctivitis that is now limited to developing countries. It is primarily seen in Africa, although it occurs in many other areas, including the Middle East, the Indian subcontinent, Burma, Vietnam, Central Asia, some areas of China, Latin America, Australia, and the Pacific Islands.[4] The disease has been linked to *Chlamydia trachomatis* serotypes A, B, Ba, and C. These serotypes are associated with classic blinding trachoma, which is the endemic form of the disease. It is typically associated with poverty, poor personal hygiene, and inadequate environmental sanitation, and it may be transmitted directly or indirectly from person to person.

Serotypes D through K may produce ocular inflammation and are associated with inclusion conjunctivitis, which is usually associated with sexually transmitted diseases and is rarely visually significant. This form will not be discussed further in this textbook

Classification of Endemic Trachoma

Several classification systems have been developed to aid in the management of patients with trachoma. From a Third World standpoint, the best classification system is simple to understand, so that, potentially, nonophthalmic personnel could stage the disease process and provide the appropriate level of treatment. WHO has developed such a simplified grading scheme for trachoma (Table 27-1)[5]:

- TF: trachomatous inflammation, follicular (Figure 27-1a);
- TI: trachomatous inflammation, intense;
- TS: trachomatous conjunctival scarring (Figure 27-1b);
- TT: trachomatous trichiasis; and
- CO: corneal opacity (Figure 27-1c).

Clinical Course

As previously mentioned, trachoma is a chronic keratoconjunctivitis. Previously it had been thought that the visual sequelae were secondary to the acute infection. However, over the years it has been found that the process of multiple reinfections is responsible for the blinding complication of trachoma.[6]

The earliest manifestation of trachoma is follicular conjunctivitis (see Figure 27-1a). The follicles are usually associated with an infiltration of lymphocytes and polymorphonuclear cells. The upper tarsus is the more common site of involvement. As the disease progresses beyond the inflammatory phase, the conjunctival tarsus becomes thickened and scarred. The classic scarring pattern produces the line of von Arlt (see Figure 27-1b), which is a distinct horizontal scar in the upper tarsus where the ascending and descending subconjunctival vessels meet. Other patterns of scarring include fine, linear scars; stellate patterns; and broad, confluent, and deeper patterns. The scarring process may extend and involve the lacrimal drainage system and produce obstruction, fistula formation, or dacryocystitis.

TABLE 27-1

WORLD HEALTH ORGANIZATION'S SIMPLIFIED TRACHOMA GRADING SYSTEM

Abbreviation	Classification	Description
TF	Follicular trachoma	The presence of five or more follicles (≥ 0.5 mm) in the upper tarsal conjunctiva (see Figure 27-1a)
TI	Trachomatous inflammation, intense	Pronounced inflammatory thickening of the upper tarsal conjunctiva that obscures more than half of the normal deep tarsal vessels
TS	Trachomatous conjunctival scarring	The presence of easily visible scarring in the tarsal conjunctiva (see Figure 27-1b)
TT	Trachomatous trichiasis	Evidence of at least one eyelash touching the globe; evidence of recent removal of inturned eyelashes is also graded as TT
CO	Corneal opacity	The presence of easily visible corneal opacity that obscures at least part of the pupillary margin (see Figure 27-1c)

Source: Munoz B, West S. Trachoma: The forgotten cause of blindness. *Epidemiol Rev.* 1997;19:205–217.

a

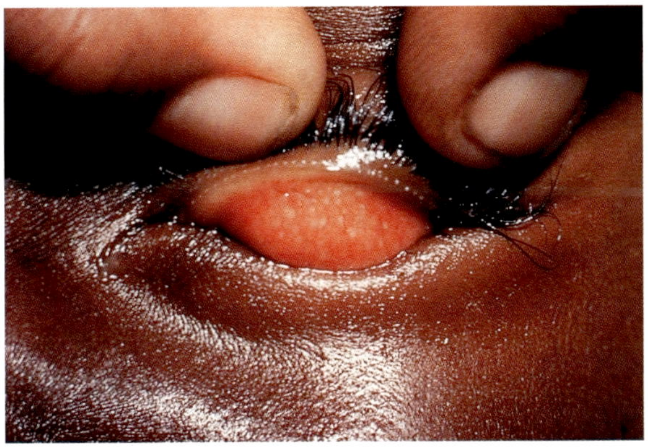

b

c

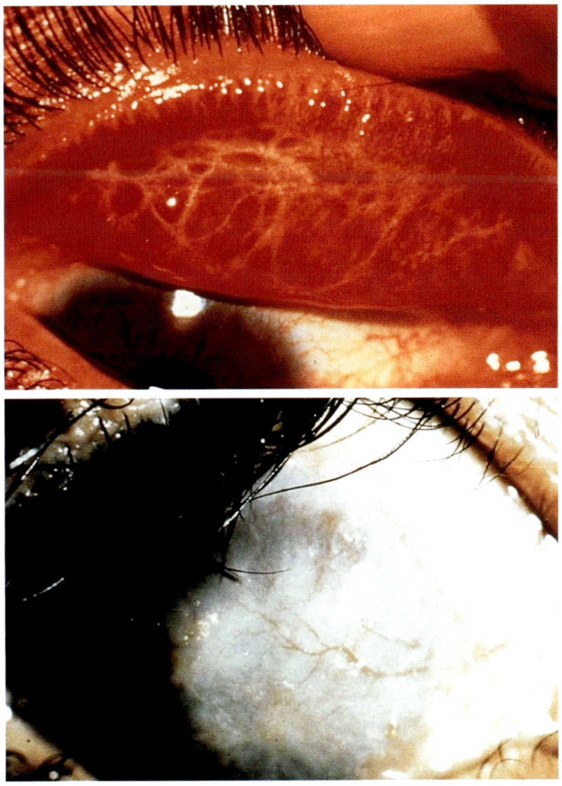

Fig. 27-1. Progression of trachoma. (**a**) Trachomatous inflammation, follicular. The palpebral conjunctiva shows early reticular scar formation with both follicular and papillary reactions. This case is consistent with the follicular trachoma (TF) stage of the World Health Organization's (WHO's) simplified grading system. (**b**) Trachomatous conjunctival scarring (line of von Arlt). In later stages of trachoma, patients develop superficial and deep scarring of the conjunctiva. Dense scar tissue near the upper eyelid margin may contract, leading to the formation of von Arlt's line. This case is consistent with the trachomatous scarring (TS) stage of WHO's simplified grading system. (**c**) Trachomatous corneal opacification. Complications of severe trachoma are the result of conjunctival contraction and deep scar tissue, which can result in cicatricial entropion, trichiasis, and lid shortening. The marked corneal scarring is associated with drying, a result of conjunctival disease. This case is consistent with the corneal opacity (CO) stage of WHO's simplified grading system. Photographs a and b: Courtesy of Sheila West, PhD, Wilmer Ophthalmological Institute, Johns Hopkins Hospital, Baltimore, Md. Photograph c: Reproduced with permission from Spalton DJ, Hitchings RA, Hunter PA. *Atlas of Clinical Ophthalmology.* Philadelphia, Pa: JB Lippincott Co; 1984: Figure 4.37.

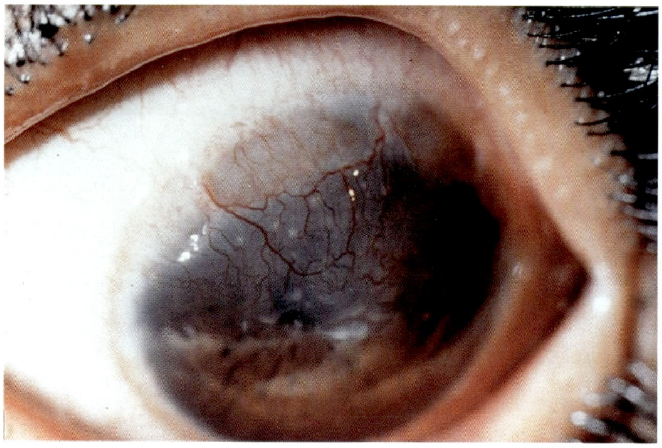

Fig. 27-2. Active trachoma with limbal follicles and an active corneal pannus (ie, dilated limbal blood vessels and diffuse infiltrate affecting the upper cornea). Reproduced with permission from Spalton DJ, Hitchings RA, Hunter PA. *Atlas of Clinical Ophthalmology*. Philadelphia, Pa: JB Lippincott; 1984: Figure 4.33.

As the conjunctival findings progress, they reach a cicatricial stage in which goblet cells are lost, which results in a loss of mucous secretion, which then produces an inadequate tear film and sets the framework for corneal complications. Corneal changes may arise at the same time as the conjunctival findings, but they are more commonly are seen after repeated bouts of the disease. The cornea may show focal inflammatory infiltrates, with histopathology similar to that seen in the conjunctival follicles. As the inflammation progresses, a superior vascular pannus usually develops (Figure 27-2). Pannus ulcers may develop anterior to the advancing border of the vascular pannus. They typically appear as horizontal-oval epithelial defects. Clinically, they may appear similar to the shield ulcer of vernal keratoconjunctivitis. The vascular pannus is most commonly located superiorly but may involve the entire limbus. Herbert's pits are also a manifestation of trachoma (Figure 27-3). The pits are most commonly found at the limbus and represent residual of inflammation.

The blinding sequelae of trachoma are usually secondary to cicatricial changes. These changes alter the normal lid position, resulting in entropion and trichiasis. The trichiasis can further compromise corneal integrity and create breakdown. Because of trachoma's association with poor hygiene, individuals afflicted with the disease are at increased risk for developing bacterial or viral superinfection, complications that can also cause blindness.

The clinical diagnosis of trachoma requires that two or more of the following findings be present:

- follicles on the upper tarsal conjunctiva,
- limbal follicles or Herbert's pits,
- typical conjunctival scarring, and
- vascular pannus, most notably involving the superior limbus.

Management

A variety of therapies have been used to treat the active infectious process. Traditional therapies have included such agents as topical tetracycline, erythromycin, and sulfa-based medications. Each of these medications, however, has problems associated with its use. The most significant limitations are the needs for multiday dosing and for prolonged treatment periods; these requirements decrease patient adherence to treatment, thereby decreasing the likelihood of eradicating the disease. Tetracycline cannot be used in the pediatric population, and trachoma predominantly affects this population. Sulfa-based medications are associated with high rates of allergic responses, the most serious being the potentially life-threatening Stevens–Johnson syndrome.

More recently, azithromycin has been used in the treatment of trachoma; it requires only a single dose but may not completely eradicate the organism. Studies are underway to determine when the medication dose needs to be repeated. Another limitation of azithromycin is its significant expense.

The lid complications of trachoma typically require surgical correction. In many Third World

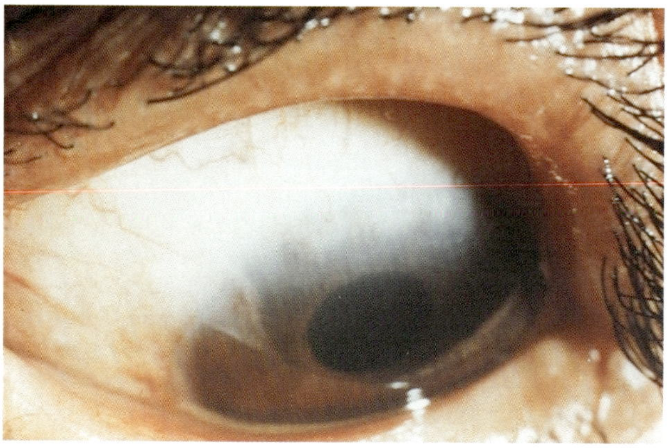

Fig. 27-3. In later stages of trachoma, patients may develop an inactive pannus (downgrowth of vessels and scarring without active inflammation) in which shallow depressions, known as Herbert's pits, can be observed. Reproduced with permission from Spalton DJ, Hitchings RA, Hunter PA. *Atlas of Clinical Ophthalmology*. Philadelphia, Pa: JB Lippincott; 1984: Figure 4.36.

countries, ophthalmic assistants are taught to perform these corrective procedures, thereby reducing the burden for the ophthalmologist.

Management of trachoma requires a multidisciplinary approach. The disease is associated with poverty, poor sanitary conditions, and poor environmental conditions with an abundance of flies and overall poor personal hygiene.[7] The populations in which trachoma is endemic must be educated about the ways they might be able to alter these factors and reduce the incidence of disease. An initiative known as "VISION 2020: Global Elimination of Avoidable Blindness 2020," is a consortium of nongovernmental developmental organizations, donor organizations, field experts, and WHO. One of the goals of this initiative is to eliminate new cases of trachomatous blindness by 2020 through public health, medical, and surgical management efforts. To this end, WHO has developed the SAFE strategy (*s*urgery, *a*ntibiotics, *f*acial cleanliness, *e*nvironmental improvement) to help fight blinding trachoma.[8] The VISION 2020 group believes that the use of the SAFE strategy in affected areas should lead to the elimination of trachoma as a blinding disease by the year 2020.[9] In addition, VISION 2020 has been working with the pharmaceutical industry to provide free azithromycin to populations in whom trachoma is endemic.

ONCHOCERCIASIS

Onchocerciasis is a parasitic disease that has ocular as well as systemic manifestations and is caused by the microfilariae of *Onchocerca volvulus*. Various estimates report approximately 18 million persons infected, 270,000 persons blinded, and 500,000 severely visually disabled.[10] The disease is commonly known as river blindness because of the disease's association with close proximity to rivers and fast-flowing streams where black flies breed.[11] Humans are the only natural host; the disease is transmitted via the bite of the black fly, *Simulium* species, which transmits infectious larvae to the human.

The disease itself is most commonly seen in the African continent with a few small foci in Central and South America. Within Africa there are varying patterns of severity of ocular disease. The most significant ocular disease may be found within the savanna woodland belt. Less-significant ocular disease is associated with the African rain forests and the highlands.

Clinical Course

The ocular and dermatological manifestations of onchocerciasis occur as a result of microfilariae deaths. The well-known Mazzotti reaction is an intense inflammatory response secondary to the deaths of millions of microfilariae in association with diethylcarbamazine (DEC) treatment.

Proposals for the route of ocular entry have included the microfilariae entering the eye through several routes[10]: along the sheaths of the posterior ciliary arteries and nerves, through the blood or cerebrospinal fluid, or via the orbital septum. Ocular onchocerciasis may involve any ocular tissue, and the manifestation of ocular disease depends on which tissue or tissues are affected.[12,13]

A relatively benign corneal manifestation takes the form of *punctate keratitis*. The dead microfilariae are surrounded by an inflammatory infiltrate and appear as ill-defined punctate opacities. Histopathologically, these are focal collections of lymphocytes and eosinophils with associated edema. Typically, the lesions clear and leave no significant visual sequelae.

A more severe corneal finding—and an important cause of blindness—is *sclerosing keratitis*.[14] This process begins peripherally, at the limbus within the interpalpebral fissure, and progresses toward the central cornea. Initially, sclerosing keratitis presents as increasing limbal haze with progressive fibrovascular pannus and an inflammatory infiltrate (Figure 27-4). The inflammation usually extends to the level of Bowman's membrane. Progressive changes

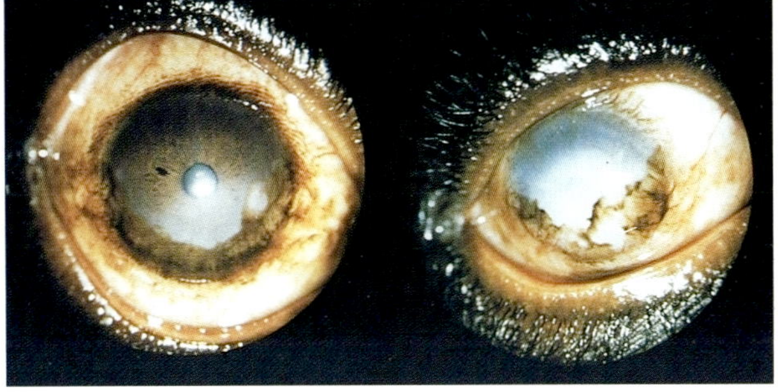

Fig. 27-4. Onchocerciasis can cause a mild (left) or severe (right) sclerosing keratitis with corneal scarring, vascularization, and pigmentary migration. Photograph: Reproduced with permission from Spalton DJ, Hitchings RA, Hunter PA. *Atlas of Clinical Ophthalmology.* Philadelphia, Pa: JB Lippincott; 1984: Figure 4.53.

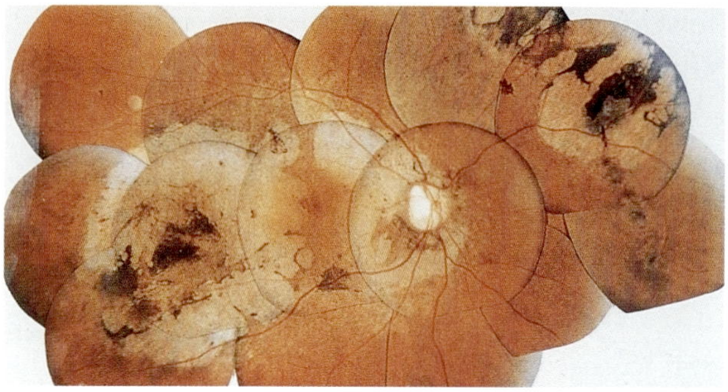

Fig. 27-5. Onchocerciasis chorioretinitis. Focal or diffuse chorioretinitis can occur, leading to a significant loss of vision. Additional findings in the posterior segment can include hemorrhage, choroidal granuloma, retinal edema, and optic atrophy.

continue in the form of advancing corneal opacification. Sclerosing keratitis is more commonly associated with regions receiving high amounts of sunlight. Microfilariae may be seen within the anterior chamber with or without an associated inflammatory component. When inflammation is present, it usually manifests as a granulomatous uveitis, which can be further complicated by secondary glaucoma and cataract.

Another leading cause of onchocercal blindness is *chorioretinitis* (Figure 27-5). The pathogenesis of the chorioretinitis is uncertain, although various mechanisms have been proposed. Such postulations include local inflammatory reaction occurring secondary to microfilariae, autoimmune response, and destruction of the retinal pigment epithelium. Clinically, retinal pigment epithelial atrophy, chorioretinal atrophy, and subretinal fibrosis can be seen. Histopathological examination has demonstrated a chronic nongranulomatous chorioretinitis with infiltration by lymphocytes, plasma cells, and eosinophils. There is a secondary degenerative change in the overlying choriocapillaris, retinal pigment epithelium, and neuroretina. Additional posterior segment findings include retinal edema, intraretinal deposits, hemorrhages, cotton wool spots, and choroidal granulomas. Patients may also present with an optic neuritis or optic atrophy; however, these findings are more common in patients who have been treated with DEC or suramin sodium.

Dermatological manifestations of onchocerciasis may also be noted by the ophthalmologist. One of the most common complaints is itching, which can be so severe that patients scratch themselves to the point of skin breakdown and develop a secondary bacterial infection. Pigmentary changes are frequently seen and produce what is known as the "leopard skin" appearance. There may be dermal scarring with loss of elasticity, and atrophy of the overlying epidermis gives the appearance of being prematurely aged. *Sowdah,* a reactive onchodermatitis, is an enhanced cell-mediated and humoral immune response. Histopathological examination shows dermal invasion with plasma cells, edema, and fibrosis. A final manifestation is an asymptomatic skin nodule (Figure 27-6). These nodules are usually located near the pelvis or joints and are firm, round masses at the dermis or deep fascial planes.

Onchocerciasis can be diagnosed in several ways. The most common is the skin-snip test. On average, six sites are biopsied (epidermis and dermis), incubated within tissue culture medium, and then examined for microfilariae. Microfilariae may also be observed within the anterior chamber of the eye and in various body fluids including urine, sputum, vaginal secretions, cerebrospinal fluid, and blood. Another diagnostic modality involves excising nodules and looking for adult worms.

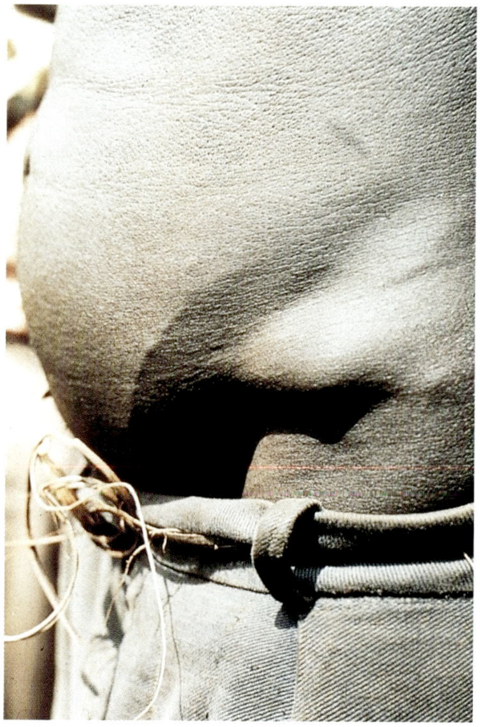

Fig. 27-6. Onchocerciasis skin nodule. The adult worm (*Onchocerca volvulus*) lives in subcutaneous nodules usually near the pelvis or joints. Reproduced with permission from Spalton DJ, Hitchings RA, Hunter PA. *Atlas of Clinical Ophthalmology.* Philadelphia, Pa: JB Lippincott; 1984: Figure 4.50.

Management

The treatment of onchocerciasis is aimed at prevention but also includes the medical management of active disease. Disease prevention needs to be geared toward preventing insect bites by avoiding breeding sites near the hours of dusk and dawn, when black fly activity is greatest. Protective clothing and insect repellents also decrease the chance of insect bites. The Onchocerciasis Control Programme[15] is focusing on vector control by spraying breeding grounds with larvicidal agents to kill the offending organism during its larval stage. This large-scale endeavor has numerous complicating factors, including expense; changes in water flow; and poorly accessible breeding grounds, which makes effective spraying difficult.

Medical management now consists of the use of ivermectin,[16–18] an agonist for the neurotransmitter γ-aminobutyric acid (GABA). Ivermectin produces a spastic paralysis of the microfilariae. This drug is associated with less-severe Mazzotti reactions than is DEC. Patients receiving ivermectin require long-term treatment at a dose of 150 μg/kg/y. It is not known, however, how many years of treatment are required. Treatment with ivermectin produces fewer side effects, compared with suramin or DEC. The latter two agents, which had been the mainstay of therapy until ivermectin became available, are now reserved for high-risk individuals facing severe infection or impending blindness. The inflammatory reaction caused by the death of the microfilariae is intense, and use of the drugs may further be complicated by optic nerve disease, which can further compromise vision.

NUTRITIONAL BLINDNESS

An aspect of ophthalmology that we are less familiar with in the developed world is nutritional blindness, most of which is caused by vitamin A deficiency.[19] In the Third World, the deficiency is most commonly associated with an inadequate dietary intake. However, other causes—all of which are associated with impaired vitamin A absorption—include lack of dietary lipids, impaired secretions of digestive enzymes, gastroenteritis, celiac sprue, and protein deficiencies. Vitamin A stores can also be depleted during febrile illnesses such as measles, severe gastroenteritis, and bronchopneumonia. The disease is seen in Asia, the Caribbean, and Central and South America, and frequently affects pregnant women and children younger than 6 years of age. Women are susceptible because of the number and frequency of their pregnancies and their suboptimal diet. Various theories have evolved regarding the high risk in the child subpopulation[2,20–22]:

- Children born to vitamin A–deficient mothers receive very little vitamin A in breast milk.
- Rapid growth during childhood creates a high demand on vitamin A stores.
- Children are fed sweetened condensed milk, which is deficient in both vitamin A and protein.
- Cultural beliefs teach the withholding of food from seriously ill children, which further exacerbates the problem.

Clinical Course

Vitamin A deficiency may manifest with numerous systemic findings, leading to a high incidence of systemic morbidity and mortality.[21] Such systemic findings include respiratory disease, diarrhea, anemia, and growth retardation.

Ocular manifestations involve mainly the conjunctiva and cornea, but posterior segment manifestations have also been documented (Table 27-2).[20,23] The earliest manifestation may be night blindness. The vitamin A–deficient state causes an alteration of dark-adapted (ie, scotopic) vision. If vitamin A therapy is instituted, then vision, specifically night vision, improves within 24 to 48 hours.

Patients with conjunctival xerosis present with patchy, granular areas of dryness that are unable to

TABLE 27-2

WORLD HEALTH ORGANIZATION CLASSIFICATION OF XEROPHTHALMIA

Abbreviation	Classification of Xerophthalmia
XN	Night blindness
X1A	Conjunctival xerosis
X1B	Bitot's spots
X2	Corneal xerosis
X3A	Corneal ulceration xerosis involving <1/3 corneal surface
X3B	Corneal ulceration xerosis involving >1/3 corneal surface
X5	Corneal scar
XF	Xerophthalmic fundus

Source: Steinkuller PG. Nutritional blindness in Africa. *Soc Sci Med.* 1983;17:1715–1721.

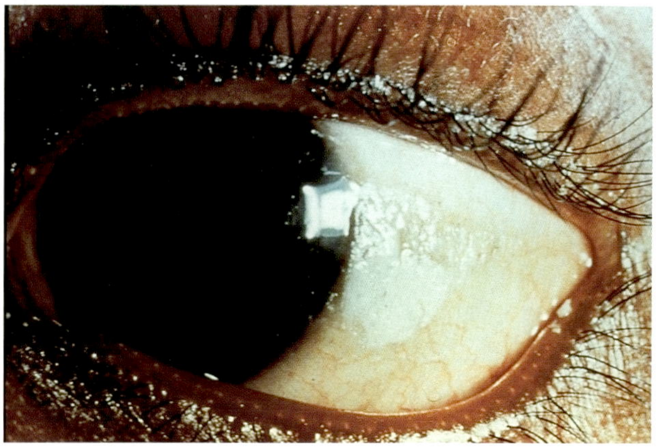

Fig. 27-7. Bitot's spots are small, white, cheeselike patches that have a foamy appearance and do not wet easily. This finding is often associated with a punctate keratopathy. Reproduced with permission from Spalton DJ, Hitchings RA, Hunter PA. *Atlas of Clinical Ophthalmology*. Philadelphia, Pa: JB Lippincott; 1984: Figure 5.42.

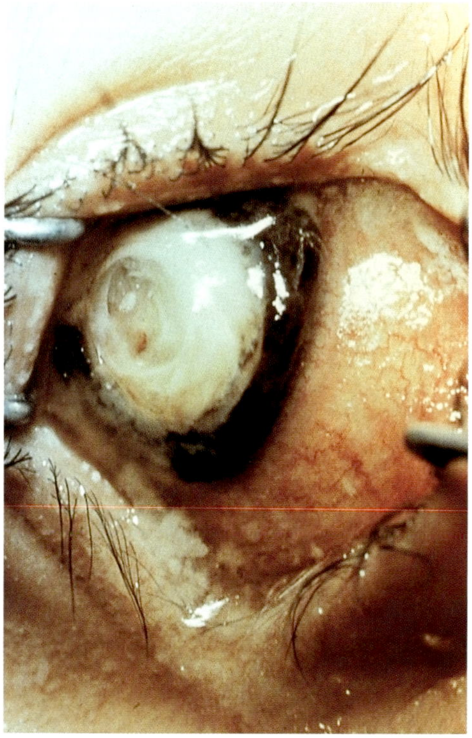

Fig. 27-8. Advanced keratomalacia associated with vitamin A–deficient xerosis can cause the entire cornea to become opacified and can also be complicated by secondary infection, perforation, and endophthalmitis. Reproduced with permission from Spalton DJ, Hitchings RA, Hunter PA. *Atlas of Clinical Ophthalmology*. Philadelphia, Pa: JB Lippincott; 1984: Figure 5.44.

be wetted. These patches are almost always seen temporally; when they are found nasally, they usually suggest vitamin A deficiency. If there is more than 180° of conjunctival xerosis, the conjunctivae take on a thickened appearance, appearing more prominent with circumferential folds. Bitot's spots are foamy, cheesy aggregations of desquamated keratin and saprophytic bacilli (Figure 27-7). They overlie areas of xerosis and will remain even after adequate vitamin A therapy.

The earliest corneal manifestation of vitamin A deficiency is xerosis, and this may present in the pattern of superficial punctate keratitis. Although the quadrant most commonly involved is the inferonasal, xerosis can be progressive with larger areas of involvement, commonly involving the interpalpebral zone. There may be stromal edema as well as keratinization. Xerosis tends to respond to vitamin A therapy. Vitamin A deficiency can also lead to xerophthalmic ulcers, which are small, sharply demarcated, punched-out lesions. The ulcers may be partial or full thickness and are most commonly found nasally and peripherally. They may advance and become complicated by secondary bacterial infection and stromal destruction and keratomalacia (Figure 27-8).

The posterior segment findings manifest as small, white blisters, appearing as intraretinal dots. These are more commonly found in the periphery and respond to vitamin A therapy.

Diagnosis

Vitamin A deficiency can be diagnosed in various ways, although these modalities may not be available in underdeveloped countries. Serum vitamin A levels may be determined with high-pressure liquid chromatography. A vitamin A level higher than 20 μg/dL is considered adequate. A second test is the determination of the level of total retinal binding protein (RBP) via an immunoassay for circulating RBP. A relative dose response may also be done; this records the changes in serum vitamin A–RBP after an oral or intravenous vitamin A test dose is administered. Lastly, conjunctival impression cytology may be evaluated. With this method, the specialist looks for evidence of squamous metaplasia, loss of goblet cells, irregularly shaped cells, enlarged cells, and keratinized epithelial cells.

Management

With nutritional blindness, the treatment goal is

to replenish vitamin A stores.[24] The patient may be administered oral vitamin A in an oil- or water-miscible form. If ocular disease does occur, the goal is to prevent blinding complications: protect the eye against secondary bacterial infection, and protect the globe when the structural integrity has been disrupted.

Prevention, once again, is an important aspect of the management of nutritional blindness (Table 27-3). The populations at risk should be identified, and treatment should begin with periodic administration of vitamin A. Within the at-risk population, the overall absorptive ability of the patient must be considered, and the patient should accordingly be dosed with vitamin A. Educational programs have been developed but as yet have not been shown to be very effective.

TABLE 27-3

WORLD HEALTH ORGANIZATION RECOMMENDATIONS FOR VITAMIN A PROPHYLAXIS

Population	Dose and Frequency
Pregnant and lactating women	20,000 IU/wk or 5,000 IU/d
Newborns	50,000 IU at birth
Children < 1 y old	100,000 IU every 4–6 mo
Children > 1 y old	200,000 IU every 4–6 mo

IU: international unit
Source: Steinkuller PG. Nutritional blindness in Africa. *Soc Sci Med.* 1983;17:1715–1721.

HANSEN'S DISEASE

Hansen's disease (leprosy) is a chronic granulomatous inflammation caused by *Mycobacterium leprae*. Worldwide, there are approximately 10 million to 12 million ocular cases, but only about half of these cases are registered.[2] Hansen's disease may be more widespread than some of the other ophthalmic diseases that have been discussed in this chapter. Areas in which ocular leprosy occurs include tropical climates, North and South Korea, Argentina, central Mexico, central Africa, the Middle East, Southeast Asia, India, and Indonesia.

Classification

Various classification schemes have been developed with a variable degree of overlap. The primary forms of disease are tuberculoid, lepromatous, borderline, and intermediate. In the tuberculoid pattern, the clinical findings may resemble those of tuberculosis. Lesions tend to be well demarcated, hypopigmented, and hypoesthetic. The histopathological findings include epithelioid cells, giant cells, and lymphocytes—findings that are commonly seen in specimens obtained from tuberculosis patients.

Multiple diffuse, less-well-defined lesions characterize the lepromatous form. The dermatological manifestations are heralded by thickening of the skin, producing leonine facies. The lepromatous form of Hansen's disease has more systemic involvement, compared with the tuberculoid form, and is also associated with a cell-mediated immune defect. Histopathological examination reveals numerous intracellular and extracellular acid-fast bacilli, lipid-laden macrophages, and histiocytes.

The borderline and intermediate categories of Hansen's disease represent mixes of the tuberculoid and lepromatous forms and will not be discussed further.

Ocular Leprosy

The ocular manifestations of Hansen's disease can involve any portion of the eye, but most findings are related to the periorbital skin region and the anterior segment. The orbicularis may be involved, particularly the pretarsal fibers, producing dermatochalasis. Similarly, there may be eyebrow loss with subsequent ptosis that typically begins temporally and may progress nasally. Atrophic changes involving the canthal tendons, the tarsal plates, or both can cause ectropion or entropion, which may further be complicated by trichiasis. In this population, tear dysfunction may develop secondary to infiltration of the meibomian glands, resulting in inadequate lipid production. The lacrimal gland may also be involved, producing dry eyes. Lacrimal gland involvement can be further complicated by recurrent dacryocystitis. Various eyelid nodules have also been reported[2] to occur.

Hansen's disease may also cause polyneuropathy. Involvement of the seventh cranial nerve typically results in lagophthalmos and ectropion, potentially compromising the ocular surface. Fifth cranial nerve involvement results in an anesthetic cornea, which, when combined with a seventh nerve palsy, greatly increases the chance that a corneal ulcer will develop.

Multiple corneal findings have been reported.[2] Individuals with these findings are at high risk for developing an exposure keratitis, particularly when there is an associated fifth and seventh cranial nerve palsy. The keratitis may subsequently become complicated by corneal ulcer, globe perforation, phthisis, and, ultimately, blindness. Affected individuals may develop an avascular or a punctate keratitis, or both, which typically begins in the superior temporal quadrant as well-defined, chalky white opacities. In time, the lesions become less-well-defined, resulting in a confluent haze with later development of a neovascular pannus.

Histopathologically, the corneal lesions represent miliary lepromas and demonstrate macrophages, lymphocytes, *M leprae* organisms, calcium deposition, and destruction of Bowman's membrane. The avascular or punctate keratitis, or both, may also be associated with an interstitial keratitis.

Ocular leprosy is one of the conditions that is associated with prominent or enlarged corneal nerves. They appear as focal beadlike swellings but are accumulations of *M leprae*. Within the Asian population, corneal lepromas may be identified. They occur more commonly at the limbus and may extend onto the cornea.

A principal cause for blindness in Hansen's disease is uveitis. The patients tend to have a chronic, low-grade uveitis in which they present with a very quiet-appearing eye. Clinically, it may be possible to identify corneal keratic precipitates, iris stromal atrophy with a moth-eaten appearance (which can progress to iris holes), hypopyon, synechiae, hyphema, elevated intraocular pressure, and small, poorly reactive pupils. The uveitis is believed to represent an antigen-antibody–mediated hypersensitivity reaction. Interestingly, this hypersensitivity may arise as a response to treatment. Iris pearls may also be identified near the papillary border. These may migrate posteriorly, producing what have been called[2] "retinal pearls."

Patients with Hansen's disease may also present with evidence of scleral inflammation. This inflammation may manifest as an episcleritis or a scleritis, which may be further subdivided into nodular and diffuse. The etiology for this inflammation is not certain. It could represent direct invasion of *M leprae*. It could be an immune-complex-mediated process, similar to the uveitis previously discussed. Scleral inflammation may be complicated by scleromalacia, staphyloma, and globe disorganization, all of which may compromise visual function. Rare posterior segment findings have been reported[2] and include uveal effusions, choroiditis, and retinal pearls.

Management

The management of Hansen's disease must focus on prevention as well as treatment of the active disease, as was also the case with onchocerciasis and vitamin A–deficiency blindness, above. Research into a vaccine is currently in progress. The treatment of active disease can be divided into medical and surgical approaches. For years, dapsone had been the treatment of choice. However, resistance to dapsone has been developing, and the treatment is beginning to incorporate other agents used in conjunction with dapsone. The other agents include rifampin, clofazimine, ofloxacin, and minocycline. Clofazimine, however, is very costly and can cause hyperpigmentary changes of the skin.

WHO's treatment recommendations divide patient groups into multibacillary and paucibacillary leprosy. The paucibacillary group is further divided into single or multiple skin lesion subtypes. In multibacillary leprosy, the medical treatment is for 12 months and consists of rifampin, dapsone, and clofazimine. Paucibacillary patients with multiple skin lesions are treated with rifampin and dapsone for 6 months. The final subtype, paucibacillary with a single skin lesion, is treated with a single dose of rifampin, ofloxacin, and minocycline.

From a surgical standpoint, eyelid deformities need to be corrected in an effort to protect the cornea. A peripheral iridectomy may be useful in patients who present with angle closure glaucoma. A sector iridectomy may be useful in patients with small pupils; it will result in a larger pupil, which may improve the patient's visual function. Patients with small pupils tend to develop cataracts at an earlier age and, therefore, require surgical correction to improve their vision.

SUMMARY

Although the ocular diseases associated with blindness and visual impairment are too numerous—and the geographical distribution of ocular disease too extensive—to be reviewed in a single chapter, a brief overview of the leading causes of preventable blindness worldwide has been presented. Military medical personnel may encounter these conditions while on deployments or in a theater of operations.

WHO has been instrumental in promoting awareness of Third World ophthalmology. This organization has been able to recruit many other organizations to work toward the goal of reducing the incidence of worldwide blindness, with the goal of reducing blindness prevalence globally to less than 0.5% and in any country to less than 1%.

Because we military ophthalmologists are not part of the ophthalmic community in Third World locations, we can easily remain ignorant of global issues that need to be addressed. Industrialized nations have tremendous resources that can help troubled and underdeveloped countries, however, including developing medications and vaccinations. Military ophthalmologists might also consider humanitarian missions that offer opportunities for engaging in ophthalmological care in the developing world.

REFERENCES

1. World Health Organization. *World Health Report 1998.* Geneva, Switzerland: WHO; 1998.
2. Taylor HR. Geographic and preventive ophthalmology. In: Tasman W, Jaeger EA, eds. *Duane's Clinical Ophthalmology.* Philadelphia, Pa: JB Lippincott; 2002: Chaps 50–63.
3. Mabey D, Bailey R. Eradication of trachoma worldwide. *Br J Ophthalmol.* 1999;83:1261–1263.
4. An B, Adamis A. Chlamydial ocular diseases. *Int Ophthalmol Clin.* 1998;38(1):221–230.
5. Munoz B, West S. Trachoma: The forgotten cause of blindness. *Epidemiol Rev.* 1997;19:205–217.
6. Ward ME. The immunobiology and immunopathology of chlamydial infections. *APMIS.* 1995;103:769–796.
7. Taylor HR. Trachoma. *Int Ophthalmol.* 1990;14:201–204.
8. Thylefors B. A global initiative for the elimination of avoidable blindness. *Am J Ophthalmol.* 1998;125:90–93.
9. World Health Organization. *VISION 2020: Global Initiative for the Elimination of Avoidable Blindness.* April 2000. Press Release WHO/27. Available at: http://www.who.int/inf-pr-2000/en/pr2000-27.html. Accessed 22 October 2001.
10. Abiose A. Onchocercal eye disease and the impact of Mectizan. *Ann Trop Med Parasitol.* 1998;92(suppl 1):S11–22.
11. Rowe S, Durand M. Blackflies and whitewater: Onchocerciasis and the eye. *Int Ophthalmol Clin.* 1998;38(1):231–240.
12. Taylor HR. Onchocerciasis. *Int Ophthalmol.* 1990;14:189–194.
13. Maertens K. Onchocerciasis in Zaire. *Int Ophthalmol.* 1990;14:181–188.
14. Berger IB, Nnadozie J. Onchocerciasis and other eye problems in developing countries: A challenge for optometrists. *J Am Optom Assoc.* 1993;64:699–702.
15. World Health Organization Expert Committee. *Epidemiology of Onchocerciasis.* Geneva, Switzerland: WHO; 1987. Technical Report Series 752.
16. Gilles HM, Awadzi K. The conquest of "river blindness." *Ann Trop Med Parasitol.* 1991;85(1):97–101.
17. Malatt AE, Taylor HR. Onchocerciasis. *Infect Dis Clin North Am.* 1992;6:963–977.
18. Kale OO. Onchocerciasis: The burden of disease. *Ann Trop Med Parasitol.* 1998;92(suppl 1):S101–115.
19. Smith GT, Taylor HR. Epidemiology of corneal blindness in developing countries. *Refract Corneal Surg.* 1991;7:436–439.
20. Steinkuller PG. Nutritional blindness in Africa. *Soc Sci Med.* 1983;17:1715–1721.
21. Sommer A. Xerophthalmia and vitamin A status. *Prog Retin Eye Res.* 1998;17:9–31.

22. Sommer A, West KP Jr. *Vitamin A Deficiency: Health, Survival and Vision.* New York, NY: Oxford University Press; 1996.

23. Khan MU, Haque E, Khan MR. Nutritional ocular diseases and their association with diarrhoea in Matlab, Bangladesh. *Br J Nutr.* 1984;52:1–9.

24. Foster A, Gilbert C. Community efforts in the reduction of corneal blindness. *Refract Corneal Surg.* 1991;7:445–448.

ABBREVIATIONS AND ACRONYMS

2-PAM Cl: pralidoxime chloride

A

ABC: airway, breathing, and circulation
AC: anterior chamber
ACLS: Advanced Cardiac Life Support
AEF: American Expeditionary Force
AFIP: Armed Forces Institute of Pathology
AMEDD: Army Medical Department
ANSI: American National Standards Institute
AP: anteroposterior
APD: afferent pupillary defect
ATH: Air Transportable Hospital
ATLS: Advanced Trauma Life Support

B

BAL: British anti-Lewisite
BLPS: ballistic and laser protective spectacle

C

C-DCR: conjunctivo-dacryocystorhinostomy
CNS: central nervous system
CONUS: continental United States
CS: 2-chlorobenzalmalonitrile (tear gas)
CSF: cerebrospinal fluid
CSH: combat support hospital
CT: computed tomography

D

DCR: dacryocystorhinostomy
DEC: diethylcarbamazine
DEPMEDS: *dep*loyable *med*ical *s*ystem
DNA: deoxyribonucleic acid
DOD: Department of Defense

E

EAU: experimental autoimmune uveitis
ECCE: extracapsular cataract extraction
EH: evacuation hospital
EMEDS: Expeditionary Medical Support
ENT: ear, nose, and throat
ERG: electroretinogram

F

FAMC: Fitzsimons Army Medical Center
FB: foreign body
FH: field hospital

G

GA: tabun
GABA: γ-aminobutyric acid
GB: sarin
GD: soman
GH: general hospital

H

HLA: human leukocyte antigen
HM: hand motions
HU: Hounsfield unit

I

ICCE: intracapsular cataract extraction
IOFB: intraocular foreign body
IOL: intraocular lens
IOP: intraocular pressure
IRBP: interstitial retinoid binding protein

K

KP: keratoprosthesis

L

LP: light perception

M

MAC: monitored anesthesia care
MACV: Military Assistance Command Vietnam
MAMC: Madigan Army Medical Center
MASH: mobile army surgical hospital
MEDCAP: Medical Civil Action Program
MEDSOM: *med*ical *s*upply, *o*ptical and *m*aintenance
MEOTS: Madigan Eye and Orbit Trauma Scale
MMART: Medical Mobilization Augmentation Readiness
MOS: military occupation specialty
MRI: magnetic resonance imaging
MUST: medical unit self-contained transportable

N

Nd:YAG: neodymium:yttrium-aluminum-garnet
NETS: National Eye Trauma System
NLP: no light perception
NOE: naso-orbital-ethmoid

O

OJT: on-the-job training
OMFS: oromaxillofacial surgery
OR: operating room
ORIF: open reduction with internal fixation
OTS: Ocular Trauma Score/ch6

P

PIP: pseudoisochromatic color plate
POE: postoperative endophthalmitis
PROFIS: *pro*fessional *fi*ller *s*ystem
PTE: posttraumatic endophthalmitis
PVR: proliferative vitreoretinopathy

R

RBP: retinal binding protein
RF: radio frequency
RPE: retinal pigment epithelium

S

SAFE: *s*urgery, *a*ntibiotics, *f*acial cleanliness, *e*nvironmental improvement
SO: sympathetic ophthalmia
SOOF: suborbicularis oculi fat
SOP: standing operating procedure
SPEARR: Small Portable Expeditionary Aeromedical Rapid Response
SPECS: special protective eyewear cylindrical surface
SPH: subperiosteal hemorrhage

T

TNT: trinitrotoluene
TO&E: Table of Organization and Equipment
TO: theater of operations
TOEC: theater of operations eye care
TPA: thromboplastin activator
tPA: tissue plasminogen activator

U

U: units
UV: ultraviolet

V

VKH: Vogt-Koyanagi-Harada syndrome
VX: no expansion, no common name

W

WDMEV: Wound Data and Munitions Effectiveness in Vietnam
WHO: World Health Organization

Z

ZA: zygomatic arch
ZF: zygomaticofrontal
ZM: zygomaticomaxillary
ZMC: zygomaticomaxillary complex
ZT: zygomaticotemporal

INDEX

C

G

H

I

M

N

O

Q

R

S

T

U

V

W

X

Y

Z

ISBN 0-16-051364-2
90000
9 780160 513640